ULTRASONOGRAPHY IN OBSTETRICS AND GYNECOLOGY

Peter W. Callen, M.D.

Professor of Radiology,
Obstetrics & Gynecology
University of California,
San Francisco
School of Medicine
San Francisco, California

SECOND EDITION

W. B. SAUNDERS COMPANY

Harcourt Brace Jovanovich, Inc.

Philadelphia / London / Toronto
Montreal / Sydney / Tokyo

W. B. SAUNDERS COMPANY
Harcourt Brace Jovanovich, Inc.

The Curtis Center
Independence Square West
Philadelphia, PA 19106

Listed here is the latest translated edition of this book together with the language of the translation and the publisher.

Spanish *(1st Edition)*—Editorial Medica Panamericana,
  Buenos Aires, Argentina

Library of Congress Cataloging-in-Publication Data

Ultrasonography in obstetrics & gynecology.

Rev. ed. of: Ultrasonography in obsetrics and gynecology. 1983.

Includes bibliographies and index.

1. Ultrasonics in obstetrics.   2. Generative organs, Female—Ultrasonic imaging.   I. Callen, Peter W. II. Ultrasonography in obstetrics and gynecology. [DNLM: 1. Fetal Diseases—diagnosis.   2. Fetal Monitoring. 3. Genital Diseases, Female—diagnosis. 4. Obstetrics. 5. Ultrasonic Diagnosis.   WQ 100 U47]

RG527.5.U48U47 1988   618   88–15862

ISBN 0–7216–2244–5

Editor: W. B. Saunders Staff
Designer: Maureen Sweeney
Production Manager: Pete Faber
Manuscript Editor: David Indest
Illustration Coordinator: Lisa Lambert
Indexer: Aja Lipavsky

Ultrasonography in Obstetrics & Gynecology   ISBN 0–7216–2244–5

Last digit is the print number: 9   8   7   6   5   4

To Karen, Brooke, Melanie, and Andy

CONTRIBUTORS

N. Scott Adzick, M.D.
Assistant Professor of Surgery, University of California School of Medicine, San Francisco, California

Geraldine Ballard, R.D.M.S.
Chief Ultrasound Technician, Health Sciences Centre, Winnipeg, Manitoba, Canada

James D. Bowie, M.D.
Chief of Ultrasound; Associate Professor of Radiology; Assistant Professor of Obstetrics and Gynecology, Duke University School of Medicine, Durham, North Carolina

Harbinder S. Brar, M.D.
Assistant Professor of Obstetrics and Gynecology, University of Southern California Medical Center, Women's Hospital, Los Angeles, California

Peter W. Callen, M.D.
Professor of Radiology and Obstetrics, Gynecology, and Reproductive Sciences, University of California School of Medicine, San Francisco, California

Daryl H. Chinn, M.D.
Staff Radiologist of Radiology, Hoag Memorial Presbyterian Hospital, Newport Beach, California

Peter L. Cooperberg, M.D.
Professor of Radiology, St. Paul's Hospital, Vancouver, British Columbia, Canada

Greggory R. DeVore, M.D.
Director of Intermountain Fetal Diagnostic and Treatment Center, Salt Lake City, Utah

Roy A. Filly, M.D.
Professor of Radiology and Obstetrics, Gynecology, and Reproductive Sciences, University of California School of Medicine, San Francisco, California

Alan W. Flake, M.D.
Research Fellow of Pediatric Surgery, University of California School of Medicine, San Francisco, California

James D. Goldberg, M.D.
Assistant Professor of Obstetrics, Gynecology, and Reproductive Sciences, University of California School of Medicine, San Francisco, California

Ruth B. Goldstein, M.D.
Assistant Professor of Radiology, University of California School of Medicine, San Francisco, California

Frank P. Hadlock, M.D.
Professor of Radiology, Jefferson Davis Hospital, Houston, Texas

Michael R. Harrison, M.D.
Associate Professor of Surgery, University of California School of Medicine, San Francisco, California

Maria R. Kidney, M.B.
Clinical Assistant Professor of Radiology, University of British Columbia, Vancouver General Hospital, Vancouver, British Columbia, Canada

Alfred B. Kurtz, M.D.
Professor of Radiology, Obstetrics and Gynecology, Thomas Jefferson University Hospital, Philadelphia, Pennsylvania

Clifford S. Levi, M.D.
Associate Director of Ultrasound, Health Sciences Centre, Winnipeg, Manitoba, Canada

Daniel J. Lindsay, M.D.
Lecturer, University of Manitoba, Health Sciences Centre, Winnipeg, Manitoba, Canada

Edward A. Lyons, M.D.
Professor of Radiology, Section of Diagnostic Ultrasound, Health Sciences Centre, Winnipeg, Manitoba, Canada

Laurence A. Mack, M.D.
Professor of Radiology; Director of Ultrasound, University Hospital, Seattle, Washington

Barry S. Mahony, M.D.
Department of Ultrasound, Swedish Hospital Medical Center, Seattle, Washington

Shirley M. McCarthy, M.D.
Assistant Professor of Diagnostic Radiology, Director of Clinical Magnetic Resonance Imaging, Yale University School of Medicine, New Haven, Connecticut

Ellen B. Mendelson, M.D.
Clinical Assistant Professor of Radiology, University of Pittsburgh School of Medicine; Chief of Women's Imaging, Director of Breast Diagnostic Imaging Center, The Western Pennsylvania Hospital, Pittsburgh, Pennsylvania

Laurence Needleman, M.D.
Associate Professor of Radiology, Division of Diagnostic Ultrasound, Thomas Jefferson University Hospital, Philadelphia, Pennsylvania

Harvey L. Neiman, M.D.
Clinical Professor of Radiology; Chairman of Radiology, University of Pittsburgh School of Medicine, The Western Pennsylvania Hospital, Pittsburgh, Pennsylvania

David A. Nyberg, M.D.
Department of Ultrasound, Swedish Hospital Medical Center, Seattle, Washington

Lawrence D. Platt, M.D.
Professor of Obstetrics and Gynecology, University of Southern California School of Medicine, San Francisco, California

Klaus G. Schmidt, M.D.
Research Fellow of Pediatric Cardiology, University of California School of Medicine, San Francisco, California

Norman H. Silverman, M.D.
Professor of Pediatrics and Radiology (Cardiology); Director of Pediatrics, Echocardiography Laboratories, University of California School of Medicine, San Francisco, California

PREFACE

It has been more than five years since the first edition of this text was written. In the interim, I determined to rewrite the entire text on the basis of recent advances in the field rather than simply revise the previous edition.

The success of this text in the past has been due to its practical nature, making it useful to both the novice and the experienced practitioner of ultrasound. Those aims have been maintained in the second edition. In addition to serving as a reference, this text should also be readable enough for each chapter to be read in its entirety. The useful comments of the readers of the first edition have been taken into consideration in the writing of this text.

This text has been enhanced in several ways. First, the number of chapters has been expanded. This allows better coverage of our improved knowledge of both normal and abnormal fetal morphology as well as the newer techniques of Doppler, computed tomography, and magnetic resonance imaging. Second, owing to the complexity and importance of neural axis abnormalities, the chapter on this subject has been significantly expanded. Third, the quality and number of illustrations and line drawings have been increased. The appendix, containing useful tables, has been expanded.

In this undertaking, there are a number of individuals who deserve recognition and my gratitude: the authors, for their excellent, timely, and well-researched contributions to this text; my family, associates, technologists, and colleagues in Obstetrics, for their understanding and support; Lisette Bralow and the people at W. B. Saunders, for their assistance in compiling this text; my secretary, Antoinette Turk, whose tireless efforts and sense of humor kept me going in moments of despair; and last but not least, you, the readers, who have encouraged me to produce this text.

PETER W. CALLEN, M.D.

CONTENTS

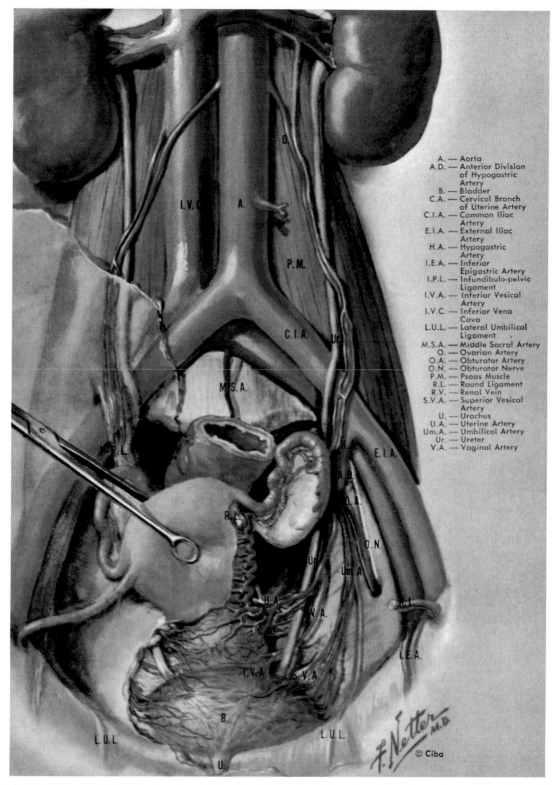

A. — Aorta
A.D. — Anterior Division of Hypogastric Artery
B. — Bladder
C.A. — Cervical Branch of Uterine Artery
C.I.A. — Common Iliac Artery
E.I.A. — External Iliac Artery
H.A. — Hypogastric Artery
I.E.A. — Inferior Epigastric Artery
I.P.L. — Infundibulo-pelvic Ligament
I.V.A. — Inferior Vesical Artery
I.V.C. — Inferior Vena Cava
L.U.L. — Lateral Umbilical Ligament
M.S.A. — Middle Sacral Artery
O. — Ovarian Artery
O.A. — Obturator Artery
O.N. — Obturator Nerve
P.M. — Psoas Muscle
R.L. — Round Ligament
R.V. — Renal Vein
S.V.A. — Superior Vesical Artery
U. — Urachus
U.A. — Uterine Artery
Um.A. — Umbilical Artery
Ur. — Ureter
V.A. — Vaginal Artery

Plate 1. Diagram of the anterior view of the abdominal and pelvic retroperitoneal structures. (*From* Netter FH: Medical Illustrations: Reproductive System; Vol 2. West Caldwell, New Jersey, CIBA-Geigy Corp, 1954, p 97. © *Copyright* 1954. CIBA-Geigy Corp. *Reproduced with permission from* THE CIBA COLLECTION OF MEDICAL ILLUSTRATIONS by Frank H. Netter, MD. All rights reserved.)

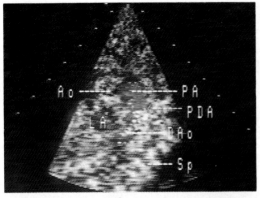

Plate 2

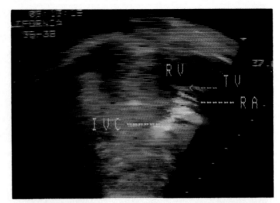

Plate 3

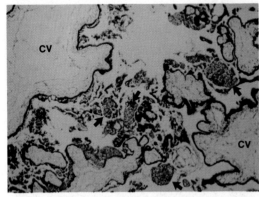

Plate 4

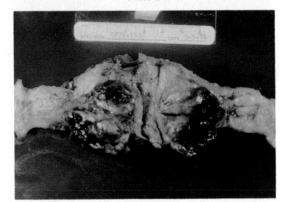

Plate 5

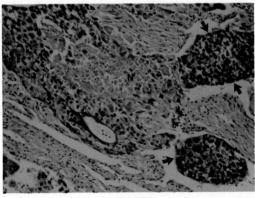

Plate 6

Plate 2. Color Doppler flow map taken in a short-axis view in a fetus of 34 weeks' gestation, with complete heart block and a structurally normal heart. The red and blue color bars indicate flow directed toward and away from the transducer, respectively. Normal flow directed away from the transducer is seen in the pulmonary artery (PA) indicated by blue color, but a change in color occurs in the ductus arteriosus (PDA) and in the descending aorta (DAo). This color change into yellow and turquoise represents a phenomenon called aliasing. Aliasing occurs when the velocity of the blood flow exceeds the equipment's ability to recognize the velocity accurately. In this case, the acceleration of the flow velocity is related to the narrowing of the ductus arteriosus that occurs as the fetus matures. Ao, aorta; LA, left atrium; Sp, spine.

Plate 3. Color Doppler flow map taken in a short-axis view of a 29 week fetus with tricuspid regurgitation due to a structural cardiac defect (univentricular atrioventricular connection, aortic arch hypoplasia). In this systolic frame, the tricuspid valve (TV) can be seen between the right ventricle (RV) and the right atrium (RA). A regurgitant jet, refluxing all the way back into the inferior vena cava (IVC), is depicted in red and yellow colors, indicating its direction toward the transducer.

Plate 4. Photomicrograph from a patient with a hydatidiform mole. Abnormal nests of trophoblastic cells (*arrows*) are seen scattered among markedly swollen chorionic villi (CV). The degree of hydropic change of the chorionic villus, in addition to the presence of trophoblastic proliferation, distinguishes this from hydropic degeneration occurring in otherwise normal pregnancies.

Plate 5. Pathologic specimen from a patient with choriocarcinoma. The bivalved uterus demonstrates a large, hemorrhagic necrotic mass involving the body of the uterus.

Plate 6. Photomicrograph from a patient with choriocarcinoma. Multiple cords (*arrows*) of malignant trophoblastic tissue infiltrate the uterine stroma. The absence of villi and the necrosis (N) of the tumor differentiate this process from invasive trophoblastic disease and a hydatidiform mole.

THE OBSTETRIC ULTRASOUND EXAMINATION

Peter W. Callen, M.D.

It has been estimated, in some countries, that as many as 90 to 100 percent of women seeking obstetric care will have at least one ultrasound examination during their pregnancy.[1,2] The increased use of ultrasound during the past several years has prompted inquiries into its safety and quality. As a result of this concern, committees from interested groups such as the National Institutes of Health, the American College of Obstetrics and Gynecology, and the American Institute of Ultrasound in Medicine have established preliminary guidelines for the obstetric ultrasound examination.[3-5]

What follows is the author's own bias as to what constitutes an appropriate ultrasound examination. In some respects, this is an expansion of the guidelines previously mentioned. As this multiauthored text is essentially a detailed review of the obstetric ultrasound examination, it is recognized that this chapter and those that follow may reflect differences of opinion.

ULTRASOUND EQUIPMENT AND SAFETY

Equipment

During the past several years, the dramatic improvements in real-time ultrasound equipment have made it indispensable in the obstetric ultrasound examination because it (1) rapidly, accurately, and safely confirms fetal life; (2) more easily images a moving target such as a fetus; and (3) with its constant feedback of the real-time images and its lesser number of controls, seems more "user-friendly" to many examiners than a static articulated-arm scanner.

With all these advantages, however, this equipment is not without some limitations, its major one being a limited field of view. The small field of view of real-time images makes it more difficult to ascertain fetal lie and presentation, placental relationships to the fetus and uterus, and estimated amniotic fluid volume. In addition, in the real-time examination, the scans tend to be more random and less reproducible than static articulated-arm scans. In an ideal world where cost is not a factor, it might be optimal to utilize both forms of equipment. There have been, however, a number of features made available on real-time scanners to compensate for these deficiencies, e.g., dual-image recording and wider field-of-view transducers.

While the debate over real-time imaging equipment versus articulated-arm scanners has lessened somewhat, there is still controversy regarding sector versus linear array transducers, mechanical versus phased-array imaging systems, and black on white versus white on black recorded images.

TRANSDUCER SELECTION. When sector transducers first became available, there were a number of problems in obtaining a distortion-free image from which measurements could be made. More recently, most of these problems have been solved. While in most cases the linear array transducer has less distortion and better resolution than sector transducers, the large surface area required for contact of the linear array transducers sometimes makes them problematic.

Phased-array imaging systems likewise suffered initially from poor image quality but now are setting the standard for high-resolution images. The lack of moving parts, and thus the infrequent downtime, as well as the ease of changing image quality by altering only the software, have made them extremely desirable. The major limitation of these systems presently is their high cost compared with mechanical sector systems; however, this is likely to decrease in the future.

The controversy over the best method to interpret images, white on black versus black on white, may never be resolved. This is obviously a matter of viewer preference, and no rigid rules exist in this area. There should be no issue, however, that documentation using "hard-copy" film occurs in every examination.

Safety

The debate over the safety of the obstetric ultrasound examination has intensified during recent years and is likely to continue. The wide and possibly excessive use of this technique has prompted questions concerning safety and the appropriateness of the ultrasound examination. This has led to numerous meetings specifically addressing these issues. Without elaborating on all of the historical background and individual studies concerning safety and efficacy, on the basis of these hearings, it is reasonable to conclude the following:

1. Despite the fact that ultrasound has been in use for over 25 years, there have been no reported instances of adverse effects to the patient or operator from commercially available equipment at diagnostic levels.[5]

2. Animal studies showing a deleterious effect of ultrasound have used energy levels higher than commonly used diagnostically, and the results of many of these studies have not been reproduced by other investigators. However, the possibility that some information from these studies may be applicable to humans makes it mandatory that well-designed long-term studies be carried out to determine absolutely the effect of in utero ultrasound exposure on the fetus.[4]

Although one may obtain some reassurance of ultrasound's safety from the above two statements, until *good* long-term studies are carried out, ultrasound, like any other medical test, should be performed only when there are sound clinical indications. The following is the list of indications for obstetric ultrasound based upon the NIH panel that convened in 1983:[4]

- *Estimation of gestational age* by ultrasound for confirmation of clinical dating for patients who are to undergo elective repeat cesarean delivery, induction of labor, or elective termination of pregnancy.
- *Evaluation of fetal growth* (when the patient has an identified etiology for uteroplacental insufficiency, such as severe preeclampsia, chronic hypertension, chronic significant renal disease, severe diabetes mellitus, or for other medical complications of pregnancy where fetal malnutrition, i.e., intrauterine growth retardation [IUGR] or macrosomia, is suspected).
- *Vaginal bleeding* of undetermined etiology in pregnancy.
- *Determination of fetal presentation* when the presenting part cannot be adequately assessed in labor.
- *Suspected multiple gestation.*
- *Adjunct to amniocentesis.*
- *Significant uterine size/clinical dates discrepancy.*
- *Pelvic mass detected clinically.*
- *Suspected hydatidiform mole.*
- *Adjunct to cervical cerclage placement.*
- *Suspected ectopic pregnancy.*
- *Adjunct to special procedures.*
- *Suspected fetal death.*
- *Suspected uterine abnormality.*
- *Intrauterine contraceptive device localization.*
- *Ovarian follicle development surveillance.*
- *Biophysical profile for fetal well-being* after 28 weeks of gestation.

- *Observation of intrapartum events (e.g., version/extraction of second twin, manual removal of placenta, etc.).*
- *Suspected polyhydramnios or oligohydramnios.*
- *Suspected abruptio placentae.*
- *Adjunct to external version from breech to vertex presentation.*
- *Estimation of fetal weight and/or presentation in premature rupture of membranes and/or premature labor.*
- *Abnormal serum alpha-fetoprotein value for clinical gestational age when drawn.*
- *Follow-up observation of identified fetal anomaly.*
- *History of previous congenital anomaly.*
- *Serial evaluation of fetal growth in multiple gestations.*
- *Estimation of gestational age in late registrants for prenatal care.*

THE FIRST TRIMESTER ULTRASOUND EXAMINATION

Identification of an Intrauterine Pregnancy

The primary goal of ultrasound evaluation in the first trimester is to determine whether the pregnancy is intrauterine and whether the embryo is living, if possible. With present-day equipment, both of these tasks should be readily accomplished at very early stages of gestation. The same care taken in concluding that a later pregnancy has a lethal malformation should be applied in deciding that an early pregnancy is nonviable. If there is a reasonable doubt about the viability, a repeat examination in as little as seven to ten days will invariably make the conclusion unequivocal.

Fetal Number

There is no question that, with a careful examination, the true number of embryos can be accurately determined in the first trimester. The literature has emphasized that it is important not to overestimate the number of developing gestations by misinterpreting findings such as a "double sac sign," fluid in the uterine cavity, or the presence of the amnion as evidence of multiple sacs and thus multiple gestations. However, one

may be just as likely to underestimate the number of developing gestations and embryos if a thorough evaluation of the gestational sac is not made for all embryos. It is the author's feeling that when multiple gestations are missed using ultrasound, it is usually from a less than optimal first trimester examination. It is for these reasons that some investigators prefer that if one ultrasound examination is to be done concentrating on fetal number, then it should be in the early to middle second trimester of pregnancy.

Estimating Gestational Age

This subject will be covered in detail in Chapter 4. Suffice it to say that some estimate of gestational age should be performed: measurement of the gestational sac in very early pregnancies and the crown-rump length thereafter. It should be emphasized that the terms "menstrual age" and "gestational age" will be used interchangeably in this text. They both represent the age of the pregnancy based on counting from the first day of the last normal menstrual period. The term "fetal age," representing the age of the fetus from the presumed day of conception (approximately two weeks less than the menstrual or gestational age), will not be used. (See below under *Assigning Gestational Age and Weight*.)

Placenta

In very early pregnancies, it may be difficult to ascertain the site of the developing placenta. If, however, one can confidently identify the site of placentation, either anterior or posterior, this information should be documented. There are a number of cases in which the early first trimester ultrasound is the only examination obtained during pregnancy. Later in pregnancy, if either an amniocentesis or a cesarean section is planned and no ultrasound equipment is available, it would be helpful to know the location of the placental site from an earlier exam.

Uterus and Adnexa

The maternal uterus should be carefully examined for evidence of uterine anomalies, particularly in high-risk patients. Late in pregnancy, these anomalies may be extremely difficult to detect. If myomas are detected, their size, site, and relationship to the cervix should be recorded. It should be remembered that transient myometrial contractions may simulate myomas.

The adnexa should be carefully searched for the presence of cysts as well as ovarian neoplasms, both benign and malignant. Again, later in pregnancy, the adnexal areas may be extremely difficult to evaluate adequately.

THE SECOND AND THIRD TRIMESTER ULTRASOUND EXAMINATION

Fetal Number and Fetal Life

Though evaluating the number of fetuses may be difficult during early pregnancy, it should be extremely easy and accurate in the second and third trimesters. The increased perinatal morbidity and mortality of multiple gestations make it mandatory that a "surprise twin" at delivery be a rare event in any patient who has had second or third trimester ultrasound. The major potential error in determining the number of fetuses is underestimation. This mistake, when made, is likely due to either not evaluating the fundal region or not making sure that the fetal head is associated with its body rather than that of a twin. When a multiple gestation is identified, it is important to determine, if possible, the number of placentas and the number of gestational sacs (the chorionicity and amnionicity). This subject will be covered in the discussion of the placenta.

In the ultrasound report, a statement should be made that the fetus was living, if this was the case, by virtue of cardiac motion being identified. Even in a setting where only static scanners are available, positioning the transducer over the thorax and observing under M-mode ultrasound will verify the presence of fetal life. The diagnosis of fetal demise ideally should be confirmed by more than one examiner based on the absence of fetal or cardiac motion for at least three minutes.

Fetal Position

Once fetal life and number have been identified, it is the task of the sonographer to determine the fetal lie and presenting part. Fetal lie refers to the relationship of the long axis of the fetus to the long axis of the uterus. Presentation defines the presenting fetal part closest to the cervix. The most common fetal lie is longitudinal, and the most common presenting part is the fetal head. Fetal lies or presentations other than these are referred to as malpresentations. Their significance lies in increased perinatal morbidity during delivery.

The advent of real-time ultrasound has placed an additional demand upon the ultrasonographer. If the people interpreting the examination have not performed it themselves, they must be able to deduce the lie and presentation from several images rather than from a single one. This may be done only by understanding the normal fetal anatomy and applying it to the scanning position (Figs. 1–1, 1–2). Likewise, congenital anomalies will be recognized only fortuitously if a structure is identified as abnormal by virtue of its abnormal position related to the lie and presentation of the fetus.

As mentioned above, the most common presenting part is the fetal head: cephalic presentation. (The author prefers the use of the term "cephalic," rather than "vertex," as "vertex" may also be used to describe a location on the fetal head.) When the head is adjacent to the lower uterine segment, it is likely that the fetus is in cephalic presentation; however, one must see all images before coming to that conclusion. The fetal body may also be low in the uterus with the fetal head, and thus the fetus would be in a transverse lie rather than in cephalic presentation.

Fetal malpresentations require that the sonographer extend the examination to answer two additional questions important to the referring obstetrician. First, what specifically is the presenting part, i.e., foot, the buttocks, or both in case of a breech presentation or a face or shoulder in the case of a fetus in longitudinal lie (Figs. 1–3, 1–4)? Second, is there an associated fetal malformation or placental abnormality that may be causally related to the abnormal lie?[6]

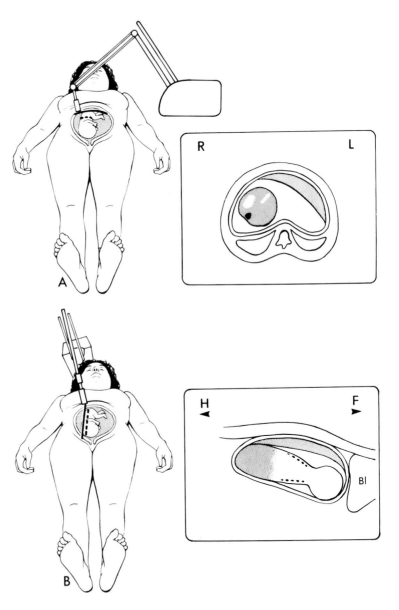

Figure 1–1. *A*, Illustration of a transverse plane of section of the gravid uterus. As the fetus is in a cephalic presentation, this scan transects the fetal abdomen transversely. *B*, Longitudinal plane of section of the same fetus. These are viewed with the maternal head to the left of the recorded image.

**A LONGITUDINAL LIE
CEPHALIC PRESENTATION**

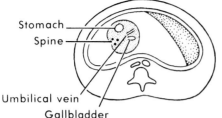

Stomach
Spine

Umbilical vein
Gallbladder

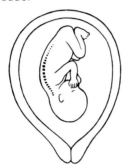

**B LONGITUDINAL LIE
BREECH PRESENTATION**

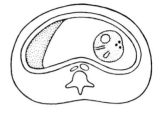

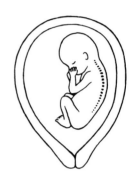

**C TRANSVERSE LIE
HEAD, MATERNAL LEFT**

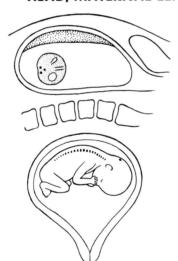

**D TRANSVERSE LIE
HEAD, MATERNAL RIGHT**

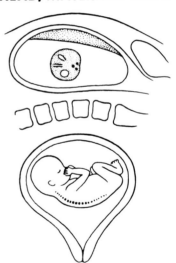

Figure 1–2. Knowledge of the plane of section across the maternal abdomen (longitudinal or transverse) as well as the position of the fetal spine and left-sided (stomach) and right-sided (gallbladder) structures can be used to determine fetal lie and presenting part. *A,* This transverse scan of the gravid uterus demonstrates the fetal spine on the maternal right with the fetus lying with its right side down (stomach anterior, gallbladder posterior). Since these images are viewed looking up from the patient's feet, the fetus must be in longitudinal lie and cephalic presentation. *B,* When the gravid uterus is scanned transversely and the fetal spine is on the maternal left with the right side down, the fetus is in a longitudinal lie and breech presentation. *C,* When a longitudinal plane of section demonstrates the fetal body to be transected transversely and the fetal spine is nearest the uterine fundus with the fetal left side down, the fetus is in a transverse lie with the fetal head on the maternal left. *D,* When a longitudinal plane of section demonstrates the fetal body to be transected transversely and the fetal spine is nearest the lower uterine segment with the fetal left side down, the fetus is in a transverse lie with the fetal head on the maternal right. Although real-time scanning of the gravid uterus quickly allows the observer to determine fetal lie and presenting part, this maneuver of identifying specific right- and left-sided structures within the fetal body forces one to determine fetal position accurately and identify normal and pathologic fetal anatomy.

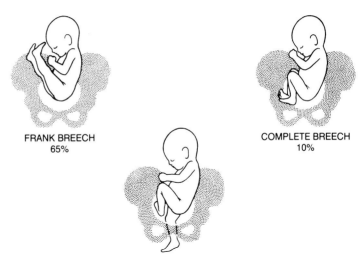

FRANK BREECH
65%

COMPLETE BREECH
10%

FOOTLING BREECH (Single or Double)
25%

Figure 1–3. Illustration of the types of breech presentations. In a frank breech presentation (the most common), the thighs are flexed at the hips with the legs and knees extended. In complete breech (the least common), the thighs are flexed at the hips, and there is flexion of the knees as well. One or both hips and knees are extended in the footling breech. The risk of cord prolapse is greatest with a footling breech and least with a frank breech.

Assigning Gestational Age and Weight

This subject will be covered in detail in Chapters 4 and 5. It is important to remember several concepts when assigning gestational age using ultrasonography. First, measurements made early in pregnancy, for the most part, are more accurate than those near term. Second, pathologic states should be taken into consideration when deciding which body parts to use in assigning gestational age or weight. The abdominal circumference measurement is likely to be inaccurate in the presence of fetal ascites and the

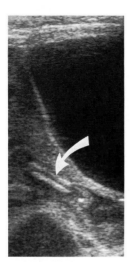

Figure 1–4. Longitudinal scan of a footling breech presentation. In this scan, the leg *(arrow)* and foot extend into the lower uterine segment and cervix.

femur length unreliable in fetuses with short-limbed dwarfism. Third, every obstetrical ultrasound report should relate the calculated sonographic age to the patient's menstrual age. Because menstrual histories are frequently inaccurate, there is often a tendency to not believe any woman's menstrual history in deference to the calculated sonographic age. In doing so, however, one runs the risk of back-dating a fetus that is in fact older but growth retarded or of back-dating a post-term pregnancy, thus placing the fetus at risk for in utero death or fetal postmaturity syndrome. Fourth, the calculated fetal weight should be stated not only in grams but also as a percentile based upon the patient's menstrual age. Again, if the patient's menstrual dates are inaccurate, the obstetrician can make the decision not to become alarmed at a reported low weight percentile. This is far better than misinterpreting a growth-retarded fetus as normal by relating only the estimated weight to the sonographic age. Last, if there has been a previous ultrasound examination, in the report, there should be some statement whether fetal growth has been normal or abnormal.

Amniotic Fluid Volume

During the past several years, there has been tremendous interest in the role of amniotic fluid on fetal development and well-being. While there is relatively good agreement on the significance of extremes of amniotic fluid volume, there is controversy over the methodology used to make the diagnosis of either too much or too little amniotic fluid. It is the author's feeling that the diagnosis of oligohydramnios and polyhydramnios can best be made subjectively. The difficulty with objective measurements is that they are often too stringent and are not gestational age related. The ability to subjectively assess amniotic fluid volume at different stages of gestation is readily learned and should not be difficult for most examiners.

In making the diagnosis of oligohydramnios, one should remember two points: (1) because, in most cases, this will imply the likelihood of a fetal renal malformation or severe growth retardation in the absence of ruptured membranes, this diagnosis should be made only when there is essentially no amniotic fluid; (2) because of the association of severe decreases in amniotic fluid with fetal demise, the obstetrician should be alerted immediately if this diagnosis is made.

The diagnosis of polyhydramnios, while seeming to be less serious, in many cases may in fact be associated with significant complications to the mother and fetus: in the mother, preterm labor and ruptured membranes; and in the fetus, fetal anomalies. Although most cases of polyhydramnios ultimately result in a normal fetus, the high number of anomalous fetuses with this condition reported in literature should alert the sonographer so that a thorough evaluation can be performed when this diagnosis is suspected.[7]

AMNIOTIC FLUID VOLUME IN MULTIPLE GESTATIONS. If one looks at a list of causes of polyhydramnios in many obstetric texts, multiple gestations will most likely appear. Although increased amniotic fluid volume may appear in twin gestations, in most cases the cause is some abnormality of pregnancy.[8] Hashimoto and associates noted that in twin pregnancies with definite persistent polyhydramnios, there was some abnormality of pregnancy in all cases.[8] In many of these, the polyhydramnios occurred in one of the amniotic sacs, while the remaining sac was in fact oligohydramniotic (stuck-twin sign).[9] In cases in which the amniotic fluid was initially thought to be increased and later thought to be normal, the misreading was likely due to the additive visual appearance of the fluid in the two sacs.

The Placenta

As mentioned earlier, whenever the placenta is identified in pregnancy, its position and relationship to the cervix should be noted in the interpretation. The literature has emphasized the large number of false-positive diagnoses of placenta previa that are made either early in pregnancy or in the face of an overdistended urinary bladder.[10, 11] Although this is true, one must not be lulled into a sense of security in thinking that all low-lying placentas will "go away" and be clinically unimportant. If one is unsure about the relationship of the edge of the placenta to the cervical os, the placenta should be interpreted as low lying, and a placenta previa cannot be excluded. These patients will therefore be followed more closely clinically.

Abruptio placentae is a diagnosis that is often difficult to make using ultrasonography. One should remember that the myometrium and its vessels, as well as a transient myometrial contraction, may simulate a hematoma and that these potential false-positive diagnoses should be avoided. As most clinicians are aware that abruptio placentae is a difficult diagnosis, they often refer patients for ultrasound to exclude a placenta previa rather than to specifically see the abruption.

Fetal Malformations

The subject of fetal malformations is among the most emotionally charged issues that either the parents or diagnostician may have to face. During the past ten years, ultrasound has undergone a transformation that has allowed us to answer not only the basic question whether the patient is pregnant but also whether a fetal anomaly is detected. As smaller and smaller abnormalities are identified, the question now becomes what degree of assurance should a patient expect from a report that no anomaly was seen during a routine ultrasound examination? This is a complex issue. The large number of anatomic structures that can be detected using ultrasound have necessitated that anomaly detection, by and large, be a *targeted* examination. To examine every patient for all anomalies would be highly impractical. Fortunately, most major anomalies will be detected as part of a routine

Table 1–1. THE ROUTINE ULTRASOUND EXAMINATION

Structure or Measurement	Abnormality
Fetal head [biparietal diameter (BPD), head circumference (HC)]	Anencephaly, hydrocephalus, encephalocele, cystic hygroma
Fetal heart	Cardiac abnormality, thoracic mass, pleural effusion
Fetal abdomen [abdominal circumference (AC)]	Esophageal atresia (absent stomach), small bowel atresias (dilated bowel), ascites, hydronephrosis, gastroschisis, omphalocele
Femur length	Skeletal dysplasias, short-limbed dwarfism
Amniotic fluid	Polyhydramnios due to gastrointestinal obstruction or oligohydramnios from urinary tract obstruction
Placenta	Placenta previa, abruptio placentae, chorioangioma

evaluation with several minor modifications. Table 1–1 provides a list of the structures or measurements visualized as part of a routine examination and of the corresponding abnormalities that *might* be detected fortuitously. The only additional modification to this would be evaluation of the fetal spine. Because neural tube defects can be devastating to the fetus and not seen as part of the routine evaluation, it is important to evaluate this area specifically.

The patient and referring obstetrician should be made aware that the obstetric "anomaly" ultrasound examination is a targeted evaluation. Except for large gross abnormalities, individual lesions are likely to be detected only when the fetus is known to be at risk for a specific malformation. Anatomic malformations are likely to grow during pregnancy just as the fetus does; a defect seen at birth may have been too small to be detected earlier in pregnancy. Last, it is important for sonographers to know the limits of their expertise. If a malformation is suspected and the examiner has had little experience with the abnormality in question, the case should be referred to a more experienced examiner. Only in this way will patients be best served.

Uterus and Adnexa

Evaluation of the uterus and adnexa becomes more difficult the later in gestation that the examination occurs. The most com-

mon abnormalities that are likely to be detected are uterine myomas. As stated earlier, it is important to measure the size, record the location, and define the relationship of the myoma to the cervix. If ovarian abnormalities are suspected and not seen, patients should have a postpartum examination.

References

1. Report of the Royal College of Obstetricians and Gynaecologists Working Party on Routine Ultrasound Examination in Pregnancy, December 1984.
2. Eik-Nes S, Okland O, Aure J, Ulstein M: Ultrasound screening in pregnancy: A randomized controlled trial. Lancet 1:1347, 1984.
3. Leopold GR: Antepartum obstetrician ultrasound examination guidelines. J Ultrasound Med 5:241, 1986.
4. The Use of Diagnostic Ultrasound Imaging in Pregnancy: US Department of Health and Human Services, Public Health Service, National Institutes of Health, NIH Publication No. 84-667, 1984.
5. AIUM: Safety statements. J Ultrasound Med 2:S19, 1983.
6. Neilson DR: Management of the large breech infant. Am J Obstet Gynecol 107:345, 1970.
7. Barkin SZ, Pretorius DH, Beckett MK, et al: Severe polyhydramnios: Incidence of anomalies. AJR 148:155, 1987.
8. Hashimoto BE, Callen PW, Filly RA, Laros RK: Ultrasound evaluation of polyhydramnios and twin pregnancy. Am J Obstet Gynecol 154:1069, 1986.
9. Mahony BS, Filly RA, Callen PW: Amnionicity and chorionicity in twin pregnancies: Prediction using ultrasound. Radiology 155:205, 1985.
10. Zemlyn S: The effect of the urinary bladder in obstetrical sonography. Radiology 128:169, 1978.
11. Laing FC: Placenta previa: Avoiding false-negative diagnoses. J Clin Ultrasound 9:109, 1981.

2

THE ROLE OF GENETIC SCREENING IN THE OBSTETRIC PATIENT

James D. Goldberg, M.D.

The availability of prenatal diagnosis for a wide range of genetic disorders represents a major advance in the area of reproductive genetics. Historically, couples at risk were informed of their chances of producing affected offspring. These couples then had the option of taking their chances or not reproducing at all. The advent of prenatal diagnosis for many genetic diseases has allowed couples at risk the option of having unaffected offspring. Progress has also been made in prospective population screening tests both to identify couples at risk for having offspring affected with a genetic disorder and to screen for abnormal fetuses.

Ultrasound has played a central role in the development of the various approaches to prenatal diagnosis. This chapter will focus on the interface between reproductive genetics and ultrasound. A brief discussion of genetic counseling principles will be presented, followed by a description of various prenatal diagnostic procedures now in use and their relationship to ultrasound. The importance of sonographic guidance will become evident as the various techniques are described. Other chapters in this book will discuss the increasing importance of ultrasound as a primary diagnostic tool for fetal structural anomalies.

PRINCIPLES OF GENETIC COUNSELING

The provision of nondirective genetic counseling is fundamental to the prenatal diagnosis of any disorder. It is essential that the couple at risk be informed of all their reproductive options. If they choose to undergo any prenatal diagnostic studies, they must understand the risks and advantages of the procedures. This is particularly important with any new procedure for which the safety and accuracy have not been adequately assessed.

Before attempting the prenatal diagnosis of any inherited disease, it is essential to establish or confirm the specific disorder under consideration. Efforts must be directed toward eliminating the possibility of misdiagnosis due to phenotypic, metabolic, or genetic heterogeneity. In the case of an enzymatic or molecular diagnosis, the precise defect must be demonstrated in the proband or affected relatives. If the proband is deceased, the heterozygosity of both parents (or of the mother for an X-linked disease) must be documented. In the case of a dysmorphic syndrome, all manifestations of the disorder must be known and looked for at the time of evaluation.

Indications for Prenatal Diagnosis

The most common indications for prenatal diagnostic studies are listed in Table 2–1. By far the most frequent indication, however, is advanced maternal age. Many studies have shown an increased incidence of chromosomal trisomy with advanced maternal age.[1] When quoting risk figures, it is important to realize that the incidence of aneuploidy at 16 weeks' gestation is approximately double that of newborns, implying a natural spontaneous-loss rate of aneuploid fetuses from 16 weeks to term. Maternal age-specific risk figures for fetal chromosomal abnormalities are listed in Table 2–2. Although the initial data suggested a paternal age effect for chromosomal aneuploidy, this has not been confirmed in later studies. Even so, a complete family history is critical, as couples with one indication for prenatal diagnosis frequently have other risk factors.

The family history of a genetic disorder is another common indication for prenatal diagnosis if a specific molecular, enzymatic, or structural defect is diagnosable in the fetus. As mentioned above, the precise diagnosis must be known to provide accurate prenatal diagnostic studies. The inheritance pattern of the disorder must also be known to provide accurate risk figures; some disorders have differing patterns of inheritance in different families. In addition, the ethnic background of a couple must be ascertained, as certain ethnic groups have an increased incidence of specific disorders, such as sick-

Table 2–2. MATERNAL AGE-SPECIFIC ANEUPLOIDY RATES AT TIME OF AMNIOCENTESIS

Maternal Age at Delivery	Aneuploidy Rate (%)
35	0.78
36	0.97
37	1.2
38	1.5
39	1.9
40	2.4
41	3.1
42	3.9
43	4.9
44	6.3
45	8.0
49	21.1

Modified from Hook EB, Cross PK, Schreinemachers DM: Chromosomal abnormality rates at amniocentesis and in live-born infants. JAMA 249:2034, 1983.

le cell disease in blacks, Tay-Sachs disease in Ashkenazi Jews, and thalassemia in Asians and individuals of Mediterranean descent.

Maternal Serum alpha-Fetoprotein Screening

Maternal serum alpha-fetoprotein (MSAFP) screening has been developed as a prenatal screening test for neural tube defects (NTD). The American College of Obstetrics and Gynecology, while not fully endorsing this test, nonetheless indicates that all health care providers should be aware of the screening procedure and suggests that such testing be offered to all pregnant patients where appropriate follow-up care is available. An understanding of the screening procedure is thus important for all who care for pregnant women.

Alpha-fetoprotein (AFP) is produced mainly in the fetal liver and is the predominant protein in fetal blood. AFP is found in the amniotic fluid at concentrations 150-fold less than in fetal blood, and at even smaller concentrations in the maternal serum, as shown in Figure 2–1. The AFP concentration in all three of these fluids increases steadily through the middle trimester of pregnancy. Elevated middle trimester AFP values, which have been found to be associated with fetal open neural tube defects, are thought to be due to transcapillary transudation of fetal proteins across the lesion. This elevation, however, is not specific, and other open

Table 2–1. INDICATIONS FOR PRENATAL DIAGNOSIS

Chromosomal Abnormality
  Advanced maternal age
  Previous child with a chromosomal disorder
  Balanced translocation carrier for a chromosomal disorder
Single Gene Defects
  Previous child with an inherited metabolic disorder
  Heterozygous couples detected prospectively by screening programs
  Previous child with a disorder detectable by ultrasound
Multifactorial Disorders
  Previous child with a neural tube defect
  Previous child with a developmental defect or malformation syndrome detectable by ultrasound
Environmental Defect
  Prenatal exposure to teratogenic drug or infectious agent

fetal defects that allow increased leakage of serum, or other disorders that interfere with swallowing, may also cause an AFP rise.

The MSAFP screening test measures the concentration of AFP in the maternal serum at 15 to 20 menstrual weeks. The MSAFP concentration, measured in nanograms per milliliter, is converted to multiples of the median (MOM) by dividing by the specific laboratory's median value for the gestational age at the time the sample was drawn. Cor-

rection factors for maternal weight, race, and insulin-dependent diabetes should also be applied.

Many large studies have shown that MSAFP screening will detect 80 to 90 percent of NTD.[2] Approximately 3 to 5 percent of screened pregnancies have an elevated (usually 2.0 to 2.5 MOM) MSAFP level and are referred for Level I ultrasound evaluation to insure accurate dating and to detect conditions that would explain the elevation, i.e., multiple gestation, anencephaly, or fetal demise. This ultrasound screening explains the elevation of AFP in about one-half of the cases. For the others, amniocentesis for amniotic fluid AFP and acetylcholinesterase measurement is offered. The NTD rate for patients undergoing amniocentesis for this purpose is approximately one in 16, or about 6 percent. In those pregnancies with an elevated MSAFP concentration in which the amniotic fluid AFP level is subsequently found to be normal, there appears to be an unexplained increased perinatal mortality of about 65 per 1000.[3]

It is important to review the outcome in cases where the amniotic fluid AFP concentration is elevated. In a review of 11,276 amniotic fluid specimens analyzed at the author's institution, 90 fetuses were found to have elevations greater than three standard deviations above the mean.[4] As shown in Tables 2–3 and 2–4, two groups were evaluated: those with elevations three to five standard deviations above the mean for gestational age and those with greater than five standard deviations. Most significant anomalies (NTD, cystic hygroma, and omphalo-

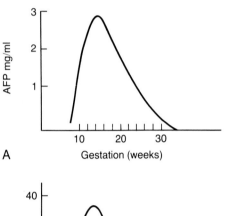

A

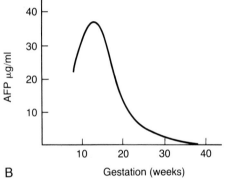

B

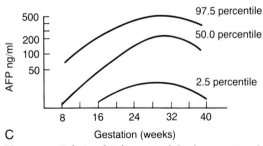

C

Figure 2–1. Relationship between alpha-fetoprotein values in A, fetal serum, B, amniotic fluid, and C, maternal serum. Note the different units for each graph. (*From* Habib A: Maternal serum alpha-fetoprotein: Its value in antenatal diagnosis of genetic disease and in obstetrical-gynecological care. Acta Obstet Gynecol Scand Suppl 61:14, 1977.)

Table 2–3. AMNIOTIC FLUID ALPHA-FETOPROTEIN 3–5 SD > MEAN

	Sonographic Diagnosis	Final Diagnosis
Normal	39	39
Normal (declined sonography)	—	5
Trisomy	—	3
Placental choroid cysts (normal at birth)	2	2
Omphalocele	2	2
Dandy-Walker syndrome	1	1
Intrauterine fetal demise (declined sonography)	—	1
Meningomyelocele	1	1
Cystic hygroma	1	1
Total	46	55

SD = Standard Deviations.

Table 2–4. AMNIOTIC FLUID ALPHA-FETOPROTEIN >5 SD OF MEAN

	Sonographic Diagnosis	Final Diagnosis
Normal	12	10
IUGR, toxemia, neonatal death		1
Pharyngeal teratoma		1
Normal with dead twin	3	3
Cystic hygroma	5	5
Anencephaly	5	5
Encephalocele	4	4
Meningomyelocele	2	2
Omphalocele	2	2
Dysplastic kidneys	1	1
Ventriculomegaly	1	1
Total	35	35

SD = Standard Deviations.

cele) occurred in the second group, and all were detected by ultrasound except for one pharyngeal teratoma noted in an otherwise healthy newborn. All fetuses predicted to be anatomically normal (with the exception of the pharyngeal teratoma) were normal at birth. In view of the increasing numbers of pregnancies found to have an elevated MSAFP concentration, the statistics above should be helpful in counseling persons studied by ultrasound after being noted to have elevated MSAFP and amniotic fluid AFP levels.

In addition to the significance of an elevated level, there appears to be an association between a low MSAFP concentration and fetal Trisomy 21.[5] Data from preliminary studies have been used to create a risk factor table based on maternal age and AFP level.[6] The "cut-off" values for AFP concentration run from about 0.3 MOM for a 20 year old woman to 0.7 MOM for a 34 year old woman and are calculated so that the woman's risk for carrying a Trisomy 21 fetus increases to that of a 35 year old woman. Early estimates suggest that 20 percent of Trisomy 21 fetuses could potentially be identified in this manner.

Techniques for Prenatal Diagnosis

AMNIOCENTESIS. The traditional approach to prenatal diagnosis has been transabdominal amniocentesis performed at approximately 16 weeks' gestation. The amniotic fluid obtained contains desquamated fetal cells that can be grown in tissue culture and karyotyped or used for a variety of metabolic assays or DNA extraction. The volume of amniotic fluid at 15 menstrual weeks has been shown to be 125 ml, which increases 50 ml per week for the next 13 weeks.[7] Initial studies indicated that procedures performed before 15 to 16 weeks' gestation resulted in a significant incidence of "dry taps." With improved ultrasound techniques, this can be minimized, and procedures can technically be performed much earlier in gestation. This provides the advantage of an earlier, safer termination of pregnancy if an affected fetus is diagnosed and the couple elects to abort the pregnancy. The safety of performing amniocentesis before 15 to 16 weeks, however, is not well documented. Preliminary studies suggest an increased fetal loss compared with the well-established loss rate of 0.5 percent at 15 to 16 weeks.[8]

The author's institution uses the following technique for midtrimester amniocentesis. Linear array real-time ultrasound is performed to assess gestational age, fetal life, fetal number, and placental location. If possible, a placental free window is located and the position marked by indenting the maternal abdomen. Increased fetal morbidity has been reported with procedures that traverse the placenta.[9] The abdomen is then prepared with an iodine antiseptic, and the skin and subcutaneous tissues are infiltrated with local anesthetic. The ultrasound transducer is then placed in a polyethylene "sandwich" bag that has been gas sterilized, and sterile gel is applied to the abdomen. The position of the amniotic fluid pocket is reconfirmed, and a 22 gauge 3½ inch spinal needle is inserted under direct ultrasound vision. It is important to maintain the ultrasound transducer in a plane as parallel as possible to the needle; this helps avoid foreshortening of the needle tip. The obturator is then removed, a syringe attached to the needle, and 24 ml of amniotic fluid withdrawn after discarding the first 0.5 ml to avoid maternal cell and blood contamination. Approximately 1.4 percent of specimens are discolored, usually because of heme pigment.[10]

The usefulness of continuous ultrasound monitoring has been debated. Although no significant decrease in fetal morbidity has been reported, a significant decrease in the incidence of bloody and dry taps of the first needle insertion and in the number of patients who required multiple needle insertions has been reported.[11] Moreover, it is extremely reassuring to the patient to know that the fetus is not in the needle's path. Also, additional information is provided to the operator in instances when fluid is not immediately obtained owing to tenting of the membranes or contraction of the uterus.

If a twin gestation is identified on ultrasound, additional counseling and a change in the amniocentesis technique are necessary. Since one-third of twin gestations are monozygotic, the increased risk of aneuploidy would be 5/3 times the maternal age-specific risk. For indications other than advanced maternal age, the specific risks for twin gestations have been determined and should be discussed with the couple.[12]

The technique for sampling a twin gestation involves first visualizing the dividing membrane and identifying an amniotic fluid pocket in both sacs. After removal of fluid from the first sac, 0.5 ml of indigo carmine dye is instilled. Methylene blue should not be used owing to reports of fetal hemolysis when it is injected intra-amniotically.[13] Aspiration of clear fluid from the second sac insures proper placement.

The finding of a single affected fetus in a twin gestation presents a significant counseling dilemma. Until recently, the couple had limited options. They could choose to do nothing and allow the pregnancy to continue with the birth of one normal and one potentially disabled infant. Otherwise, they could choose to abort the pregnancy, thus terminating both a normal and an abnormal fetus. A third alternative has been reported: selective termination of the affected fetus.[14] Initial reports described the use of cardiac puncture and air injection to terminate the affected fetus. The author has found fetal intracardiac injection of potassium chloride to be effective.

CHORIONIC VILLUS SAMPLING. As described above, amniocentesis at 16 weeks' gestation, followed by culture and analysis of the obtained amniocytes, frequently results in a prenatal diagnosis at 19 to 20 weeks' gestation. If an affected fetus is diagnosed and the couple elects to abort the pregnancy, a second trimester termination procedure is necessary, with its increased medical and psychologic risks as compared with a first trimester termination. Because of this, research efforts have been directed toward developing an early first trimester diagnostic procedure.

The first attempt to obtain chorionic villus cells was reported by Hahnemann and Mohr in 1968.[15] These and other investigators were able to obtain trophoblast by transcervical hysteroscopy of women undergoing midtrimester termination of pregnancy. The yield of tissue, however, was extremely low, and there was difficulty culturing what little they had. The first series of chorionic villus sampling (CVS) in ongoing pregnancies was reported in a Chinese study in 1975.[16] One hundred patients underwent transcervical CVS without ultrasound guidance for the diagnosis of fetal sex. Only four spontaneous losses were noted; however, the induced termination rate was high.

The use of ultrasound to guide the sampling catheter has resulted in a markedly increased success rate in obtaining villi. Ward and colleagues reported up to a 90 percent success rate using ultrasound guidance in obtaining trophoblast.[17] Rodeck and associates described a single operator technique in which one hand holds the ultrasound transducer and the other controls the sampling catheter.[18] Other investigators have described similar high success rates in obtaining chorionic villi with ultrasound guidance, and this has become the most commonly used CVS technique.[19–22]

In addition to guiding the catheter into the trophoblast, ultrasound provides many other advantages for CVS. One of the most important is verifying that a fetus is alive before sampling is performed. Studies have shown that over 10 percent of women presenting for CVS have nonviable gestations.[23] Moreover, multiple gestations can be identified in most instances. It must be recognized, however, that a proportion of multiple gestations observed in the first trimester will revert to a single gestation as pregnancy progresses.[24] Ultrasound also identifies local uterine variations such as fibroids and uterine contractions that can interfere with insertion and placement of the sampling catheter.

The technique of transcervical chorionic villus sampling is described below. Using a sector scanner, fetal life is documented, multiple gestations are sought, the trophoblast is localized, and the sampling path is estimated. Alteration of the bladder's volume frequently helps optimize the sampling position. The patient is then put in the lithotomy position, a speculum inserted, and the vagina prepared with an iodine antiseptic. Under direct ultrasound visualization, the sampling catheter, a 16 gauge polyethylene catheter with a malleable stainless steel obturator, is inserted into the area of the trophoblast as shown in Figure 2–2. A 20 ml syringe is then attached to the catheter and with 5 to 10 ml of negative pressure, the sample is aspirated as the catheter is removed. The sample is immediately examined under a low-power dissecting microscope to determine its adequacy. A tenaculum is occasionally needed to stabilize the cervix. As many as three passes of the catheter are performed, if necessary, with a new catheter used each time. No anesthesia is necessary; frequently, however, a cramping sensation is reported by the patient as the catheter passes through the internal os of the cervix.

In some instances, with a fundal implantation or an extremely anteflexed or retroflexed uterus, it has been impossible to reach the trophoblast with the transcervical approach. An alternative transabdominal approach has been used by some investigators in these cases. The technique is similar to ultrasound-guided amniocentesis, but the needle is guided into the trophoblast only and a sample aspirated as the needle is withdrawn. This appears to be a useful alternative to the transcervical approach, but further evaluation will be necessary before a final assessment is made.

The primary concern with any new technique is its safety. This has been particularly difficult to assess with CVS because of the significant baseline fetal loss rate associated with the gestational age at which it is performed (nine to 11 menstrual weeks). Until recently, the fetal loss rate after demonstrated heart activity at eight to nine menstrual weeks was unknown. Two studies address this and reveal an increasing fetal loss rate with increasing maternal age.[25, 26] In the maternal age range where CVS is most commonly performed (≥35 years), the baseline fetal loss rate was 4.1 to 4.5 percent.

These baseline loss figures must be compared with the fetal loss rate after CVS. To date, the most comprehensive collection of fetal loss data has been detailed in the CVS Latest News, which is edited by Jackson.[27] This newsletter reports results from contributors worldwide and currently lists over 20,000 procedures. The overall loss rate has remained stable at approximately 3.5 to 4 percent. Comparing this with the baseline loss rate of 4.1 to 4.5 percent results in a very small procedure-related loss rate. An increased number of cases will be needed to assess more accurately this risk.

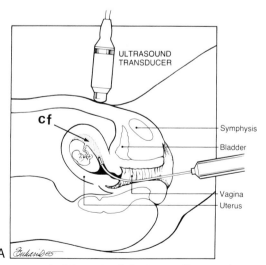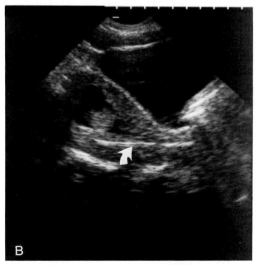

Figure 2–2. *A*, Schematic of chorionic villus sampling procedure. cf, chorion frondosum. (*Reprinted by permission from* Simpson JL: Genetic counseling and prenatal diagnosis. *In* Gabbe SG, Niebyl JR, Simpson JL (eds): Obstetrics: Normal and Problem Pregnancies. New York, Churchill Livingstone, 1986, pp 211–244.) *B*, Sonographic image of a chorionic villus catheter *(arrow)* in a posteriorly implanted trophoblast.

To assess this loss rate in a more controlled manner, several countries have undertaken studies to compare the safety and accuracy of CVS with that of amniocentesis. One of these is a seven-center collaborative investigation sponsored by the National Institute of Child Health and Human Development and designed as a case control study to assess both the accuracy and safety of CVS as compared with amniocentesis. Other studies under way in Canada and several Scandinavian and European centers are being conducted in a randomized manner and will provide valuable safety information.

RHESUS SENSITIZATION. The risk of Rhesus sensitization following amniocentesis or CVS is controversial. Several studies have suggested an increased risk based on the discovery of fetal red cells in the maternal circulation after the procedure or on an increase in maternal serum alpha-fetoprotein.[28, 29] Two large retrospective studies, however, found no increase in isoimmunization in women not receiving Rh prophylaxis after amniocentesis.[30, 31] In addition, it has been suggested that if early prophylaxis is given, it should be repeated at regular intervals during the pregnancy to avoid an enhancement phenomenon.[29]

FETAL BLOOD SAMPLING. As listed in Table 2–5, there are many indications that require gaining access to the fetal circulation and sampling the fetal blood. The most common indication is the confirmation of abnormal findings from amniocentesis or chorionic villus sampling. Another frequent indication is the need for a rapid chromosomal diagnosis. Analysis of fetal blood requires 48 to 72 hours compared with two to three weeks for amniocentesis. An increasingly common indication is the finding of a structural anomaly on ultrasound. In a report by Ni-

Table 2–6. INCIDENCE OF CHROMOSOMAL ANEUPLOIDY

Nonimmune hydrops fetalis (12/37)	32%
Omphalocele (8/12)	67%
Duodenal atresia (1/3)	33%
Obstructive uropathy (9/39)	23%
Unilateral pleural effusion (1/3)	33%
Severe IUGR and oligohydramnios (2/10)	20%
Hydrocephalus (2/9)	22%
Choroid plexus cyst (3/4)	75%

Modified from Nicolaides KH, Rodeck CH, Gosden CM: Rapid karyotyping in non-lethal fetal malformations. Lancet 1:283, 1986.

colaides and associates summarized in Table 2–6, a significant number of fetuses found to have a structural anomaly on ultrasound were aneuploid.[32]

Until recently, fetal blood sampling was performed by fetoscopic-guided puncture of the umbilical vessels. The first prenatal diagnosis by fetoscopy was reported in 1974 by Hobbins and colleagues.[33] The procedure involved transabdominal insertion of a 1.7 mm endoscope through an approximately 3.2 mm trocar. The fetal vessels were then visualized on the placental surface and needled under direct vision for a fetal blood sample. Samples obtained in this way were frequently mixed with maternal blood. A significant advance in the fetoscopic procedure was reported by Rodeck and Campbell.[34] Under direct vision, the umbilical cord was punctured near its insertion into the placenta. This resulted in pure fetal samples in almost all cases. This highly specialized technique was available only at a limited number of centers around the world. A 5 percent fetal loss rate was reported for patients undergoing fetoscopy at these centers.[35]

A new approach to fetal blood sampling was recently reported by Daffos and associates.[36] This involves percutaneous umbilical blood sampling (PUBS) under sonographic guidance. They reported over 600 cases of fetal blood sampling with a fetal loss rate less than 1 percent. This approach has become the method of choice for fetal blood sampling and fetal intravascular transfusion.

The procedure is described below. The area of umbilical cord insertion into the placenta is visualized by a sector scanner. This is the optimal area for sampling as the cord is fixed at this location. The umbilical cord insertion site into the fetus or a free loop of cord may be used; however, this

Table 2–5. INDICATIONS FOR FETAL BLOOD SAMPLING

Confirm chromosomal mosaicism found on
   amniocentesis
Rapid karyotyping
Fetal blood grouping
Assessment of fetal anemia or thrombocytopenia
Hemoglobinopathies
Hemophilia A or B and other clotting disorders
Imunodeficiencies and other white cell disorders
Inborn errors of metabolism

approach is frequently more difficult because of cord movement. The mother is then given parenteral sedation both for her comfort and to decrease fetal movements. The use of intramuscular or intravenous fetal injections of curare pancuronium bromide (Pavulon) has been reported to eliminate fetal movement during the longer intravascular transfusion procedures.[37, 38] The long-term effects of temporary fetal paralysis are unknown. The abdomen is then prepared and draped, and the insertion site and subcutaneous tissues are infiltrated with local anesthetic. While infiltrating the subcutaneous tissue, one can check the angle of the needle insertion with ultrasound. Under ultrasound guidance, a 22 or 25 gauge 3½ inch spinal needle is advanced into the umbilical circulation as shown in Figure 2–3. Samples of fetal blood are then aspirated into preheparinized syringes.

The fetal blood sample is immediately analyzed using a Coulter cell sizer to verify a fetal origin. The fetal red cell size is plotted against a maternal sample and will show a larger size distribution. Betke-Kleihauer staining may also be performed for further verification. The ability to analyze the sample immediately makes it possible to obtain a second one if a maternal specimen has been obtained.

FETAL TISSUE SAMPLING. Some inherited diseases are expressed only in a specific tissue and thus sampling of that tissue is necessary if a prenatal diagnosis is to be made. Both fetal liver and fetal skin have been obtained by ultrasonically guided biopsy.[39, 40] These procedures are performed at only a few referral centers.

DNA METHODOLOGY. As progress is made in the elucidation of the specific molecular defect in an ever increasing number of genetic diseases, prenatal diagnosis will be possible by DNA analysis. Since DNA is present in every nucleated cell, minimally invasive techniques, such as amniocentesis or chorionic villus sampling, may replace the more invasive procedures, such as fetal blood sampling or fetal liver biopsy, for the prenatal diagnosis of many diseases. The list of diseases diagnosable by DNA analysis is continually expanding; thus, before attempting a prenatal diagnosis, a current compendium or a geneticist should be consulted.

Safe and reliable access to the fetal circulation is ushering in a new era in fetal

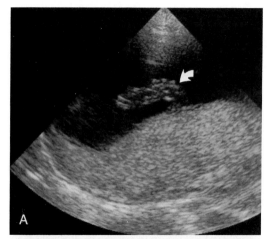

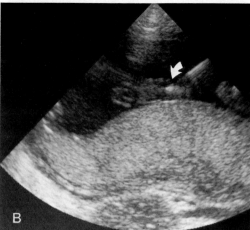

Figure 2–3. A, Sonographic image of posterior insertion of the umbilical cord into the placenta (arrow). B, Sonographic image of a sampling needle in the umbilical cord at the insertion site (arrow).

prenatal diagnosis and therapy. Initial reports of fetal intravascular transfusion of red cells or platelets for isoimmunization appear promising.[41, 42] In addition, the availability of early first trimester diagnosis may provide opportunities for prenatal therapy for certain disorders by replacement of missing enzymes or cofactors, by somatic gene replacement, or by stem cell transplantation. Ultrasound will continue to play a critical role in the development of these new approaches to fetal prenatal diagnosis and therapy.

References

1. Hook EB, Cross PK, Schreinemachers DM: Chromosomal abnormality rates at amniocentesis and in live-born infants. JAMA 249:2034, 1983.

2. Simpson JL, Nadler HL: Maternal serum alpha-fetoprotein screening in 1987. Obstet Gynecol 69:134, 1987.
3. Macri JN, Weiss RR: Prenatal serum alpha-fetoprotein for neural tube defects. Obstet Gynecol 59:663, 1982.
4. Anderson RL, Goldberg JD, Golbus MS: Findings at sonography in evaluation of elevated amniotic fluid alpha-fetoprotein. Proceedings 7th International Congress of Human Genetics, Berlin, 1986.
5. Cuckle HS, Wald NJ, Lindenbaum RH: Maternal serum alpha-fetoprotein measurement: A screening test for Down syndrome. Lancet 1:926, 1984.
6. Martin AO, Liu K: Implications of "low" maternal serum alpha-fetoprotein levels: Are maternal age risk criteria obsolete? Prenat Diag 6:243, 1986.
7. Fuchs F: Volume of amniotic fluid at various stages of pregnancy. Clin Obstet Gynecol 9:449, 1966.
8. Hanson FW, Zorn EM, Tennant FR, et al: Amniocentesis before 15 weeks gestation: Outcome, risks, and technical problems. Am J Obstet Gynecol 156:1524, 1987.
9. Kappel B, Nielsen J, Brongaard-Hansen K, et al: Spontaneous abortion following mid-trimester amniocentesis: Clinical significance of placental perforation and blood-stained amniotic fluid. Br J Obstet Gynaecol 94:50, 1987.
10. Hess LW, Anderson RL, Golbus MS: Significance of opaque discolored amniotic fluid at second trimester amniocentesis. Obstet Gynecol 67:44, 1986.
11. Romero R, Jeanty P, Reece EA, et al: Sonographically monitored amniocentesis to decrease intraoperative complications. Obstet Gynecol 65:426, 1985.
12. Hunter AGW, Cox DM: Counselling problems when twins are discovered at genetic amniocentesis. Clin Genet 16:34, 1979.
13. McEnerney JK, McEnerney LN: Unfavorable neonatal outcome after intraamniotic injection of methylene blue. Obstet Gynecol 61 (Suppl):35, 1983.
14. Kerenyi TD, Chitkara U: Selective birth in twin pregnancy with discordancy for Down's syndrome. N Engl J Med 304:1525, 1981.
15. Hahnemann N, Mohr J: Genetic diagnosis in the embryo by means of biopsy from extraembryonic membranes. Bull Eur Soc Hum Gen 2:23, 1968.
16. Department of Obstetrics and Gynecology, Tietung Hospital, Anshan Iron and Steel Company: Fetal sex prediction by sex chromatin of chorionic villi cells during early pregnancy. Clin Med J 1:117, 1975.
17. Ward RHT, Modell B, Petrou M, et al: Method of sampling chorionic villi in first trimester of pregnancy under guidance of real time ultrasound. Br Med J 286:1542, 1983.
18. Rodeck CH, Morsman JM, Gosden CM, et al: Development of an improved technique for first-trimester microsampling of chorion. Br J Obstet Gynaecol 90:1113, 1983.
19. Old JM, Ward RHT, Karagozlu F, et al: First trimester fetal diagnosis for haemoglobinopathies: Three cases. Lancet 2:1413, 1982.
20. Grebner EE, Wapner RJ, Barr MA, et al: Prenatal Tay-Sachs diagnosis by chorionic villi sampling. Lancet 2:286, 1983.
21. Pergament E, Ginsberg N, Verlinsky Y, et al: Prenatal Tay-Sachs diagnosis by chorionic villi sampling. Lancet 2:286, 1983.
22. Simoni G, Brambati B, Danesino C, et al: Efficient direct chromosome analyses and enzyme determinations from chorionic villi samples in the first trimester of pregnancy. Hum Genet 63:349, 1983.
23. Jones, S, Dorfmann A, Patton L, et al: Non-viable pregnancy in patients anticipating chorionic villus sampling. Am J Hum Gen 34:A257, 1986.
24. Landy HL, Weiner S, Corson SL, et al: The "vanishing twin": Ultrasonographic assessment of disappearance in the first trimester. Am J Obstet Gynecol 155:14, 1986.
25. Gilmore DH, McNay MB: Spontaneous fetal loss rate in early pregnancy. Lancet 1:107, 1985.
26. Wilson RD, Kendrick V, Wittmann BK, et al: Risk of spontaneous abortion in ultrasonically normal pregnancies. Lancet 2:920, 1984.
27. Jackson L (ed): CVS Latest News, Jefferson Medical College, Philadelphia, May 28, 1987.
28. Blakemore KJ, Baumgarten A, Schoenfield-Dimaio M, et al: Rise in maternal serum alpha-fetoprotein concentration after chorionic villus sampling and the possibility of isoimmunization. Am J Obstet Gynecol 155:988, 1986.
29. Bowman JM, Pollack JM: Transplacental fetal hemorrhage after amniocentesis. Obstet Gynecol 66:749, 1985.
30. Golbus MS, Stephens JD, Cann HM, et al: Rh isoimmunization following genetic amniocentesis. Prenat Diag 2:149, 1982.
31. Tabor A, Jerne S, Boeck JE: Incidence of rhesus immunisation after genetic amniocentesis. Br Med J 293:533, 1986.
32. Nicolaides KH, Rodeck CH, Gosden CM: Rapid karyotyping in non-lethal fetal malformations. Lancet 1:283, 1986.
33. Hobbins JC, Mahoney MJ: In utero diagnosis of hemoglobinopathies: Technique for obtaining fetal blood. N Engl J Med 290:1065, 1974.
34. Rodeck CH, Campbell S: Umbilical-cord insertion as source of pure fetal blood for prenatal diagnosis. Lancet 1:1244, 1979.
35. The status of fetoscopy and fetal tissue sampling. The results of the first meeting of the International Fetoscopy Group. Prenat Diagn 4:79, 1984.
36. Daffos F, Capella-Pavlovsky M, Forestier F: Fetal blood sampling during pregnancy with use of a needle guided by ultrasound: A study of 606 consecutive cases. Am J Obstet Gynecol 153:665, 1985.
37. de Crespigny LC, Robinson HP, Quinn M, et al: Ultrasound-guided fetal blood transfusion for severe rhesus isoimmunization. Obstet Gynecol 66:529, 1985.
38. Seeds JW, Bowes WA: Ultrasound-guided fetal intravascular transfusion in severe rhesus immunization. Am J Obstet Gynecol 154:1105, 1986.
39. Holzgreve W, Golbus MS: Prenatal diagnosis of ornithine transcarbamylase deficiency utilizing fetal liver biopsy. Am J Hum Genet 36:320, 1984.
40. Esterly NB, Elias S: Antenatal diagnosis of genodermatoses. J Am Acad Dermatol 8:655, 1983.
41. Berkowitz RL, Chitkara U, Goldberg JD: Intrauterine intravascular transfusions for severe red blood cell isoimmunization: Ultrasound-guided percutaneous approach. Am J Obstet Gynecol 155:574, 1986.
42. Daffos F, Forrestier F, Muller JY, et al: Prenatal treatment of alloimmune thrombocytopenia. Lancet 2:632, 1984.
43. Habib A: Maternal serum alpha-fetoprotein: Its value in antenatal diagnosis of genetic disease and in obstetrical-gynecological care. Acta Obstet Gynecol Scand Suppl 61:14, 1977.

THE FIRST TRIMESTER

Roy A. Filly, M.D.

In the past decade, a wealth of new information has become available regarding the first trimester of pregnancy, particularly its earliest beginnings. Programs of in vitro fertilization have caused physicians to see the first trimester in a new light. This perception has been greatly augmented by powerful new tools, such as high-resolution real-time sonography and radioimmune assays (RIA) to detect extremely small quantities of human chorionic gonadotropin (hCG). Newer sonographic systems enable visualization of early embryonic structures as early as six weeks after the last normal menstrual period (LNMP) or four weeks after conception. Another relatively new program, chorionic villus sampling, is gathering a great deal of sonographic and chromosomal information from pregnancies of seven to ten menstrual weeks.

Sonographers have long recognized their potential contribution to the evaluation of early pregnancy. Ian Donald, the early pioneer of obstetric sonography, stated in his Gold Medal address: "We are particularly interested in studying the first 12 weeks of uterine development, which are even more interesting than the last 12 weeks. It is surely the most crucial period in any being's existence. . . ."[1]

From the perspective of the sonographer, we are at the dawn of the widespread use of intracorporeal transducers. Very-high-frequency transducers, painlessly introduced into the vagina, yield a view of early pregnancy likely to impress even classically trained embryologists. Intravaginal scanning also serves as an "equalizer"; those sonographers with practices too small to offset the cost of selectively focused, phased-array ultrasound systems will be able to substantially improve their ability to image early pregnancies by availing themselves of this powerful "add-on" to existing lower resolution systems.

The sonographic approach recommended in this chapter is one of pragmatism. There is a widely held belief that the way to proceed in sonographically suspected abnormal first trimester pregnancies is to subject the patient to a seemingly endless sequence of follow-up examinations. Although all diagnosticians recognize the value of adding the dimension of time and serial observation to particularly difficult cases, this philosophy should not become so pervasive that one virtually abdicates diagnostic responsibility. A number of extremely reliable indicators of a nonviable pregnancy have been described; once these have been observed, nothing is gained by prolonging the pregnancy.

WHAT IS A PREGNANCY?

With the advent of in vitro fertilization programs and in view of both moral and ethical questions surrounding legal therapeutic abortion, gynecologists are re-examining the fundamental concept of pregnancy. Is a fertilized ovum (zygote) a pregnancy? Is an implanted blastocyst a pregnancy? What should in vitro fertilization programs, charging women thousands of dollars per attempt, claim as their "pregnancy rate"?[2]

Researchers can now detect the presence of a recently implanted pregnancy at a very early age. Human chorionic gonadotropin is first elaborated after implantation of the blastocyst into the decidualized endometrium of the uterus. The hormone is produced by the trophoblastic cells of the developing chorionic villi. Extraordinarily low levels of this hormone (< 1 ng/ml) can be detected by RIA techniques, making it possible for investigators to confidently detect a pregnancy before a woman misses her first menstrual period.

Numerous studies have addressed the issue of early pregnancy identification and have recorded a surprisingly high loss rate.[2-4] Of 100 ova exposed to fertilization, 16 will fail to be fertilized.[3] Of the 84 that become zygotes, a further 15 will fail to implant. Thus, 69 blastocysts actually implant in the uterus and result in detectable levels of hCG (chemical pregnancy). However, 27 of these (39 percent) will abort very near the expected onset of the ensuing menstruation. In this manner, the developing gestation is lost (menstrual abortion) before the woman recognizes even the possibility that she is pregnant. It is not until a woman has missed a menstrual period and consults a physician who confirms a positive pregnancy test that an entity exists that can be termed a clinical pregnancy. By this point, only 42 of the original 100 exposed ova have survived to become recognized pregnancies, even though 84 became embryos. Simply put, one-half of the embryos are lost before they are recognized by the mother or a clinician.

Even amongst clinically recognized pregnancies, the difficult journey is far from complete. Within this group, one-fourth will threaten to abort, and fully one-half of these will indeed be lost (recognized abortion). Recall that up to this point, the obstetrician has yet to have an opportunity to influence the final outcome. It is only among the remaining 30 potentially viable fetuses that modern obstetrics can begin to make an impact, and even then a further small percentage will be lost, and some viable outcomes will be less than desirable.

These figures become somewhat less de-pressing when one realizes that the bulk of these losses are not random "bad luck" but rather "nature's way" of eliminating anomalous fetuses. The frequency of chromosomal anomalies in abortuses up to six weeks is very high, approximately 70 percent.[5] Over 99 percent of chromosomally anomalous fetuses are eliminated during the course of pregnancy. It is difficult to accept that the unfortunate newborns we sometimes encounter with chromosomal anomalies are, in fact, the "cream of the chromosomally abnormal crop." Their counterparts could not survive the arduous process of pregnancy and birth.

NORMAL EARLY EMBRYONIC DEVELOPMENT*

A zygote is formed when an oocyte unites with a sperm cell; development begins at that moment.[6] Cleavage occurs in the fallopian tube and commences approximately one day after fertilization (Fig. 3–1). Subsequent divisions occur rapidly, such that after three days a small solid ball of cells (approximately 16) is produced. This entity is called a morula, the structure that enters the uterine cavity.

Fluid promptly passes into the morula from the endometrial cavity. This fluid separates the embryonic cells (blastomeres) into two layers. The outer layer or trophoblast eventually becomes the chorionic membrane and the fetal contribution to the placenta, while the inner cell mass gives rise to the embryo, amnion, cord, and secondary yolk sac. This cystic structure is called the blastocyst (Fig. 3–1).

The blastocyst remains within the endometrial cavity approximately two days and then attaches to the decidualized endometrial wall. It is the trophoblast immediately adjacent to the embryo (inner cell mass) that attaches to and begins to invade the endometrial epithelium. By the end of the first week of development, some three weeks after the onset of LNMP, the blastocyst is implanted. As further invasion of the endo-

---

*The following section was largely excerpted from Dr. Keith Moore's excellent embryologic textbook (Moore KL: The Developing Human: Clinically Oriented Embryology, 4th Ed. Philadelphia, WB Saunders Co, 1988).[6-8]

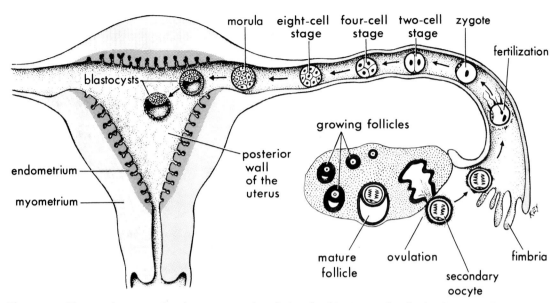

Figure 3–1. Diagram demonstrating the sequence of ovulation, fertilization, and early development of the embryo. The morula is the structure that enters the endometrial cavity. Fluid rapidly enters the morula, creating the blastocyst. The blastocyst is the embryonic structure that implants into the decidualized endometrium. (*From* Moore KL: The Developing Human: Clinically Oriented Embryology, 4th Ed. Philadelphia, WB Saunders Co., 1988.)

metrium occurs, early chorionic villi develop. These cells elaborate hCG, a substance that can now be measured in a minute quantity, i.e., the "pregnancy test" becomes positive.

The blastocyst continues to invade the endometrium until it is virtually submerged, and indeed, the breeched surface heals over the blastocyst (Fig. 3–2A, B).[7] As the blastocyst cavity expands, a layer of cells separates from the blastocyst wall, forming Heuser's membrane, the exocoelomic membrane, thus creating the primitive or primary yolk sac that occupies the bulk of the early blastocyst cavity. Simultaneously, the smaller amniotic cavity begins to form. Lying between the amniotic cavity and the primary yolk sac is the embryonic disc.

The primitive yolk sac shrinks as the secondary yolk sac takes shape. The embryonic disc now lives between the forming amniotic cavity and the secondary yolk sac (Fig. 3–3A). At the end of the second week of development (four weeks since beginning of the LNMP), the blastocyst cavity has attained a size of only 1 mm. Within a few days, the blastocyst cavity has attained a mean diameter of 2 to 3 mm; thereafter, high-resolution sonography can begin to detect the presence of a gestation.

By the end of the third week (five LNMP weeks), the chorionic cavity is well developed and contains the bulk of the fluid that sonographers call the gestational sac (Figs. 3–2C, 3–3A, B). The amniotic sac, at this stage, is much smaller than the chorionic cavity. The edges of the amnion are fused with the embryonic disc (Fig. 3–3A). Enlargement and folding of the embryo cause it to come to lie within the enlarging amniotic cavity (Fig. 3–3B). As the embryo folds, the dorsal curvature bows into the amniotic sac. The attachment of the amnion to the embryo thus comes to be along its ventral aspect; in fact, the amnion envelops the umbilical cord (Figs. 3–3C, 3–4). The yolk sac's communication with the embryo is progressively "pinched" off and comes to lie within the chorionic cavity. The yolk stalk maintains a connection between the yolk sac and the embryo.

The amniotic cavity progressively enlarges until it obliterates the chorionic cavity toward the end of the first trimester. At the end of the eighth embryonic week (ten weeks since the beginning of the LNMP), the embryo "officially" becomes a fetus. Thus, the sonographically favored term of "fetal pole" is inappropriate, since it is usually employed to refer to embryos.

An equally vital structure, the placenta, is developing in parallel with the early embryo.[8] Recall that the developing blastocyst is entirely embedded in the endometrial sur-

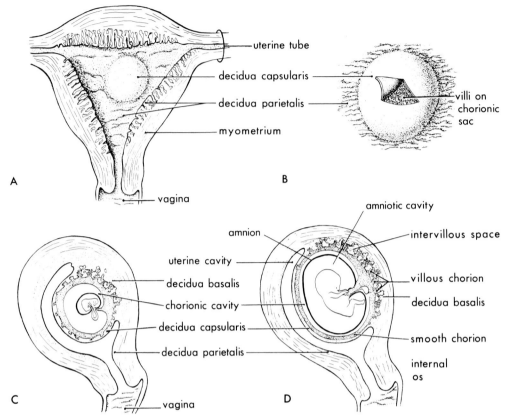

Figure 3–2. A, The implanted blastocyst is entirely covered by the decidua capsularis. B, Reflection of the decidua capsularis shows multiple chorionic villi covering the chorionic sac. C, D, Progressive growth brings the decidua capsularis in contact with the decidua parietalis. (*From* Moore KL: The Developing Human: Clinically Oriented Embryology, 4th Ed. Philadelphia, WB Saunders Co, 1988.)

face, and the decidualized endometrium has healed over it by the end of the second week (four LNMP weeks) (Fig. 3–2A, B). The decidua that heals over and covers the surface of the blastocyst is termed the *decidua capsularis*. At three weeks of development (five LNMP weeks), chorionic villi (tertiary type) developing from the trophoblastic layer have proliferated extensively and cover the surface of the blastocyst entirely and equally (Fig. 2–2B, 3–3A, B). However, as the sac grows and expands into the endometrial cavity, the villi adjacent to the decidua capsularis become compressed and begin to degenerate, producing a bare area of chorion, the *chorion laeve* (Figs. 3–2C, D, 3–3C, 3–4). This structure eventually becomes the chorionic membrane. As growth continues, the enlarging gestational sac fills the endometrial cavity, bringing the decidua capsularis, which covers the chorion laeve, into intimate and full contact with the decidua lining the remainder of the uterine cavity

(the *decidua parietalis*). The decidua capsularis is now greatly attenuated and eventually fuses with the decidua parietalis, obliterating the endometrial cavity. The decidua capsularis then degenerates and disappears. After the disappearance of the decidua capsularis, the chorion (from the chorion laeve) in turn fuses with the decidua parietalis. This fusion can be separated and usually is when bleeding occurs. The blood pushes the chorion away from the decidua parietalis, re-establishing the potential space of the endometrial cavity.

Conversely, the portion of the chorionic sac known as the *chorion frondosum* demonstrates progressive villus formation and forms the fetal component of the placenta. The chorion frondosum develops around the most deeply imbedded section of the blastocyst, that portion immediately adjacent to the inner cell mass (early embryo). The maternal component of the placenta arises from the *decidua basalis* (the decidua adjacent to

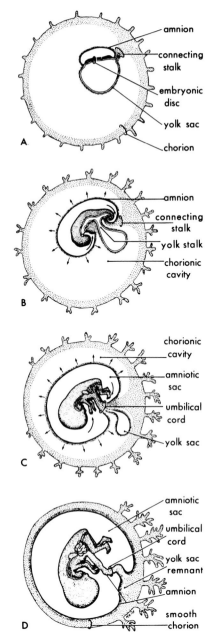

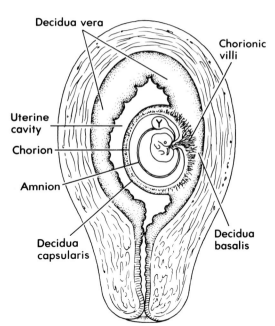

Figure 3–4. Diagram of an early gestation. The embryo lies entirely within the amnion. The amnion has not yet fused with the chorion. Chorionic villi (the chorion frondosum) are intermingled with the decidua basalis. The decidua capsularis covers the smooth chorion. The decidua capsularis is not yet in apposition with the decidua vera. The decidua capsularis (and smooth chorion) and decidua vera form the reflective margins of the double decidual sac sign.

the chorion frondosum). So-called anchoring villi cause firm adherence to the maternal and fetal components. Therefore, by inference, the center of the early placenta marks the site of implantation; the *center* of the fluid in the gastrointestinal sac *does not* mark the relative position of implantation (Figs. 3–2*A*, *C*). Since the chorionic membrane (from the chorion laeve) and the fetal placenta (from the chorion frondosum) develop from the same layer of cells, they are firmly attached at the edges.

NORMAL SONOGRAPHIC ANATOMY IN THE FIRST TRIMESTER

There is a natural tendency to relate sonographically observed landmarks in the first trimester of pregnancy to menstrual age. However, from a clinical perspective, it is more practical to relate observations seen on early pregnancy sonograms to the size of the gestational sac rather than to the menstrual or embryonic age of the pregnancy. This is

Figure 3–3. *A*, Early blastocyst showing the beginning development of the amnion and the secondary yolk sac. The embryonic disc lies between. This structure is attached to the chorion by the connecting stalk. Note that villi are equally distributed around the periphery of the chorion. *B*, The dorsal aspect of the embryo begins to fold into the amnion. This infolding begins to constrict the attachment of the yolk sac to the embryo, forming the yolk stalk. The chorionic villi at the base of the yolk stalk are more prolific than those along the opposite pole of the blastocyst. *C*, The amnion now is enfolding the developing umbilical cord, pushing the yolk sac into the chorionic cavity. A smooth area of chorion is now easily seen. *D*, The smooth chorion is now well developed. The amnion is fused to the smooth chorion, and the early placenta is well established. (*From* Moore KL: The Developing Human: Clinically Oriented Embryology, 4th Ed. Philadelphia, WB Saunders Co, 1988.)

particularly true since an abnormal gestational sac may be discordant (usually smaller) with dates, or the dates may be inaccurate. Because pressure from the urinary bladder or focal myometrial contractions (FMC) commonly cause mild to moderate distortions in sac shape, it is best to judge sac size by estimating a mean sac diameter (MSD).[9-13] The MSD equals the length (craniocaudal dimension), plus the width (transverse dimension), plus the height (anteroposterior dimension) of the gestational sac, divided by three. These measurements are obtained from the chorionic tissue-fluid interface. Only the width is measured on transverse scans. Longitudinal scans are required to obtain the craniocaudal and anteroposterior dimensions.

Occasionally, with modern equipment, especially instruments equipped with intravaginal transducers, one can detect a gestational sac when it has only a 2 to 3 mm MSD (approximately four weeks, three days since the LNMP).[14] With most high-resolution scanners, even employing a transabdominal approach, one can consistently detect a gestational sac when the MSD equals approximately 5 mm (35 days: five menstrual weeks).* It appears as an intrauterine fluid collection surrounded by a rim of moderate echoes (Fig. 3–5).[10] At this point in gestation, the hCG will measure approximately 1800 mIU/ml (Second International Standard). Unfortunately, a variety of other conditions may result in intrauterine fluid collections that may have a similar appearance to early gestational sacs. These include bleeding, endometritis, cervical stenosis, and the pseudogestational sac of ectopic pregnancy, to name the most common.[18] However, only the pseudogestational sac of

---

*There is some controversy in the literature regarding the precise age at which ultrasound can first detect a gestational sac, estimates ranging from 3.5 to five weeks.[9, 10, 14-16] There is less controversy regarding the size of the gestational sac when it is first observed.[14] This is now thought to be approximately 2 to 3 mm in mean sac diameter. Similarly, most observers agree that the MSD increases about 1 mm per day in early gestation.[9, 10, 12, 16, 17] Controversy returns when one looks at age estimates of mean sac diameter by various authors.[9, 10, 15, 16] Embryologic data and recent data gathered by de Crespigny and colleagues leave little doubt that the MSD is 2 to 3 mm at four weeks and three to four days.[6, 14] It is reasonably safe to assume that a gestational sac reaches 5 mm at five weeks.[10] Thus, until a mean sac diameter of 25 mm is reached, gestational age in days can be calculated by adding 30 to the MSD; i.e., the MSD at five weeks is 5 mm.[10, 17]

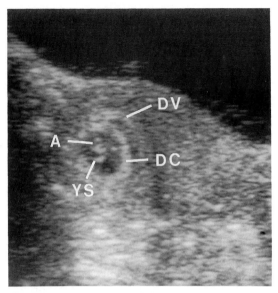

Figure 3–5. Transabdominal high-resolution real-time sonogram of an early gestation, demonstrating the decidua vera (DV), decidua capsularis (DC), yolk sac (YS), and amnion (A). The margin of the gestational sac includes not only the decidua capsularis but the chorionic tissue as well. Compare Figure 3–3A.

ectopic pregnancy is also associated with detectable circulating levels of hCG (Fig. 3–6).[19-22]

Sonographic visualization of early pregnancies has progressively improved since the first observations were made.[1, 9, 16, 23-30] Pregnancies can be observed within 14 days of implantation. Occasionally, sacs smaller than 5 mm in MSD are observed by using the classical transabdominal method of uterine visualization through the distended urinary bladder. This method allows a distance of approximately 10 to 15 cm from the transducer surface to the gestational sac. Intravaginal transducers shorten this distance by a factor of five, enabling one to employ higher frequency transducers and to image in an area of the beam much easier to focus.[14] One may reasonably anticipate that this trend of obtaining clearer and clearer images of early embryos will continue (Fig. 3–7).

The early normal gestational sac is filled predominantly with chorionic fluid.[6] Since the surrounding rim of trophoblastic and decidual tissue is not included in the measurement of the MSD, the actual complex of echoes identified in early pregnancy is, in fact, more prominent and thus easier to see than is suggested by the MSD. This tissue is seen as an echogenic rim of moderate-am-

Figure 3–6. Two patients with similar-sized intraendometrial fluid collections. *A,* Longitudinal sonogram through the uterus of a patient with a true intrauterine pregnancy. The double decidual sac sign is well demonstrated. Bl, bladder. *B,* Parasagittal sonogram through the uterus in a patient whose intraendometrial fluid collection is surrounded by a single rim of echoes. This fluid collection is a pseudogestational sac (PGS) from an ectopic pregnancy. F, fluid in cul-de-sac.

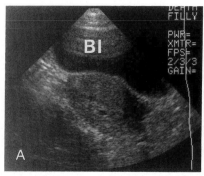
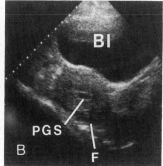

plitude echoes surrounding the echolucent chorionic cavity (Figs. 3–5 to 3–7).

The earliest embryonic structures are not usually seen until the gestational sac reaches approximately 10 mm in MSD and are not consistently seen until the sac reaches a mean diameter of 15 mm (40 to 45 days since the LHMP).[11, 23] The first such structure to be seen is a combination of the yolk sac and the developing amniotic sac.[23] This "double bubble" makes a distinctive pattern within the chorionic cavity (Figs. 3–3, 3–8 to 3–10). The primitive embryonic disc is the line of echoes dividing these minute fluid-containing sacs. The entire echo complex is only a few millimeters in diameter, but the surrounding chorionic fluid provides the background contrast against which the

beginnings of human life are observed with high-resolution real-time sonography.

The yolk sac grows slowly, and its wall appears to thicken (Figs. 3–11, 3–12), yet the amnion expands quickly, thinning the amniotic membrane. At this point, the yolk sac dominates the interior of the gestational sac (Fig. 3–11).[23–25] The embryo, lying in close contiguity with the yolk sac, measures only 2 to 3 mm in length and, as such, is less readily visible than the yolk sac itself (Fig. 3–7). Interestingly, Cadkin pointed out that an embryonic marker is more clearly seen at this stage of development than the corpus of the embryo.[11] This marker is the tiny pulsation of the forming embryonic heart, so unmistakable on the screen of the sonographic device. It is, of course, artificial

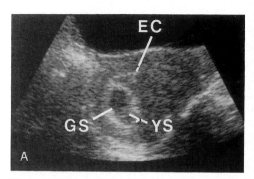
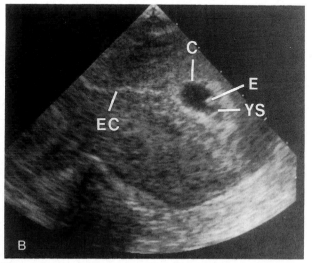

Figure 3–7. Transabdominal *(A)* and intravaginal *(B)* sonograms of the same patient. This patient was obese and difficult to examine. The transabdominal sonogram demonstrates a gestational sac (GS) and a probable yolk sac (YS). EC, endometrial cavity. In *B,* the endometrial cavity (EC), the margin of the chorion (C), the yolk sac (YS), and indeed a small embryo (E), lying in immediate contiguity with the yolk sac, are identified. Although the embryo cannot yet be morphologically identified on the basis of its appearance, its heartbeat leaves no doubt that this small reflection is truly the embryo.

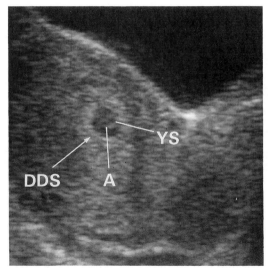

Figure 3–8. Longitudinal high-resolution sonogram of a very early intrauterine pregnancy. The chorionic cavity contains two tiny cystic structures representing the amniotic sac (A) and the yolk sac (YS). The linear echo between these tiny fluid collections is the embryonic disc. The chorionic cavity is surrounded by two layers of echoes representing a double decidual sac (DDS) sign. The inner layer of decidua, which represents both the decidua capsularis and the chorion, defines the chorionic cavity. Compare Figure 3–3A.

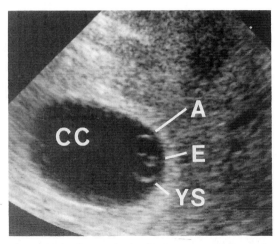

Figure 3–10. Intravaginal ultrasonogram of the early gestational sac, clearly showing the chorionic cavity (CC), amnion (A), early folding embryo (E), and yolk sac (YS). Compare Figure 3–3A, B.

to segregate "the embryo" from the yolk sac, the amnion, or certainly its own heartbeat. These distinctions are drawn only to sequence properly sonographic observations.

When the embryo achieves a crown-rump length (CRL) of 5 mm, it can be consistently seen as a discrete structure separable from the wall of the yolk sac and within which one or several echoes pulsate (Fig. 3–13).[27] At this point, the MSD is usually 15 to 18 mm, and the menstrual age is approximately 6.5 weeks. It is not possible even to discrim-

inate which end of the embryo is its crown and which is its rump, but the unmistakable cardiac pulsations confirm without doubt that this small "clump" of echoes is a living human embryo. From this point forward, visualization of the embryo itself dominates the sonographic observations. Intraembryonic structures become progressively clearer. When an embryo reaches approximately 10 mm in CRL, the head can be discriminated from the torso (Fig. 3–14). Remember, the embryo's head will constitute fully one-half of its total volume. Pro-

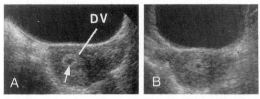

Figure 3–9. Longitudinal (A) and transverse (B) sonograms of an early gestational sac. The mean sac diameter is 5 to 6 mm. The double decidual sac sign, composed of the decidua capsularis (arrow) and decidua vera (DV), is clearly seen. The mean sac diameter measures only the fluid-containing sac. Obviously, the entire gestational complex (sac plus surrounding double decidual sac sign) is a much larger and more readily recognized entity.

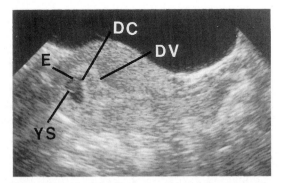

Figure 3–11. Longitudinal sonogram of the uterus obtained transabdominally. There is an early gestational sac demonstating the double decidual sac sign defined by the decidua capsularis (DC) and the decidua vera (DV). Note that the gestation bulges into the endometrial cavity. The yolk sac (YS) dominates the interior of the chorionic cavity. The early embryo (E) is a vague complex of echoes adjacent to the yolk sac. However, at real time, the easily identified heartbeat clearly documents the embryonic position.

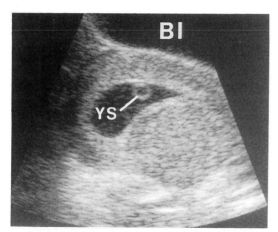

Figure 3–12. High-resolution real-time sonogram of an eight week gestation, demonstrating the yolk sac (YS). When compared with Figures 3–10 and 3–11, the yolk sac wall has considerably thickened by this stage of development. Thus, it has higher subjective contrast and is more readily seen. Bl, urinary bladder.

gressively, one visualizes the limb buds, the umbilical cord, and then the primary ossification centers of the maxilla, mandible, and clavicle (Figs. 3–15, 3–16).[28] Thereafter, the gamut of visible anatomy rapidly unfolds as the embryo (through the eighth week of development: ten menstrual weeks) becomes the fetus (beginning of the ninth week of development: 11 menstrual weeks). This transition occurs when the CRL reaches approximately 30 to 35 mm.

AMNIOTIC AND CHORIONIC MEMBRANES

Recall that the amnion was amongst the earliest visible embryonic structures (Figs. 3–7 to 3–9).[23] As it rapidly expands, it passes

through a stage of relative "invisibility." During this brief period, our observations center next on the yolk sac, and promptly thereafter on the embryo. However, the amnion quickly "reappears" as a much larger sac with an extremely thin wall (Fig. 3–17).[26] Still, its thinness is no match for the resolving capacity of modern instruments, although one commonly resolves only segments of the amnion. Now, the embryo lies entirely within the confines of the amniotic membrane; the yolk sac is excluded and lies within the chorionic cavity, usually between the amniotic membrane and the fetal surface of the developing placenta. Where just two weeks before the bulk of the fluid within the gestational sac resided within the chorionic cavity (the amniotic sac being minute), now the bulk of visible fluid is amniotic. The chorionic cavity diminishes progressively until ultimately the amnion "fuses" to the chorion and obliterates this cavity.*

One can usually continue to observe the yolk sac well into the late stages of the first trimester. A bright curvilinear echo is commonly observed extending toward the yolk sac (Fig. 3–15).[23] Unlike the amnion, this structure is not a sheet and is usually a brighter reflector (compare Figs. 3–15 and 3–17). Logically, this reflector represents the yolk stalk.

An understanding of the points of attachment of the chorion and amnion is important

---

*In fact, in mid-trimester, puncture of these membranes during amniocentesis commonly allows quantities of amniotic fluid to leak into the chorionic cavity and re-establish this potential space, a so-called chorioamniotic (CA) separation. A CA separation has no deleterious effect on a pregnancy and should not be considered evidence for the presence of the amniotic band syndrome.

Figure 3–13. Longitudinal (A) and transverse (B) sonograms of an early gestational sac. The decidua vera (DV) and decidua capsularis (DC) are clearly identified. (Recall that the echo complex of the decidua capsularis includes the smooth chorion.) The yolk sac (YS) is identified in A, while the early embryo, demarcated by the measurement cursors, is clearly seen in B. This embryo measures approximately 5 mm. Embryos

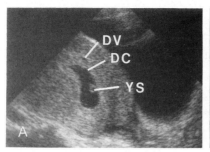
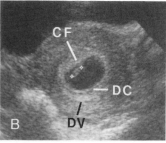

can be consistently seen when they achieve a crown-rump length of 5 mm. Note the thickened area of chorion adjacent to the embryo. This represents the chorion frondosum (CF). Again, a component of the echo complex of the chorion frondosum is contributed by the decidua basalis.

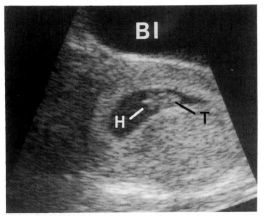

Figure 3–14. Longitudinal sonogram of an early pregnancy. A 13 mm embryo is seen within the gestational sac. Note that the head (H) and torso (T) can be discriminated in embryos of this size. Bl, bladder.

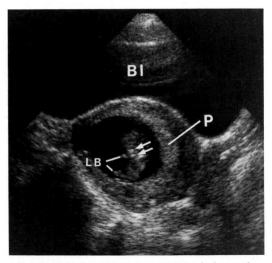

Figure 3–15. High-resolution sonogram of a late embryo demonstrating the limb buds (LB) and the ossification centers of the maxilla *(upper arrow)* and mandible *(lower arrow)*. P, placenta; Bl, bladder.

in order to characterize accurately the location of various fluid collections during pregnancy.[29] Recall, the placenta and chorion had identical origins and are inseparably fused (Figs. 3–2 to 3–4). The chorion always leads to the edge of the placenta (Fig. 3–3D). By contrast, the amnion surrounds the fetus and is continuous with and covers the umbilical cord where it joins the placenta (Figs. 3–3C, D, 3–4). Thus, the amnion can be separated from the fetal surface of the placenta (unlike the chorion) but cannot be separated from its junction point with the cord insertion site into the placenta.

Although the chorion cannot be separated from the placental edge, it is easily separated from the endometrial lining (decidua parietalis), to which it is supposedly "fused," by *any* intraendometrial cavity fluid collection. Physicians sometimes inject saline into the endometrial cavity during chorion villus sampling to separate the chorion from the decidua parietalis; this allows them to locate precisely the junction of the developing placental edge.[30] The only commonly occurring

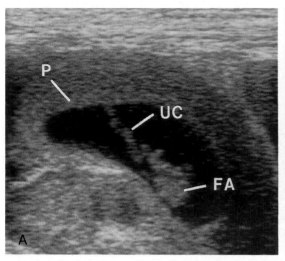

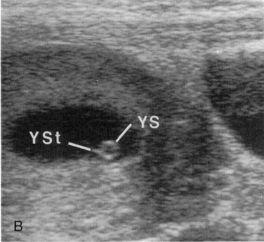

Figure 3–16. Sequential longitudinal sonograms of a late first trimester pregnancy. In *A*, the umbilical cord (UC) is seen coursing from the placenta (P) to the fetal abdomen (FA). In *B*, the yolk sac (YS) is noted, and a short segment of the terminal yolk stalk (YSt) is seen leading to the yolk sac.

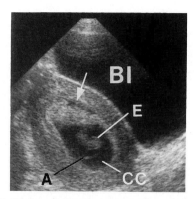

Figure 3–17. Longitudinal sonogram through the uterus of a patient experiencing first trimester bleeding. An embryo (E) is clearly identified. However, no heartbeat was identified, confirming nonviability. A small accumulation of blood *(arrow)* is seen lying between the chorion frondosum and the uterine wall; this indicates an abrupting early placenta. Bl, bladder; A, amnion; CC, chorionic cavity.

natural (albeit pathologic) fluid collection within the endometrial cavity during early pregnancy is blood, seen in women who are in danger of aborting. This is a so-called "subchorionic" collection (of blood) (Fig. 3–18). It would be preferable to abandon this confusing term in favor of the term "intraendometrial" cavity collection, which accurately describes the anatomic location of the fluid.

Similarly a "chorioamniotic" accumulation is a somewhat confusing term. This simply refers to fluid in the chorionic cavity, a normal and universal finding prior to "fusion" of the chorion and amnion (Fig. 3–19). Such a collection can be accurately localized because the fluid lies between the fetal surface of the placenta and the membrane (amnion) forming its contralateral boundary (an impossibility for fluid contained in the endometrial cavity [subchorionic collection]).[29] After "fusion," fluid may reappear in this space after needle puncture that allows amniotic fluid to leak into the chorionic cavity and re-establish this potential space by "stripping away" the amniotic membrane. The "trauma" of midtrimester amniocentesis commonly causes this inconsequential chorioamniotic separation; however, amniocentesis may result in true hemorrhagic complications. The hemorrhage may be either fetal blood (usually devastating) or, more commonly, maternal blood, and may accumulate behind the placenta (abruption) (Fig. 3–17), in the endometrial cavity (subchorionic) (Fig. 3–18), in the chorionic cavity (chorioamniotic), or in the amniotic cavity itself. While all such occurrences are best avoided, an intra-amniotic or chorioamniotic accumulation of blood is not specifically harmful to a fetus.

EVALUATION OF GESTATIONAL AGE

The first trimester is an opportune time to employ the sonographic parameters of pregnancy dating in patients with an uncertain menstrual history. In the first trimester, as throughout the remainder of pregnancy, menstrual age is estimated by measuring the size of a structure. Prior to embryonic visualization, one can measure the size of the gestational sac (Figs. 3–5, 3–6, 3–8, 3–9, 3–11).[9, 10, 16, 17] After embryonic visualization, the embryo itself can be measured, at first in toto (the so-called "crown-rump" length) (Figs. 3–20, 3–21); later, as specific fetal

Figure 3–18. Longitudinal *(A)* and transverse *(B)* sonograms of a patient experiencing bleeding in the first trimester. A so-called "subchorionic" hemorrhage has accumulated between the chorion (C) and the decidua vera (DV). Note that the chorion extends circumferentially to meet the edges of the developing placenta *(arrowheads)*. Note as well that the margins of the placenta are separated from the uterine wall, i.e., marginal abruption. The embryo (E) demonstrated an active heartbeat, indicating that this pregnancy should be observed expectantly. *Arrows,* amniotic membrane nearly opposed to the chorion.

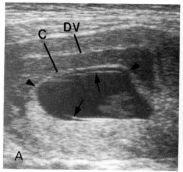
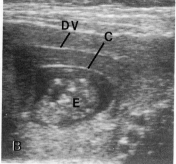

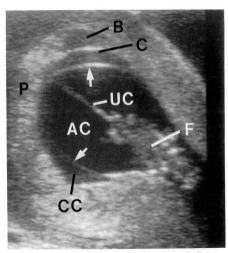

Figure 3–19. Longitudinal sonogram through the uterus of a patient experiencing first trimester bleeding. The fetus (F) is readily identified dangling from its umbilical cord (UC). No fetal heartbeat was identified, confirming nonviability. All of the potential spaces are noted in this case. The amnion *(arrows)* defines the amniotic cavity (AC). Note that the amnion extends to the base of the umbilical cord. The chorionic cavity (CC) lies between the amnion and the chorion (C). The chorion extends to the edge of the placenta (P). Blood (B) has accumulated in the endometrial cavity, i.e., external to the chorion. This blood represents a so-called "subchorionic" hemorrhage.

parts become visible, the individual fetal parameters can be measured.[27, 31-34] These are the same in the first trimester as during the remainder of pregnancy (biparietal diameter, head circumference, femur length, and abdominal circumference).

From a philosophic perspective, estimation of menstrual age by any biometric measurement is a trade-off between two competing problems. The first is the measurement's accuracy and the second is the measurement's predictive validity for age. The feature that most influences the latter is biologic variation. Inexorably, throughout pregnancy, biologic variation in size increases. Thus, without question, an individual measurement is more likely to predict the gestational age accurately the earlier in pregnancy it is measured. The opposing feature is ease and accuracy of measurement. Obviously, measurements that result in large inter- or intraobserver variations manifest significant predictive inaccuracy even though they can be measured at a gestational stage when biologic variation is small.

One might therefore reason that the most accurate prediction of menstrual age would

be obtained by measuring the gestational sac (the earliest sonographically visible structure in pregnancy) between five and 6.5 weeks (Figs. 3–5, 3–6). It is easily and accurately measured and biologic variation should be quite small. Although no one has ever tested this notion, it is likely true. The fallacy of this concept, of course, is that there is such a narrow window in which to apply it. Furthermore, if the pregnancy dates were known with sufficient accuracy to schedule the examination within this narrow time window, it is unlikely that a mechanism to further improve the dating would be necessary.

After 6.5 weeks, the gestational sac can still be measured, but now there is an alternative measurement, the CRL.[27, 31-34] The embryo is as yet too small to have its individual parts measured, but its length can be estimated (Fig. 3–13). There are, unfortunately, some pitfalls in the estimation of the CRL. Since no anatomic marker exists at the tip of the crown or the rump, one must always assume that the "longest" CRL is the most accurate. This, however, can be influenced by beam divergence, beam splitting, side lobe artifacts, the erroneous inclusion of extraneous structures (most notably the yolk sac) (Figs. 3–20, 3–21),[24] or a change in the resting position of the embryo. The embryo normally rests with a kyphotic curvature, but within a few weeks of its visualization, the embryo can begin to extend and straighten itself, "altering" its crown-rump length.

Indeed, Robinson, in his original description of CRL measurement, noted the potential for some of the above-described inaccuracies.[31] The literature is now replete with manuscripts that document beyond any reasonable doubt that early CRL measurement (between 6.5 and ten menstrual weeks) is the single most accurate method of pregnancy dating.[31-34] The size of the gestational sac, of course, can still be measured accurately during the same time frame; however, available evidence strongly indicates that the measurement of a fetal parameter (CRL) is more accurate than the measurement of any general feature of a pregnancy (sac or uterine size).[9]

After the tenth week, it is possible to measure specific fetal parts. These specific structures are more accurately measurable than the CRL; moreover, the CRL begins to

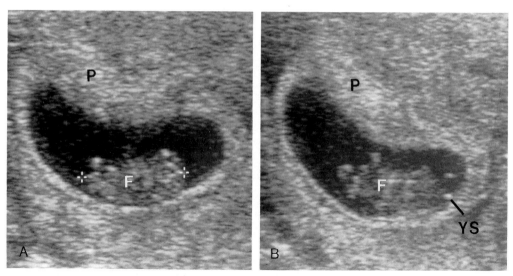

Figure 3–20. *A*, Scan appropriately oriented through a 32 mm fetus (F) to obtain a proper crown-rump length. P, placenta. *B*, Scan demonstrating that an inadvertent addition of the yolk sac (YS) to the crown-rump length of the fetus would erroneously increase the length by approximately 5 mm.

show a substantial increase in biologic variation toward the beginning of the second trimester. Thus, once visible for measurement, the head and femur become the preferred biometric parameters for estimating gestational age.

It is important to remember that the methods used in research experiments conducted by highly motivated examiners may not translate into equivalent predictive accura-

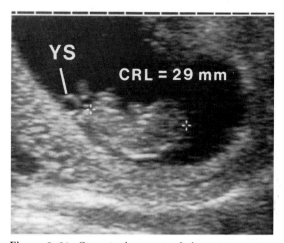

Figure 3–21. Correct placement of the measurement cursors to obtain a proper crown-rump length (CRL). The yolk sac (YS) should be excluded from the measurement. Note that the embryo has a lordotic curvature, the amount of which affects the crown-rump length measurement. One must assume that all embryos and fetuses have the same lordotic curvature, an assumption that is not always valid.

cies when practiced in the general community or even at other research centers.

Campbell and associates investigated this problem, and the results were enlightening.[35] These authors reviewed more than 4500 consecutive pregnancy sonograms and compared the accuracy of a CRL prediction of the estimated date of confinement (EDC) with that of a biparietal diameter (BPD) obtained before the 18th week. CRL correctly predicted EDC ($\pm$ 14 days) in 85 percent of cases. Interestingly, BPD predicted EDC ($\pm$ 14 days) in 89 percent of cases. Even a BPD between 18 to 22 weeks matched the prediction by the CRL. Of further interest, LMP predicted EDC ($\pm$ 14 days) in 85 percent of cases if an optimal history could be obtained. An optimal history was defined as certainty of the first day of the LNMP, regular cycles, no exposure to birth control pills for at least two months, and no unusual bleeding. Unfortunately, such a history was only available in 55 percent of the patient group.

Despite Campbell's study, the weight of evidence suggests that pregnancies are most accurately dated by sonographic parameters measured in the first trimester.[31–34] The CRL is the most accurate measurement, but an early MSD is also highly accurate. Still, even among those studies documenting improved accuracy of the CRL over a BPD performed at about 18 weeks, the demonstrated improvement in predictive accuracy is only slightly greater than one-half week.

Simply because a pregnancy can be more accurately dated in the first than in the early second trimester does not mean that it should. Too high a price is paid to gain a small advantage in age estimation. At 18 weeks, one can characterize a large number of important pregnancy parameters that cannot be judged at all in early pregnancy. The placental position can be accurately judged, amniotic fluid volume can be estimated, early shortening of the cervix can be recognized, and numerous fetal anomalies can be detected. Despite the somewhat improved accuracy of pregnancy dating in the first trimester, one is ill advised to pursue pregnancy dating early unless there are other mitigating circumstances besides an uncertain menstrual history. Furthermore, when the menstrual history is optimal, as it is in most pregnant women, ultrasound is not likely to offer any significant clinical benefit in defining gestational age, even if performed in the first trimester.[35] Table 3–1 briefly lists the indications for sonography in the first trimester.

THREATENED ABORTION

One could not begin to write about the sonographic diagnosis of abnormal first trimester pregnancies without recognizing the pioneering work of Dr. Hugh Robinson.[1, 16, 27, 31, 36, 37] Not only did he set the stage and

Table 3–1. INDICATIONS FOR SONOGRAPHY IN THE FIRST TRIMESTER

Common
  Threatened abortion
  Suspected ectopic pregnancy
  Size and date discrepancy (or uncertain dates)
  Evaluation for associated masses
Less Common
  Guidance for chorionic villus sampling
  Assessment of success of ovulation indication
    pregnancies (± in vitro fertilization)
  Assessment for multiple pregnancies
  Uterine anomalies
  Retained IUD and pregnancy
  Assessment of pregnancy "health" before cervical
    cerclage
  Adjunct to therapeutic abortion
  Evaluation of completeness of abortion
  Failure to obtain chorionic villi during an abortion

The above list is not meant to be all-inclusive, nor does the appearance on this list insure the validity of the indication. The diagnosis of ectopic pregnancy is considered in detail in Chapter 22.

define the goals, but his papers also directed the course of the decade's subsequent research, which simply validated his original observations.[38–44] "The primary objective," said Dr. Robinson, "is to formulate criteria for the sonar [identification] of abnormal pregnancies such that these diagnoses [can] be applied prospectively and with complete reliability in the active management of established early pregnancy failures."[1]

Dr. Robinson's objective has largely been achieved, and sonographic diagnosis can now be appropriately applied in threatened abortion, the major indication for ultrasonography in the first trimester. Threatened abortion is a clinically descriptive term that applies to women who have vaginal spotting or bleeding, mild uterine cramping, and a closed cervical os during the first 20 weeks of pregnancy. The following discussion will involve women in the first 13 weeks of pregnancy.

Threatened abortion is a common complication that occurs in approximately 25 percent of clinically apparent pregnancies.[45–47] Despite efforts to alter the outcome, about one-half of these pregnancies ultimately abort. In such cases, the embryo is most often already dead and usually has been dead for some time. Thus, the administration of progestational drugs is ineffective and only prolongs the natural course of abortion. Although the embryo is dead, chorionic tissue may still be functional, resulting in a persistently positive pregnancy test.

While nearly all nonviable gestations eventually abort, spontaneous expulsion is frequently delayed for weeks after the onset of clinical symptoms.[45, 47] This may lead to prolonged vaginal bleeding, infection, and patient anxiety. Although none of these are life threatening, their seriousness should not be underestimated. Clinical management depends on whether or not the embryo is living. Therefore, the reliable identification of nonviable gestations is important for determining which patients merit uterine evacuation; potentially viable, living embryos, on the other hand, are observed expectantly.

Methods to assess embryonic life include hormonal assays (human chorionic gonadotropin, estrogen, progesterone, human placental lactogen, pregnancy-specific β-glycoprotein, and alpha-fetoprotein) and sonography.[34, 45, 48–52] Among the hormonal studies, progesterone and hCG levels are more accurate than the others. Falling hCG levels predict pregnancy failure quite accurately.[45] Unfortunately, serial hCG determinations are not uncommonly equivocal. Cases of blighted ovum and embryonic demise may demonstrate normal hCG levels even when villi appear abnormal by gross and microscopic evaluation. It is an attractive hypothesis to assume that low hCG levels are related to the abnormal histology of chorionic villi. Unfortunately, this is not necessarily so.[49]

While such determinations are useful, sonography is the pivotal examination in this clinical setting. Recall that when the patient presents, she has about a 50/50 chance of the pregnancy ending in abortion. However, numerous studies now document that ultrasonic demonstration of a living embryo alters these statistics dramatically and favorably. When a living embryo is identified, 90 to 97 percent continue.[49, 53-56] Therefore, once an embryonic heartbeat is seen, the clear course of action is to observe the patient expectantly. Indeed, so important is the observation of a fetal heartbeat that it overrides any simultaneous finding, e.g., dead twin, subchorionic hemorrhage, sac too large, or sac too small (Fig. 3–22). This is not to say that a large subchorionic (endo-

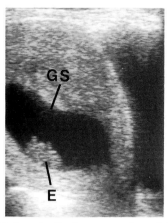

Figure 3–22. Longitudinal sonogram through the uterus of a patient with a threatened abortion. An embryo (E) is seen that is clearly too small for the size of the gestational sac (GS). Additionally, the chorionic and decidual tissues surrounding the gestational sac are poorly developed. However, the embryo has a visible heartbeat. Although one would expect this to be an abnormal gestation, the presence of the heartbeat overrides the other features, and the pregnancy is observed expectantly. As might be anticipated, the embryo did not survive.

metrial) blood accumulation will not influence the pregnancy's outcome (Fig. 3–18); however, it does not sufficiently alter its management.[55, 56]

Among embryos in which a heartbeat is seen, what are the reasons for subsequent abortion? As previously noted, the background loss rate of very early pregnancies is quite high. There is, of course, a further background loss rate in all subsequent stages of pregnancy that falls progressively throughout the gestational period. Considerable interest currently exists in establishing the background loss rate of living embryos in the range of seven to 12 menstrual weeks since this figure impacts quite directly on the reported procedure-related pregnancy loss rate from chorion villus sampling.

There are several studies addressing this issue.[53, 54] A comprehensive evaluation in 1986[53] found that among living embryos from seven to 12 menstrual weeks, the overall abortion rate was 2.3 percent. The risk decreased following the tenth week, i.e., the abortion rate from seven to nine weeks was 5 percent but dropped to 1 to 2 percent between ten and 12 weeks. Further subdivision of this group showed a loss rate of 1.3 percent if the mother was not spotting. However, if spotting was present, 5.4 percent aborted. Furthermore, the risk of abortion increased with maternal age, presumably in relation to the increased risk of chromosomal anomalies in older mothers.

Maternal factors may influence a woman's propensity to lose a pregnancy with a living embryo. These most commonly include numerous or submucous myomas, uterine anomalies (didelphic or bicornuate uteri), and a mother who was exposed to diethylstilbestrol during pregnancy (being a DES daughter).

Sonographic demonstration of an embryo that lacks cardiac motion is the most specific evidence of embryonic demise (Figs. 3–23, 3–24). This statement, though well documented in the literature, requires some discussion.[49, 56] Not the least reason is that several years ago, there was evidence suggesting that visualization of the embryonic corpus preceded visualization of the embryonic heartbeat.[57] Now, in fact, exactly the opposite is true.[11] Before the corpus of the embryo is visible, the embryonic heartbeat is seen as a discrete pulsation adjacent to the yolk sac. The literature still contains

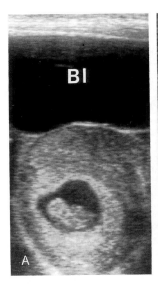 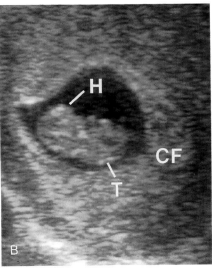

Figure 3–23. Unmagnified *(A)* and magnified *(B)* sonograms of a 25 mm embryo. In an embryo of this size, the head (H) and torso (T) are easily discriminated. The precise location for a heartbeat can be determined. In this case, no heartbeat was identified, confirming a nonviable pregnancy. Note that the chorion frondosum (CF) has an abnormal echotexture, a common associated finding in abnormal pregnancies but clearly of lesser importance than the absence of cardiac activity. Bl, bladder.

some admonitions regarding the inability to see the embryonic heartbeat sonographically when it is actually present (prior to the seventh week or in embryos less than 10 mm in size), but the author judges such statements to be erroneous.[55] The evidence strongly indicates that the heartbeat is more conspicuous and thus more easily recognized than the embryonic corpus.[11, 49, 56]

Nonetheless, experienced imaging specialists know that negative observations (no heartbeat observed) are fraught with more problems than positive observations (heart-

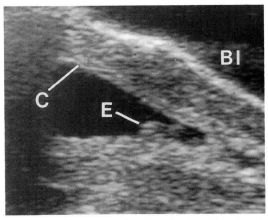

Figure 3–24. Sonogram of a patient with a threatened abortion. An embryo (E) is clearly identified but measures only 6 mm. Despite the embryo's small size, the inability to see a heartbeat in a technically high-quality scan is conclusive evidence of embryonic demise. Note in addition that the chorionic (C) and decidual tissues are much less echogenic than the interface between the bladder (Bl) and the uterus.

beat observed), and caution is certainly appropriate when evaluating a patient who is threatening to abort. There are three precautions that should be taken. The first of these is by far the most important: *be sure you are looking at the embryo before you search the entity for a heartbeat.* This is a trivially simple exercise when the embryo exceeds 10 mm in CRL since it has a discernible head and torso by that time (Fig. 3–23). However, between 5 and 10 mm in CRL, the embryo has no morphologically recognizable structure other than its heartbeat, which, of course, will not be available for inspection if it is dead. The 5 to 10 mm embryo is seen only as a globular collection of echoes (Fig. 3–24). Still, there are reasonable criteria of observation that can be applied. A recognizable early embryo is at least 4 to 5 mm long and has a reasonable width in proportion to its length (Figs. 3–13, 3–25). It usually lies near the yolk sac and may be seen to be surrounded by amnion (Fig. 3–17).

Once one is certain that the structure being investigated for the presence of a heartbeat is indeed the embryo, the second precaution loses significance, although at first glance it appears to be the pivotal point. This precaution is simply to *observe the embryo thoroughly for evidence of a heartbeat.* No one fears this problem when looking at larger embryos, but confidence wanes when looking at smaller ones. In fact, simple logic tells us that the smaller the volume that must be searched for a heartbeat, the less likely one is to overlook it. Missing the heartbeat in a

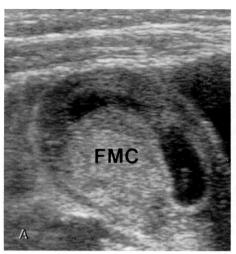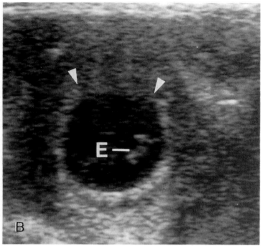

Figure 3–25. Longitudinal *(A)* and magnified *(B)* views of a pregnancy that is threatening to abort. A focal myometrial contraction (FMC) distorts the contours of the gestational sac. Note that this contraction does not affect the serosal contour of the uterus. The margins of the gestational sac are poorly developed. Indeed, segments of the choriodecidual reaction are clearly absent *(arrowheads)*. Still, the most convincing evidence that the pregnancy is nonviable is the inability to identify a heartbeat in the tiny, 8 mm embryo (E).

tiny living embryo is not the problem, but searching a structure that is not an embryo for a heartbeat is. Nonetheless, for many years, the author has imposed the following rule in his own clinical scanning area: before an embryo is judged to be dead, it is viewed by two independent examiners (usually a technologist and a physician), each for a three-minute period. To the inexperienced sonographer, six minutes may seem a treacherously short time to make such a weighty decision, but the experienced examiner knows that six minutes is a painfully long time to view a dead embryo with a real-time sonographic device.

The final precaution cannot be simply taught, but all sonographers recognize its importance not only in the situation under consideration but in all scanning circumstances. We must *judge the technical adequacy of the examination.* If the technical quality is significantly and adversely affected by either a maternal factor or an instrumental factor, extraordinary caution must be used. With the advent of intravaginal transducers, adverse maternal factors, such as obesity or uterine retroflexion, can be readily overcome.

When an embryo is identified, the sonographer's task is relatively straightforward: if no heartbeat is seen, the gestation can be safely evacuated; whereas, if an embryonic heartbeat is seen, the gestation clearly must

be observed expectantly. Unfortunately, most abnormal gestations cease development before a recognizable embryo is formed, in which case sonographic assessment is considerably more difficult.[1, 48, 58] Difficulty arises because normal gestational sacs can be identified sonographically before the embryo can be detected. It becomes incumbent on the examiner to discriminate a normal early pregnancy from an abnormal anembryonic pregnancy.

Despite the frequency with which "empty" gestational sacs are encountered, the literature is sparse regarding the sonographic features that can be said to discriminate normal from abnormal gestations on a single examination. One method that has been suggested is to demonstrate that the gestational sac is small for the menstrual dates.[1, 40, 48, 50] This approach, however, relies on an accurate menstrual history, which is often lacking.

Sonographers are constantly asked to examine women with "poor dates." What are "good" dates, and what deficiencies change dates to "poor" ones? This analysis will be confined to those situations in which a sonographer, seeing a patient for the first time and performing the examination in the first trimester, must decide whether or not to employ the patient's dates when judging the normalcy of the pregnancy.

As a general rule, one is always better off

excluding the patient's dates from considerations about potential viability of an early pregnancy. Note that throughout the discussion of the sonographic features of threatened abortion, the patient's dates are never considered. Only independently judged sonographic parameters are employed. However, some patients have unambiguously reliable dates and in such circumstances, the addition of this factor to the analysis can be pivotal in determining that a gestation is no longer viable.

Patients undergoing ovulation induction, artificial insemination, or in vitro fertilization know precisely the date of conception. Indeed, in this unfortunately small group, one would be ill advised to ignore the patient's dates. In many patients, a "minimal" length of gestation can be calculated. This can be done by knowing the date that the pregnancy test became positive and the type and sensitivity of the test employed. For example, if a patient had a "serum" pregnancy test that was positive four weeks ago, one can very safely assume that she is at least 7.5 menstrual weeks into the pregnancy (four weeks since the test and a minimum of 3.5 weeks for the test to become positive). The probabilities, of course, favor that she is even further along.

Other than these circumstances, one imposes an element of risk when "factoring" in a patient's dates in the sonographic analysis of a threatened abortion. This is not to say that most pregnant women are unreliable historians; it is strictly a safety feature. The following features positively influence the validity of dates: infrequent exposure to intercourse, recording the basal body temperature, noting the first day of the last normal menstrual period on a calendar, a history of regular periods, an absence of recent exposure to birth control pills, and an absence of unusual episodes of bleeding.[35]

A second method used to identify abnormal pregnancies is to evaluate the appearance of the gestational sac. Some observers have found the anomalous sonographic appearance of a gestational sac, when present, to be reliable evidence of an abnormal pregnancy.[40, 48, 58-60] Others have concluded that, in the absence of an embryo, serial examinations are required to confirm abnormal growth and development prior to definitive treatment.[13] Anomalous morphologic features that suggest nonviability include a bizarre or irregular sac shape (Figs. 3-26, 3-27), an unusually large sac size that lacks an embryo (Figs. 3-28, 3-29), an incompletely or poorly formed decidual reaction (Figs. 3-29, 3-30), the absence of a double decidual sac finding (Fig. 3-30), or the presence of a fluid level (Fig. 3-31).[1, 40, 48, 50, 60]

Sonography can frequently distinguish abnormal from normal "empty" gestational sacs on a single examination, independent of the menstrual history.[60] Among the potential abnormal features listed above, one might well expect that some are more predictive than others (Table 3-2).[60] Certain sonographic criteria are virtually 100 percent specific and accurately predict an abnormal outcome. One such criterion is an "abnormally" large sac (greater than 25 mm in mean sac diameter) that lacks an embryo (Figs. 3-13, 3-14, 3-29, 3-32) or a gestational sac (greater than 20 mm in mean sac diameter) that lacks a yolk sac (Figs. 3-7 to

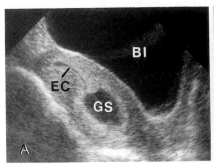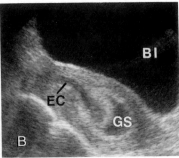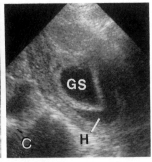

Figure 3-26. Sequential longitudinal sonograms (A and B) with the urinary bladder (Bl) distended. Longitudinal sonogram (C) with the urinary bladder empty. This sequence of images demonstrates a markedly distorted gestational sac (GS), which is low lying in the endometrial cavity (EC). Additionally, an endometrial accumulation of blood (H) surrounds a substantial percentage of the gestational sac (i.e., "subchorionic" hemorrhage). Such a gestation is clearly being evacuated by normal processes and can be judged as nonviable with certainty.

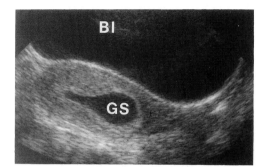

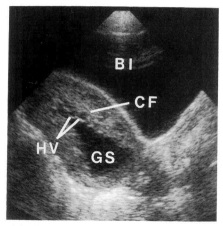

Figure 3–27. Longitudinal sonogram of the uterus in a patient who has a threatened abortion and also is considered at risk for ectopic pregnancy. A large, distorted gestational sac (GS) is identified. The choriodecidual reactions surrounding the gestational sac are poorly echogenic compared with the bladder (Bl) and myometrial interface reflection, and there is no double decidual sac finding. The mean sac diameter exceeds 25 mm, and no embryo is identified. In the absence of definitive criteria for an intrauterine pregnancy, such a patient must be considered at risk for ectopic gestation. However, if this intraendometrial fluid collection is indeed a gestational sac, one can be confident that it is nonviable (i.e., fulfills a major criterion). Therefore, the initial management decision is straightforward: evacuate the uterus and search for chorionic villi. If they are identified, the suspected nonviable gestation has been adequately treated, and the ectopic pregnancy has been excluded.

Figure 3–28. Longitudinal sonogram of the uterus in a patient who has a threatened abortion. Unlike most nonviable first trimester gestations (compare Figs. 3–22, 3–24, 3–29, and 3–30), the chorion frondosum (CF) in this one is markedly thickened instead of thinned. Small hydropic villi (HV) are noted. This constitutes a separate pattern of anomalous development of first trimester pregnancies, somewhat akin to partial moles but having a more viable abnormal fetal karyotype (so-called "hydropic" degeneration of the placenta). Bl, bladder; GS, gestational sac.

3–12, 3–30, 3–33). Also, a grossly distorted sac shape invariably predicts an abnormal outcome (Fig. 3–26). Since these figures are easily recognized and uniformly predict an abnormal outcome, they should be considered *major criteria* for diagnosing a nonviable gestation.

Pathologic correlation suggests that large gestational sacs that lack an embryo are always abnormal and are usually caused by a blighted ovum (anembryonic pregnancy).[44, 45, 48, 49, 58] Blighted ova are common in first trimester abortion and often demonstrate chromosomal anomalies. In these patients, trophoblastic activity may continue despite the absence of a developing embryo.[45] The trophoblastic cells continue to elaborate the pregnancy hormone, although usually at a much reduced rate, attempting to perpetuate this already lost gestation.

Recall that embryos can be consistently

Figure 3–29. Sequential (A and B) longitudinal sonograms through the uterus of a patient who has a threatened abortion. A typical abnormal gestational sac of a so-called "blighted ovum" is seen. The gestational sac (GS) is quite large. A fetus should be clearly identified, yet none is seen. The yolk sac (YS) is readily noted. The margins of the gestational sac are nearly devoid of chorionic and decidual tissues. There can be no question, based on a single examination, that this pregnancy is nonviable. Bl, bladder.

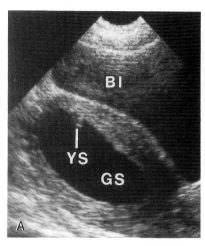

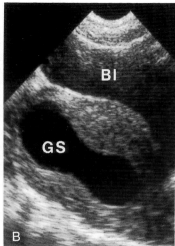

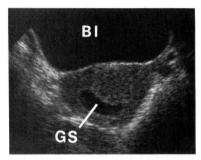

Figure 3–30. Transverse sonogram through the uterus of a patient who has a threatened abortion. An abnormal gestational sac (GS) is noted. The mean sac diameter is 22 mm, yet a yolk sac cannot be identified. Additionally, the choriodecidual reaction is thin, is weakly echogenic, and fails to disclose a double decidual sac sign (three minor criteria and one major criterion). Most experienced examiners would confidently and correctly conclude that this pregnancy is nonviable. Bl, bladder.

detected when they achieve a CRL of 5 mm or more. Within a 25 mm sac, one expects to encounter an embryo that has a CRL of 14 mm (Fig. 3–32). Volumetrically, a 12 mm embryo is substantially larger than a 5 mm embryo (compare Figs. 3–13 and 3–14). Even relatively inexperienced examiners are unlikely to fail to identify an embryo of this size. Thus, one may confidently employ the criterion to establish nonviability. Remember, this criterion is independent of the patient's dates.

That a yolk sac should be visible when the gestational sac has attained a mean diameter of 20 mm or greater, i.e., before one can consistently demonstrate an embryo, is in keeping with normal embryologic development and sonographic observations of

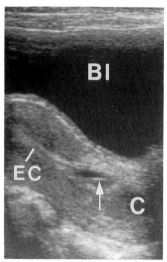

Figure 3–31. Longitudinal sonogram through the uterus of a patient who has a threatened abortion. All observers would agree that the small gestational sac located near the cervix (C) of the uterus is unambiguously nonviable. Although an uncommon finding, the presence of a fluid level (*arrow*) in such a gestational sac is conclusive evidence of nonviability. The low position does not signify a low implantation but, rather, the process of abortion. This pregnancy will not be in the uterus long enough for a "follow-up examination" to be performed. Bl, bladder; EC, endometrial cavity.

normal pregnancies (see above).[13, 60] The early yolk sac, a more conspicuous structure than the small adjacent embryo, is detectable at an earlier stage of pregnancy because of two features (Figs. 3–7, 3–11). First, it is volumetrically larger than the early embryo. Second, it is a fluid-containing sac, therefore possessing a relatively high subject contrast. Application of this criterion requires more

Table 3–2. SENSITIVITY, SPECIFICITY, AND PREDICTIVE VALUES FOR SONOGRAPHIC CRITERIA OF ABNORMAL GESTATIONAL SACS

Sonographic Criterion of Abnormal Sac	Sensitivity (%)*	Specificity (%)†	Positive Predictive Value (%)
Major			
≥ 25 mm without embryo	29	100	100
≥ 20 mm without yolk sac	41	100	100
Minor‡			
Thin decidual reaction (≤ 2 mm)	28	99	96
Weak decidual amplitude	53	99	98
Irregular contour	37	99	97
Absent DDS	37	98	94
Low position	20	99	94

*Abnormal outcome, n = 83.

†Normal outcome, n = 85.

‡Specificity and positive prediction of an abnormal outcome increase to 100 percent when three or more minor criteria are identified.

From Nyberg DA, Laing FC, Filly RA: Threatened abortion: Sonographic distinction of normal and abnormal gestation sacs. Radiology 158:397, 1986.

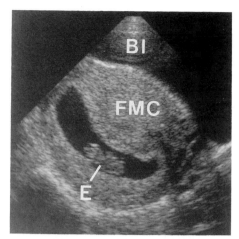

Figure 3–32. Transverse sonogram of the uterus in a patient who has a threatened abortion. A gestational sac with a mean diameter of 29 mm is identified. Notice how easily the embryo (E) is identified in a sac of this size. A heartbeat was easily seen in the embryo. A focal myometrial contraction (FMC) mildly distorts the gestational sac. Note that the FMC affects the endometrial surface of the uterus more than the serosal surface. Note as well that the echogenicity of the FMC is equivalent to the adjacent normal myometrium. Bl, bladder.

experience than the identification of an embryo in a 25 mm sac. With intravaginal ultrasound transducers becoming more widely available, even relatively inexperienced observers will likely adopt this crite-

rion (Fig. 3–7). Still, the greatest value of the above two criteria is that they are not subjective. The MSD is easily measured, and the yolk sac and embryo are either observed or they are not.

The third major criterion that is uniformly reliable for predicting an abnormal outcome is a distorted sac shape.[60] Although the shape of a normal gestational sac may vary somewhat depending predominantly upon the degree of bladder distention, grossly aberrant shapes are readily recognized by experienced sonographers and reliably predict an abnormal outcome (Fig. 3–26). Unfortunately, only about 10 percent of abnormal gestations meet this criterion. Thus, this criterion, although useful, suffers from two problems: it is somewhat subjective and relatively insensitive.

The remaining criteria are more subjective, are less than 100 percent specific for diagnosing abnormal gestations, and should be considered *minor criteria* (Table 3–2).[60] Minor criteria include a thin, weakly echogenic, or irregular choriodecidual reaction; the absence of a double decidual sac; and a low position of the gestational sac. Although diagnostic accuracy employing these criteria will undoubtedly vary with the experience of the interpreter, recent studies indicate that each minor criterion has a relatively high specificity (98 percent or greater) and

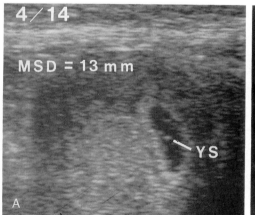
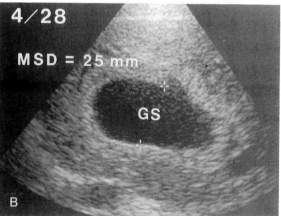

Figure 3–33. Longitudinal sonograms of the uterus (*A* and *B*) in a patient who had a threatened abortion. The examinations were performed two weeks apart. On the early sonogram (*A*), the mean sac diameter (MSD) was 13 mm, and a yolk sac (YS) was identified. However, no embryonic heartbeat was detected. Still, these features are within normal limits. Bleeding persisted, and a subsequent sonogram demonstrated nearly normal interval growth of the gestational sac (GS), now with a mean diameter of 25 mm. At this time, however, neither a yolk sac nor an embryo was visible. Thus, conclusive evidence of nonviability was confirmed despite nearly normal interval growth of the gestational sac lumen. Note that the surrounding chorionic tissue appears relatively normal (compare Figs. 3–29 and 3–30). Recall that gestational sac growth is more dependent on the chorionic tissue than on the presence of the embryo.

positive predictive accuracy (94 to 98 percent) for diagnosing an abnormal outcome. Importantly, specificity and predictive accuracy for an abnormal outcome increase to 100 percent when three or more minor criteria are present.

Of the above-described five minor criteria for identifying abnormal gestations, four relate to the appearance of the "choriodecidual" tissue surrounding the sac fluid. As a rule, normal small sacs have less surrounding chorionic and decidual tissue than larger sacs (compare Figs. 3–5, 3–7, 3–13, and 3–14). Although choriodecidual tissue is normally somewhat variable in appearance, clearly deficient choriodecidual tissue is easily noted (Figs. 3–29, 3–30). Abnormally thin or weakly echogenic choriodecidual tissues reliably correlate with abnormal gestational development. However, special note should be made that some first trimester nonviable pregnancies instead show dramatic thickening of the chorionic tissue secondary to hydropic degeneration of villi (Figs. 3–28 to 3–34).

Absence of a double decidual sac (DDS) (see Chap. 22) suggests nonviability of an early pregnancy (Figs. 3–27, 3–30). The DDS probably disappears when decidual necrosis occurs. Importantly, the presence of a DDS was originally described to discriminate early intrauterine pregnancies from other intrauterine fluid collections not representing true pregnancies. Use of this sign for distinguishing normal from abnormal early pregnancies is a secondary feature and must be judged in concert with other findings of abnormal gestational sac development. Occasionally, a DDS is not visible for small (less than 10 mm) normal gestational sacs.

The fifth, and final, minor criterion used to identify an abnormal gestation is a low position of the gestational sac (Fig. 3–31). This feature has been previously reported as useful by some observers, but not by others. Low position of the gestational sac is a stage rather than a cause of abortion. Thus, one would expect this feature to be highly reliable for predicting subsequent pregnancy loss. A low position of the gestational sac, situated in whole or in part within the lower uterine segment, is seen in only 20 percent of abnormal pregnancies and predicts an abnormal outcome in 94 percent of cases (Table 3–2).

CORRELATION OF GESTATIONAL SAC SIZE AND hCG

Since the "minor criteria" involve relatively subjective judgments, it would be helpful to have a less subjective criterion for evaluating gestational sacs less than 20 mm in MSD (above this MSD, of course, the major criteria can be employed). Correlating the sonographic examination of intrauterine contents simultaneously with serum hCG determinations has proved to be a useful method for evaluating early normal intrauterine pregnancies.[10, 61] A close relationship between ultrasound findings and quantitative serum hCG levels normally exists during early pregnancy (Fig. 3–35). Gestational sac size and hCG levels increase proportionately until eight menstrual weeks, at which time the gestational sac is approximately 25 mm in MSD, and an embryo should be easily detected.[10, 61, 62] After eight weeks, the hCG

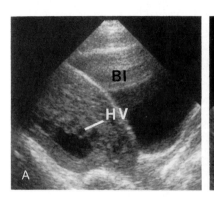
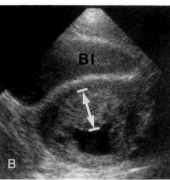

Figure 3–34. Longitudinal (A) and transverse (B) sonograms of the uterus in a patient who has a threatened abortion. Unlike the situation in Figures 3–27, 3–29 to 3–31, and 3–33, the chorionic tissue is markedly thickened (double-headed arrow) and demonstrates hydropic villi (HV). This pattern, seen also in Figure 3–28, is a less common manifestation in early embryonic demise, associated with villus hydrops rather than atrophy. Hydropic degeneration of the placenta is likely a part of the syndrome called partial mole. Bl, bladder.

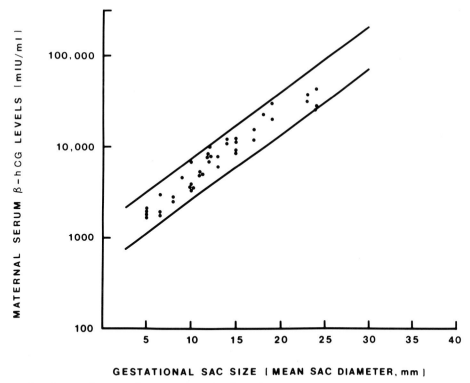

Figure 3–35. Correlation of maternal serum β-hCG levels with gestational sac size in normal pregnancies in the first trimester. (*From* Nyberg DA, Filly RA, Filho DLD, et al: Abnormal pregnancy: Early diagnosis by US and serum chorionic gonadotropin levels. Radiology 158:393, 1986.)

levels plateau and subsequently decline while the gestational sac continues to grow.

As noted above, quantitative hCG levels strongly correlate with gestational sac size in normal pregnancies. This enables one to employ a quantitative serum hCG level as an additional, less subjective feature to ensure the normality or abnormality of pregnancies less than 20 mm in MSD. A small gestational sac is the most difficult to evaluate for potentially abnormal features. Evidence indicates that a normal gestational sac can be consistently demonstrated when the hCG level is 1800 mIU/ml (2nd IS) or greater (Table 3–3).[10, 62] The relationship between quantitative serum hCG levels and sac size is not unexpected since both sac development and hCG production are a function of trophoblastic activity. Both gestational sac size and hCG determinations accurately predict menstrual age. A normal gestational sac grows approximately 1.1 mm per day while hCG levels rise exponentially, doubling every two to three days.[17]

The expected relationship between sonographic findings and simultaneous hCG levels is not observed in many abnormal gestations (Fig. 3–36).[62] This augments the reliability of identifying abnormal gestations on the basis of a single examination despite the absence of a detectable embryo (Figs. 3–37, 3–38). Again, correlation with the menstrual history is not required; women with an uncertain last menstrual period and women with irregular vaginal bleeding can be accurately evaluated by this method.

Table 3–3. DETECTION OF GESTATIONAL SAC COMPARED WITH hCG LEVEL FOR NORMAL GESTATIONS

	Normal Outcome (N = 76)	
hCG Level (2nd IS)	No Sac	Sac
< 1800	19	2*
> 1800	0	55

*1750 mIU/ml and 1620 mIU/ml.
NOTE: all prior to embryonic visualization.

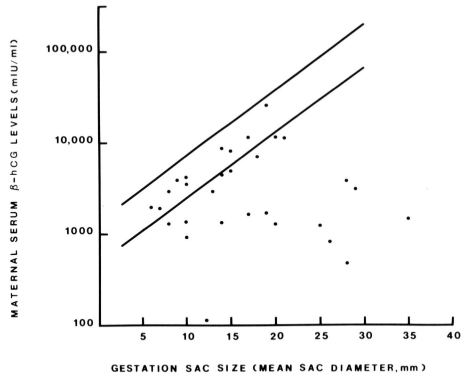

Figure 3–36. Correlation of maternal serum β-hCG levels and gestational sac size in abnormal gestations in the first trimester. Compare Figure 3–35. Note that a substantial percentage of abnormal gestations have low hCG levels compared with equivalent-sized normal gestations. (*From* Nyberg DA, Filly RA, Filho DLD, et al: Abnormal pregnancy: Early diagnosis by US and serum chorionic gonadotropin levels. Radiology 158:393, 1986.)

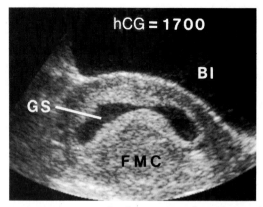

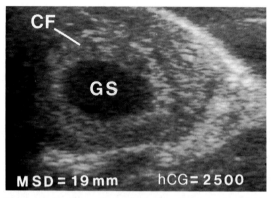

Figure 3–37. Longitudinal sonogram of an abnormal gestational sac (GS) in a patient who has a threatened abortion. One would have to rely on minor morphologic criteria to confirm this pregnancy as abnormal. However, the hCG level is very low (1700 mIU/ml). Ordinarily, one would not even identify a normal gestation when the hCG level is this low. Bl, bladder; FMC, focal myometrial contraction.

Figure 3–38. Magnified sonogram of an abnormal-appearing gestational sac (GS). Note the abnormal echotexture of the chorion frondosum (CF). The mean sac diameter (MSD) of 19 mm does not correlate with the simultaneous hCG level of 2500 mIU/ml. One would have expected the hCG to be greater than 5000 mIU/ml. This helps substantially in confirming this pregnancy as an abnormal gestation, despite the inability to use morphologic major criteria.

Almost without exception, abnormal pregnancies demonstrate a low hCG level relative to gestational sac development.[51, 61, 62] Comparison of the hCG levels with the gestational sac size demonstrated proportionately low levels for 65 percent of abnormal gestational sacs (Table 3–4, Fig. 3–36).[62] These data support prior results indicating that hCG levels frequently fall before the spontaneous expulsion of nonviable gestations.[61, 63] Simultaneous hCG levels are less likely to be useful for diagnosing abnormal pregnancies when the sonographic examination fails to detect a gestational sac. In this situation, the major competing pathologic diagnosis is ectopic pregnancy, which is covered in detail in Chapter 22.

There is bound to be some overlap between the purely sonographic findings of an abnormal sac and the correlation of sac size with quantitative hCG levels. Indeed, initial experience suggests that these two methods identify similar groups of patients.[58] When hCG levels are disproportionately low, the gestation usually demonstrates abnormal sonographic features, including a weak or irregular choriodecidual reaction. This is not unexpected since the chorionic tissue elaborates hCG. However, these sonographic criteria are subjective and require an experienced sonographer for their correct interpretation. Quantitative hCG levels and the mean sac size are more easily assessed and may be objectively compared with normal data. When the sonographic findings alone are uncertain or when confirmation is desired, a disproportionately low hCG level is supportive evidence for an abnormal pregnancy.

Table 3–4. CORRELATION OF SAC SIZE WITH hCG LEVEL

	Abnormal	Normal
Does not correlate	21*	0
Correlates	10	39
Prevalence:	31/70 =	44%
Sensitivity:	21/31 =	68%
Specificity:	39/39 =	100%
Positive Accuracy:	21/21 =	100%
Negative Accuracy:	39/49 =	80%

*Twenty cases had disproportionately low hCG levels, and one case (molar pregnancy) had an elevated hCG level.

From Nyberg DA, Filly RA, Filho DLD, et al: Abnormal pregnancy: Early diagnosis by US and serum chorionic gonadotropin levels. Radiology 158:393, 1986.

This section appropriately began with a quote from Donald regarding the goals and objectives in the evaluation of pregnancy failure, and it can appropriately end with an admonition from Robinson: "Any other worker wishing to provide [this service] must be prepared to establish these techniques in his own hands with a period of nonintervention and with good lines of communication [with the referring clinicians]."[1]

EVALUATION OF MASSES IN EARLY PREGNANCY

There are two relatively common pathologic masses seen in early pregnancy and one very common "physiologic" mass. The pathologic masses are uterine myomas and ovarian corpus luteum cysts (CLC); the physiologic mass is the so-called "focal myometrial contraction" (FMC). The myomas must be distinguished from focal myometrial contractions, a sometimes difficult task, and the CLC must be distinguished from ovarian neoplastic cysts, e.g., cystadenomas, cystadenocarcinomas, and cystic teratomas, an always important task.

Distinguishing between a myoma and an FMC (Figs. 3–25, 3–32, 3–37) is occasionally difficult, but the following rules usually result in an accurate discrimination. Recall that the following are tendencies, and both overlap and variations exist.

1. A myoma tends to be hypoechoic relative to the adjacent myometrium, but an FMC tends to be isoechoic with the adjacent myometrium.

2. A myoma attenuates the acoustic beam, but an FMC does not.

3. The mass effect of a myoma tends to distort both the serosal and endometrial contours of the uterus, but that from an FMC tends to distort only the endometrial surface.

4. An FMC is virtually always homogeneous; a myoma is sometimes heterogeneous in echo texture.

If necessary, a patient can always be reexamined after a short interval to distinguish between a contraction and a myoma. It is rarely necessary to delay a patient for this purpose since segregating these two entities is hardly a critical distinction. Occasionally, an exophytic area of myometrial tissue is neither an FMC nor a myoma but a nongravid horn of a bicornuate uterus. This is usually readily recognized since there is decidualized endometrium centrally positioned within the observed tissue.

The major problem caused by myomas in early pregnancy is related to the spontaneous abortion of otherwise normal embryos.[64] This is particularly true of submucous myomas and numerous myomas that distort the uterus. Although myomas may grow to a very large size during pregnancy, undergo necrosis, precipitate preterm labor, or interfere with vaginal delivery, none of these situations pertain to the first trimester.[64]

The life cycle of the corpus luteum begins with rupture of the graafian follicle. The follicle wall collapses, and the cells lining the follicle undergo proliferation and alteration to lutein cells.[65] These cells elaborate progesterone to support any possible pregnancy. Morphologically, a corpus luteum is a thick-walled, noncystic structure that may attain a size up to 2 cm. The corpus luteum continues to enlarge if pregnancy occurs. This structure may now occupy as much as half of the ovary. Normally, the corpus luteum of pregnancy begins to regress after ten weeks; its function is gradually taken over by the developing placenta. From a practical pathologic perspective, the corpus luteum is called "cystic" when it exceeds 3 cm.[66] It is the central zone that organizes into a cyst; the gelatinous liquid contained therein is fibrin. Occasionally, these cysts become quite large, at times exceeding 10 cm.

Although any type of ovarian tumor may complicate early pregnancy, unilocular cysts, even those with somewhat thickened walls, that are discovered in the first trimester should be assumed to represent corpus luteum cysts and should be observed (Fig. 3–39). These lesions are so common during this stage of pregnancy that it would be impractical to proceed with invasive diagnostic procedures, such as laparoscopy, or to elect to excise the lesion before sufficient time has been allotted to examine the mass serially. Corpus luteum cysts, like the corpus

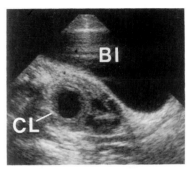

Figure 3–39. Longitudinal sonogram of the left ovary in a patient with a normal, ongoing first trimester pregnancy. A typical corpus luteum cyst (CL) is identified. Notice the thick wall and echolucent center. Bl, bladder.

luteum of pregnancy, tend to regress as the end of the first trimester nears.

Follow-up at the beginning of the second trimester (14 menstrual weeks) usually shows the lesion to be regressing or gone.[64–66] Furthermore, laparotomy for ovarian masses is usually not conducted until the middle second trimester (after the 18th week), provided, of course, that the operation can be postponed until then.[64] This is a period of quiescence of the uterine muscle; thus laparotomy is unlikely to precipitate abortion. This additional time can be used to advantage for further follow-up since, occasionally, these lesions do not regress until later than ordinarily expected. Despite all these precautions and the long period available to follow these masses for regression, corpus luteum cysts occasionally disobey all the rules and continue to expand, and thus become suspect as true ovarian neoplasms.

The decision to remove an asymptomatic ovarian mass is a clinical one.[64] Malignant tumors of the ovary are exceedingly rare complications of pregnancy. Even though sonography may be unable to exclude a malignancy on the basis of observed morphology of the lesion, one should not employ this deficiency as evidence that the mass must be excised.

Glossary

1. **Abortion:** The premature expulsion from the uterus of the products of conception—of the embryo, or of a nonviable fetus.

2. **Viable:** Capable of living, especially said of a fetus that has reached such a stage of development that it can live outside the uterus.

3. **Fetus:** The developing young in the human uterus after the end of the eighth menstrual week. Before this, it is called an embryo; it becomes an infant when it is completely outside the body of the mother, even before the cord is cut.

4. **Complete Abortion:** An abortion in which all the products of conception have been expelled from the uterus and identified.

5. **Imminent Abortion:** An impending abortion in which the bleeding is profuse, the cervix is softened and dilated, and the cramps approach the character of labor pains.

6. **Inevitable Abortion:** An abortion in progress.

7. **Missed Abortion:** The retention of a dead pregnancy for at least two months.

8. **Blighted Ovum:** A fertilized ovum in which development has become arrested.

References

1. Robinson HP: The diagnosis of early pregnancy failure by sonar. Br J Obstet Gynaecol 82:849, 1975.
2. Soules MR: The in vitro fertilization pregnancy rate: Let's be honest with one another. (Editorial.) Fertil Steril 43:511, 1985.
3. Jones HW, Acosta AA, Andrews MC, et al: What is a pregnancy? A question for programs of in vitro fertilization. Fertil Steril 40:728, 1983.
4. Edmonds DK, Linday KS, Miller JR, et al: Early embryonic mortality in women. Fertil Steril 38:447, 1982.
5. Schlesselman JJ: How does one assess the risk of abnormalities from human in vitro fertilization? Am J Obstet Gynecol 135:135, 1979.
6. Moore KL: The beginning of human development: The first week. In Moore KL: The Developing Human: Clinically Oriented Embryology, 4th Ed. Philadelphia, WB Saunders Co, 1988.
7. Moore KL: Formation of the bilaminar embryo: The second week. In Moore KL: The Developing Human: Clinically Oriented Embryology, 4th Ed. Philadelphia, WB Saunders Co, 1988.
8. Moore KL: The placenta and fetal membranes. In Moore KL: The Developing Human: Clinically Oriented Embryology, 4th Ed. Philadelphia, WB Saunders Co, 1988.
9. Hellman LM, Kobayashi M, Fillisti L, et al: Growth and development of the human fetus prior to the twentieth week of gestation. Am J Obstet Gynecol 103:789, 1969.
10. Nyberg DA, Filly RA, Mahony BS, et al: Early gestation: Correlation of hCG levels and sonographic identification. AJR 144:951, 1985.
11. Cadkin AV, McAlpin J: Detection of fetal cardiac activity between 41 and 43 days of gestation. J Ultrasound Med 3:499, 1984.
12. Batzer FR, Weiner S, Corson SL, et al: Landmarks during the first forty-two days of gestation demonstrated by the beta-subunit of human chorionic gonadotropin and ultrasound. Am J Obstet Gynecol 146:973, 1983.
13. Bernard KG, Cooperberg PL: Sonographic differentiation between blighted ovum and early viable pregnancy. AJR 144:597, 1985.
14. DeCrispigny LC, Cooper D, McKenna M: Early detection of intrauterine pregnancy with ultrasound. J Ultrasound Med 7:7, 1988.
15. Yeh HC, Goodman JD, Carr L, Rabinowitz JG: Intradecidual sign: A US criterion of early intrauterine pregnancy. Radiology 161:463, 1986.
16. Robinson HP: "Gestation sac" volumes as determined by sonar in the first trimester of pregnancy. Brit J Obstet Gynaecol 82:100, 1975.
17. Nyberg DA, Mack LA, Laing FC, Patten RM: Distinguishing normal from abnormal gestational sac growth in early pregnancy. J Ultrasound Med 6:23, 1987.
18. Lang FC, Filly RA, Mark W, et al: Ultrasonic demonstration of endometrial fluid collections unassociated with pregnancy. Radiology 137:471, 1980.
19. Nyberg DA, Laing FC, Filly RA, et al: Ultrasonographic differentiation of the gestational sac of early intrauterine pregnancy from the pseudogestational sac of ectopic pregnancy. Radiology 146:755, 1983.
20. Cadkin AV, McAlpin J: The decidua-chorionic sac: A reliable sonographic indicator of intrauterine pregnancy prior to detection of a fetal pole. J Ultrasound Med 3:539, 1984.
21. Marks WM, Filly RA, Callen PW, et al: The decidual cast of ectopic pregnancy: A confusing ultrasonographic appearance. Radiology 133:451, 1979.
22. Bradley WG, Fiske CE, Filly RA: The double sac sign of early intrauterine pregnancy: Use in exclusion of ectopic pregnancy. Radiology 143:223, 1983.
23. Yeh HC: Anatomy of early pregnancy. Presented at the Annual Meeting of the Society of Radiologists in Ultrasound, Chicago, 1986.
24. Sauerbrei E, Cooperberg PL, Poland JB: Ultrasound demonstration of the normal fetal yolk sac. J Clin Ultrasound 8:217, 1980.
25. Mantoni M, Pederson JF: Ultrasound visualization of the human yolk sac. J Clin Ultrasound 7:459, 1979.
26. Jeanty P, Renoy P, vanKerkem J, et al: Ultrasonic

demonstration of the amnion. J Ultrasound Med 1:243, 1982.

27. Robinson HP, Fleming JEE: A critical evaluation of sonar "crown-rump length" measurements. Br J Obstet Gynaecol 82:702, 1975.

28. Mahony BS, Filly RA: High resolution sonographic assessment of the fetal extremities. J Ultrasound Med 3:489, 1984.

29. Burrows PE, Lyons EA, Phillips HJ, Oates I: Intra-uterine membranes: Sonographic findings and clinical significance. J Clin Ultrasound 10:1, 1982.

30. Lofberg L, Iosif CS, Edvall H, Gustavii B: Direct vision sampling of chorionic villi during extra-amniotic instillation of physiologic saline. Am J Obstet Gynecol 152:591, 1985.

31. Robinson HP: Sonar measurement of the fetal crown-rump length as a means of assessing maturity in the first trimester of pregnancy. Br Med J 4:28, 1973.

32. Kurjak A, Cecuk S, Breyer B: Prediction of maturity in the first trimester of pregnancy by ultrasonic measurement of fetal crown-rump length. J Clin Ultrasound 4:83, 1976.

33. Drumm JE: The prediction of delivery date by ultrasonic measurement of fetal crown-rump length. Br J Obstet Gynaecol 84:1, 1977.

34. Chervenak FA, Brightman RC, Thornton T, et al: Crown-rump length and serum human chorionic gonadotropin as predictors of gestational age. Obstet Gynecol 67:210, 1986.

35. Campbell S, Warsof SL, Little D, Cooper DJ: Routine ultrasound screening for the prediction of gestational age. Obstet Gynecol 65:613, 1985.

36. Robinson HP: Detection of fetal heart movement in the first trimester of pregnancy using pulsed ultrasound. Br Med J 4:466, 1972.

37. Robinson HP: Sonar in the management of abortion. J Obstet Gynaecol Br Commonw 79:90, 1972.

38. Levi S: Diagnostic use of ultrasonics in abortion: A study of 250 patients. Int J Gynecol Obstet 11:195, 1973.

39. Kohorn E, Kaufman M: Sonar in the first trimester of pregnancy. Obstet Gynecol 44:473, 1974.

40. Duff GB: The prognosis in threatened abortion: A comparison between predictions made by sonar, urinary hormone assays and clinical judgement. Br J Obstet Gynaecol 82:858, 1975.

41. Drumm J, Clinch J: Ultrasound in management of clinically diagnosed threatened abortion. Br Med J 2:424, 1975.

42. Jouppila P: Diagnostics in threatened abortion: A study by ultrasonic, clinical, hormonal and histopathological methods. Ultrasound Med 3A:595, 1976.

43. Smith C, Gregori C, Breen J: Ultrasonography in threatened abortion. Obstet Gynecol 51:173, 1978.

44. Young GB, McDicken WN: Signs of fetal death in early pregnancy. J Clin Ultrasound 6:244, 1978.

45. Hertz JB: Diagnostic procedures in threatened abortion. Obstet Gynecol 66:223, 1984.

46. Fantel AG, Shepard TH: Basic aspects of early (first trimester) abortion. In Iffy L, Kaminetsky HA (eds): Principle and Practice of Obstetrics and Perinatology, Vol 1. New York, John Wiley & Sons, 1981, p 553.

47. Cavanagh D, Comas MR: Spontaneous abortion. In Danforth DN (ed): Obstetrics and Gynecology. Philadelphia, Harper & Row Pubs, 1982, p 378.

48. Donald I, Morley P, Barnett E: The diagnosis of blighted ovum by sonar. Br J Obstet Gynaecol 79:304, 1972.

49. Jouppila P, Huhtaniemi I, Tapanainen J: Early pregnancy failure: Study by ultrasonic and hormonal methods. Obstet Gynecol 55:42, 1980.

50. Anderson SG: Management of threatened abortion with real-time sonography. Obstet Gynecol 55:259, 1980.

51. Braunstein GD, Karow WG, Gentry WC, et al: First trimester chorionic gonadotropin measurements as an aid in the diagnosis of early pregnancy disorders. Am J Obstet Gynecol 131:25, 1978.

52. Ericksen PS, Philipsen T: Prognosis in threatened abortion evaluated by hormone assays and ultrasound scanning. Obstet Gynecol 55:435, 1980.

53. Wilson RD, Kendrick V, Wittman BK, McGillivray B: Spontaneous abortion and pregnancy outcome after normal first trimester ultrasound examination. Obstet Gynecol 67:352, 1986.

54. Christiaens GC, Stoutenbeek P: Spontaneous abortions in proven intact pregnancies. Lancet 2:57, 1984.

55. Mantoni M: Ultrasound signs of threatened abortion and their significance. Obstet Gynecol 65:471, 1985.

56. Goldstein SR, Subramanyan BR, Raghavendra BN, et al: Subchorionic bleeding in threatened abortion: Sonographic findings and significance. AJR 141:975, 1983.

57. Ghorashi B, Gottesfeld KR: The gray scale appearance of the normal pregnancy from 4 to 16 weeks of gestation. J Clin Ultrasound 5:195, 1977.

58. Jouppila P, Herva T: Study of blighted ovum by ultrasonic and histopathologic methods. Obstet Gynecol 55:574, 1980.

59. Young GB, McDicken WN: Signs of fetal death in early pregnancy. J Clin Ultrasound 6:1244, 1978.

60. Nyberg DA, Laing FC, Filly RA: Threatened abortion: Sonographic distinction of normal and abnormal gestation sacs. Radiology 158:397, 1986.

61. Batzer FR, Weiner S, Corson SL, et al: Landmarks during the first 42 days of gestation demonstrated by the beta-subunit of human chorionic gonadotropin and ultrasound. Am J Obstet Gynecol 146:9733, 1983.

62. Nyberg DA, Filly RA, Filho DLD, et al: Abnormal pregnancy: Early diagnosis by US and serum chorionic gonadotropin levels. Radiology 158-393, 1986.

63. Yuen BH, Livingston JE, Poland BJ, et al: Human chorionic gonadotropin, estradiol, progesterone, prolactin, and B-scan ultrasound monitoring of complications in early pregnancy. Obstet Gynecol 57:207, 1981.

64. Nesbitt REL, Abdul-Karim RW: Coincidental disorders complicating pregnancy. In Danforth DN (ed): Obstetrics and Gynecology, 4th Ed. Harper & Row Pubs, Philadelphia, 1982, pp 542–543.

65. Blaustein A: Anatomy and histology of the human ovary. In Blaustein A (ed): Pathology of the Female Genital Tract. New York, Springer-Verlag, 1977, pp 378–383.

66. Kraus FT: Female genitalia. In Anderson WAD, Kissane JM (eds): Pathology, 7th Ed. St. Louis, CV Mosby Co, 1977, p 1731.

ULTRASOUND ASSESSMENT OF FETAL AGE

Alfred B. Kurtz, M.D.
Laurence Needleman, M.D.

Accurate knowledge of fetal age is important. It helps the pregnant woman, her family, the obstetrician, and the radiologist in the planning of the pregnancy, in the prediction of maturity, and in the detection of growth retardation. The gestational age, a term used interchangeably with menstrual age, is taken from the first day of the woman's last menstrual period prior to the onset of the pregnancy.

Before the advent of ultrasound, the gestational age had to be established by a combination of history (menstrual dates) and physical examination (uterine fundal height). Both of these contain inaccuracies, even in the best of circumstances (Table 4–1). It has been estimated that menstrual history is not reliable in at least 20 percent of women for reasons that may include oligomenorrhea, bleeding in the first trimester, and becoming pregnant in the postpartum period or after the use of oral contraceptives or intrauterine devices.[1, 2] In women with optimal menstrual histories, only 85 percent delivered within ± two weeks of their estimated date of confinement (EDC), decreasing to 70 percent in women uncertain of their dates.[1] The physical examination is also inaccurate, an inaccuracy that increases toward term. Although in the first trimester,

the physical examination may predict gestational age to within ± two weeks, by the third trimester, the fundal height may vary by as much as 7 inches (17.5 cm). This is equivalent to 14 gestational weeks (Table 4–1).[3]

The advent of ultrasound has allowed a more direct evaluation of the structure and

Table 4–1. GESTATIONAL AGE PREDICTORS

Clinical and Ultrasound Parameters	Estimated Range for 95% of Cases
In vitro fertilization	± 1 day
Ovulation induction	± 3 days
Recorded basal body temperature	± 4 to 5 days
Crown-rump length	± 5 to 7 days
Biparietal diameter—second trimester	± 5 to 7 days
Gestational sac (average diameter)	± 7 days (?)
First trimester physical examination	± 2 weeks
Optimal menstrual history	± 2.5 weeks
Biparietal diameter—third trimester	± 2 (?) to 4 weeks
Fundal height measurement—before 28 weeks	± 4 weeks
Suspect menstrual history	± more than 4 weeks
Fundal height measurement—after 28 weeks	± 4 to 6 weeks

development of the fetus. Measurements of a wide variety of parameters have been devised to establish gestational age. In the first trimester, the gestational sac and crown-rump length (CRL) have become the primary means of establishing gestational age. In the second and third trimester, the fetus is large enough for specific anatomic structures to be routinely identified. The major fetal parameters that can be used to establish gestational age are the head, body, extremities, and their ratios. Internal fetal parts, such as the lateral ventricles, liver and kidneys, and more recently, the fetal heart and cerebellum, are also consistently imaged. These will not be evaluated further since their measurements do not add to the accuracy of establishing fetal age. The outer orbital (binocular) diameter, helpful at times in establishing fetal age, particularly when the fetal head is in a difficult position to measure or when there is a head to body discrepancy, is not used routinely and will not be discussed further. Fetal weight is commonly calculated using multiple parameters; although it is helpful in assessing growth retardation and macrosomia, it is not a primary measurement in the prediction of gestational age.

At the present time, there are over 400 articles in the English-speaking literature bombarding the radiologist, obstetrician, and sonographer with a myriad of parameters and measurement tables. In general, it is not necessary to measure every identifiable fetal parameter. In addition, the measurement of more and more parameters, each establishing a gestational age, frequently leads to confusion. It is therefore the purpose of this chapter to discuss the most widely used and accepted parameters, showing the correct anatomic places to measure, the pitfalls in measurements, and their accuracies. An approach to the establishment of gestational age will be discussed.

FIRST TRIMESTER (3 TO 12 GESTATIONAL WEEKS)

In the first trimester, the gestational sac and crown-rump length are used to establish fetal age. Both parameters are useful because each measures a different aspect of the first trimester pregnancy. The gestational sac parameter is a measure of the anechoic space containing the fluid, embryo, and extraembryonic structures. It is routinely identified by transabdominal scanning as early as five gestational weeks. The crown-rump length is a measurement of the embryo and is usually not identified transabdominally until one to two weeks later, at seven gestational weeks. With the recent advent of endovaginal scanning, the early pregnancy can be imaged in greater detail so that the gestational sac and the embryo are identified earlier. Preliminary work suggests that both parameters can be routinely measured one to two weeks earlier; however, this has not yet been completely accepted.

Gestational Sac

The gestational sac is the first identifiable structure routinely imaged in the first trimester. Almost all of the articles on gestational sac measurements were written prior to 1975. Although the statistical analyses in these articles were primitive and the exact methods were vague, continued use has established guidelines for measurement of the gestational sac. The sac is measured inside the hyperechoic rim, including only the anechoic space (Fig. 4–1). If the sac is round, only one dimension is needed; if ovoid, usually caused by compression from the filled maternal urinary bladder, three measurements are taken and an average diameter calculated (Fig. 4–1). It is important that the long axis and anteroposterior measurements be obtained from the sagittal image, the long-axis measurement taken first and the anteroposterior dimension measured perpendicular to it. The transverse image, obtained at the level of the anteroposterior measurement, provides the width measurement.

The authors recommend Table 4–2, which compares the gestational age from five to 12 weeks with the mean gestational sac size.[4] The accuracy of gestational sac size as a predictor of gestational age has been evaluated in only one article and found to be approximately ± one week (Table 4–1).[5]

Crown-Rump Length

The embryo is measured along its longest axis (Fig. 4–2). Initially, distinct landmarks cannot be identified so that the embryo appears hyperechoic and ill defined, with heart

Figure 4–1. Measurement of the gestational sac. A, Ultrasound long axis scan of the uterus, imaging a slightly ovoid sac. The anechoic space is measured first in long axis, along the long axis of the uterus *(solid line)*. The anteroposterior measurement is taken perpendicular to the long axis measurement *(solid line)*. B, Ultrasound transaxial scan of the uterus is obtained at the point where the anteroposterior measurement had been taken. The transverse measurement is then obtained *(solid line)*.

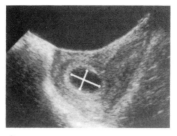

A

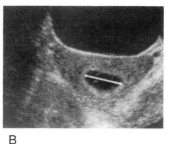

B

Mean Sac Diameter = L + W + H / 3

* *Measurements from inner to inner sac*

motion centrally. As the pregnancy continues, by approximately nine to ten weeks the head can be differentiated from the rump. The crown-rump length measurement is still used during this time since internal anatomy is not consistently demonstrated (Fig. 4–2). However, by 12 weeks, when the internal structures of the fetal head are routinely identified, its measurement is used to obtain a gestational age.

Table 4–2. GESTATIONAL SAC MEASUREMENT TABLE

Mean Predicted Gestational Sac (cm)	Gestational Age (weeks)	Mean Predicted Gestational Sac (cm)	Gestational Age (weeks)
1.0	5.0	3.6	8.8
1.1	5.2	3.7	8.9
1.2	5.3	3.8	9.0
1.3	5.5	3.9	9.2
1.4	5.6	4.0	9.3
1.5	5.8	4.1	9.5
1.6	5.9	4.2	9.6
1.7	6.0	4.3	9.7
1.8	6.2	4.4	9.9
1.9	6.3	4.5	10.0
2.0	6.5	4.6	10.2
2.1	6.6	4.7	10.3
2.2	6.8	4.8	10.5
2.3	6.9	4.9	10.6
2.4	7.0	5.0	10.7
2.5	7.2	5.1	10.9
2.6	7.3	5.2	11.0
2.7	7.5	5.3	11.2
2.8	7.6	5.4	11.3
2.9	7.8	5.5	11.5
3.0	7.9	5.6	11.6
3.1	8.0	5.7	11.7
3.2	8.2	5.8	11.9
3.3	8.3	5.9	12.0
3.4	8.5	6.0	12.2
3.5	8.6		

$$\text{Gestastional Age (weeks)} = \frac{\text{Gestational Sac (cm)} + 2.543}{0.702}$$

From Hellman LM, Kobayashi M, Fillisti L, et al: Growth and development of the human fetus prior to the twentieth week of gestation. Am J Obstet Gynecol 103:784, 1969.

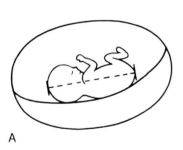

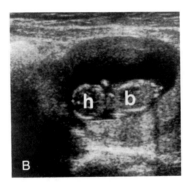

Figure 4–2. Measurement of the crown-rump length. *A, diagram, Dotted line* shows the measurement from the top of the crown (head) to the bottom of the rump. *B,* Ultrasound scan of the pregnant uterus, showing the longest length of a 9 week fetus. While the fetal head (h) can be differentiated from the body (b), the internal anatomy cannot be clearly distinguished.

The authors recommend Table 4–3, which compares the crown-rump length with the gestational age from six to 14 weeks.[6] This table should be used only until the fetal head is identified. As the fetus continues to grow beyond 12 weeks, it is more likely to flex and extend, making the crown-rump length measurement less accurate.

The initial accuracy of the crown-rump length was felt to be extremely high, approaching ± 2.7 days, and therefore was recommended as the best measurement to establish the gestational age.[6] Since then, other observers have evaluated the crown-rump length and found it to be somewhat less accurate. Although still one of the best estimates, with an accuracy of ± five to seven days (Table 4–1), the crown-rump length is comparable with a second trimester biparietal diameter measurement.[7, 8]

Table 4–3. CROWN-RUMP LENGTH MEASUREMENT TABLE

Mean Predicted Crown-Rump Length (mm) "Regression Analysis"	Gestational Age (weeks)	Mean Predicted Crown-Rump Length (mm) "Regression Analysis"	Gestational Age (weeks)
		34.0	10.1
6.7	6.3	35.5	10.3
7.4	6.4	36.9	10.4
8.0	6.6	38.4	10.6
8.7	6.7	39.9	10.7
9.5	6.9	41.4	10.9
10.2	7.0	43.0	11.0
11.0	7.1	44.6	11.1
11.8	7.3	46.2	11.3
12.6	7.4	47.8	11.4
13.5	7.6	49.5	11.6
14.4	7.7	51.2	11.7
15.3	7.9	52.9	11.9
16.3	8.0	54.7	12.0
17.3	8.1	56.5	12.1
18.3	8.3	58.3	12.3
19.3	8.4	60.1	12.4
20.4	8.6	62.0	12.6
21.5	8.7	63.9	12.7
22.6	8.9	65.9	12.9
23.8	9.0	67.8	13.0
25.0	9.1	69.3	13.1
26.2	9.3	71.8	13.3
27.4	9.4	73.9	13.4
28.7	9.6	76.0	13.6
30.0	9.7	78.1	13.7
31.3	9.9	80.2	13.9
32.7	10.0	82.4	14.0

From Robinson HP, Fleming JEE: A critical evaluation of sonar "crown-rump length" measurements. Br J Obstet Gynaecol 82:702, 1975.

SECOND AND THIRD TRIMESTER MEASUREMENTS (FROM 12 GESTATIONAL WEEKS)

Head Measurements

BIPARIETAL DIAMETER. The biparietal diameter (BPD) is the most discussed and documented obstetric ultrasound measurement. To date, over 60 articles have been published comparing it with the gestational age. The biparietal diameter is taken in the transaxial plane at the widest portion of the skull, with the thalamus positioned in the midline.[9, 10] A leading edge to leading edge measurement is obtained from the first echo of the closer temporoparietal calvarial table to the first echo of the farther temporoparietal calvarial table (Fig. 4–3).

The most appropriate method for analyzing gestational age for each biparietal diameter is with a table encompassing both the mean gestational age and the range of gestational ages (Table 4–4). The mean gestational age is important because it most likely represents the fetal age. The range of gestational ages is also important since the fetus cannot be assigned a single gestational age on the basis of a biparietal diameter measurement. Instead, a single biparietal diameter encompasses a range of ages in which most fetuses of that size are most likely to fall. A composite range table, obtained by combining the results of a number of investigators into one table, is recommended (Table 4–4).[11] Its advantage is the large number of subjects and consequent better statistical analysis.

The range table can be used to establish the EDC. For example, a fetal biparietal diameter of 40 mm corresponds to a mean gestational age of 17.6 weeks. Since the average fetus would be delivered at 40 weeks, the mean EDC is 22.4 weeks after the ultrasound examination. Although this is the most likely gestational age, many normals are not at the mean. Instead, 90 percent of normal fetuses will actually be 16.4 to 18.8 weeks old so that the EDC is 21.2 to 23.6 weeks after the ultrasound study.

There are technical factors involved in the biparietal diameter measurement. Once the correct anatomic position to obtain the measurement has been found, the major factor is placing the calipers in the correct position. It has been estimated that even the most experienced observer has a measurement error of at least 1 mm, and perhaps as high as 2 mm, when measuring a biparietal diameter.[12–14]

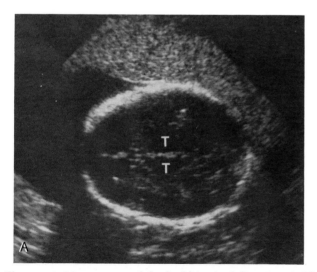

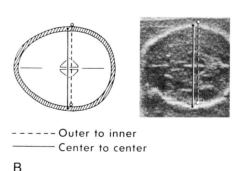

- - - - - - Outer to inner
———— Center to center

B

Figure 4–3. Measurement of the fetal biparietal diameter. *A,* Ultrasound transaxial image of the fetal head, taken with the thalami (T) imaged in the midline, equidistant from the temporoparietal tables of the calvarium. This, or a slightly lower level at the midbrain, is acceptable for obtaining a correct biparietal diameter. *B,* Diagram and image showing the leading edge (outer) to leading edge (inner) measurement of the fetal head, taken at the level of the thalami. While these images also show a center to center measurement, which would give the same value, the boundary echoes of leading edge measurements are slightly more precise.

Table 4–4. COMPOSITE BIPARIETAL DIAMETER TABLE

Biparietal Diameter (cm)	Gestational Age (weeks)		Biparietal Diameter (cm)	Gestational Age (weeks)	
	Mean*	Range 90% Variation†		Mean*	Range 90% Variation†
2.0	12.0	12.0			
2.1	12.0	12.0	6.1	24.2	22.6 to 25.8
2.2	12.7	12.2 to 13.2	6.2	24.6	23.1 to 26.1
2.3	13.0	12.4 to 13.6	6.3	24.9	23.4 to 26.4
2.4	13.2	12.6 to 13.8	6.4	25.3	23.8 to 26.8
2.5	13.5	12.9 to 14.1	6.5	25.6	24.1 to 27.1
2.6	13.7	13.1 to 14.3	6.6	26.0	24.5 to 27.5
2.7	14.0	13.4 to 14.6	6.7	26.4	25.0 to 27.8
2.8	14.3	13.6 to 15.0	6.8	26.7	25.3 to 28.1
2.9	14.5	13.9 to 15.2	6.9	27.1	25.8 to 28.4
3.0	14.8	14.1 to 15.5	7.0	27.5	26.3 to 28.7
3.1	15.1	14.3 to 15.9	7.1	27.9	26.7 to 29.1
3.2	15.3	14.5 to 16.1	7.2	28.3	27.2 to 29.4
3.3	15.6	14.7 to 16.5	7.3	28.7	27.6 to 29.8
3.4	15.9	15.0 to 16.8	7.4	29.1	28.1 to 30.1
3.5	16.2	15.2 to 17.2	7.5	29.5	28.5 to 30.5
3.6	16.4	15.4 to 17.4	7.6	30.0	29.0 to 31.0
3.7	16.7	15.6 to 17.8	7.7	30.3	29.2 to 31.4
3.8	17.0	15.9 to 18.1	7.8	30.8	29.6 to 32.0
3.9	17.3	16.1 to 18.5	7.9	31.1	29.9 to 32.5
4.0	17.6	16.4 to 18.8	8.0	31.6	30.2 to 33.0
4.1	17.9	16.5 to 19.3	8.1	32.1	30.7 to 33.5
4.2	18.1	16.6 to 19.8	8.2	32.6	31.2 to 34.0
4.3	18.4	16.8 to 20.2	8.3	33.0	31.5 to 34.5
4.4	18.8	16.9 to 20.7	8.4	33.4	31.9 to 35.1
4.5	19.1	17.0 to 21.2	8.5	34.0	32.3 to 35.7
4.6	19.4	17.4 to 21.4	8.6	34.3	32.8 to 36.2
4.7	19.7	17.8 to 21.6	8.7	35.0	33.4 to 36.6
4.8	20.0	18.2 to 21.8	8.8	35.4	33.9 to 37.1
4.9	20.3	18.6 to 22.0	8.9	36.1	34.6 to 37.6
5.0	20.6	19.0 to 22.2	9.0	36.6	35.1 to 38.1
5.1	20.9	19.3 to 22.5	9.1	37.2	35.9 to 38.5
5.2	21.2	19.5 to 22.9	9.2	37.8	36.7 to 38.9
5.3	21.5	19.8 to 23.2	9.3	38.8	37.3 to 39.3
5.4	21.9	20.1 to 23.7	9.4	39.0	37.9 to 40.1
5.5	22.2	20.4 to 24.0	9.5	39.7	38.5 to 40.9
5.6	22.5	20.7 to 24.3	9.6	40.6	39.1 to 41.5
5.7	22.8	21.1 to 24.5	9.7	41.0	39.9 to 42.1
5.8	23.2	21.5 to 24.9	9.8	41.8	40.5 to 43.1
5.9	23.5	21.9 to 25.1			
6.0	23.8	22.3 to 25.5			

*From weighted least mean square fit equation: $Y = -3.45701 + 0.50157x - 0.00441x^2$
†For each biparietal diameter, 90% of gestational age data points fell within this range.
From Kurtz AB, Wapner RJ, Kurtz RJ, et al: Analysis of biparietal diameter as an accurate indicator of gestational age. J Clin Ultrasound 8:319, 1980. Copyright 1980, John Wiley & Sons.

The accuracy of the biparietal diameter, a reflection of the accuracy of all fetal measurements in the second and third trimester, has been extensively studied. In the second trimester, up to 24 weeks, the biparietal diameter's accuracy is as good as that of the crown-rump length, ± five to seven days (Table 4–1).[7, 8] Some observers have stated that this accuracy may be extended into the beginning of the third trimester, to 30 weeks.[15, 16] Later in the third trimester, however, all observers state that the range of the biparietal diameter, as of all other measurements, becomes wider (Table 4–1). This increased variation is thought to be caused by the increased differences between fetal size and fetal age, which in turn is caused by normal genetic and environmental influences. One observer evaluating the crown-rump length in the first trimester, the biparietal diameter in the second trimester, and the biparietal diameter measurement at 30 to 33 weeks (in the middle of the third trimester) found the accuracy of the mid-third trimester biparietal diameter to be ± two weeks.[7] This study, however, was not continued to term. Most authors, evaluating the entire third trimester, find the inaccuracies were even greater, as much as ± 3.5 to 4 weeks at term.[9, 17, 18] At the present time, it is the authors' viewpoint that the accuracy is closer to ± 2 weeks (Table 4–1). This issue is still debated and needs further work before final resolution.

HEAD SHAPE DETECTION AND CORRECTION. Since the biparietal diameter is a linear measurement taken from one temporoparietal table to the other, it is only accurate if the head is the appropriate ovoid shape. If the head is unusually rounded (brachycephalic) or unusually elongated (scaphocephalic or dolichocephalic), the standard biparietal diameter measurement would over- or underestimate the head size. To determine whether the head shape is appropriate, two measurements are needed: the biparietal diameter (short axis) and the fronto-occipital diameter (long axis), calculated as a ratio with a formula called the cephalic index (Fig. 4–4, Table 4–5). The

Table 4–5. CEPHALIC INDEX FORMULA*

$$\text{Cephalic Index} = \frac{\text{Short Axis (Biparietal Diameter)}}{\text{Long Axis (Fronto-occipital Diameter)}} \times 100 = 78.3$$

Normal Range
At 2 Standard Deviations = 70 to 86

*Measurements of short and long axis taken from outer to outer margins of head.
From Hadlock FP, Deter RL, Carpenter RJ, Park SK: Estimating fetal age: Effect of head shape on BPD. AJR 137:83, 1981. Copyright by The American Roentgen Ray Society, 1981.

cephalic index had been previously used in the newborn child. One observer decided to use the same index in fetuses and found it to be almost identical, with a mean value of 78.3 and a 2 SD range of 70 to 86.[19] It is important to note that measurements are taken from outer edge to outer edge for both diameters.

If the cephalic index is abnormal (greater than 86 or less than 70), two types of corrections are possible. The head size can be measured in a transaxial view as a circumference, or the head shape can be "corrected" to an optimized biparietal diameter. The formula to correct the head shape to a

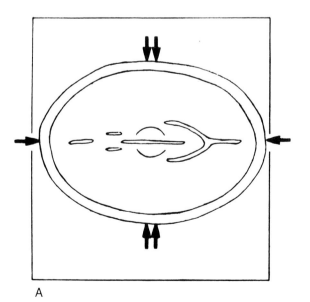

A

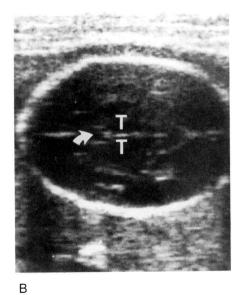

B

Figure 4–4. Measurement of the cephalic index. *A,* The short axis (the biparietal diameter), denoted by *double arrows,* and the long axis (the fronto-occipital diameter), denoted by *single arrows,* are both taken outer edge to outer edge. A ratio of the two gives the cephalic index. *B,* Ultrasound transaxial scan of the fetal head, at the level of the thalami (T) and cavum septi pellucidi *(curved arrow).*

cephalic index of 78 is called an area-corrected biparietal diameter (Table 4–6).[20] Some observers feel that all fetal head measurements should be corrected to the ideal shape prior to the use of the biparietal diameter table.

HEAD CIRCUMFERENCE. The head circumference measurement can be substituted for the biparietal diameter. Although its mean gestational age numbers are equally reliable, the range of gestational ages is larger (Table 4–7).[21] This increased variation is probably due to the much smaller sample size used in making the head circumference tables. Regardless, the circumference measurement

Table 4–6. CORRECTED BIPARIETAL DIAMETER (BPD)

Area-Corrected BPD (BPDa)

$$BPDa = \sqrt{(BPD \times FOD)/1.265}$$

FOD, fronto-occipital diameter.

From Doubilet PM, Greenes RA: Improved prediction of gestational age from fetal head measurements. AJR, 142:797, 1984. *Copyright by* The American Roentgen Ray Society, 1984.

of the head is a substitute for the biparietal diameter. Even though a digitizer or map reader tracing the outer perimeter of the head is the most reliable (Fig. 4–5), certain

Table 4–7. HEAD CIRCUMFERENCE MEASUREMENT TABLE

Head Circumference (cm)	Gestational Age (weeks) Predicted Mean Values	Head Circumference (cm)	Gestational Age (weeks) Predicted Mean Values
8.0	13.4	23.0	24.9
8.5	13.7	23.5	25.4
9.0	14.0	24.0	25.9
9.5	14.3	24.5	26.4
10.0	14.6	25.0	26.9
10.5	15.0	25.5	27.5
11.0	15.3	26.0	28.0
11.5	15.6	26.5	28.1
12.0	15.9	27.0	29.2
12.5	16.3	27.5	29.8
13.0	16.6	28.0	30.3
13.5	17.0	28.5	31.0
14.0	17.3	29.0	31.6
14.5	17.7	29.5	32.2
15.0	18.1	30.0	32.8
15.5	18.4	30.5	33.5
16.0	18.8	31.0	34.2
16.5	19.2	31.5	34.9
17.0	19.6	32.0	35.5
17.5	20.0	32.5	36.3
18.0	20.4	33.0	37.0
18.5	20.8	33.5	37.7
19.0	21.2	34.0	38.5
19.5	21.6	34.5	39.2
20.0	22.1	35.0	40.0
20.5	22.5	35.5	40.8
21.0	23.0	36.0	41.6
21.5	23.4		
22.0	23.9		
22.5	24.4		

Gestational Age (weeks)	Variability (weeks) at 95% Confidence Limits
12 to 18	± 1.3
18 to 24	± 1.6
24 to 30	± 2.3
30 to 36	± 2.7
36 to 42	± 3.4

From Hadlock FP, Deter RL, Harrist RB, Park SK: Fetal head circumference: Relation to menstrual age. AJR 138:649, 1982. *Copyright by* The American Roentgen Ray Society, 1982.

Figure 4–5. Measurement of the head circumference. *A,* Diagram showing a *dotted line* outlining the head, the correct place to take a circumference measurement. *B,* Ultrasound transaxial scan showing the thalami *(arrowheads),* well positioned in the midline. A *dotted line,* created by a digitizer, outlines the correct perimeter, just outside the hyperechoic calvarium, to obtain a circumference measurement.

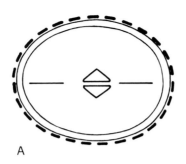

A

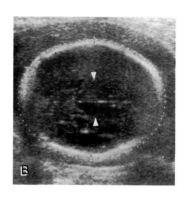

formulas have been shown to have almost the same accuracy. The use of an equation for the circumference of a circle (Table 4–8), initially but incorrectly called an equation for the circumference of an ellipse, has a maximal error of 6 percent near term. This is an acceptable inaccuracy if a digitizer or map reader is not available.[22, 23] Other, more complicated formulas have also been proposed but have not been shown to have greater reliability.[23]

The accuracy of head circumference measurements has been compared with that of biparietal diameter measurements. In general, the head circumference is no more accurate than the biparietal diameter as a predictor of gestational age.[21] However, when unusual head shapes occur, the head circumference may be of greater value.

Fetal Body Measurements

The measurements of the thorax and abdomen have been obtained primarily in a transaxial view. In the thorax, the only consistent landmark is the heart. This type of measurement may be potentially valuable in the analysis of thoracic disproportions.

The abdomen, on the other hand, has been extensively evaluated. Most measurements have been obtained at the level of the fetal liver, using the umbilical portion of the left portal vein as a landmark. To obtain a correct measurement, this vessel is imaged within the liver, equidistant from the lateral walls. Unlike the measurement of the head, there is no outer edge to inner edge (leading edge to leading edge) measurement. Rather, all measurements are taken from the outermost aspects of the soft tissues. The value of the abdominal measurements is twofold: to establish gestational age (no more accurate, however, than that determined by the head measurement) and to evaluate head to body disproportions.

ABDOMINAL DIAMETER. The measurement of the abdominal diameter depends upon the configuration of the fetal body. If the abdomen is round, only one outer edge to outer edge measurement is necessary. If ovoid, two measurements perpendicular to one another, preferably anteroposterior and transverse, are obtained, and the average of the two is used as the linear dimension (Fig. 4–6). A comparison of the biparietal diameter with the average body diameter approximates 1:1 throughout the second trimester.[24] A further study showed that the two measurements are within 5 mm of each other from 13 to 33 gestational weeks. After 33 weeks, the fetal abdomen becomes progressively larger and by term, because of increased body fat, may be as much as 15 mm larger than the head (Table 4–9).[25]

ABDOMINAL CIRCUMFERENCE. The measurement of the abdominal circumference is performed the same way as that of the head circumference, either by using a digitizer or a map reader to trace the outer limits of the fetal body (Fig. 4–7) or by using the same equation for the circumference of a circle (Table 4–7). Both have been found to be accurate, with inaccuracies no greater than 6 percent at term (Table 4–10).[11, 21]

Table 4–8. CIRCUMFERENCE COMPUTATIONS

1. Planimetry:
   Map measurer, digitizer,
   computer-generated "best fit"
2. Equation for a Circle:

$$\frac{D_1 + D_2}{2} \pi = (D_1 + D_2) \times 1.57$$

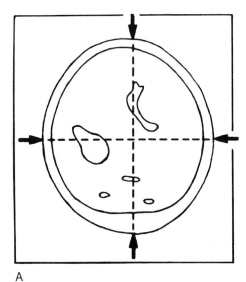

A

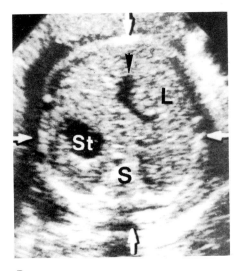

B

Figure 4–6. Measurement of the abdominal diameter. *A,* The abdominal measurements are taken outer edge to outer edge. If the body is round, as in this case, only one measurement is needed. If ovoid, two measurements perpendicular to one another are averaged. *B,* Ultrasound transaxial image of the upper abdomen, showing the umbilical portion of the left portal vein *(arrowhead)* positioned correctly within the liver, equidistant from the lateral walls. L, liver; St, stomach; S, spine. *Arrows* denote outer margins of the abdomen.

It has been proposed that the abdominal circumference is the most accurate determination of asymmetric fetal growth retardation.[26] Although this may be correct, the abdominal measurement is no more accurate than a head measurement in establishing fetal age. However, since the abdomen is most affected in asymmetric growth retar-

Table 4–9. ABDOMINAL DIAMETER MEASUREMENT TABLE

Gestational Age (weeks)	Predicted Mean Biparietal Diameter (mm)	Predicted Mean Average Abdominal Diameter (mm)
13	25.6	22.7
14	28.5	26.4
15	31.5	30.1
16	34.6	33.7
17	37.7	37.3
18	40.9	40.9
19	44.1	44.5
20	47.4	48.0
21	50.6	51.4
22	53.9	54.9
23	57.1	58.3
24	60.4	61.7
25	63.5	65.0
26	66.6	68.4
27	70.0	71.7
28	72.6	74.9
29	75.4	78.2
30	78.1	81.4
31	80.7	84.6
32	83.1	87.7
33	85.4	90.8
34	87.5	93.9
35	89.4	97.0
36	91.1	100.1
37	92.6	103.1
38	93.8	106.1
39	94.8	109.0
40	95.5	112.0

From Eriksen PS, Sechor NJ, Weis-Bentzon M: Normal growth of the fetal biparietal diameter and the abdominal diameter in a longitudinal study: An evaluation of the two parameters in predicting fetal weight. Acta Obstet Gynecol Scand 64:65, 1985.

dation, a ratio of the head to the abdominal circumference should be useful as an accurate predictor of head to abdomen symmetry and asymmetry (Table 4–11).[26, 27]

Fetal Extremities

With real-time ultrasound, all the fetal long bones can be adequately examined and measured. A large number of tables have been published evaluating the growth of these bones, correlating them with either the gestational age or the biparietal diameter measurements. The femur is the largest of the long bones, least movable, and easiest to image. Its measurement is as accurate as that of any other long bone. It is an excellent

Figure 4–7. Measurement of the abdominal circumference. *A,* The abdominal circumference is shown as a *dotted line* traced at the outer margin of the abdomen. *B,* Ultrasound trans-axial image showing the umbilical portion of the left portal vein *(arrowheads)* correctly positioned within the liver and equidistant from the lateral walls. s, spine; L, liver; st, stomach. A *dotted line,* created by a digitizer, outlines the outer margins of the abdomen, the correct place to obtain an abdominal circumference measurement.

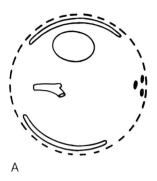

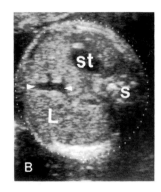

Table 4–10. ABDOMINAL CIRCUMFERENCE MEASUREMENT TABLE

Abdominal Circumference (cm)	Gestational Age (weeks) *Predicted Mean Values*	Abdominal Circumference (cm)	Gestational Age (weeks) *Predicted Mean Values*
10.0	15.6		
10.5	16.1	25.5	29.7
11.0	16.5	26.0	30.1
11.5	16.9	26.5	30.6
12.0	17.3	27.0	31.1
12.5	17.8	27.5	31.6
13.0	18.2	28.0	32.1
13.5	18.6	28.5	32.6
14.0	19.1	29.0	33.1
14.5	19.5	29.5	33.6
15.0	20.0	30.0	34.1
15.5	20.4	30.5	34.6
16.0	20.8	31.0	35.1
16.5	21.3	31.5	35.6
17.0	21.7	32.0	36.1
17.5	22.2	32.5	36.6
18.0	22.6	33.0	37.1
18.5	23.1	33.5	37.6
19.0	23.6	34.0	38.1
19.5	24.0	34.5	38.7
20.0	24.5	35.0	39.2
20.5	24.9	35.5	39.7
21.0	25.4	36.0	40.2
21.5	25.9	36.5	40.8
22.0	26.3		
22.5	26.8		
23.0	27.3		
23.5	27.7		
24.0	28.2		
24.5	28.7		
25.0	29.2		

Gestational Age (weeks)	Variability (weeks) at 95% Confidence Limits
12 to 18	± 1.9
18 to 24	± 2.0
24 to 30	± 2.2
30 to 36	± 3.0
36 to 42	± 2.5

From Hadlock FP, Deter RL, Harrist RB, Park SK: Fetal abdominal circumference as a predictor of menstrual age. AJR 139:367, 1982. *Copyright by* The American Roentgen Ray Society, 1982.

Table 4–11. HEAD TO ABDOMEN CIRCUMFERENCE RATIO TABLE

Gestational Age (weeks)	Ratio of Head Circumference/ Abdominal Circumference		
	5th Percentile	Mean	95th Percentile
13 to 14	1.14	1.23	1.31
15 to 16	1.05	1.22	1.39
17 to 18	1.07	1.18	1.29
19 to 20	1.09	1.18	1.29
21 to 22	1.06	1.15	1.25
23 to 24	1.05	1.13	1.21
25 to 26	1.04	1.13	1.22
27 to 28	1.05	1.13	1.22
29 to 30	0.99	1.10	1.21
31 to 32	0.96	1.07	1.17
33 to 34	0.96	1.04	1.11
35 to 36	0.93	1.02	1.11
37 to 38	0.92	0.98	1.05
39 to 40	0.87	0.97	1.06
41 to 42	0.93	0.96	1.00

From Campbell S, Thoms A: Ultrasound measurement of the fetal head to abdomen circumference in the assessment of growth retardation. Br J Obstet Gynaecol 84:165, 1977.

parameter to confirm the accuracy of the head and body diameters. The femur measurement is also of value in the detection of fetal skeletal dysplasias since its length will be abnormal in all types of this significant deformity.

The femur is measured along the long axis of the diaphysis, the osseous portion of the shaft (Fig. 4–8). The normal diaphysis has a straight lateral and a curved medial border.[28]

A straight measurement of the femur is taken from one end to the other, disregarding the curvature. The proximal and distal epiphyseal cartilages are not ossified and are excluded from the measurement.[29] Infrequently, a hyperechoic "distal femoral point" is imaged (Fig. 4–8). This is a nonosseous extension that continues from the distal end of the diaphysis. It is part of the smooth surface of the distal epiphyseal cartilage[29] and if included in the femoral length could falsely overestimate it by as much as three weeks.[30] After 30 weeks, a punctate hyperechoic distal femoral epiphysis may be observed.[31] This is separated from the distal end of the diaphysis and should also be excluded from the femoral length measurement.

A potential source of error in the measurement of the long bones is the effect of the type of transducer on the measurement. The transducers used in mechanical sector scanners are sometimes incorrectly calibrated, a problem that tends to affect certain transducers more than others, especially with increased age. The magnitude of the error has varied in different reports. Two studies[32, 33] have stated that a horizontal image of the femur had an error of up to 8 mm in the focal zone, increasing up to 26 mm or 47 percent outside the focal zone. These inaccuracies were worse in the far field and at the lateral margins of the image. Two other investigators[34, 35] found no significant measurement error when the femur was horizon-

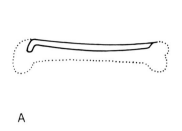

A

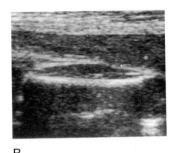

B

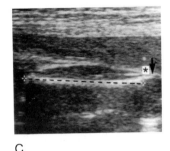

C

*The reflection from the distal femoral cartilage is not included.

Figure 4–8. Measurement of the femur length. *A, diagram* and *B, ultrasound image.* The hyperechoic line is the ossified lateral margin of the femoral diaphysis. The ends of the bone are the epiphyseal cartilages that have not yet calcified and are therefore hypoechoic. *C,* The hyperechoic diaphysis is measured from one end to the other, denoted by the cursors and a *dotted line.* The "distal femoral point" (* and *arrow*) is a nonossified extension of the distal epiphyseal cartilage. It should not be included in the measurement.

tally positioned. None of the articles noted a significant error on a vertically positioned femur. In contradistinction, the linear array and phased-array scanners gave consistently accurate measurements and are therefore preferable. If a mechanical sector scanner is used, the most accurate measurements will be made when the extremity is close to the transducer, within the focal zone, and in the middle of the image.

A femur length table is recommended (Table 4–12)[38] Its accuracy has been extensively studied. In general, most observers consider the femur measurement to be as accurate as that of the biparietal diameter.[36, 37] It can,

therefore, be used to predict fetal age, particularly when the head is in a difficult position to be adequately measured. In addition, the femur length can be compared with other parameters to evaluate for fetal disproportion, frequently a sign of abnormality. A ratio of the femur to the head, compared both with the biparietal diameter,[39] as an age independent ratio, and with the head circumference,[40] has allowed the diagnosis of such entities as microcephaly or skeletal dysplasia.

The femur and the abdomen have also been compared. Two articles[26, 41] proposed the femur length to abdominal circumfer-

Table 4–12. FEMUR MEASUREMENT TABLE

Bone Length (mm)	Gestational Age (weeks)			Bone Length (mm)	Gestational Age (weeks)		
	5th Percentile	Predicted Mean Value	95th Percentile		5th Percentile	Predicted Mean Value	95th Percentile
10	10.4	12.6	14.9				
11	10.7	12.9	15.1	46	23.1	25.4	27.6
12	11.1	13.3	15.6	47	23.6	25.9	28.0
13	11.4	13.6	15.9	48	24.0	26.1	28.4
14	11.7	13.9	16.1	49	24.4	26.6	28.9
15	12.0	14.1	16.4	50	24.9	27.0	29.1
16	12.4	14.6	16.9	51	25.1	27.4	29.6
17	12.7	14.9	17.1	52	25.6	27.9	30.0
18	13.0	15.1	17.4	53	26.0	28.1	30.4
19	13.4	15.6	17.9	54	26.4	28.6	30.9
20	13.7	15.9	18.1	55	26.9	29.1	31.3
21	14.1	16.3	18.6	56	27.2	29.6	31.7
22	14.4	16.6	18.9	57	27.7	29.9	32.1
23	14.7	16.9	19.1	58	28.1	30.3	32.6
24	15.1	17.3	19.6	59	28.6	30.7	32.9
25	15.4	17.6	19.9	60	28.9	31.1	33.3
26	15.9	18.0	20.1	61	29.4	31.6	33.9
27	16.1	18.3	20.6	62	29.9	32.0	34.1
28	16.6	18.7	20.9	63	30.1	32.4	34.6
29	16.9	19.0	21.1	64	30.7	32.9	35.1
30	17.1	19.4	21.6	65	31.1	33.4	35.6
31	17.6	19.9	22.0	66	31.6	33.7	35.9
32	17.9	20.1	22.3	67	32.0	34.1	36.4
33	18.3	20.6	22.7	68	32.4	34.6	36.9
34	18.7	20.9	23.1	69	32.6	35.0	37.1
35	19.0	21.1	23.4	70	33.3	35.6	37.7
36	19.4	21.6	23.9	71	33.7	35.9	38.1
37	19.9	22.0	24.1	72	34.1	36.4	38.6
38	20.1	22.4	24.6	73	34.6	36.9	39.0
39	20.6	22.7	24.9	74	35.1	37.3	39.6
40	20.9	23.1	25.3	75	35.6	37.7	39.9
41	21.3	23.6	25.7	76	36.0	38.1	40.4
42	21.7	23.9	26.1	77	36.4	38.6	40.9
43	22.1	24.3	26.6	78	36.9	39.1	41.3
44	22.6	24.7	26.9	79	37.3	39.6	41.7
45	22.9	25.0	27.1	80	37.9	40.0	42.1

From Jeanty P, Rodesch F, Delbeke D, Dumont JE: Estimation of gestational age from measurements of fetal long bones. J Ultrasound Med 3:75, 1984.

ence ratio as a valuable age-independent variable. Elevated ratios were suggested as a means of diagnosing growth retardation, and low ratios, macrosomia. Follow-up studies,[42–45] however, have shown that these values overlap too much with normal ones for accurate prediction of either.

Multiple Parameters

Hadlock and coworkers[46, 47] decided to combine several measurements in the hope of increasing gestational age accuracy. This group measured the biparietal diameter, head circumference, abdominal circumference, and femoral length. They then took the mean gestational age of from two to four of these parameters and averaged them together to obtain a mean gestational age. They found that the accuracy of predicting a fetal age near term using the biparietal diameter alone was ± four weeks. The use of multiple parameters had an accuracy of ±2.3 to 2.4 weeks after 30 gestational weeks.

It is undoubtedly correct that averaging up to four parameters would eliminate a maximal error created by a discrepancy in any one or two of the measurements. It is questionable, however, whether this type of accuracy could really be obtained unless the biparietal diameter itself were more accurate than these authors stated. Reasons for inaccuracies in the biparietal diameter measurement after 30 weeks could be statistical or technical rather than real. There were relatively few cases that could cause a large standard deviation (statistical inaccuracy). Failure to calculate a cephalic index would lead to using biparietal diameters of the wrong shape (technical inaccuracy). Not unexpectedly, the head circumference was found to be the best single parameter.[46] In addition, to obtain head and abdomen circumferences, the outer limits of the head and abdomen were measured in two directions perpendicular to each other, and the circumference was calculated by using the circle circumference equation. Since only linear array scanners were used, there would have been many cases, particularly in the late third trimester, in which the outer margins of the head and body could not have been completely imaged so that these margins would have had to be estimated. This too could have led to a significant technical error.

Therefore, until larger studies confirm their value, the use of multiple parameters is recommended only for select cases in which it is not certain that the head measurement is accurate or in which one parameter is markedly discrepant from the others.

Interval Growth

When the pregnancy is evaluated by serial ultrasound examinations, interval growth can be analyzed. This concept is not new. In the pediatric literature, interval growth is used as an important means of evaluating a child's normal development. The same concept applies in utero. A fetus that is growing at or above the tenth percentile would be expected to be normal, and a fetus growing below the tenth percentile is suspected of having growth retardation.[48] In fact, approximately one-half of the fetuses with growth below the tenth percentile will turn out to be growth retarded, but the rest will be normal. The concept of interval growth makes the following two assumptions: (1) a fetus should hold at a certain percentage of growth throughout gestation;[49] and (2) the growth of the fetus is faster in the beginning of the pregnancy, gradually slowing in a linear fashion toward the end of the pregnancy.

At present, only the biparietal diameter has been adequately analyzed for interval growth (Table 4–13).[48] Two examples of how this table is used follow. A woman presents for the first time with a 22 week old fetus having a biparietal diameter that measures 54 mm; ten weeks later, at 32 gestational weeks, it has a biparietal diameter measurement of 84 mm. There has been 30 mm of fetal head growth in a ten week period equaling an interval growth rate of 30 mm per 10 weeks or 3 mm per week. This rate reflects the growth throughout the ten week period, initially fast and then slowing. The fetal age used to reflect the growth between the two studies is the mean:

$$\frac{22 + 32 \text{ weeks}}{2} = 27 \text{ weeks}$$

For 27 weeks and 3 mm per week, the interval growth is normal, greater than the 80th percentile (line 13 of Table 4–13). If instead the same fetus presented at 22 weeks with the same biparietal diameter of 54 mm but at 32 weeks had a biparietal diameter of

Table 4–13. BIPARIETAL DIAMETER GROWTH RATE TABLE

Gestational Age (weeks)	Mean Biparietal Diameter (mm)	Predicted Interval Growth (mm/week)				
		10%	*20%*	*50%*	*80%*	*90%*
15	32	—	—	3.88	—	—
16	36	—	—	3.20	—	—
17	39	—	2.86	3.20	3.44	—
18	41	—	2.85	3.05	3.85	—
19	44	—	2.80	3.25	3.90	—
20	48	2.56	2.69	3.15	3.33	3.63
21	50	2.56	2.70	3.10	3.70	3.89
22	54	2.50	2.78	3.09	3.43	3.90
23	57	2.31	2.58	2.85	3.31	3.49
24	59	2.32	2.56	2.85	3.20	3.47
25	63	2.41	2.55	2.74	3.06	3.36
26	66	2.26	2.34	2.58	3.01	3.21
27	68	2.16	2.33	2.57	2.97	3.22
28	71	2.12	2.25	2.47	2.76	3.06
29	75	2.06	2.17	2.42	2.68	2.93
30	78	1.86	2.00	2.30	2.64	2.90
31	80	1.69	1.87	2.16	2.42	2.68
32	82	1.56	1.78	2.02	2.37	2.61
33	84	1.17	1.45	1.92	2.32	2.56
34	85	1.15	1.39	1.85	2.23	2.60
35	87	0.95	1.21	1.67	1.95	2.25
36	89	0.90	1.10	1.56	1.95	2.44
37	90	0.76	0.91	1.40	1.91	2.25
38	92	0.69	0.89	1.45	1.92	2.36
39	93	0.43	0.85	1.38	1.94	2.88
40	94	0.57	0.87	1.38	2.35	2.91
41	94	0.63	0.87	1.57	2.86	2.93
42	95	0.62	0.87	1.38	1.19	1.95

Adapted from Levi S, Smets P: Intrauterine fetal growth studied by ultrasonic biparietal measurements. Acta Obstet Gynecol Scand 52:193, 1973.

74 mm, there would have been only 20 mm of growth in the same ten week period or a 2 mm per week growth rate. At a mean of 27 weeks, the growth would be below the tenth percentile (line 13 of Table 4–13), and the fetus would be at risk for growth retardation.

The use of interval growth has been carefully evaluated in one article.[50] Five types of fetal growth patterns were detected. Normal growth that maintained the same percentile throughout pregnancy, and growth that started low and then rose into the normal range, were both found to be normal. Growth retardation was rare in these two groups (three of 95 fetuses or 3 percent). In two other groups, a single subnormal growth profile and a uniformly low growth profile, all below the 10th percentile, growth retardation was correctly predicted in eight of 17 fetuses or 47 percent. In the last group,

consisting of only eight fetuses, the growth pattern started within the normal range and then decreased rapidly. Although this could have been an abnormal type of growth, only one of these fetuses was growth retarded.

Errors could potentially double when two measurements are taken to calculate an interval growth rate. As previously stated, the biparietal diameter has an error of up to 2 mm per examination. When two examinations are performed, this error could be as large as 4 mm. Therefore, when evaluating the interval growth of the biparietal diameter, enough real growth must have occurred to make the potential measurement error insignificant. It is, therefore, suggested that at least 8 mm of growth should occur between the two studies. In the second trimester, when the fetus is growing fast, two to three weeks between examinations will suffice. In the third trimester, and particularly near term, as much as four to five weeks would be necessary. This interval is not always possible. If growth retardation is suspected in the third trimester, the obstetrician needs to know as soon as possible. Waiting for a repeat study to show low growth while the fetus remains in a potentially "hostile environment" may be impractical. Nevertheless, this interval between examinations should be sought whenever possible.

Multiple Gestations

Twin gestations occur once in every 85 births. Larger numbers of multiple gestations are relatively rare, with triplets and quadruplets presenting once in 7600 and once in 70,000 births, respectively. As a result, biometric studies have been performed only on twins.

The detection of twin gestations is important since twins are at greater risk for many complications, particularly growth disturbances. This risk increases depending upon whether the twins are (1) totally in separate sacs (the least risk), called dichorionic-diamniotic; (2) partially share the same environment but each still within its amniotic sac, called monochorionic-diamnionic; or (3) completely sharing the same sac (the highest risk), called monochorionic-monoamnionic.[51]

In general, measurement tables made for singleton gestations can be used accurately on twin gestations at least until 31 to 33 weeks, depending upon the measurement.[52] In the last two months of the pregnancy, there is some decrease in the size of the fetuses toward the lower tenth percentile.[52] Of interest, an article[52] showed that while the biparietal diameter and abdomen circumference decreased within these last two months, the femur continued to grow normally throughout the pregnancy (the study ended at 37 weeks).[52] As a result, when there are any discrepancies in the head and body measurements of twins, the femurs should be measured using a singleton gestational table.

It would be anticipated that the growth of one twin could serve as a marker for the growth of the other, and if the growth of one fetus did not closely parallel that of the other, growth retardation might be suggested in the smaller one. It has, therefore, been suspected that the biparietal diameters of the twins should be within 5 mm or 5 percent of each other and that any discrepancy that might exist should not increase by greater than 3 mm over a two week period.[53-55] Although this would seem to make sense and be a good diagnostic tool, one article[54] detected only 77 percent of growth-retarded fetuses using these criteria. It is possible that using the interval growth of the femurs might be of greater value. To date this method has not been investigated.

A simple but uniform approach to the evaluation of gestational age should be performed in all fetuses. In addition to the measurements presented in this chapter, many other measurement parameters, including ratios and weights, could be added. Although this may look very erudite and impress both the clinicians and the patient, multiple numbers rarely, if ever, add to the accuracy of gestational dating.

As a rule, we base the gestational age on the crown-rump length or on the head (biparietal diameter, corrected biparietal diameter, or circumference) measurement. If a pathologic condition is suspected in the fetal head, another measurement, usually the abdominal circumference or femur length, is used instead. Both the mean and the range in weeks are reported.

The fetal age is preferably based on the earliest study, as long as the measurements were technically adequate. The earliest study is used because the fetal measurements have the least variability in the first and second trimester. On each subsequent examination, the fetal age is calculated by adding the number of interval weeks to the original fetal age. For example, if an initial biparietal diameter measured 22 mm for a mean of 12.7 and a range of 12.2 to 13.2 weeks, 23 weeks later the fetal age would have a mean of 35.7 and a range of 35.2 to 36.2 weeks. The follow-up biparietal diameter measurement would be used to evaluate its proportion to the body and femur and to calculate an interval growth rate, not to establish the gestational age. If the first study were in the first trimester, the tables for the crown-rump length and gestational sac provide only a mean gestational age. Since it has been shown that the first trimester measurements have a range of approximately seven days (Table 4–1), a crown-rump length of 11 mm, for example, would be equivalent to a gestational age of 7.1 ± 1 weeks.

Any time a biparietal diameter is measured and the head shape appears abnormal, the cephalic index should be obtained. If the cephalic index is normal, the biparietal diameter should be compared with the average body diameter. If the head is abnormal in shape, or if the observer prefers to use a head circumference, an abdominal circumference should also be performed and a ratio of the head to the abdominal circumference be obtained. The femur should be measured and its range compared with those of the head and body measurements in order to evaluate for asymmetry and dwarfism. Furthermore, when there is more than one study, the interval growth of the biparietal diameter should be added to these measurements.

References

1. Campbell S, Warsof SL, Little D, Cooper DJ: Routine ultrasound screening for the prediction of gestational age. Obstet Gynecol 65:613, 1985.
2. Dewhurst CJ, Beazley JM, Campbell S: Assessment of fetal maturity and dysmaturity. Am J Obstet Gynecol 113:141, 1972.
3. Beazley JM, Underhill RA: Fallacy of the fundal height. Br Med J 4:404, 1970.
4. Hellman LF, Kobayashi M, Fillisti L, Lavenhar M: Growth and development of the human fetus prior to the twentieth week of gestation. Am J Obstet Gynecol 103:784, 1969.
5. Jouppila PC: Length and depth of the uterus and the diameter of the gestation sac in normal gravidas

during early pregnancy. Acta Obstet Gynecol Scand 50(15 Suppl):29, 1971.

6. Robinson HP, Fleming JEE: A critical evaluation of sonar "crown-rump length" measurements. Br J Obstet Gynaecol 82:702, 1975.

7. Smazal SF, Weisman LE, Hoppler KD, et al: Comparative analysis of ultrsonographic methods of gestational age assessment. J Ultrasound Med 2:147, 1983.

8. Kopta MM, May RR, Crane JP: A comparison of the reliability of the estimated date of confinement predicted by crown-rump length and biparietal diameter. Am J Obstet Gynecol 145:562, 1983.

9. Shepard M, Filly RA: A standardized plane for biparietal diameter measurement. J Ultrasound Med 1:145, 1982.

10. Hadlock FP, Deter RL, Harrist RB, Park SK: Fetal biparietal diameter: Rational choice of plane of section for sonographic measurement. AJR 138:871, 1982.

11. Kurtz AB, Wapner RJ, Kurtz RJ, et al: Analysis of biparietal diameter as an accurate indicator of gestional age. J Clin Ultrasound 8:319, 1980.

12. Cooperberg PL, Chow T, Kite V, Austin S: Biparietal diameter: A comparison of real time and conventional B-scan techniques. J Clin Ultrasound 4:421, 1976.

13. Lunt RM, Chard L: Reproducibility of measurement of fetal biparietal diameter by ultrasonic cephalometry. J Obstet Gynaecol Br Commonw 81:682, 1974.

14. Davison JM, Lind T, Farr V, Whittingham TA: The limitations of ultrasonic fetal cephalometry. J Obstet Gynaecol Br Commonw 80:769, 1981.

15. Campbell S: The prediction of fetal maturity by ultrasonic measurement of the biparietal diameter. J Obstet Gynaecol Br Commonw 76:603, 1969.

16. Sabbagha RE, Turner H, Rockett H, et al: Sonar BPD and fetal age: Definition of the relationship. Obstet Gynecol 43:7, 1974.

17. Campbell S, Newman GB: Growth of the fetal biparietal diameter during normal pregnancy. J Obstet Gynaecol Br Commonw 78:518, 1971.

18. Sabbagha RE, Hughey M: Standardization of sonar cephalometry and gestational age. Obstet Gynecol 52:402, 1978.

19. Hadlock FP, Deter RL, Carpenter RJ, Park SK: Estimating fetal age: Effect of head shape on BPD. AJR 137:83, 1981.

20. Doubilet PM, Greenes RA: Improved prediction of gestational age from fetal head measurements. AJR 142:797, 1984.

21. Hadlock FP, Deter RL, Harrist RB, Park SK: Fetal head circumference: Relation to menstrual age. AJR 138:649, 1982.

22. Hadlock FP, Kent WR, Loyd JL, et al: An evaluation of two methods for mesuring fetal heads and body circumferences. J Ultrasound Med 1:359, 1982.

23. Shields JR, Medearis AL, Bear MB: Fetal head and abdominal circumferences: Ellipse calculations versus planimetry. J Clin Ultrasound 15:237, 1987.

24. Sarti DA, Crandall BF, Winter J, et al: Correlation of biparietal and fetal body diameters: 12–26 weeks gestation. AJR 137:87, 1981.

25. Eriksen PS, Secher NJ, Weis-Bentzon M: Normal growth of the fetal biparietal diameter and the abdominal diameter in a longitudinal study. Acta Obstet Gynecol Scand 64:65, 1985.

26. Hadlock FP, Deter RL, Harrist RB, et al: A date-independent predictor of intrauterine growth retar-

27. dation: Femur length/abdominal circumference ratio. AJR 141:979, 1983.

27. Campbell S, Thoms A: Ultrasound measurement of the fetal head to abdomen circumference ratio in the assessment of growth retardation. Br J Obstet Gynaecol 84:165, 1977.

28. Abrams SL, Filly RA: Curvature of the fetal femur: A normal sonographic finding. Radiology 156:490, 1985.

29. Jeanty P, Kirkpatrick C, Dramaix-Wilmet M, Struyven J: Ultrasonographic evaluation of fetal limb growth. Radiology 140:165, 1981.

30. Goldstein RB, Filly RA, Simpson G: Pitfalls in femur length measurements. J Ultrasound Med 6:203,1987.

31. Chinn DH, Bolding DB, Callen PW, et al: Ultrasonographic identification of fetal lower extremity epiphyseal ossification centers. Radiology 147:815, 1983.

32. Winter J, Kimme-Smith C, King W: Measurement accuracy of sonographic sector scanners. AJR 144:645, 1985.

33. Gamba JL, Bowie JD, Dodson WC, Hedlund LW: Accuracy of ultrasound in fetal femur length determination. Ultrasound phantom study. Invest Radiol 20:316, 1985.

34. Pretorius DH, Nelson TR, Manco-Johnson ML: Fetal age estimation by ultrasound: The impact of measurement errors. Radiology 152:763, 1984.

35. Jeanty P, Beck GJ, Chervenak FA, et al: A comparison of sector and linear array scanners for the measurement of the fetal femur. J Ultrasound Med 4:525, 1985.

36. Hadlock FP, Harrist RB, Deter RL, Park SK: A prospective evaluation of fetal femur length as a predictor of gestational age. J Ultrasound Med 2:111, 1983.

37. Wolfson RN, Peisner DB, Chik LL, Sokol RJ: Comparison of biparietal diameter and femur length in the third trimester: Effects of gestational age and variation in fetal growth. J Ultrasound Med 5:145, 1986.

38. Jeanty P, Rodesch F, Delbeke D, Dumont JE: Estimation of gestational age from measurements of fetal long bones. J Ultrasound Med 3:75, 1984.

39. Hohler CW, Quetel TA: Comparison of ultrasound femur length and biparietal diameter in late pregnancy. Am J Obstet Gynecol 141:759, 1981.

40. Hadlock FP, Harrist RB, Shah Y, Park SK: The femur length/head circumference relation in obstetric sonography. J Ultrasound Med 3:439, 1984.

41. Hadlock FP, Harrist RB, Fearneyhough TC, et al: Use of femur length/abdominal circumference ratio in detecting the macrosomic fetus. Radiology 154:503, 1985.

42. Ott WJ: Fetal femur length, neonatal crown-heel length, and screening for intrauterine growth retardation. Obstet Gynecol 65:460, 1985.

43. Vintzileos AM, Neckles S, Campbell WA, et al: Three fetal ponderal indexes in normal pregnancy. Obstet Gynecol 6:807, 1985.

44. Benson CB, Doubilet PM, Saltzman DH, Jones TB: FL/AC ratio: Poor predictor of intrauterine growth retardation. Invest Radiol 20:727, 1985.

45. Benson CB, Doubilet PM, Saltzman DH, et al: Femur length/abdominal circumference ratio. Poor predictor of macrosomic fetuses in diabetic mothers. J Ultrasound Med 5:141, 1986.

46. Hadlock FP, Deter RL, Harrist RB, Park SK: Esti-

mating fetal age: Computer-assisted analysis of multiple fetal growth parameters. Radiology 152:497, 1984.

47. Hadlock FP, Harrist RB, Shah YP, et al: Estimating fetal age using multiple parameters: A prospective evaluation in a racially mixed population. Am J Obstet Gynecol 156:955, 1987.

48. Levi S, Smets P: Intra-uterine fetal growth studied by ultrasonic biparietal measurements: The percentiles of biparietal distribution. Acta Obstet Gynecol Scand 52:193, 1973.

49. Sabbagha RE, Hughey M: Standardization of sonar cephalometry and gestational age. Obstet Gynecol 52:402, 1978.

50. Sholl JS, Woo D, Rubin JM, et al: Intrauterine growth retardation risk detection for fetuses of unknown gestational age. Am J Obstet Gynecol 144:709, 1982.

51. Naeye RL, Tafari N, Judge D, Marboe CC: Twins: Causes of perinatal death in 12 United States cities and one African city. Am J Obstet Gynecol 131:267, 1978.

52. Grumbach K, Coleman BG, Arger PH, et al: Twin and singleton growth patterns compared using US. Radiology 158:237, 1986.

53. Crane JF, Tomich PG, Kopta M: Ultrasonic growth patterns in normal and discordant twins. Obstet Gynecol 55:678, 1980.

54. Houlton MCC, Marivate M, Philpott RH: The prediction of fetal growth retardation in twin pregnancy. Br J Obstet Gynaecol 88:264, 1981.

55. Haney AF, Crenshaw MC, Dempsey PJ: Significance of biparietal diameter differences between twins. Obstet Gynecol 51:609, 1978.

FETAL GROWTH

James D. Bowie, M.D.

The problem of assessing fetal growth in utero remains one of the most difficult ones for obstetricians and sonographers despite the multitude of publications, the numerous ultrasound measurements, and the complex theories of fetal growth. Why is there this concern for fetal growth? Recognizing the extremes of fetal growth is one way of identifying some of the fetuses that have a higher risk for perinatal morbidity or mortality. There is considerable evidence that optimal survival rates occur among infants who are several hundred grams above mean birthweight, but neonatal death rates actually do not vary much across the birthweights between 3000 and 4000 gm. The greatest neonatal losses occur in infants below 2000 gm and in those approaching 5000 gm (Fig. 5–1).[1]

With no fetal monitoring and few therapeutic tools available, for a long time these problems of growth were looked upon in a very uncritical manner. The development of fetal monitoring techniques, stress and nonstress testing, and effective agents for delaying labor, along with the improved survival of premature infants, has directed interest into the problem of fetal growth. Current theories propose that the birthweight distribution is nongaussian, with a significant portion of newborns falling outside the "expected" distribution at its extremes. This residual outside the distribution represents the highest risk newborn, and presumably if these could be identified in utero, the actual outcome would improve.[2] Thus, several

large programs have been instituted for the ultrasonic screening of pregnancies to detect abnormal growth. Much of the information regarding sonographic screening comes from programs in Great Britain and Scandinavia,[3–5] where the sonographic screening of fetuses that are either small or large for their gestational age is considered far superior to clinical screening.[6] It is important for American readers to recognize that the situation in the United States is not analogous; here ultrasound is not commonly used as a primary screening tool but is reserved for pregnancies with specific indications of a possible problem. This produces a subtle but important shift in emphasis. In situations where sonography is used as a systematic screening device, its sensitivity to the presence of disease is of the greatest value, whereas in a preselected (high-risk) population, its specificity for certain diseases becomes important.

Closer examination of the smallest babies suggests that they are indeed a heterogeneous group and do not all have the same clinical problems. It has been hypothesized that very-low-birthweight infants include those who are small because of prematurity, those who are small because of poor growth, and those who are small because of both prematurity and poor growth. Originally this idea was postulated with the hope that such distinctions would help management decisions and permit clinicians to decide which fetuses would best benefit from expeditious

65

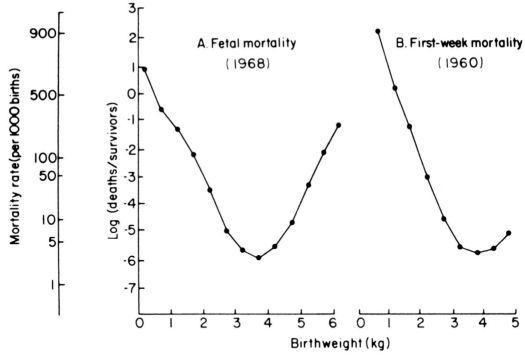

Figure 5–1. Birthweight-specific mortality curves (United States whites, 1968 and 1960). The left-hand vertical scale is in mortality rate per 1000 births. The right-hand vertical scale is expressed as the log (deaths/survivors). This figure shows clearly how the extremes of birthweight are related to increased mortality. (*From* Wilcox AJ, Russell IT: Birthweight and perinatal mortality: II. On weight-specific mortality. Int J Epidemiol 12:319, 1983.)

delivery and which ones would better be kept in utero with continuation of the pregnancy.

Although these ideas are appealing, and the measurement of birthweight as a predictor of outcome seems simple, there is increasing dissatisfaction with this approach. The basis of this dissatisfaction is that birthweight represents a "risk" factor but not a specific disease or condition that is the direct cause of the increased perinatal mortality or morbidity that we wish to prevent. At this time, increased efforts to identify a group at risk because of abnormal size do not seem to have as much potential for improved fetal outcome as does identification of factors more directly related to the underlying fetal condition, such as congenital abnormalities, fetal hypoxia, or fetal acidosis.[7]

An explanation of why this topic of fetal growth remains so difficult would require an equally confusing review. It is enough to state that "intrauterine growth retardation" and "macrosomia" have no universally accepted definitions based on clinical conditions.[8] Therefore, most published materials

use a weight for age basis when defining these conditions. Thus, intrauterine growth retardation (IUGR) becomes a weight below the tenth percentile for age (small for gestation age [SGA]), and macrosomia becomes a weight above the 90th percentile, or in some cases the 95th, for age (large for gestational age [LGA]). Such simplistic definitions are yet a further step away from identifying specific fetal conditions or etiologies (Table 5–1)[9] that represent a threat to a specific fetus' well-being.

Even such simplistic definitions create major problems. The standard curves for fetal "growth" and relative size must be based on cross-sectional data. That is, these curves are generated by observations of individuals only once and consist of a great many such individual observations at different (estimated) times in gestation. This is not at all the same as longitudinal data, which actually measure the growth of a group of fetuses as they progress through gestation. The importance of this distinction is that if, for any reason, there is a tendency for either smaller or larger fetuses to be born prior to the end of the expected gestational

Table 5–1. ETIOLOGY OF IUGR

Environmental
  Malnutrition
  Drugs and substance abuse
    Aminopterin
    Alcohol
    Hydantoins
    Narcotics
    Prednisone
    Trimethadione
    Smoking
    Antihypertensives

Uterine and placental anomalies and abnormalities
  Uterine
    Bicornuate uterus
    Septate uterus
    Uterine myomas
  Placental
    Circumvallation
    Abruption and circulatory disturbances
    Placental infection—villitis
    Hemangiomatous placental tumors
    Twin to twin transfusion syndrome
    Abnormal cord insertion
    Multiple gestations

Fetal infections
  Protozoan
    Malaria
    Toxoplasmosis
  Viral
    Rubella
    Cytomegalovirus
    Varicella-zoster
    Other viruses, including mumps, herpes simplex,
      vaccinia hepatitis A, and poliomyelitis

Maternal conditions, diseases (genetic and
    nongenetic)
  Abnormal maternal nutrient metabolism
  Cyanotic heart disease
  Folate deficiency anemia
  Severe (iron deficiency) anemia
  Sickle cell disease

Gastrointestinal diseases (ulcerative colitis, Crohn's
    disease, pancreatitis, and malabsorption states)
Maternal vascular disease
  Chronic hypertension
  Collagen vascular diseases
  Diabetes mellitus, Classes D, F, R
  Renal disease
  Preeclampsia
Reduced maternal plasma volume
Neurofibromatosis (maternal), ad (IUGR, HTN)
Phenylketonuria (maternal), ar
Schmidt's syndrome
High altitudes

Fetal genetic disorders
  Single gene disorders
    Placental sulfatase deficiency, X-linked
    Dubowitz' syndrome, ar
    Dwarfism
      Levi-Logi, ar
      Snubnosed, ad
    Lissencephaly, ar
    Meckel's syndrome, ar
    Potter's syndrome, ad/multifactorial
    Robert's syndrome, ar
    Russell-Silver syndrome, ad/sporadic
  Chromosomal disorders
    XO—Turner's syndrome
    Trisomies
      21—Down's syndrome
      18—Edwards' syndrome
      13—Patau's syndrome
    Deletion syndromes
      4p—short arm
      5p—cri du chat
      18p
      18q

Congenital anomalies
  Gastroschisis
  Duodenal atresia
  Pancreatic agenesis
  Osteogenesis imperfecta (congenital)
  Omphalocele: noted, not seen
  Congenital heart disease

ad, autosomal dominant inheritance; ar, autosomal recessive inheritance.
From Lockwood CJ, Weiner S: Assessment of fetal growth. Clin Perinatol 13:3, 1986.

duration, these groups are being removed from the cross-sectional data pool, and the resulting curve may not be representative of the actual growth of the remaining individuals.

Other factors influence published growth curves, such as inclusion of abnormal babies, stillborns, racial groups, location (usually altitude), sex, and birth order.[10] Thus, while mean birthweights given by published curves vary, the lower and upper percentiles may differ even more. For example, the tenth percentile for 36 weeks may be as high as 2330 gm in one curve and as low as 2050 gm in another.[11] One published chart, the "Lubchenco" curve, has received much criticism as being representative of only the population delivered in some U.S. hospitals, yet it continues to be widely used. The use of menstrual history for growth charts has been questioned, and at least one exists based on ultrasound data (Table 5–2).[12]

Establishing an appropriate growth curve and distribution of newborn weights for gestational age is not the only problem with the weight for age approach. The basis for establishing gestational age must also be questioned. If we consider conceptional age to

Table 5–2. BIRTHWEIGHT STANDARDS BASED ON ULTRASOUND DATING: Estimated 10th, 50th, and 90th percentiles for females and males in the third trimester

| Gestation | | Estimated Percentile Birthweight (gm) | | | | | |
| | | Females | | | Males | | |
Weeks	Days	10TH	50TH	90TH	10TH	50TH	90TH
27	189	708	840	997	726	852	999
28	196	869	1031	1223	896	1051	1232
29	203	1030	1222	1450	1065	1250	1466
30	210	1191	1413	1676	1235	1448	1699
31	217	1352	1604	1903	1404	1647	1932
32	224	1513	1795	2129	1574	1846	2166
33	231	1674	1986	2356	1744	2045	2399
34	238	1835	2177	2582	1913	2244	2632
35	245	1996	2367	2809	2083	2443	2865
36	252	2156	2558	3035	2252	2642	3099
37	259	2317	2749	3262	2422	2841	3332
38	266	2478	2940	3488	2591	3040	3565
39	273	2639	3131	3715	2761	3238	3798
40	280	2800	3322	3941	2931	3437	4032
41	287	2961	3513	4168	3100	3636	4265
42	294	3122	3704	4394	3270	3835	4498
43	301	3283	3895	4621	3439	4034	4732

From Secher NJ, Hansen PK, Lenstrup C, et al: Birth weight standards based on early ultrasound estimation of gestational age. Br J Obstet Gynecol 93:128, 1986.

be the time from the day of conception, and gestational age to be this time plus two weeks to correspond to the first day of the last menstrual period (LMP) (a hypothetical time in many cases), then the evidence suggests that while the usual clinical estimators of gestational age, the LMP and the Dubowitz evaluation, are representative of mean ages for large groups of subjects, the range associated with their predictions of gestational age are unacceptably wide to evaluate individual cases.

The variation resulting from estimation of gestational age by LMP is no surprise to clinicians and has received much documentation in the literature.[13, 14] The variation associated with the Dubowitz evaluation is not well established. Relatively few studies have been published that evaluate the Dubowitz since, until recently, no "gold standard" has been available with which to compare this clinical evaluation. One study based on "good" menstrual history indicated that for 95 percent of the measured cases, the gestational age estimated by the Dubowitz varied by three weeks for babies over 38 weeks, and only 87 percent were correctly dated plus or minus three weeks if the known gestational age was less than 38 weeks.[15] There is also evidence that the Dubowitz score is influenced by birthweight, independent of the actual gestational age,

larger babies being scored as more mature than smaller ones.[16] These results are not surprising since the Dubowitz signs were originally based on menstrual history, and only seven babies under 32 weeks were included in the data base for the evaluation.[17]

Although the sonographic evaluation of abnormal growth may be supplanted by more useful direct measures of fetal well-being, and the clinical definitions of abnormally large and small babies remain vague, there are nevertheless good reasons for the sonographer to be familiar with methods of estimating fetal age and size.

It is important for the sonographer to know that while clinical determinants of gestational age are likely to be insufficiently accurate for our purpose,[13, 14] there are some indicators that should not be ignored. These include a history of ovulation induction, in vitro fertilization, single intercourse, and similar events. In the absence of these special clinical determinants, the ultrasonically obtained crown-rump length (CRL) is the most accurate determinant of gestational age if measured between six and 12 weeks.[18] Other ultrasound measurements are possibly slightly less accurate but acceptable up to about 20 weeks of gestation.[19] These include, but are not limited to, the biparietal diameter (BPD), the head circumference (HC), and the femur length (FL). The author recommends averaging the BPD and FL between 15 and 20 weeks, the optimal time to establish gestational age.

Having estimated gestational age, the remaining tasks are to estimate size and to determine whether the size is extremely large or small for the estimated age. There is fairly consistent agreement that measurements of the size of the fetal trunk correlate most strongly with the overall size of the fetus.[3, 19] There have been a variety of approaches suggested for this measurement that has been variously called an "abdominal" or a "chest" measurement. No clear superiority has been shown for any of these separate approaches since they all are attempts to do the same thing. In the author's opinion, the most reproducible and systematic of these measurements is the "abdominal diameter" (AD) or "abdominal circumference" (AC) when it represents a true cross section of the upper fetal abdomen at the level of the fetal liver. Anatomically, this level has been defined as one that includes the fetal portal venous system, both the ascending and transverse portions of the left portal vein and, ideally, the right portal vein as well (Fig. 5–2). No clear advantage has been shown in using an outer circumference, a cross-sectional area, or a circumference calculated from two orthogonal outer to outer diameters.[20, 21] This last approach is

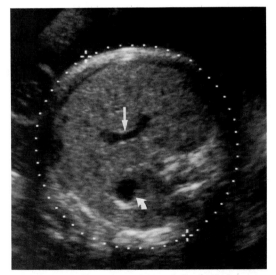

Figure 5–2. In this cross-section of the fetal abdomen, the ascending and transverse portions of the left portal vein are seen (arrow). The stomach is on the fetal left (curved arrow).

the one used by the author only because it is simple to do with his equipment.

This measurement can be used to calculate a fetal weight or compared directly with a standard chart to estimate whether the fetus is unusually large or unusually small. However, this calculated abdominal circumference is not a direct measure of size and, thus, only estimates whether the fetus is large or small. These estimations are far from perfect. The sensitivity of this parameter to identify babies that at birth are below the tenth percentile for weight varies from 64 to 82 percent when the lower 25th percentile cutoff is used for all fetuses after 25 weeks.[3] Both the sensitivity and predictive value of a positive test increases with gestational age, the latter growing from 24 percent at 25 weeks to 55 percent at 38 weeks.[3] For clinical management, earlier recognition of SGA babies is important. Thus the optimal time for screening is probably 34 ± 1 weeks.[3] Using the 15th percentile for a low-risk population, the predictive value of the test is about 20 percent at 32 weeks, but the sensitivity approaches 90 percent.[5] In a higher risk population, a lower threshold (tenth percentile) can be used with approximately a 70 to 75 percent sensitivity and a 70 percent predictive value for a positive test at 33 to 36 weeks' gestation.[4, 22] These numbers are greatly influenced by the incidence of low birthweight babies in the population studied, as well as by the average interval between the sonogram and delivery. Corresponding numbers for detecting large babies are not available.

A suggested approach to the actual use of the AC is to employ the 15th percentile cutoff as a screening level for low-risk populations between 28 and 34 weeks of gestation, but in order to reduce the number of false positives, the tenth percentile can be used for high-risk pregnancies or those near term, i.e., after 36 weeks.

Because use of the calculated or measured AC requires rather accurate knowledge of fetal gestational age, which usually means an ultrasound study prior to 20 weeks of gestation, this simple measure is not always useful in screening for fetuses that are small for their gestational age. As a result, two age-independent ratios have been proposed. The first was the ratio of femur length to abdominal circumference. This ratio has been shown to stabilize after 24 weeks of gestation and remain about 22 ± 2 percent (for two standard deviations [SD].)[23] Despite 24 percent being the upper second standard deviation, 23.5 percent has been suggested as the threshold for identifying SGA babies.[23] Subsequent studies at this threshold suggest that the sensitivity is only 60 percent and the predictive value of a positive test only 20 percent.[24] Although these results are disappointing, they are better than the clinical identification of SGA fetuses and may be the only established sonographic measurement that can be used when the gestational age of the fetus is unknown.

It has been suggested that low FL/AC ratios identify macrosomic fetuses; for a lower threshold of 20.5 percent, 86 percent of LGA babies fall below this level, with a 68 percent predictive value for a positive test.[25] In this study, LGA was defined as weight above the 90th percentile for age, with actual weights from 3900 to 5046 gm. In a subsequent study, when the FL/AC threshold was 20 percent, the sensitivity was 64 percent for identifying babies above 4000 gm, the predictive value of a positive test being 36 percent.[26]

The other ratio that has been proposed actually has two separate forms. These are the ratios of femur length to thigh circumference (or diameter) and tibial length to calf circumference.[27] The techniques for making these measurements are not as clear-cut as those for the FL/AC. The problem is that of standardizing the level at which to obtain thigh or calf circumference measurements. One proposal is to measure the thigh at the level at which the cross-sectional shape of the femur changes from round to oval.[28] Preliminary reports suggest this ratio may be superior to the FL/AC in identifying both unusually large and small babies, but until additional data is available, this ratio is not suggested as part of routine screening for fetal size.

A third ratio deserves mention. This is the head circumference (HC) to abdominal circumference (AC) ratio.[29] This ratio must be considered separate from the previously mentioned ones because it is not an age-independent one. As such, it seems to offer little additional information over evaluation of the AC alone for screening for the extremes of fetal size. The literature is unclear as to whether this is an acceptable screening measure, and generally HC/AC ratios have been suggested as an adjunct to classify the type of "growth retardation." The typing of growth retardation itself has recently come into question, and it is no longer clear that the physical proportions of small babies are easily divided into either symmetric or asymmetric groups.[30, 31] This topic merits some discussion, but the reader is referred to the literature; with no good definition of IUGR and no evidence of a bimodal distribution of proportions of low birthweight infants, the only possible practical use of the HC/AC is to explain why some fetuses had normal BPD growth yet were SGA at delivery. Since it is no longer suggested that serial BPDs alone be used to identify potential SGA babies,[3] this topic is not of much practical concern today.

In another sense, head measurements do continue to have value in evaluation for fetal growth. These measurements contribute to most formulas that attempt to derive an estimated fetal size. Use of such formulas has an intuitive appeal. If what we wish to predict is whether the fetal weight (size) is above or below a certain percentile for fetal age, the task could be viewed as one of estimating first the gestational age then the fetal weight. Although our limitations and capabilities of estimating gestational age are fairly well known, the problems of fetal weight estimations are not so clear. The literature seems to be growing at a fairly steady rate, yet the ultimate formula eludes us. The simplest formula uses the AC alone.[32] The BPD and AC can be combined into a table form; however, there is some suggestion that the more complex formulas that include femur length may give the best results.[33, 34] The author suspects that there are inherent limitations of the mathematical modeling approach that do not account for variations in fetal proportions, densities, and perhaps alterations that occur in the transition from the intrauterine to extrauterine environment. One study showed that even direct measurements of multiple physical dimensions in newborn babies, including limb lengths and diameters and trunk lengths and diameters, produced an 8 percent error (2 SDs) when converted to weight, and this error doubled when the measurements were made sonographically in utero.[35]

Despite the limitations of predicting fetal weight, a formula similar to the most popular fetal weight formula,[36] which uses the BPD and AC, has been shown to have a sensitivity only moderately less than the AC alone, but with a much higher predictive value for a positive test. Using the lower fifth percentile as the threshold, Selbing and associates were able to detect 75 percent of SGA babies with a 40 percent predictive value for a positive test in a low-risk population, whereas the AC alone had only a 20 percent predictive value.[5] This argues that the fetal weight for gestational age approach should improve the predictive value of ultrasound measurements by eliminating some of the false-positive cases the AC alone will identify. Similar standards for the popular Warsof and Shepard weight curves have been published.[37]

Although initial reports of the ultrasonic determination of oligohydramnios as a predictor of IUGR were promising,[38] subsequent studies indicated a 40 percent predictive value for a positive test in a high-risk population and, in an unselected population, only a 16 percent sensitivity.[39] A major problem with this approach is the lack of an objective definition of oligohydramnios. The initial suggested definition, the absence of at least one pocket of fluid measuring 1 cm in its greatest diameter, has been viewed as too restrictive,[40] yet such observations as subjective lack of amniotic fluid, poor definition of the fetal surface, increased uterine/fetal contact, or marked crowding of fetal small parts seem even more subjective. In post-term babies, a fluid index, calculated as the length multiplied by the height by the width of the largest fluid pocket, was strongly associated with the postmaturity syndrome if the index was less than 60.[41] It remains to be seen if establishing appropriate thresholds of this index at earlier gestational ages would permit recognition of fetal distress or IUGR.

Most of the data given thus far have been concerned with the detection of SGA babies. Macrosomic babies have received less attention, not because of a lack of concern, but simply because this condition is even more vaguely defined than IUGR. There is no consistent definition of macrosomia;[42] 4000 gm is commonly used, but the highest risk is over 4500 gm.[43] Both these numbers apply to term infants, without adjustment for gestational age, and the concern is largely for mechanical problems, such as postpartum hemorrhage, shoulder dystocia, and tears of the birth canal. However, these problems of delivery are determined not only by fetal

size but by such other factors as the baby's body shape (especially shoulder width),[44] the force and duration of labor, and the size of the maternal pelvis. Deter and Hadlock[42] have suggested that the use of weight formulas is not adequate for detecting this group. The use of ratios has been suggested by some, but the sensitivity and specificity are relatively low, resulting in poor predictive values for the test unless there is a high incidence of macrosomia in the population being studied. In diabetic patients, when the chest diameter minus the BPD was 1.4 cm or greater, about 90 percent of macrosomic babies (over 4000 gm) were detected with an approximately 60 percent predictive value for a positive test.[45] These figures have not been confirmed by enough investigators for the reader to accept them as final.

What can be said in summary? Despite the many doubts raised, it is evident that the sonographic evaluation of fetal morphology and estimation of fetal age are sufficiently accurate and useful to justify the liberal monitoring of pregnancy by ultrasound. In one study, even among women with early prenatal care, regular cycles, and reliable menstrual history, almost 20 percent had unacceptably inaccurate clinical estimations of gestational age when compared with the ultrasound crown-rump length.[46] Routine early ultrasound determination of gestational age reduced postmature deliveries from one in 15 to one in 300. Beyond the gathering of more basic knowledge of fetal growth, however, the value of the sonographic monitoring of growth parameters in the absence of a systematic screening program is more doubtful. Nevertheless, since the extremes of the birthweight distribution curve represent definite risk groups, there remains an impetus to identify them in utero. Of the sonographic measures available, the AC is the single most useful measure for identifying these groups. Fetal weight calculations in utero may offer improved specificity over the AC for low birthweight babies, but its role in large babies is uncertain. The FL/AC ratio has many false positives but may be the only screening tool for SGA babies in the third trimester without a known gestational age. Its role in detecting macrosomia is less clear. Other ratios, such as femur length to thigh circumference or abdominal diameter to BPD, may have value for finding either small (FL/TC) or unusually large (TC/BPD) babies, but we await more independent confirmations to establish this. All of these suggested approaches are limited by low predictive values for positive tests, and none can be said to "diagnose" IUGR.[47] Thus, while much of this topic can be easily summarized, little can be concluded since our understanding of fetal growth is far from complete. Rather than leave the reader with the same confusion the author has when reviewing this topic, he offers the following guidelines that provide a practical but unfortunately nonscientific approach to this problem.

STEP BY STEP APPROACH TO IDENTIFICATION OF THE IUGR FETUS

Considering the difficulties in defining intrauterine growth retardation (IUGR) and the inadequacies of the literature, any practical approach to this problem is an arbitrary one. The following is a brief description of one such approach. It should be emphasized that it is based on assumptions that have not been proved. It is also likely that some other approaches will be more effective and useful; certainly the author hopes so.

The first practical step is to make the best estimation of fetal gestational age (BEGA). The amount of confidence that can be placed in this estimation is the major limiting factor for all subsequent steps. The best estimations are from especially good historical information (see Table 5–3) and sonographic measurements up to 20 weeks' gestation. Other data are less reliable and certainly compromise the approach to recognition of IUGR. The measurements we use sonographically are the CRL up to 12 weeks and the

Table 5–3. ESPECIALLY GOOD HISTORICAL EVIDENCE FOR THE BEGA

1. Single episode of intercourse
2. In vitro fertilization
3. Artificial insemination
4. Ovulation induction
5. Basal body temperature monitoring

In the author's practice, he includes this list as part of a questionnaire given to patients that, in addition to asking information about menstrual history and other prenatal care, asks if they have special reasons for knowing their date of conception.

BPD and FL in combination from 12 to 20 weeks. HC could be used in place of the BPD, but it is often difficult to obtain early in pregnancy for technical reasons; thus, we use it in place of the BPD only after 20 weeks. There has been proposed a relatively sophisticated way of combining BPD and FL to improve age estimation,[48] but we simply average these two results to use for the BEGA.

The CRL is found in Table 5–4, the BPD in Table 5–5, and the FL in Table 5–6. A variety of tables exist, and the ones chosen by the author match his technique. In selecting a table for use in the laboratory, it is important to recognize that slight differences in technique will produce systematic variation in measurements. It is, therefore, important to select a group of patients with "known" dates and determine that the mean values for this group in the laboratory match the values in the table selected.

Once a BEGA is made, this plus the expected range for 2 SDs should be given. For estimations of 20 weeks or less, this is generally plus or minus one week or less. After 20 weeks, the range rather rapidly increases so that by 28 weeks, it is generally plus or minus four weeks or more. This rapid alteration of the expected range later in pregnancy makes it difficult to specify the gestational age since the increasing uncertainty of the estimation compounds the uncertainty of the range.

Once the BEGA has been made, it remains the best estimation for subsequent studies unless an error is discovered in the original calculation or some new historical information is uncovered that takes precedence over previous information. Using the established BEGA, "reverse" tables are important in subsequent studies to determine if, given the gestational age, the measurements obtained are unusually large or small. Reverse tables are most useful for the AC (Table 5–7) but are also useful for the HC (Table 5–8) and FL (Table 5–9). Note that in some cases, the limits are given in standard deviations and in others in percentiles.

There is considerable evidence that the AC is the most sensitive indicator of fetal size and that if the gestational age is reasonably well known (that is, equivalent to ultrasound measurement prior to 20 weeks), a low AC is the most sensitive indicator of the presence of an SGA fetus. Various thresholds

Table 5–4. FETAL CROWN-RUMP LENGTH COMPARED WITH GESTATIONAL AGE

CRL	Gestational Age (weeks)			CRL	Gestational Age (weeks)		
	Mean	− 2 SD	+ 2 SD		Mean	− 2 SD	+ 2 SD
7	6.25		7.15	39	10.65	10.00	11.35
8	6.45		7.30	40	10.75	10.10	11.45
9	6.70		7.55	41	10.80	10.20	11.55
10	6.90	6.25	7.70	42	10.90	10.30	11.65
11	7.10	6.50	7.90	43	11.05	10.40	11.70
12	7.25	6.60	8.10	44	11.10	10.45	11.80
13	7.45	6.85	8.25	45	11.20	10.55	11.90
14	7.60	7.00	8.45	46	11.30	10.66	12.00
15	7.75	7.15	8.60	47	11.35	10.70	12.05
16	7.90	7.30	8.70	48	11.45	10.80	12.15
17	8.10	7.45	8.90	49	11.55	10.90	12.25
18	8.20	7.60	9.00	50	11.60	10.95	12.30
19	8.40	7.75	9.15	51	11.70	11.10	12.40
20	8.50	7.90	9.30	52	11.80	11.15	12.50
21	8.60	8.05	9.40	53	11.85	11.20	12.55
22	8.80	8,15	9.55	54	11.95	11.30	12.65
23	8.90	8.30	9.65	55	12.05	11.40	12.75
24	9.05	8.40	9.80	56	12.10	11.50	12.80
25	9.15	8.55	9.90	57	12.20	11.55	12.90
26	9.30	8.70	10.00	58	12.30	11.65	12.95
27	9.40	8.80	10.10	59	12.35	11.70	13.05
28	9.50	8.90	10.25	60	12.45	11.80	13.15
29	9.65	9.05	10.35	61	12.50	11.85	13.20
30	9.70	9.15	10.45	62	12.60	11.90	13.30
31	9.85	9.25	10.55	63	12.65	12.00	13.40
32	9.95	9.35	10.65	64	12.75	12.50	13.45
33	10.05	9.45	10.75	65	12.85	12.10	13.55
34	10.15	9.55	10.85	66	12.90	12.20	13.60
35	10.20	9.60	10.95	67	12.95	12.30	13.70
36	10.35	9.70	11.05	68	13.05	12.35	13.75
37	10.40	9.80	11.15	69	13.10	12.45	13.80
38	10.55	9.90	11.25	70	13.15	12.50	13.90

From Robinson H, Fleming J: A critical evaluation of sonar crown-rump length measurements. Br J Obstet Gynaecol 82:702, 1979.

Table 5–5. CONVERSION FROM BPD IN MM TO MENSTRUAL AGE IN WEEKS

BPD (mm)	Menstrual Age (weeks)	90% Range	BPD (mm)	Menstrual Age (weeks)	90% Range
22	12.7	12.2–13.2	61	24.2	22.6–25.8
23	13.0	12.4–13.6	62	24.6	23.1–26.1
24	13.2	12.6–13.8	63	24.9	23.4–26.4
25	13.5	12.9–14.1	64	25.3	23.8–26.8
26	13.7	13.1–14.3	65	25.6	24.1–27.1
27	14.0	13.4–14.6	66	26.0	24.5–27.5
28	14.3	13.6–15.0	67	26.4	25.0–27.8
29	14.6	13.9–15.2	68	26.7	25.3–28.1
30	14.8	14.1–15.5	69	27.1	25.8–28.4
31	15.1	14.3–15.9	70	27.5	26.3–28.7
32	15.3	14.5–16.1	71	27.9	26.7–29.1
33	15.6	14.7–16.5	72	28.3	27.2–29.4
34	15.9	15.0–16.8	73	28.7	27.6–29.8
35	16.2	15.2–17.2	74	29.1	28.1–30.1
36	16.4	15.4–17.4	75	29.5	28.5–30.5
37	16.7	15.6–17.8	76	30.0	29.0–31.0
38	17.0	15.9–18.1	77	30.3	29.2–31.4
39	17.3	16.1–18.5	78	30.8	29.6–32.0
40	17.6	16.4–18.8	79	31.2	29.9–32.5
41	17.9	16.5–19.3	80	31.6	30.2–33.0
42	18.2	16.6–19.8	81	32.1	30.7–33.5
43	18.5	16.8–20.2	82	32.6	31.2–34.0
44	18.8	16.9–20.7	83	33.0	31.5–34.5
45	19.1	17.0–21.2	84	33.5	31.9–35.1
46	19.4	17.4–21.4	85	34.0	32.3–35.7
47	19.7	17.8–21.6	86	34.5	32.8–36.2
48	20.0	18.2–21.8	87	35.0	33.4–36.6
49	20.3	18.6–22.0	88	35.5	33.9–37.1
50	20.6	19.0–22.2	89	36.1	34.6–37.6
51	20.9	19.3–22.5	90	36.6	35.1–38.1
52	21.2	19.5–22.9	91	37.2	35.9–38.5
53	21.5	19.8–23.2	92	37.8	36.7–38.9
54	21.9	20.1–23.7	93	38.3	37.3–39.3
55	22.2	20.4–24.0	94	39.0	37.9–40.1
56	22.5	20.7–24.3	95	39.7	38.5–40.9
57	22.8	21.1–24.5	96	40.3	39.1–41.5
58	23.2	21.5–24.9	97	41.0	39.9–42.1
59	23.5	21.9–25.1	98	41.8	40.5–43.1
60	23.9	22.3–25.5			

From Kurtz AB, Wapner RJ, Kurtz RJ, et al: J Clin Ultrasound 8:319, 1980. © Copyright 1980, John Wiley & Sons. Reprinted by permission.

Table 5–6. PREDICTED MENSTRUAL AGE FOR
FEMUR LENGTHS

Femur Length (mm)	Menstrual Age (weeks)	Femur Length (mm)	Menstrual Age (weeks)
10	12.8	45	24.5
11	13.1	46	24.9
12	13.4	47	25.3
13	13.6	48	25.7
14	13.9	49	26.1
15	14.2	50	26.5
16	14.5	51	27.0
17	14.8	52	27.4
18	15.1	53	27.8
19	15.4	54	28.2
20	15.7	55	28.7
21	16.0	56	29.1
22	16.3	57	29.6
23	16.6	58	30.0
24	16.9	59	30.5
25	17.2	60	30.9
26	17.6	61	31.4
27	17.9	62	31.9
28	18.2	63	32.3
29	18.6	64	32.8
30	18.9	65	33.3
31	19.2	66	33.8
32	19.6	67	34.2
33	19.9	68	34.7
34	20.3	69	35.2
35	20.7	70	35.7
36	21.0	71	36.2
37	21.4	72	36.7
38	21.8	73	37.2
39	22.1	74	37.7
40	22.9	75	38.3
41	22.5	76	38.8
42	23.3	77	39.3
43	23.7	78	39.8
44	24.1	79	40.4

From Hadlock FP, Harrist RB, Deter RL, Park SK: Fetal femur lengths as a predictor of menstrual age: sonographically measured. AJR 138:875, 1982. *Copyright by* The American Roentgen Ray Society.

have been proposed for the AC, and there is currently no clear answer since such things as the risk status of the patient and the interval from sonography to delivery influence the selection of an optimal cutoff between normal and suspicous groups. Generally, the higher the level used to separate the two groups, the greater is the sensitivity but also the number of false-positive cases. Early in pregnancy (28 to 34 weeks), and in low-risk groups, the lower 15th percentile appears to be a good cutoff. Later in pregnancy, or in high-risk groups, the 10th percentile appears better. Remember that percentiles are not standard deviations; see Table 5–10 to relate these two measures. Using these thresholds, sensitivities in the

order of 90 percent, with 20 to 50 percent predictive values, should be achieved once the gestational age has been established.[22]

Although it is unlikely that using a calculated fetal weight as a screen for SGA babies is as sensitive as using the AC alone, it may have a greater predictive power by eliminating false-positive cases. Using a formula taken from the BPD and AC, the calculated fetal "weight" is obtained.[36] The author uses what has been referred to as the "Shepard formula" because it has been studied extensively and the evidence suggests it is no worse than most of the other formulas that have been published. Table 5–11 is a chart giving the calculated weight by this formula from a table of BPD and AC values; it produces approximately a ± 12 to 15 percent error in the weight estimations, with a slight tendency to overestimate fetal weights,[37] and is least accurate when the estimations are over 4000 gm. When the weight estimation is given, it is considered abnormal if below the fifth percentile (Table 5–12). The prenatal identification of SGA babies probably has a significantly lower sensitivity with this approach but produces relatively fewer false-positive tests.

If the gestational age is not known and cannot be reasonably established, screening for SGA babies is very difficult. Lack of appropriate interval growth is suggestive, but thresholds, sensitivities, and specificities for interval growth are not well established. There have been attempts to find age-independent ratios to assist in the screening of these patients. One of these is the ratio of the FL to the AC (in centimeters) expressed as a percentage (i.e., multiplied by 100). The mean is 22 with a range of 20 to 24 for two standard deviations.[23] The suggested threshold for SGA is 23.5 or above. Using this, the sensitivity is about 60 percent, with a predictive value for a positive test near 20 percent. Despite these numbers, the FL/AC ratio proves useful because after about 24 weeks, it is not necessary to know the gestational age. A similar approach can be taken with the TC/FL; preliminary results with this measure are promising but await confirmation since it appears to vary greatly.[27]

The HC/AC is not age independent and therefore, is not a substitute for the FL/AC. The HC/AC was first proposed as a screen for IUGR but more recently has generally been used as a measure of disproportion,

Table 5–7. FETAL ABDOMINAL CIRCUMFERENCE COMPARED WITH GESTATIONAL AGE

Gestational Age (weeks)	Abdominal Circumference				
	− 2 SD	10th Percentile	15th Percentile	Mean	+ 2 SD
14	6.6	7.0	7.6	8.7	11.0
15	7.5	8.0	8.6	9.7	12.0
16	8.6	9.0	9.6	10.7	12.0
17	9.6	10.1	10.7	11.8	14.1
18	10.6	11.2	11.7	12.9	15.2
19	11.7	12.2	12.8	14.0	16.4
20	12.8	13.3	14.0	15.2	17.6
21	13.8	14.4	15.0	16.4	18.8
22	14.9	15.5	16.1	17.5	20.0
23	16.0	16.6	17.3	18.7	21.4
24	17.0	17.6	18.3	19.8	22.5
25	18.0	18.6	19.4	21.0	24.0
26	19.0	19.6	20.5	22.1	25.1
27	20.0	20.6	21.6	23.3	26.3
28	21.0	21.6	22.6	24.4	27.6
29	22.0	22.6	23.7	25.5	28.8
30	23.0	23.7	24.7	26.5	30.0
31	24.1	24.7	25.8	27.7	32.2
32	25.2	25.7	26.9	28.6	32.4
33	26.2	26.7	27.8	29.6	33.5
34	27.2	27.7	28.9	30.7	34.6
35	28.1	28.7	29.8	31.7	35.6
36	29.0	29.8	30.8	32.8	36.5
37	29.9	20.6	31.7	33.7	37.3
38	30.8	31.4	32.6	34.5	37.9
39	31.6	32.2	33.4	35.4	38.4
40	32.4	33.0	34.1	36.0	38.8
41	33.2	33.8	34.8	36.6	39.2

From Campbell S, Metreweli C (ed): Practical Abdominal Ultrasound. Chicago, Year Book Medical Publishers, 1978. Reprinted with the permission of Heinemann Medical Books.

Table 5–8. FETAL HEAD CIRCUMFERENCE COMPARED WITH GESTATIONAL AGE

Gestational Age (weeks)	Head Circumference		
	− 2 SD	Mean	+ 2 SD
14	8.6	11.0	13.6
15	9.6	12.2	14.7
16	10.8	13.3	15.8
17	12.0	14.4	16.9
18	13.2	15.5	18.0
19	14.3	16.7	19.1
20	15.5	18.0	20.3
21	16.6	19.2	21.5
22	17.9	20.3	22.7
23	19.0	21.5	23.8
24	20.2	22.7	24.9
25	21.4	23.8	26.0
26	22.5	25.0	27.1
27	23.6	26.0	28.2
28	24.6	27.0	29.2
29	25.6	27.9	30.2
30	26.5	28.8	31.1
31	27.3	29.6	32.0
32	28.0	30.4	32.9
33	28.8	31.1	33.6
34	29.2	31.8	34.4
35	29.9	32.5	35.0
36	30.2	33.0	35.7
37	30.8	33.6	36.2
38	31.2	34.0	36.7
39	31.5	34.5	37.2
40	31.8	34.8	37.5
41	32.0	35.1	37.8

From Campbell S, Metreweli C (ed): Practical Abdominal Ultrasound. Chicago, Year Book Medical Publishers, 1978. *Reprinted with the permission of* Heinemann Medical Books.

Table 5–9. FEMUR LENGTH COMPARED WITH GESTATIONAL AGE

Gestational Age (weeks)	Femur Length (percentiles)		
	5th	50th	95th
11		6	
12		9	
13	6	12	19
14	5	15	19
15	11	19	26
16	13	22	24
17	20	25	29
18	19	28	31
19	23	31	38
20	22	33	39
21	27	36	45
22	29	39	44
23	35	41	48
24	34	44	49
25	38	46	54
26	39	49	53
27	45	51	57
28	45	53	57
29	49	56	62
30	49	58	62
31	53	60	67
32	53	62	67
33	56	64	71
34	57	65	70
35	61	67	73
36	61	69	74
37	64	71	77
38	62	72	79
39	64	74	83
40	66	75	81

From Jeanty P: Letter to the editor. Radiology 147:602, 1983.

Table 5–10. RELATIONSHIP BETWEEN STANDARD DEVIATIONS AND PERCENTILES

Percentiles	Standard Deviations
25th	(−) 0.68
20th	(−) 0.84
15th	(−) 1.04
10th	(−) 1.28
5th	(−) 1.64
2.28	(−) 2.00

Remember that this relationship assumes a normal or gaussian population distribution, which can be assumed if a table is published as standard deviations but cannot be assumed if it is published as percentiles, since this expression can be used in nongaussian population distributions.

Table 5–11. ESTIMATED FETAL WEIGHTS IN "ESTIMATED GRAMS," DERIVED FROM THE SHEPARD FORMULA

Abdominal Circumference (mm) — Biparietal diameter (mm)

Biparietal diameter 30–39 mm

BPD	40	45	50	55	60	65	70	75	80	85	90	95	100	105	110	115	120	125	130	135	140	145	150
30	80	83	87	91	95	99	104	108	113	118	123	129	135	141	147	154	161						
31	83	86	90	94	98	103	107	112	117	122	128	133	139	145	152	159	166	173	181				
32			93	97	102	106	111	116	121	126	132	138	144	150	157	164	171	178	186				
33			97	101	105	110	115	120	125	130	136	142	148	155	162	169	176	184	192				
34			100	104	109	114	119	124	129	135	141	147	153	160	167	174	182	190	198	206	215		
35					113	118	123	128	134	139	145	152	158	165	172	180	187	195	204	213	222		
36					117	122	127	132	138	144	150	157	163	170	178	185	193	202	210	219	229		
37					121	126	131	137	143	149	155	162	169	176	183	191	199	208	217	226	235	245	256
38							136	142	148	154	160	167	174	182	189	197	206	214	223	233	243	253	263
39							141	146	153	159	166	173	180	187	195	203	212	221	230	240	250	260	271

Biparietal diameter 40–49 mm

BPD	70	75	80	85	90	95	100	105	110	115	120	125	130	135	140	145	150	155	160	165	170	175	180
40	145	152	158	164	171	178	186	193	202	210	219	228	237	247	257	268	279						
41			163	170	177	184	192	200	208	217	226	235	245	255	265	276	288	299	312				
42			169	176	183	190	198	206	215	223	233	242	252	262	273	284	296	308	321				
43			174	182	189	197	205	213	222	231	240	250	260	270	281	293	305	317	330				
44			180	188	195	203	211	220	229	238	247	257	268	279	290	302	314	326	340	353	368		
45					202	210	218	227	236	245	255	265	276	287	299	311	323	336	349	363	378		
46					208	217	225	234	244	253	263	274	285	296	308	320	333	346	359	374	389		
47					215	224	233	242	251	261	271	282	293	305	317	329	342	356	370	384	400	415	432
48							240	250	259	269	280	291	302	314	326	339	352	366	381	395	411	427	444
49							248	258	268	278	289	300	312	324	336	349	363	377	392	407	422	439	456

Biparietal diameter 50–59 mm

BPD	100	105	110	115	120	125	130	135	140	145	150	155	160	165	170	175	180	185	190	195	200	205	210	215	220
50	256	266	276	287	298	309	321	334	346	360	374	388	403	418	434	451	468	486	505						
51		276	285	296	307	319	331	344	357	370	385	399	414	430	447	464	481	500	519						
52			294	305	317	329	341	354	368	381	396	411	426	443	459	477	495	513	533						
53			304	315	327	339	352	365	379	393	408	423	439	455	472	490	508	527	547	568	589				
54					337	350	363	376	390	405	420	435	451	468	486	504	522	542	562	583	605				
55					348	360	374	388	402	417	432	448	464	482	499	518	537	557	577	598	620				
56					359	372	385	399	414	429	445	461	478	495	513	532	552	572	593	614	637	660	684		
57							397	412	426	442	458	474	492	509	528	547	567	587	609	631	654	677	702		
58							409	424	439	455	471	488	506	524	543	562	583	604	625	648	671	695	720		
59									453	469	485	503	520	539	558	578	599	620	642	665	689	713	739	765	792

Biparietal diameter 60–62 mm

BPD	140	145	150	155	160	165	170	175	180	185	190	195	200	205	210	215	220	225	230	235	240	245	250
60	466	483	500	517	536	554	574	594	615	637	659	683	707	732	758	784	812						
61	480	497	514	532	551	570	590	611	632	654	677	701	725	751	777	804	832						
62			530	548	567	587	607	628	650	672	696	720	745	770	797	825	853	883	913				

Table of estimated fetal weight (grams). Row values (63–100) and column headings represent fetal measurements; cell values are estimated weights.

Rows 63–69

	170	175	180	185	190	195	200	205	210	215	220	225	230	235	240	245	250	255	260	265	270	275	280	285	290
63			545	564	583	603	624	645	668	691	714	739	764	790	818	846	875	905	936						
64			561	580	600	621	642	664	686	709	734	759	784	811	839	867	897	927	959						
65					617	638	660	682	705	729	753	779	805	832	860	889	919	950	982	1.015	1.050				
66					635	657	678	701	725	749	774	800	826	854	882	912	942	974	1.006	1.040	1.075				
67					654	675	698	721	745	769	795	821	848	876	905	935	966	998	1.031	1.065	1.100	1.137	1.174		
68							717	741	765	790	816	843	870	899	928	959	990	1.023	1.056	1.091	1.127	1.164	1.202		
69							738	762	786	812	838	865	893	922	952	983	1.015	1.048	1.082	1.117	1.154	1.191	1.230		

Rows 70–79

	175	180	185	190	195	200	205	210	215	220	225	230	235	240	245	250	255	260	265	270	275	280	285	290	295
70	758	783	808	834	861	888	917	946	977	1.008	1.041	1.074	1.109	1.144	1.181	1.219	1.258	1.299	1.340						
71		808	830	857	884	912	941	971	1.002	1.034	1.067	1.101	1.136	1.172	1.209	1.248	1.287	1.328	1.371						
72			853	880	908	936	966	996	1.028	1.060	1.094	1.128	1.164	1.200	1.238	1.277	1.317	1.359	1.402						
73					932	958	987	1.022	1.054	1.087	1.121	1.156	1.192	1.229	1.268	1.307	1.348	1.390	1.433	1.478	1.524				
74						983	1.013	1.049	1.081	1.115	1.149	1.185	1.221	1.259	1.298	1.338	1.379	1.422	1.466	1.511	1.558				
75								1.076	1.109	1.143	1.178	1.214	1.251	1.290	1.329	1.370	1.411	1.455	1.499	1.545	1.592	1.641	1.691		
76								1.104	1.138	1.172	1.208	1.244	1.282	1.321	1.361	1.402	1.444	1.488	1.533	1.579	1.627	1.676	1.727		
77								1.133	1.167	1.202	1.238	1.275	1.313	1.353	1.393	1.435	1.478	1.522	1.568	1.615	1.663	1.713	1.764		
78								1.163	1.197	1.233	1.269	1.307	1.346	1.385	1.426	1.469	1.512	1.557	1.603	1.651	1.700	1.750	1.802	1.855	1.910
79									1.228	1.264	1.301	1.339	1.379	1.419	1.461	1.503	1.547	1.593	1.639	1.688	1.737	1.788	1.840	1.894	1.950

Rows 80–89

	210	215	220	225	230	235	240	245	250	255	260	265	270	275	280	285	290	295	300	305	310	315	320	325	330
80	1.260	1.296	1.334	1.373	1.412	1.453	1.495	1.539	1.583	1.629	1.677	1.725	1.775	1.827	1.880	1.934	1.990								
81			1.367	1.407	1.447	1.488	1.531	1.575	1.620	1.667	1.715	1.764	1.814	1.866	1.920	1.975	2.032	2.090	2.150						
82					1.482	1.524	1.568	1.612	1.658	1.705	1.753	1.803	1.854	1.907	1.961	2.017	2.074	2.133	2.193						
83					1.519	1.561	1.605	1.650	1.697	1.744	1.793	1.843	1.895	1.948	2.003	2.059	2.117	2.176	2.237	2.300	2.365				
84					1.556	1.599	1.643	1.689	1.736	1.784	1.834	1.885	1.937	1.991	2.046	2.103	2.161	2.221	2.282	2.346	2.411				
85					1.594	1.638	1.683	1.729	1.776	1.825	1.875	1.927	1.979	2.034	2.090	2.147	2.206	2.266	2.328	2.392	2.458				
86							1.723	1.770	1.818	1.867	1.918	1.970	2.023	2.078	2.134	2.192	2.252	2.313	2.375	2.440	2.506	2.574	2.644		
87							1.764	1.811	1.860	1.910	1.961	2.014	2.068	2.123	2.180	2.238	2.298	2.360	2.423	2.488	2.555	2.623	2.694		
88							1.806	1.854	1.903	1.954	2.005	2.059	2.113	2.169	2.227	2.286	2.346	2.408	2.472	2.538	2.605	2.674	2.745	2.817	2.892
89									1.947	1.998	2.051	2.104	2.160	2.216	2.274	2.334	2.395	2.457	2.522	2.588	2.656	2.725	2.797	2.870	2.945

Rows 90–100

	250	255	260	265	270	275	280	285	290	295	300	305	310	315	320	325	330	335	340	345	350	355	360	365	370
90	1.993	2.044	2.087	2.151	2.207	2.264	2.323	2.383	2.445	2.508	2.573	2.639	2.707	2.778	2.849	2.923	2.999								
91			2.145	2.199	2.256	2.313	2.372	2.433	2.495	2.559	2.624	2.692	2.760	2.831	2.903	2.977	3.054	3.132	3.212						
92			2.193	2.249	2.305	2.364	2.423	2.484	2.547	2.611	2.677	2.745	2.814	2.885	2.958	3.033	3.109	3.188	3.268						
93			2.243	2.299	2.356	2.415	2.475	2.537	2.600	2.665	2.731	2.799	2.869	2.941	3.014	3.089	3.166	3.245	3.326	3.409	3.494				
94					2.408	2.467	2.528	2.590	2.654	2.719	2.786	2.855	2.925	2.997	3.071	3.147	3.224	3.304	3.385	3.468	3.554				
95					2.461	2.521	2.582	2.645	2.709	2.775	2.842	2.912	2.982	3.055	3.129	3.205	3.283	3.363	3.445	3.528	3.614				
96							2.645	2.701	2.765	2.832	2.900	2.969	3.041	3.114	3.188	3.265	3.343	3.423	3.505	3.590	3.676	3.764	3.854		
97							2.701	2.757	2.823	2.890	2.958	3.028	3.100	3.173	3.248	3.325	3.404	3.485	3.567	3.652	3.738	3.827	3.918		
98							2.757	2.814	2.881	2.949	3.018	3.088	3.160	3.234	3.310	3.387	3.466	3.547	3.630	3.715	3.802	3.891	3.982	4.075	4.170
99									2.941	3.009	3.078	3.149	3.222	3.296	3.372	3.450	3.530	3.611	3.695	3.780	3.867	3.956	4.047	4.141	4.236
100									3.002	3.071	3.141	3.212	3.285	3.360	3.436	3.514	3.594	3.676	3.760	3.845	3.933	4.022	4.114	4.207	4.303

From Jeanty P, Cantraine F, Romero R, et al: A longitudinal study of fetal weight growth. J Ultrasound Med 3:321, 1984. Copyright 1984, The American Institute of Ultrasound in Medicine.

Table 5–12. THE SHEPARD FORMULA—
WEIGHT COMPARED WITH GESTATIONAL
AGE

Gestational Age (weeks)	Weight (percentile)		
	5th	*50th*	*95th*
9	44	45	46
10	46	48	51
11	50	54	59
12	57	63	71
13	67	77	90
14	81	96	116
15	100	122	151
16	125	155	196
17	155	197	253
18	192	247	322
19	237	307	404
20	288	377	499
21	346	456	607
22	411	545	728
23	484	644	862
24	563	753	1010
25	650	871	1172
26	745	1000	1347
27	847	1139	1536
28	957	1288	1740
29	1074	1448	1958
30	1199	1618	2189
31	1331	1798	2434
32	1468	1984	2688
33	1608	2176	2950
34	1750	2369	3213
35	1888	2557	3469
36	2017	2734	3711
37	2131	2890	3925
38	2221	3016	4100
39	2276	3099	4225
40	2287	3131	4290

From Jeanty P, Cantraine F, Romero R, et al: A longitudinal study of fetal weight growth. J Ultrasound Med 3:321, 1984. Copyright 1984, The American Institute of Ultrasound in Medicine.

Table 5–13. HEAD CIRCUMFERENCE/
ABDOMINAL CIRCUMFERENCE RATIO
COMPARED WITH GESTATIONAL AGE

Gestational Age (weeks)	Head Circumference		
	− 2 SD	*Mean*	*+ 2 SD*
14	1.085	1.230	1.375
15	1.080	1.225	1.365
16	1.075	1.215	1.350
17	1.070	1.205	1.340
18	1.065	1.195	1.330
19	1.060	1.185	1.320
20	1.055	1.178	1.305
21	1.050	1.177	1.295
22	1.045	1.165	1.285
23	1.040	1.155	1.275
24	1.030	1.145	1.265
25	1.025	1.135	1.255
26	1.020	1.125	1.245
27	1.010	1.120	1.235
28	1.000	1.110	1.225
29	0.990	1.095	1.215
30	0.975	1.085	1.200
31	0.965	1.075	1.190
32	0.945	1.060	1.175
33	0.935	1.045	1.165
34	0.925	1.030	1.150
35	0.915	1.020	1.135
36	0.910	1.005	1.120
37	0.905	0.995	1.100
38	0.900	0.980	1.085
39	0.896	0.970	1.065
40	0.895	0.965	1.046
41	0.894	0.960	10.25

From Campbell S, Metreweli C (ed): Practical Abdominal Ultrasound. Chicago, Year Book Medical Publishers, 1978. Reprinted with the permission of Heinemann Medical Books.

Table 5–14. SAMPLE FORM USED TO COLLECT DATA FOR OB ULTRASOUND EXAMINATION

Name: _____   Hx No.: _____   Req No.: _____

Physician: _____   Clinic/Ward: _____

Current date: _____

LMP: _____   EGA by LMP: _____

Date of prior U/S: _____   BEGA—Then: _____   Now: _____

Special reason to know dates: _____   Dates by this: _____

History: _____

No. of fetuses: _____   Living?: _____

Fetal position: _____   Fluid: _____

Placental location _____   Previa: _____

Measurements   Range

    CRL _____ → _____ Weeks ± _____

    BPD _____ → _____ Weeks ± _____

    HC _____ → _____ Weeks ± _____ → _____ Percentile

    FL _____ → _____ Weeks ± _____ → _____ Percentile

    AC _____ → _____ Weeks → _____ Percentile

EGA by LMP: _____

EGA by prior U/S: _____

EGA by measurements: _____

BEGA: _____   By prior U/S: (Yes)   (No)

AC = _____ Percentile   *if ≤15th percentile

Calc weight = _____ Percentile   *if ≤5th percentile

FL/AC = _____ (Normal = 20.5 to 23.5)   *if ≤20.5 or ≥23.5

HC/AC = _____ SD _____   *if 95th percentile or ≥ + 1.64 SD

IMPRESSION: _____

Resident: _____   Staff: _____

which some observers feel is useful in classifying the type of IUGR. Asymmetry is suggested when the HC/AC is above the 95th percentile (Table 5–13).

Finally, the author presents a worksheet for reviewing most of this data (Table 5–14). The material above acts as a general guide for the worksheet but is certainly not an exhaustive treatment of the problem of IUGR.

References

1. Wilcox AJ, Russell IT: Birthweight and perinatal mortality: II. On weight-specific mortality. Int J Epidemiol 12:319, 1983.
2. Wilcox AJ, Russell IT: Birthweight and perinatal mortality: I. On the frequency distribution of birthweight. Int J Epidemiol 12:314, 1983.
3. Warsof SL, Cooper DJ, Little D, et al: Routine ultrasound screening for antenatal detection of intrauterine growth retardation. Obstet Gynecol 67:33, 1986.
4. Geirsson RT, Patel NB, Christie AD: Intrauterine volume, fetal abdominal area and biparietal diameter measurements with ultrasound in the prediction of small-for-dates babies in a high-risk obstetric population. Br J Obstet Gynaecol 92:936, 1985.
5. Selbing A, Wichman K, Gunnar R: Screening for detection of intra-uterine growth retardation by means of ultrasound. Acta Obstet Gynecol Scand 63:543, 1984.
6. Wladimiroff JW, Laar J: Ultrasonic measurement of fetal body size. Acta Obstet Gynecol Scand 59:177, 1980.
7. Hughey MJ: Routine ultrasound for detection and management of the small-for-gestational-age fetus. Obstet Gynecol 64:101, 1984.
8. Read MS, Catz C, Grave G, et al: Introduction: Intrauterine growth retardation—identification of research needs and goals. Semin Perinatol 8:2, 1984.

9. Lockwood CJ, Weiner S: Assessment of fetal growth. Clin Perinatol 13:3, 1986.
10. Miller HC: Intrauterine growth retardation. An unmet challenge. Am J Dis Child 135:944, 1981.
11. Keirse MJ: Epidemiology and aetiology of the growth retarded baby. Clin Obstet Gynaecol 11:415, 1984.
12. Secher NJ, Hansen PK, Lenstrup C, et al: Birthweight standards based on early ultrasound estimation of gestational age. Br J Obstet Gynaecol 93:128, 1986.
13. Andersen HF, Johnson TRB, Barclay ML, et al: Gestational age assessment. I. Analysis of individual clinical observations. Am J Obstet Gynecol 139:173, 1981.
14. Beazley JM, Underhill RA: Fallacy of the fundal height. Br Med J 4:404, 1970.
15. Latis GO, Simionato L, Ferraris G: Clinical assessment of gestational age in the newborn infant. Comparison of two methods. Early Hum Dev 5:29, 1981.
16. Ounsted MK, Chalmers CA, Yudkin PL: Clinical assessment of gestational age at birth: The effects of sex, birthweight, and weight for length of gestation. Early Hum Dev 2:73, 1978.
17. Dubowitz LMS, Dubowitz V, Goldberg L: Clinical assessment of gestational age in the newborn infant. J Pediatr 77:1, 1970.
18. Selbing A, Fjällbrant B: Accuracy of conceptual age estimation from fetal crown-rump length. JCU 12:343, 1984.
19. Dubowitz LMS, Goldberg C: Assessment of gestation by ultrasound in various stages of pregnancy in infants differing in size and ethnic origin. Br J Obstet Gynaecol 88:255, 1981.
20. Shields JR, Medearis AL, Bear MB: Fetal head and abdominal circumferences: Effect of profile shape on the accuracy of ellipse equations. JCU 15:241, 1987.
21. Shields JR, Medearis AL, Bear MB: Fetal head and abdominal circumferences: Ellipse calculations versus planimetry. JCU 15:237, 1987.
22. Ferrazzi E, Nicolini V, Kustermann A, et al: Routine obstetric ultrasound: Effectiveness of cross-sectional screening for fetal growth retardation. JCU 14:17, 1986.
23. Hadlock FP, Deter RL, Harrist RB, et al: A date independent predictor of intrauterine growth retardation: Femur length/abdominal circumference ratio. AJR 141:979, 1983.
24. Benson CB, Doubilet PM, Saltzman DH, et al: FL/AC ratio: Poor predictor of intrauterine growth retardation. Invest Radiol 20:727, 1985.
25. Hadlock FP, Harrist RB, Fearneyhough TC, et al: Use of femur length/abdominal circumference ratio in detecting the macrosomic fetus. Radiology 154:503, 1985.
26. Benson CB, Doubilet PM, Saltzman DH, et al: Femur length/abdominal circumference ratio: Poor predictor of macrosomic fetuses in diabetic mothers. J Ultrasound Med 5:141, 1986.
27. Vintzileos AM, Neckles S, Campbell WA, et al: Ultrasound fetal thigh-calf circumferences and gestational age—independent fetal ratios in normal pregnancy. J Ultrasound Med 4:287, 1985.
28. Warda A, Deter RL, Duncan G, et al: Evaluation of fetal thigh circumference measurement: A comparative ultrasound and anatomical study. JCU 14:99, 1986.
29. Campbell S, Thoms A: Ultrasound measurement of the fetal head to abdomen circumference ratio in the assessment of growth retardation. Br J Obstet Gynaecol 84:165, 1977.
30. Woo JSK, Wan CW, Fang A, et al: Is fetal femur length a better indicator of gestational age in the growth-retarded fetus as compared with biparietal diameter? J Ultrasound Med 4:139, 1985.
31. Crane JP, Kopta MM: Comparative newborn anthropometric data in symmetric versus asymmetric intrauterine growth retardation. Am J Obstet Gynecol 138:518, 1980.
32. Campbell S, Wilkins D: Ultrasonic measurement of fetal abdomen circumference in the estimation of fetal weight. Br J Obstet Gynaecol 82:689, 1975.
33. Hill LM, Breckle R, Gehrking WC, et al: Use of femur length in estimation of fetal weight. Am J Obstet Gynecol 152:847, 1985.
34. Yarkoni S, Reece EA, Wan M, et al: Intrapartum fetal weight estimation: A comparison of three formulae. J Ultrasound Med 5:707, 1986.
35. Thompson TR, Manning FA: Estimation of volume and weight of the perinate: Relationship to morphometric measurement by ultrasonography. J Ultrasound Med 2:113, 1983.
36. Shepard MJ, Richards VA, Berkowitz RL: An evaluation of two equations for predicting fetal weight by ultrasound. Am J Obstet Gynecol 142:47, 1982.
37. Jeanty P, Cantraine F, Romero R, et al: A longitudinal study of fetal weight growth. J Ultrasound Med 3:321, 1984.
38. Manning FA, Hill LM, Platt LD: Qualitative amniotic fluid volume determination by ultrasound: Antepartum detection of intrauterine growth retardation. Am J Obstet Gynecol 139:254, 1981.
39. Philipson EH, Sokol RJ, Williams T: Oligohydramnios: Clinical assocations and predictive value for intrauterine growth retardation. Am J Obstet Gynecol 146:271, 1983.
40. Hoddick WK, Callen PW, Filly RA, et al: Ultrasonographic determination of qualitative amniotic fluid volume in intrauterine growth retardation. Am J Obstet Gynecol 149:758, 1984.
41. Hashimoto B, Filly RA, Belden C, et al: Objective method of diagnosing oligohydramnios in postterm pregnancies. J Ultrasound Med 6:81, 1987.
42. Deter RL, Hadlock FP: Use of ultrasound in the detection of macrosomia: A review. JCU 13:519, 1985.
43. Lazer S, Biale Y, Mazor M, et al: Complications associated with macrosomatic fetus. J Reprod Med 31:501, 1986.
44. Modanlou HD, Komatsu G, Dorchester W: Large-for-gestational-age neonates: Anthropometric reasons for shoulder dystocia. Obstet Gynecol 60:417, 1982.
45. Eliott JP, Garite TJ, Freeman RK, et al: Ultrasonic prediction of fetal macrosomia in diabetic patients. Obstet Gynecol 60:159, 1982.
46. Selbing A: The pregnant population and a fetal crown-rump length screening program. Acta Obstet Gynecol Scand 62:161, 1983.
47. Benson CB, Doubilet PM, Saltzman DH: Intrauterine growth retardation: Predictive value of US criteria for antenatal diagnosis. Radiology 160:415, 1986.
48. Yagel S, Adoni A, Oman S, et al: A statistical examination of the accuracy of combining femoral length and biparietal diameter as an index of fetal gestational age. Br J Obstet Gynaecol 93:109, 1986.

ULTRASOUND EVALUATION OF THE FETAL NEURAL AXIS

Roy A. Filly, M.D.

Among the various fetal anomalies that can be diagnosed by sonography, probably none are more devastating and therefore more important for early clinical recognition than central nervous system (CNS) abnormalities. Each year in the United States, approximately 6000 newborn infants are afflicted with one of these congenital anomalies.[1] Early in its development, prenatal sonography could detect only defects producing gross anatomic distortions.[2] More recent rapid technologic advances now allow the early and accurate diagnosis of numerous CNS malformations.[3–7] As a result, the sonographer, by observation and diagnosis, frequently initiates the obstetrician and prospective parents into a decision-making process involving difficult options. Consequently, it is incumbent upon the sonographer to provide accurate and reliable information on which these decisions can be based. Knowledge of normal and abnormal developmental neuroanatomy is essential to discriminate specific malformations.

With the widespread use of prenatal sonography, increasing numbers of fetal CNS anomalies are currently being detected.[3–6] In certain circumstances, a patient may be referred for the detection of a specific anatomic malformation; an example would be a pregnant woman who had previously delivered a child with an open neural tube defect. Her present fetus now has an increased risk for the same or a similar anomaly. However, in most cases, fetal neural defects are identified serendipitously during examinations performed for obstetric indications. Although it is uncertain whether the diagnosis of a CNS defect in utero can influence the eventual outcome for the fetus, the recognition of structural abnormalities before birth provides time to counsel the family and significantly affects obstetric management.[7]

When severe anomalies that are incompatible with postnatal survival are diagnosed in utero, e.g., anencephaly, the parents may elect pregnancy termination. When lesions that require surgical correction at or soon after birth are diagnosed, e.g., myelomeningocele, arrangements can be made for delivery at a hospital where immediate repair is possible. Hydrocephalus and certain other CNS anomalies frequently cause dystocia, therefore requiring either planned cesarean section or cephalocentesis to effect a vaginal delivery. Worsening hydrocephalus may cause progressive neurologic damage that may necessitate early delivery to hasten treatment in an ex utero environment. Finally, some abnormalities may cause progressive harm or interfere with normal development before fetal viability, e.g., some cases of progressive hydrocephalus. In this latter circumstance, sonographically guided techniques are available for intervention before birth.[8]

There is still a great deal to be learned regarding the natural history of certain CNS anomalies diagnosed prenatally. Furthermore, the area of sonographic CNS diagnosis is in its infancy, and the most experienced sonographers realize that despite the sophisticated techniques available, it is still quite possible to miss subtle but life-threatening anomalies that could alter the expected outcome and make certain treatment choices inappropriate. Therefore, as our knowledge of these disorders increases and our techniques for their diagnosis and management become more reliable, the decision-making process preceding and following diagnosis will undoubtedly change. In this chapter, the normal anatomy of the fetal brain and spinal cord, as well as the diagnosis of CNS anomalies, will be discussed in detail.

THE CENTRAL NERVOUS SYSTEM

Embryologic Development of the Brain*

Sonographers have an opportunity to visualize the developing brain with some degree of clarity from the latter portion of the first trimester onward. Despite this long period of observation and the ability to examine the human brain earlier than with any other available modality, it is important to recall that most specific brain structures have already developed before sonographers have an opportunity to begin observations.

The central nervous system develops from a thickened area of embryonic ectoderm, the neural plate. The neural plate develops at approximately 18 to 20 days after conception or 4.5 weeks after the beginning of the last normal menstrual period (LNMP). Promptly thereafter, the neural plate begins to alter, forming both the neural tube and crest (Fig. 6–1). The neural tube differentiates into the central nervous system, consisting of both

the brain and spinal cord. The neural crest gives rise to most of the structures in the peripheral nervous system.

The neural tube is temporarily opened at both the cranial and caudal ends (Fig. 6–1). The cranial opening, the rostral neuropore, closes about 24 days after conception (38 days after the LNMP). The caudal neuropore closes slightly later, 26 days after conception (40 days after the LNMP). The walls of the tube thicken to form various portions of the brain and spinal cord. The lumen of the neural tube becomes the ventricular system of the brain cranially and the central canal of the spinal cord caudally.

Growth and differentiation of the neural tube are greatest at the cranial end. Toward the end of the fourth postconception week (six LNMP weeks), the cranial end of the neural tube differentiates into three primary brain vesicles (Fig. 6–2). These consist of the prosencephalon (forebrain), the mesencephalon (midbrain), and the rhombencephalon (hindbrain). Over the ensuing week, the forebrain further differentiates into the telencephalon (endbrain), which is the most rostral portion of the embryonic brain, and the diencephalon (intermediate brain). Similarly, the hindbrain divides into the metencephalon and myelencephalon. As a result of these partial divisions, there now exist five secondary brain vesicles. In addition to the above process of diverticulation, flexion of the developing brain further differentiates these discrete areas of early brain morphology.

The diencephalon is centrally positioned, whereas the telencephalon consists of lateral expansions, the right and left cerebral vesicles (Fig. 6–2). The diencephalon develops from the tissues of the walls of the third ventricle that forms three discrete swellings; the epithalamus, the thalamus, and the hypothalamus. The thalamus is the dominant portion of the diencephalon and rapidly enlarges. As this enlargement occurs, the thalami bulge into the cavity of the third ventricle and reduce the ventricular lumen to a narrow cleft; this occurs before sonographers can visualize the developing brain with any degree of clarity. Indeed, the thalami usually meet and fuse in the midline, forming the bridge called the massa intermedia. The hypothalamus gives rise to the adult structure of the same name, whereas the epithalamus gives rise predominantly to the pineal gland.

---

*This section has been excerpted, in large part, from Moore's excellent textbook of embryology. (Moore KL: The Developing Human: Clinically Oriented Embryology, 4th Ed. Philadelphia, WB Saunders Co, 1988)

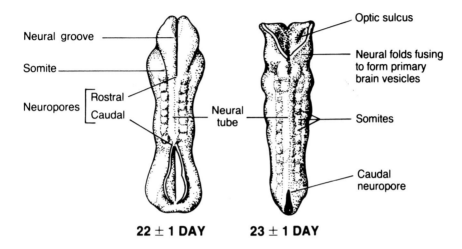

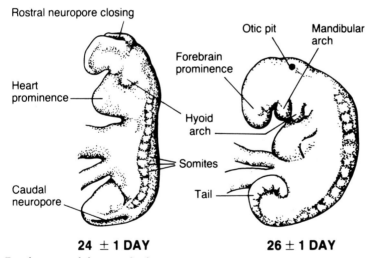

Figure 6–1. Development of the neural tube (22 to 26 days). (*From* Moore KL: The Developing Human: Clinically Oriented Embryology, 4th Ed. Philadelphia, WB Saunders Co, 1988.)

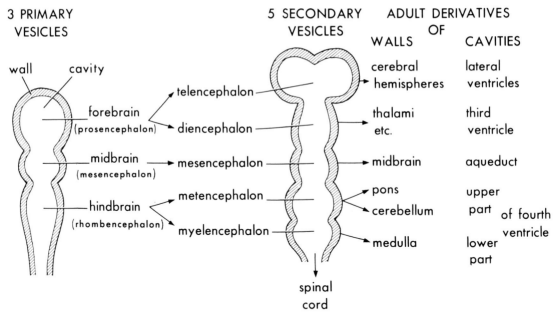

Figure 6–2. Early development of the human fetal brain, with the adult derivatives of the fetal precursors. (*From* Moore KL: The Developing Human: Clinically Oriented Embryology, 4th Ed. Philadelphia, WB Saunders Co, 1988.)

The telencephalic or cerebral vesicles, when these first arise, communicate widely with the cavity of the third ventricle (Fig. 6–2). Along the choroidal fissure, the medial wall of the developing cerebral hemisphere becomes thin. It is at this site that invaginations of vascular pia form the choroid plexus of the lateral ventricles. The expanding hemispheres progressively cover the surfaces of the diencephalon, the midbrain, and ultimately, the hindbrain (Fig. 6–3). As the hemispheres grow and meet in the midline, mesenchyme is trapped and gives rise to the falx cerebri. This sequence discretely separates the lateral ventricles from the third ventricle. At this early stage, only the frontal horns, bodies, and atria of the lateral ventricles exist (Fig. 6–4). Growth of the temporal and occipital lobes eventuates in the formation of discrete occipital and temporal horns.[10] These are not clearly demarcated until 16 to 18 weeks.

In the sixth week of development (eight weeks since the LNMP), a swelling appears in the floor of each cerebral vesicle. This structure is known as the corpus striatum. As the cerebral cortex develops further, fibers pass to and from the developing hemispheres through the corpus striatum, dividing it into the caudate and lentiform nuclei. This fiber path is the internal capsule.

The mesencephalon undergoes less change than other parts of the developing brain. The lumen of this vesicle narrows to form the sylvian aqueduct. Four large groups of neurons, known as the superior and inferior colliculi (quadrigeminal body), form in the roof of the midbrain. In the basal portion of the midbrain, fibers passing from the growing cerebrum form the cerebral peduncles. A broad layer of gray matter adjacent to these large fiber tracts is known as the substantia nigra.

The rhombencephalon undergoes flexion (the pontine flexure) that divides the hindbrain into the metencephalon and myelencephalon. The myelencephalon changes little and becomes the medulla, whereas the metencephalon changes dramatically and gives rise to the pons and cerebellum. The cerebellum originates from paired symmetric swellings dorsally positioned. The fourth ventricle forms from the cavity of the hindbrain and, like the lateral and third ventricles, contains choroid plexus derived from an invagination of vascular pia into the ependyma-lined cavity of the hindbrain.

A substantial number of brain anomalies are already present when the early process of brain development is complete (anencephaly, holoprosencephaly, Dandy-Walker malformation, encephalocele, and others)

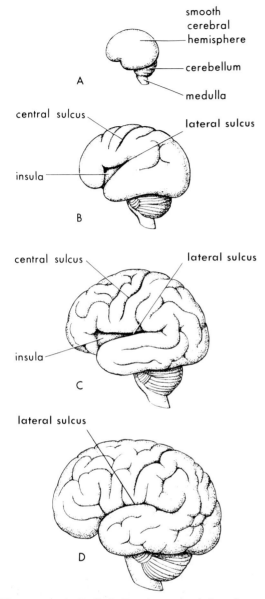

Figure 6–3. *A, B, C, D,* Development of the telencephalon, demonstrating dramatic growth with progressive development of the fissures and sulci. The open lateral sulcus matures into the sylvian cistern. The exposed insula "disappears" behind the temporal and parietal opercula. (*From* Moore KL: The Developing Human: Clinically Oriented Embryology, 4th Ed. Philadelphia, WB Saunders Co, 1988.)

Normal Sonographic Anatomy of the Fetal Brain

The fetal brain was one of the first areas of investigational interest in the diagnosis of fetal anomalies.[2] This was a result of two factors: the fetal head was imaged routinely to obtain a biparietal diameter for the determination of gestational age, and CNS anom-

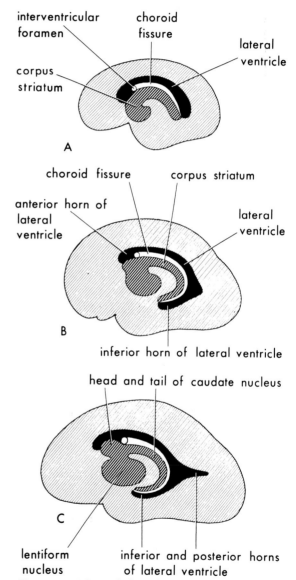

Figure 6–4. The early lateral ventricle *(A)* consists of the frontal horn, body, and atrium. Later, temporal *(B)* and occipital *(C)* horns develop; sonography can visualize the fetal ventricular system before these structures develop. (*From* Moore KL: The Developing Human: Clinically Oriented Embryology, 4th Ed. Philadelphia, WB Saunders Co, 1988.)

but are usually not recognizable on sonograms until later in gestation. Further growth of the calvarium and progressive aberration of brain development do, however, enable sonographers to recognize some of these abnormalities near the end of the first and beginning of the second trimester.

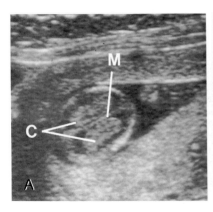

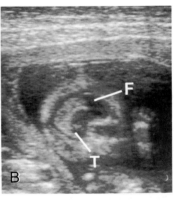

Figure 6–5. *A*, Transverse axial sonogram through the calvarium of a 12 week fetus (19 mm BPD). The division (M) of the hemispheres is well seen. The brightly echogenic choroid (C) dominates the hemisphere, filling nearly the entire ventricle, except the frontal horn. The relatively lucent brain parenchyma is only a thin rim about the ventricles. *B*, Parasagittal sonogram shows the choroid plexus filling the early ventricle. The frontal horn (F) is demarcated by specular reflectors. The early temporal horn (T) is seen.

alies are among the most common birth defects. At first, only gross morphologic aberrations, such as anencephaly or advanced hydrocephalus, were discovered prenatally. As instrumentation has improved to its present state, many malformations of the brain can now be diagnosed with accuracy even before 20 weeks of development.[1, 3–7]

The path to the diagnosis of anomalous development, as always, begins with thorough understanding of normal developmental neuroanatomy. Initially, many errors were made when normal fetal intracranial anatomy was interpreted sonographically.[14, 19, 22] This was due to the unusual circumstance that "fluid" and "solid" areas of the brain did not behave in an anticipated fashion. It was initially expected that the sono-

graphic appearance of the lateral ventricles would be dominated by cerebrospinal fluid (CSF) that would render them echolucent. Instead, their appearance was dominated by highly echogenic choroid plexus (Fig. 6–5).[17, 26] Conversely, the bulk of neural tissue, the telencephalon, diencephalon, and mesencephalon, is quite echopenic compared with other solid tissues in the human body (Fig. 6–6).[11, 17] The more recent entrant into the area of diagnostic sonography can well imagine the potential for misinterpretation among early researchers when the largest fluid-containing areas of the brain yielded the greatest amplitude echoes while the solid tissue yielded the lowest. To further complicate matters, dramatic changes occur as brain development progresses that result

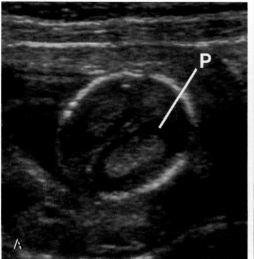

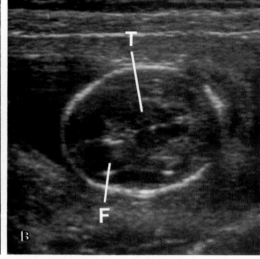

Figure 6–6. *A*, Axial scan at the level of the lateral ventricular atria. The brain parenchyma (P) is very lucent. *B*, Slightly lower scan demonstrates the well-developed thalami (T) and midbrain (27 mm BPD = 14 weeks). The frontal horns (F) are large and filled with CSF.

in ever-changing positions of certain "land-marks" (Fig. 6–3). These changes had never been observed in vivo, and a postmortem examination of the brain can be at variance with its appearance during life.

A series of key observations led to the clear delineation of normal developmental neuroanatomy as viewed by ultrasound. These observations included recognition of the fetal third ventricle, the brightly echogenic choroid plexus,[17] and the pulsating vasculature in several cisterns;[11] the first two identified the supratentorial ventricular system, whereas the last enabled identification of the sylvian cistern (middle cerebral artery pulsation), interpeduncular cistern (basilar artery pulsation), and ambient cisterns (posterior cerebral artery pulsations). The landmarks established by these observations provided a framework for subsequent identification of other specific neural structures.

Later in the course of the development of sonography, the neonatal brain came under study.[26–28] Interestingly, this resulted in much greater understanding of the appearance of the *fetal* brain since examination of "newborn children" now commonly begins at 25 to 26 weeks of development (essentially a second trimester fetus). Investigators then began to apply neuroanatomy as learned from the neonatal brain, which was imaged with great clarity through the anterior fontanelle, to the developing fetal brain. The following analysis of fetal intracranial anatomy is presented on the basis of these observations.

The fetal head can be clearly discriminated from the fetal torso when an embryo reaches a crown-rump length of approximately 10 to 15 mm. By the tenth to 11th weeks after the LNMP, one can already begin to appreciate symmetric anatomy inside the developing fetal calvarium. At this point, the intracranial tissue components consist almost entirely of the thalamus and corpus striatum that yield the symmetric appearance of the brain, as these structures narrow the developing third ventricle into a midline specular reflector.

By the end of the first trimester, the thalamus, third ventricle, midbrain, brainstem, and cerebellar hemispheres have achieved an appearance that will remain largely unchanged, other than progressively enlarging, throughout the remaining period of sonographic observation of the fetus (Fig. 6–7).

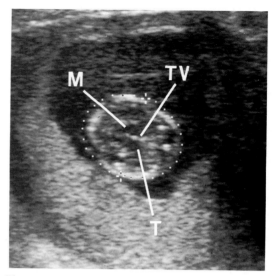

Figure 6–7. Transverse axial sonogram of a 12.5 week fetus (22 mm BPD) already demonstrates the thalami (T), third ventricle (TV), and midbrain (M).

Therefore, the vast majority of the changes that are observed (and they are substantial) relate to the growth and development of the telencephalon. As mentioned, by the end of the first and beginning of the second trimester, the sonographic appearance of the telencephalon is dominated by the lateral ventricles (Figs. 6–5, 6–6). These, in turn, are dominated by the brightly echogenic choroid plexus. By 12 to 13 weeks, the lateral ventricles are clearly seen, appear ovoid in shape, and are largely filled with choroid plexus. Only the frontal horns are devoid of choroid plexus, as they are throughout life (Figs. 6–5, 6–6). At this stage of development, only the rudiments of a temporal (Fig. 6–5B) and an occipital horn are present. The frontal horn, body of the ventricle, and atrium of the ventricle are large and easily detected. The choroid is the easiest structure to recognize because of its size and high-amplitude echogenicity. Conversely, the mantle of developing cerebral cortex surrounding the lateral ventricle is more difficult to delineate because of its low-amplitude echogenicity, but a demarcation between the lateral ventricle and the cerebral mantle can be appreciated from specular reflections arising from the walls of the lateral ventricle (Figs. 6–5B, 6–6B). These, of course, are seen where the acoustic beam intersects the ventricular wall perpendicularly. By 18 weeks, the mantle of developing cortical tissue has thickened appreciably (Fig. 6–8).

The relative echogenicity of structures, which will be viewed throughout the remainder of gestation, is largely established at this time. Two types of tissues are brightly echogenic and are therefore most easily seen during the examination of the fetal brain. These tissues are the choroid plexus, as noted above, and the brain coverings, the dura (pachymeninx) and pia-arachnoid (leptomeninx). Interestingly, the choroid develops from the vascular pia. The leptomeninges demarcate the edges of the brain with a brightly reflective margin of echoes (Figs. 6–9, 6–10). Peripheral to this echogenic margin are the subarachnoid spaces that contain CSF. A feature that confounds the inexperienced sonographer is the relative lack of change in echogenicity between the peripheral, i.e., cortical brain, tissue and the CSF space as seen across the brightly reflecting marginal echo from the pia-arachnoid; indeed, the CSF-containing space may be more echogenic (Fig. 6–11). This perceptual problem originates from the anticipation that the subarachnoid spaces should be anechoic whereas the brain parenchyma should be echogenic. This reasonable assumption is untrue in many instances. Recall that these spaces have both CSF and pia-arachnoid tissue within them. *It is the relative amount of these two components that determines*

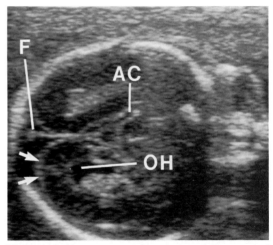

Figure 6–9. Transverse axial sonogram of the occipital lobes and occipital horns (OH). The brain edge is marginated by bright echoes, the pia-arachnoid *(arrows)*. The cisterns over the brain surface have visible CSF. F, falx; AC, ambient cistern.

the sonographic appearance of the subarachnoid spaces. Small subarachnoid cisterns, such as the basal and perimesencephalic cisterns, have an appearance dominated by pia-arachnoid and thus are seen as brightly echogenic spaces (Fig. 6–11). This is not to say that these cisterns are devoid of CSF, but the fluid does not signif-

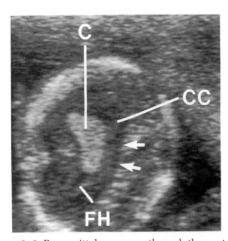

Figure 6–8. Parasagittal sonogram through the ventricle of an 18 week fetus. The choroid (C) defines the ventricular size. Note the substantial increase in cortical brain (CC) thickness compared with that of fetuses only a few weeks younger (see Fig. 6–5B). Bright echoes marginate the edge of the telencephalon *(arrows)*. FH, frontal horn.

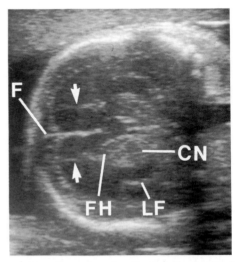

Figure 6–10. Coronal section through the heads of the caudate nuclei (CN). The frontal horn (FH), not well seen, drapes over the caudate. Extending between the ventricular margin and the edge of the brain are linear echoing structures previously mistaken for ventricles *(arrows)*. Also seen are bridging strands of pia-arachnoid through the cisterns over the convexities (probably bridging veins convered with pia-arachnoid). F, falx; LF, lateral fissure.

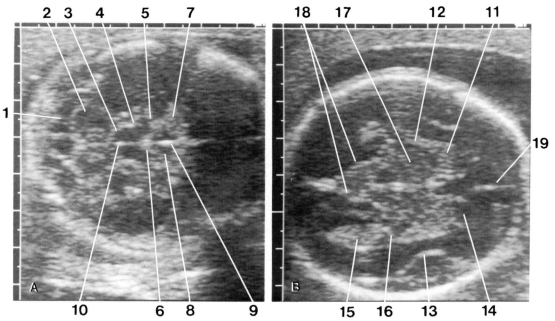

Figure 6–11. *A, B,* Transverse axial sonograms demonstrating many discrete neural structures. Note the varying echogenicities of the cisterns. Large cisterns (1 = cisterna magna) have an appearance dominated by CSF. Small cisterns (7 = basal cisterns) are dominated by pia-arachnoid. 2 = cerebellar hemisphere; 3 = quadrigeminal cistern; 4 = ambient cistern; 5 = crural cistern; 6 = interpeduncular cistern (note the walls of the basilar artery centrally in this cistern); 8 = hypothalamus; 9 = inferior recess of third ventricle; 10 = sylvian aqueduct; 11 = head of caudate; 12 = lentiform nuclei; 13 = lateral fissure; 14 = frontal horn; 15 = atrial choroid; 16 = posterior limb of internal capsule; 17 = thalamus; 18 = tentorial hiatus; 19 = falx.

icantly influence their sonographic appearance. Conversely, larger subarachnoid spaces, such as those over the convexities of the hemispheres (Fig. 6–9) and the cisterna magna (Fig. 6–11), have an appearance dominated by CSF. Thus, they behave sonographically as one would expect a fluid-containing cavity to behave. Intermediate-sized subarachnoid spaces will have both anechoic zones from visible CSF and brightly echogenic zones from visible pia-arachnoid tissues (Fig. 6–10).

As noted above, brightly reflecting structures dominate the appearance of the fetal brain as seen by the sonographer. The choroid plexus and brain coverings (pia-arachnoid and dura) are the two major components within the developing calvarium that produce bright reflections. The important dural structures from the perspective of sonographic fetal brain anatomy are the falx and tentorium (Figs. 6–10, 6–11). However, the choroid and meninges are not exclusively the bright reflectors. An occasional neural structure generates high-amplitude reflections, most commonly the cerebellar vermis.

Specular reflections from the walls of the ventricular system are also important high-amplitude echoing structures (Figs. 6–9 to 6–11). Such reflections occur when the ultrasonic beam strikes the smooth ventricular wall perpendicularly or nearly so. Thus, one would assume that points and lines of brightness so produced might vary from moment to moment, depending on the direction the transducer was pointed. This, however, is not the case for two reasons. First, fetal brain images are predominantly produced in transverse axial planes (appropriate for both BPD and head circumference measurements) and less commonly in coronal planes. In both these planes, the beam tends to intersect the ventricular system perpendicularly at the same interfaces. Second, the curvature of the bony calvarium limits the number of axial and coronal planes that can be achieved because of significant beam divergence when curved portions of the calvarium are intersected by the beam. Thus, the specular reflections from the ventricular walls tend to be seen in stable locations and can be employed as important and reproducible anatomic landmarks.

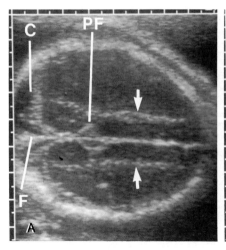

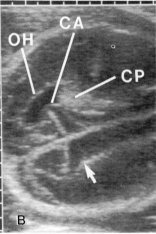

Figure 6–12. A, Transverse axial sonogram near the vertex. Bright linear echoes (arrows), often mistaken for lateral ventricles, are clearly seen. Note that these extend to the brain edge. PF, parieto-occipital fissure; F, falx; C, convexity cistern with CSF. B, Off-axis scan through both the lateral ventricle and the linear echo (arrow) seen in A. The occipital horn (OH) is now well seen. Note again that the linear echo extends to the brain edge but the occipital horn is entirely marginated by brain tissue. CP, choroid plexus; CA, calcar avis.

Additionally, within the substance of the brain, most notably in the region of the cerebral white matter tracks, other bright reflections are noted (Figs. 6–12, 6–13). Earlier, these reflectors were mistaken for the lateral ventricular walls, with which they are contiguous.[11, 22, 23] The exact origin of these reflections remains undecided, but the most likely candidates are blood vessels supplying the deeper white matter regions, particularly venous structures.

The sonographic "skeleton" of the developing fetal brain originates from the brightly reflective structures considered in Table 6–1. With these structures serving as a framework, numerous discrete neural tissue areas are discernible sonographically.[27, 28] As the brain develops, multiple areas of the telencephalon, diencephalon, midbrain, pons, and cerebellum become anatomically identifiable. These are recognized by variations in the echogenicity of specific nuclei and tracts that pass through these zones. Several brain nuclei, as well as some other areas of neural tissue, demonstrate a moderate increase in echo amplitude compared with surrounding brain elements. These nuclei demonstrate lower amplitude signals than choroid or leptomeninges. Among these structures are the caudate and lenticular nuclei, separated by the internal capsule. Less commonly, the claustrum, marginated

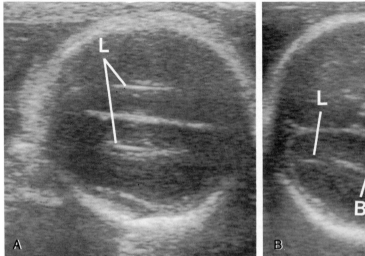

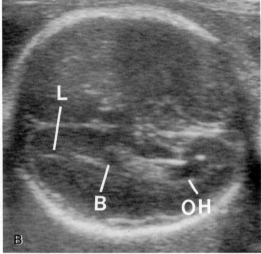

Figure 6–13. A, Transverse axial scan demonstrates linear echoes (L) in the white matter. B, Slightly lower, the body (B) and occipital horn (OH) are clearly seen. The linear echoes (L) in the white matter are clearly not the wall of the ventricle.

Table 6–1. BRIGHTLY REFLECTIVE STRUCTURES IN THE DEVELOPING FETAL BRAIN

1. Choroid plexus
2. Pia-arachnoid (leptomeninges)
3. Dura (pachymeninges)
4. Cerebellar vermis
5. Specular reflections from ventricular walls
6. Deeply penetrating veins?

by the extreme and external capsules, is visible. Similarly, the substantia nigra in the midbrain and the dentate nuclei of the cerebellum are discernible. Also, the pars ventralis (belly) of the pons is seen as a zone of moderate echogenicity, as opposed to the pars dorsalis (tegmentum), which returns low-amplitude echoes.[27] Specific structures are illustrated in Figures 6–9 to 6–11 and 6–14 to 6–19.

It is important for sonographers to be familiar with the appearance of the lateral ventricles as they change throughout growth and development of the fetal brain. By 18 to 20 weeks, easily recognizable occipital and temporal horns are visible; the lateral ventricles have achieved their adult components. From this point onward, the lateral ventricles change in shape and proportion as influenced by neural tissues growing adjacent to their walls. For example, the growth of the caudate nucleus markedly reshapes the lateral ventricles.[10] However,

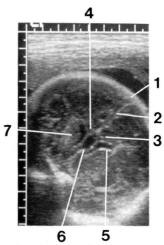

Figure 6–15. Anterior coronal sonogram. 1 = superior sagittal sinus; 2 = falx; 3 = cingulate gyrus; 4 = corpus callosum; 5 = frontal horn; 6 = cavum septi pellucidi; 7 = caudate head.

throughout the period of observation of fetal lateral ventricles, from 13 to 40 weeks, the size of the atria remains largely unchanged. The transverse diameter of the ventricular atrium at the level of the glomus of the choroid plexus shows an average dimension of 8 mm and a range of 6 to 10 mm throughout the second and third trimesters.[29] This is the most convenient area to recognize fetal ventricular enlargement, as will be discussed in detail in the section on ventriculomegaly.[17, 26, 29] It is important to note that

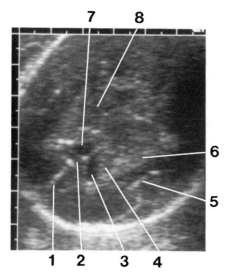

Figure 6–14. Transverse axial sonogram. 1 = falx; 2 = corpus callosum; 3 = frontal horn; 4 = caudate nucleus; 5 = lateral fissure; 6 = lentiform nuclei; 7 = cavum septi pellucidi; 8 = thalamus.

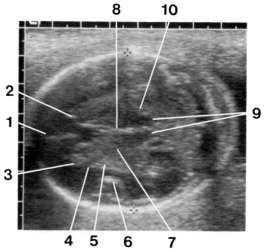

Figure 6–16. Transverse axial sonogram. 1 = falx; 2 = frontal horn; 3 = caudate head; 4 = anterior limb of internal capsule; 5 = lentiform nuclei; 6 = lateral sulcus; 7 = thalamus; 8 = third ventricle; 9 = quadrigeminal bodies; 10 = ambient cistern.

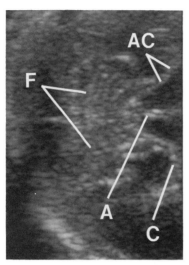

Figure 6–17. Posterior fossa view (axial) demonstrating the folia (F) of the cerebellum. AC, ambient cistern; A, sylvian aqueduct; C, choroidal fissure.

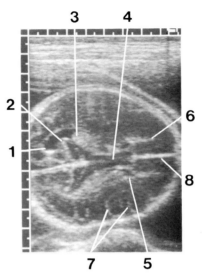

Figure 6–19. Transverse axial sonogram. 1 = occipital horn; 2 = calcar avis; 3 = atrial choroid; 4 = corpus callosum; 5 = frontal horn; 6 = linear echo in white matter (see Fig. 6–12); 7 = sulci; 8 = falx.

the anterior and occipital horns of the lateral ventricles do not possess choroid plexus. Between 24 weeks and term, the telencephalon undergoes little structural change other than increased cortical growth and the consequent increase in convolutions (and thus sulcal markings) that can be recognized adjacent to the convexities (Fig. 6–19).[20] The increase in brain volume causes the lateral ventricles, which are more stable in volume, to become progressively less conspicuous.

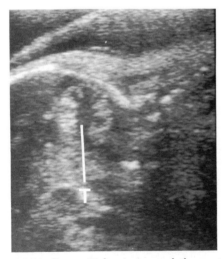

Figure 6–18. Parasagittal sonogram of the posterior fossa. Cerebellar white matter tracts (T) are well seen. The bright margin is most likely due to reflections from the folia. Gray matter is hypoechoic.

As opposed to sulci, which are narrow and develop later as gyri form, fissures are present earlier in development and can be seen before 20 weeks. Of the two that are commonly seen, the parieto-occipital fissure is smaller and less important (Fig. 6–12). The lateral fissure is a deep groove in the margin of the developing telencephalon.[19] This important fissure creates frequent confusion since it causes a portion of the brain surface to be invaginated deeply into the hemisphere (Figs. 6–10, 6–11, 6–14). The pia-arachnoid on the surface of the insula, the tissue at the base of the lateral fissure, generates a curvilinear reflection that appears to lie within the brain substance rather than at its "edge." This echo is often mistaken for a specular reflection from the lateral wall of the lateral ventricle, an error leading to misdiagnoses of hydrocephalus. With progressive growth of the temporal and parietal lobes, this fissure progressively closes, burying the previously exposed insular cortex behind the developing temporal and parietal opercula (Fig. 6–3). By term (38 to 42 weeks), the lateral fissure closes and ultimately becomes the sylvian cistern complex.

One of the difficulties in mastering the sonographic anatomy of intracranial structures is the usual inability to see both hemispheres of the brain simultaneously.[21] The hemisphere nearest to the transducer is virtually always "clouded" over by reverberation artifacts generated as the acoustic beam passes through the near calvarial wall. Calvarial ossification appears to be at the root of this problem since the artifact is markedly reduced in fetuses with recessive osteogenesis imperfecta or other bone dysplasias wherein calvarial ossification is nearly absent (Figs. 6–12, 6–20). Unfortunately, essentially all other fetuses possess calvarial ossification. The following rule should always be applied: *the sonographer must assume that a fetus' intracranial anatomy is symmetric, whether normal or abnormal, unless images document an asymmetry.*

Fetal Spine

The fetal spine is seen well from 15 to 16 weeks onward. However, evaluation for a suspected myelomeningocele is often delayed until 18 to 22 weeks of gestation. This is due to significant and favorable maturational changes in the spine that occur during this period. The fetal vertebra is composed of three ossification centers (Fig. 6–21). The anterior center generates the vertebral body, while the posterior ossification centers (POC) form the neural arch. The POC begin at the base of the transverse processes (Fig. 6–21). As ossification progresses, the laminae become visible (Fig. 6–22A, B). The inward angulation of the normal laminae is the opposite of the outward splaying of the

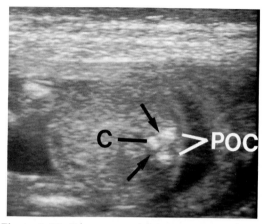

Figure 6–21. Transverse axial sonogram through the lumbar spine of an 18 week fetus. The three ossification centers of the vertebra are well seen: C, centrum; POC, posterior ossification centers; *arrows*, neurocentral synchondrosis.

laminae seen in spina bifida (see the section on myelomeningocele—spina bifida), an optimal situation for detecting this anomaly. Spina bifida, of course, is the bone anomaly seen in all myelomeningoceles. The spinal cord neural tissue, like that of most brain tissue, is echopenic (Figs. 6–22C, D, 6–23). The conus medullaris (Fig. 6–22D) and the craniocervical junction (Fig. 6–23) can be seen, albeit inconsistently, in older fetuses. The tissues surrounding the cord (leptomeninges) are brightly echogenic as are those that surround the brain, and the dura is usually also seen discretely as a linear bright reflector (Fig. 6–22C, D).

INFRATENTORIAL ANOMALIES

Dandy-Walker Syndrome

The Dandy-Walker syndrome (DWS) is a spectrum of disorders resulting from abnormal development of the cerebellum with associated maldevelopment of the fourth ventricle.[30, 31] The fundamental features include enlargement of the fourth ventricle, atresia of the Luschka and Magendie foramina (although these may be patent), agenesis or hypoplasia of the cerebellar vermis, and hydrocephalus of a variable degree.

The enlargement of the fourth ventricle is often dramatic, such that a large cyst occupies and expands the posterior fossa (the Dandy-Walker cyst) (Fig. 6–24). The expan-

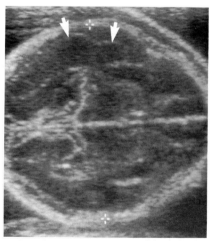

Figure 6–20. Transverse axial sonogram in a fetus with little calcification of the calvarium (recessive osteogenesis imperfecta). Note the lack of a near calvarial reverberation artifact. *Arrows*, near edge of the temporal lobe.

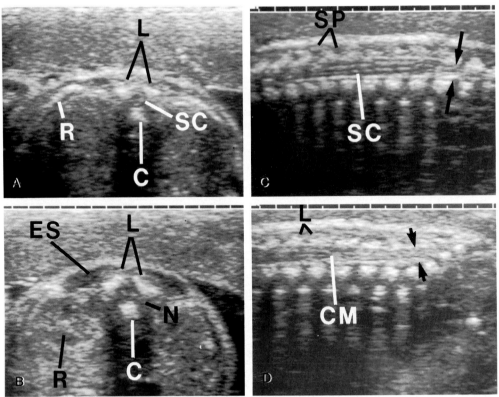

Figure 6–22. A, B, Axial sections of a 27 week fetus' lumbar spine. L, laminae; SC, spinal canal; C, centrum; N, neurocentral synchondrosis; R, rib; ES, erector spinus muscle. C, D, Longitudinal scans of the thoracolumbar (C) and lumbosacral (D) spines. SP, spinous process (in cartilage); L, laminae; SC, spinal cord (note the bright linear echo from the central canal); CM, conus medullaris; *arrows*, dura. (*From* Filly RA, Simpson GF, Linkowski GD: Fetal spine morphology and maturation during the second trimester. J Ultrasound Med 6:631, 1987.

sion elevates the tentorium and torcula.[30, 31] The former can be easily seen sonographically, the latter cannot. The cyst covering is the posterior medullary vellum, which bulges upward in the presence of the vermal defect. Thus, the inner cellular layer of the cyst is ependyma and the outer layer is pia-arachnoid.[31] There is a potential for great variation in both the size of the fourth ventricle and the degree of dysgenesis of the vermis, features that obviously affect the ease of detection of this anomaly in utero. This anomaly is established early in the development of the fetus and can often be detected early (Fig. 6–25).

DWS is commonly associated with hydrocephalus (Fig. 6–26) and agenesis of the corpus callosum (ACC) (Fig. 6–27).[30, 31] Hydrocephalus may dominate the dysmorphic appearance. Importantly, colpocephaly, associated with callosal agenesis, may be misinterpreted as a Dandy-Walker malformation (DWM) (Fig. 6–27) (see the section on agenesis of the corpus callosum). The degree of

supratentorial ventricular enlargement does not correlate with patency of the foramina, vermal hypoplasia, or size of the fourth ventricular cyst (Fig. 6–26). When the defect in the vermis is small (usually inferior), the

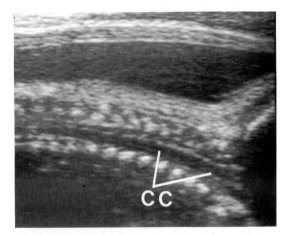

Figure 6–23. Longitudinal sonogram at the craniocervical junction, demonstrating the cervical cord (CC).

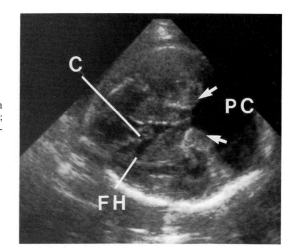

Figure 6–24. Transverse axial sonogram of a fetus with Dandy-Walker syndrome (DWS). PC, posterior fossa cyst; FH, frontal horn; C, cavum septi pellucidi; *arrows*, cerebellar hemispheres.

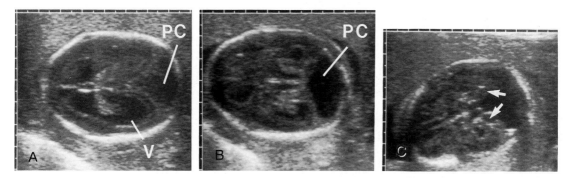

Figure 6–25. *A*, Transverse axial sonogram demonstrates a posterior fossa cyst (PC) and ventricular enlargement (V). *B*, Large posterior fossa cyst (PC). *C*, Small and separated cerebellar hemispheres (*arrows*).

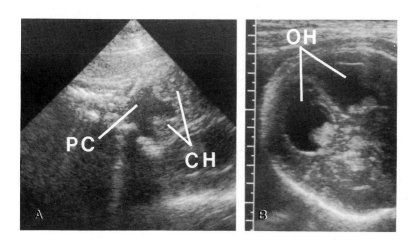

Figure 6–26. *A*, Sonogram of the posterior fossa. PC, relatively small posterior fossa cyst; CH, cerebellar hemisphere. *B*, Note the marked dilatation of the occipital horns (OH). Compare with Figure 6–24.

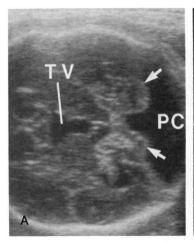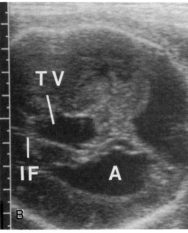

Figure 6–27. A, Transverse axial sonogram of a fetus with a Dandy-Walker malformation (DWM) and callosal agenesis. A large posterior fossa cyst (PC) insinuates itself between the cerebellar hemispheres (arrows). TV, enlarged and abnormally shaped third ventricle. B, Transverse axial sonogram showing colpocephaly (enlarged atrium [A]). The third ventricle (TV) lies high and insinuates itself into the interhemispheric fissue (IF).

fourth ventricle bulges into the void provided by the cisterna magna. Indeed, this space may only appear somewhat larger than average under these circumstances, the enlarged fourth ventricle generating no mass effect. Evaluation of the "large" cisterna magna is discussed in detail subsequently.

It is difficult to ignore that the structures involved in this complex malformation include the vermis, posterior medullary velum, fourth ventricle, and corpus callosum. All are midline structures. This anomaly appears to be most appropriately categorized with other midline anomalies; however, since the major dysmorphic features reside in the posterior fossa, it tends to be treated independently in differential diagnostic considerations.

Although the features of this malformation are often "classic" and easily recognized,[33, 39] its differential diagnosis from other posterior fossa aberrations is extremely important since prognosis varies from normal to marked disability, depending on the severity of brain malformation and the association of anomalies outside the CNS.[30, 31] The sine qua non for firm diagnosis of DWS is separation of the cerebellar hemispheres by the enlarged fourth ventricle (Figs. 6–24 to 6–27). Thus, it is not the presence of the large posterior fossa fluid collection that enables the diagnosis but the effect of the fluid collection on the cerebellum. When the DW cyst is large, the cerebellar hemispheres are widely displaced and compressed against the tentorium (Figs. 6–24, 6–25). Additionally, the hemispheres are small both in absolute mass from compression by the cyst. Therefore, they must be carefully sought.

The major competing diagnosis when a large posterior fossa cyst is seen is that of an arachnoid cyst (Figs. 6–28, 6–29).[33] A retrocerebellar arachnoid cyst is a less common and more benign abnormality than DWS since the underlying brain is normally formed. This lesion always generates a mass effect, but instead of the cystic mass separating the cerebellar hemispheres, it displaces these en bloc (Figs. 6–28, 6–29). Such a mass may well elevate the tentorium (Fig. 6–28). Thus, this feature is not differentially diagnostic.

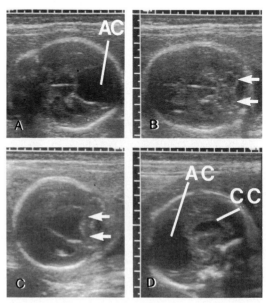

Figure 6–28. Axial (A, B), coronal (C), and midsagittal (D) sonograms of a fetus with a retrocerebellar arachnoid cyst (AC). Note that the cerebellar hemispheres (arrows) are not separated. CC, corpus callosum.

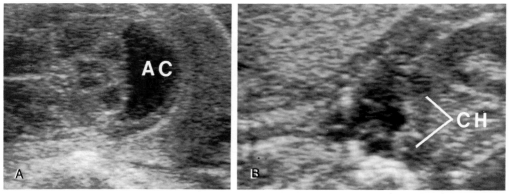

Figure 6–29. Transverse axial *(A)* and coronal *(B)* scans of a retrocerebellar arachnoid cyst (AC) versus a large cisterna magna. Note that the fluid collection does not affect the junction of the cerebellar hemispheres (CH).

It is important in the evaluation of a fetus with a posterior fossa cyst to carefully examine the supratentorial compartment. As noted above, ventriculomegaly may be present and may represent true hydrocephalus or colpocephaly associated with ACC. The features of ACC should be sought, as discussed in a later section. Large retrocerebellar arachnoid cysts may also produce ventricular enlargement by compression but are not associated with ACC or colpocephaly.

Other Infratentorial Abnormalities

In the preceding section, the diagnosis of DWS and its distinction from a retrocerebellar arachnoid cyst were considered. These entities have a similar appearance when a large cyst is generated by the underlying abnormality. However, the most difficult situation arises when the cisterna magna appears large.[40, 42] Since several congenital posterior fossa lesions alter the size of the cisterna magna, evaluation of this structure is of paramount importance in assessing fetal infratentorial anatomy and pathology.[18, 40] The cisterna magna constitutes a portion of the subarachnoid space that bathes the posterior fosssa with CSF. It arches around the cerebellum posteriorly and is normally deepest in the midline, where invagination of the space occurs between the two cerebellar hemispheres. Antenatal sonography readily demonstrates the cisterna magna, especially between 16 to 28 menstrual weeks (Fig. 6–30). Evaluation of the cisterna magna in utero has documented that its depth measures 5 ± 3 mm; the largest one measured was 10 mm in depth.[18, 40] However, the overzealous inclination of the plane of section through the posterior fossa can increase this measurement to 13 or 14 mm. As expected, this is not significantly different from that in preterm newborns.[32]

When the cisterna magna appears enlarged, it becomes incumbent upon the examiner to distinguish between the competing diagnoses of normal variant, communicating hydrocephalus, cerebellar hypoplasia, and DWS, and retrocerebellar arachnoid cyst (Figs. 6–29, 6–31). Cerebellar hypoplasia can be excluded by measuring the diameter of the cerebellar hemispheres

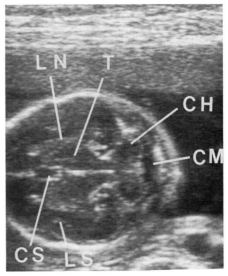

Figure 6–30. Normal cisterna magna (CM). CH, cerebellar hemispheres; T, thalamus; LN, lentiform nuclei; CS, cavum septi pellucidi; LS, lateral sulcus.

and comparing this measurement with published standards of size versus menstrual age (Fig. 6–31, Table 6–2).[41] Exclusion of this entity is important since it is associated with chromosomal anomalies; therefore, when its presence is suspected, karyotyping is indicated.

Communicating hydrocephalus is rare in fetuses, and its presence is promptly excluded when the absence of ventricular dilatation is noted. Usually, in the circumstance under consideration, only the enlarged cisterna magna is evident. Finally, close examination of the junction of the cerebellar hemispheres is indicated to look for clefting, as may been seen with small DWMs. An enlarged cisterna magna (Fig. 6–31), as a normal variant, or a small retrocerebellar arachnoid cyst is thus a diagnosis of exclusion. Since it is essentially impossible to exclude subtle vermal dysgenesis with in utero sonography alone, these benign presumptive diagnoses are unsettling. Some consolation may be taken from the relatively benign course of mild cases of DWS; patients

Table 6–2. GESTATIONAL AGE VERSUS CEREBELLAR DIAMETER

Gestational Age (weeks)	Cerebellum (mm)				
	Percentiles				
	10	25	50	75	90
15	10	12	14	15	16
16	14	16	16	16	17
17	16	17	17	18	18
18	17	18	18	19	19
19	18	18	19	19	22
20	18	19	20	20	22
21	19	20	22	23	24
22	21	23	23	24	24
23	22	23	24	25	26
24	22	24	25	27	28
25	23	21.5	28	28	29
26	25	28	29	30	32
27	26	28.5	30	31	32
28	27	30	31	32	34
29	29	32	34	36	38
30	31	32	35	37	40
31	32	35	38	39	43
32	33	36	38	40	42
33	32	36	40	43	44
34	33	38	40	41	44
35	31	37	40.5	43	47
36	36	29	43	52	55
37	37	37	45	52	55
38	40	40	48.5	52	55
39	52	52	52	55	55

(*From* Goldstein I, Reece A, Pilu G, et al: Cerebellar measurements with ultrasonography in the evaluation of fetal growth and development. Am J Obstet Gynecol 156:1065, 1987.)

so affected may develop normally. Indeed, inferior vermal agenesis may be an entity entirely different from DWS.

SUPRATENTORIAL ANOMALIES

Agenesis of the Corpus Callosum

The corpus callosum is the largest fiber tract within the central nervous system.[43–45] The fetal corpus callosum is much smaller than the adult one. However, sonographic resolution is sufficiently good that this structure can occasionally be detected in fetuses of less than 20 weeks' gestational age (Figs. 6–14, 6–15, 6–28). This fiber tract is composed of commissural fibers that radiate between symmetric regions of the cerebral cortex and serves a function, in both learning and memory, that is shared between cerebral hemispheres.[43]

Development of the corpus callosum does not begin until the 8th week and remains

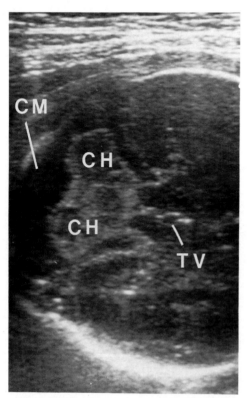

Figure 6–31. Transverse axial sonogram of a large cisterna magna (CM). Note the normal-sized and normally jointed cerebellar hemispheres (CH). TV, normal third ventricle.

incomplete until the 17th week.[46] Therefore, by comparison with most CNS structures, its development is extraordinarily late. Development begins anteriorly (genu) and proceeds posteriorly (splenium). Partial interruption of callosal development therefore tends to affect the posterior aspect of this large fiber tract. The septum pellucidum, which forms concomitantly with the corpus callosum, stretches between the corpus callosum and the fornices, a feature important in the sonographic exclusion of anomalous development of this structure.

Dysgenesis of the corpus callosum ranges from complete absence to partial absence. When partially absent, as noted above, the abnormality usually lies in the region of the splenium (most dorsal portion).[43–46] Thus far, only complete agenesis of the corpus callosum (ACC) has been diagnosed in utero by sonography.[47] The appearance of complete ACC is typical on sectional imaging studies of the newborn, such as computed tomography, transfontanelle ultrasonography, and magnetic resonance imaging.[48–52] The characteristic features seen at birth extrapolate appropriately to the fetus.

The striking dysmorphic features relate to the changed appearance of the supratentorial ventricular system when the corpus callosum fails to develop. Indeed, the presence of the corpus callosum does much to shape the ventricles, as they are seen in normal fetuses. When the corpus callosum is agenetic, the fibers that were destined to cross in this tract still have developed, although now these fibers run in thick longitudinal (Probst) bundles along the medial walls of the lateral ventricles.[44] These bundles affect the appearance of the lateral ventricles in two ways: first, the ventricles are "displaced" more laterally; and second, the medial walls are "indented," resulting in the characteristic shape seen on coronal sections when this anomaly is present (Fig. 6–32). This latter appearance causes the ventricles to be crescentic in shape, and this appearance has been likened to the horns of a steer, especially when viewed on coronal planes in the frontal regions.

The absence of the large callosal tract over the roof of the ventricles allows them to extend more cranially. This is most evident when viewing the third ventricle but is true of the lateral ventricles as well (Fig. 6–33). Indeed, the third ventricle may, in some instances, expand dramatically, herniating upward between the hemispheres. This produces the so-called "interhemispheric" cyst, not infrequently seen in this anomaly.

Deep white matter of the cerebrum is poorly developed in this condition. This results in the feature that first draws the examiner's attention to possible maldevelopment of the brain. The poorly developed white matter surrounding the atria and occipital horns of the lateral ventricles causes a measurable enlargement of these portions of the lateral ventricles, termed colpocephaly (Fig. 6–27). This type of ventriculomegaly is important for two reasons: first, it initiates a critical evaluation of the CNS anatomy, hopefully ending in the correct diagnosis of ACC; and second, it is an excellent example that ventricular enlargement does not always equate with ventricular ob-

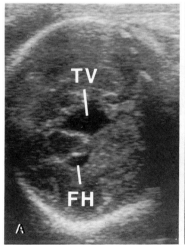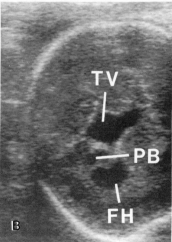

Figure 6–32. *A, B,* Anterior coronal sonograms of a fetus with agenesis of the corpus callosum. TV, enlarged and high-riding third ventricle. The frontal horns (FH) are indented medially by the Probst bundle (PB).

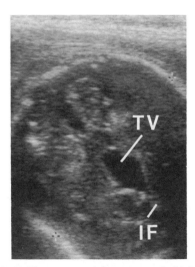

Figure 6–33. Transverse axial sonogram of a high-riding third ventricle (TV) insinuating itself into the interhemispheric fissure (IF).

struction. Although fetuses with ACC may develop true hydrocephalus, colpocephaly is not aided by shunting procedures.[45] When ventriculomegaly is noted in the atrial and occipital regions, i.e., possible colpocephaly, the association of midline developmental anomalies should be promptly excluded. Ordinarily, if one suspects ACC, an attempt should be made to demonstrate the corpus callosum. Unfortunately, this is a difficult structure to document consistently. Recall, however, that the development of the corpus callosum is integrally related to the development of the septum pellucidum and thus the cavum septi pellucidi.[43, 46] The latter is readily demonstrated in all fetuses with normal development of midline structures (Figs. 6–14 to 6–16). Thus, documentation of the cavum septi pellucidi excludes complete ACC.

The previously described elevation of the third ventricle, the medial indentation of the frontal horns, and the abnormal axis of the lateral ventricles should be sought sonographically to confirm the diagnosis of ACC. Finally, the missing corpus callosum creates an abnormal pattern of gyral development along the interhemispheric fissure that can be seen sonographically.[43] The sulci radiate toward the third ventricle, creating a wavy appearance of the midline in axial planes of section. Unfortunately, since gyri do not develop until late in pregnancy, this feature is not useful in the early diagnosis of ACC.

Although ACC may be seen as an isolated lesion, it is also associated with a variety of other central nervous system malformations and syndromes.[43] Associated CNS malformations include lobar through alobar holoprosencephaly. In alobar forms, ACC does not dominate the appearance of the CNS malformation, although it is always present. Conversely, in the lesser (lobar) forms of holoprosencephaly, this feature may dominate the sonographic picture. Interestingly, fetuses with isolated ACC may have the same type of central clefting of the lip that is commonly associated with lesser forms of holoprosencephaly. As noted in the preceding section, ACC is a common accompaniment to the DWM (Fig. 6–27). Other CNS malformations that may be present include dysgenesis or hypoplasia of the falx, cranial lipoma, and heterotopic gray matter. Importantly, as with holoprosencephaly, Trisomy 13 to 15 may be present, and karyotyping is indicated. Also Trisomy 8 and 18 have been recorded with ACC. Female fetuses with ACC are at risk for Aicardi's syndrome, which includes mental retardation and chorioretinopathy.

It is obvious that the prognosis in ACC may depend far more on the associated abnormalities than on the callosal agenesis itself. Sonography may overlook some of these important associated malformations. Although it is true that isolated agenesis may be asymptomatic, low intelligence occurs in 70 percent and seizures in 60 percent of cases.[43] Hydrocephalus requiring shunting, distinct from colpocephaly, may develop. There may be disturbances of hypothalamic function, as well.

Isolated complete ACC and minor forms of holoprosencephaly have some obvious similarities. Although they can be distinguished pathologically, one must assume, at present, that they cannot be accurately distinguished in utero. Thus, features suggesting one should result in a differential diagnosis that includes both. Pathologically, ACC has an absence of the lamina terminalis, but fornices are usually present; whereas in lobar holoprosencephaly, the lamina terminalis is thickened, and fornices are never present. In ACC the thalami are separated, usually more so than normal (i.e., enlarged third ventricle), whereas in lobar holoprosencephaly, they may be fused as in higher grades of holoprosencephaly (semilobar and alobar forms). Most of these discriminatory features cannot be seen in utero sonograms. However, fusion of the thalami may be discernible and, in some cases, may segregate these anomalies.

Holoprosencephaly

The term holoprosencephaly refers to a group of disorders stemming from a failure of normal forebrain development during early embryonic life.[53-56] The reported incidence of holoprosencephaly is approximately 0.6 per 1000 live births. Indeed, the term holoprosencephaly includes a series of complex disorders that range broadly in severity. In these disorders, a single embryologic defect affects the development of both the brain and face.[53] Normally, as discussed above, the processes of cleavage and diverticulation divide the prosencephalon into the diencephalon and telencephalon (cerebral vesicles). The latter eventually grow to meet in the midline, forming the falx and interhemispheric fissure. The optic vesicles and olfactory bulbs that evaginate from the prosencephalon early in development are frequently abnormal in the entity. In the most severe form of this disease (alobar holoprosencephaly), none of these processes have taken place.

The degree of disordered prosencephalic development determines the classification and, indeed, the clinical severity of holoprosencephaly.[53-56] In the most devastating lesion (alobar type), no cleavage of the prosencephalon has occurred.[55] The brain is small. Instead of a ventricular system with distinct lateral and third ventricles, a monoventricular cavity communicating with a dorsal sac is present. The thalamus and corpus striatum are fused. The corpus callosum, fornix, falx cerebri, optic tracts, and olfactory bulbs are absent. The midbrain, brainstem, and cerebellum are structurally normal. However, if hydrocephalus ensues, the significant mass effect of the large monoventricular cavity and dorsal sac may cause the posterior fossa contents to be hypoplastic.

With less severe developmental abnormalities of the prosencephalon, an intermediate form, semilobar holoprosencephaly, results.[53-56, 62] A monoventricular cavity with rudimentary occipital horns is present. A rudimentary falx and interhemispheric fissure form caudally, resulting in the partial formation and separation of discrete occipital lobes. The olfactory bulbs and corpus callosum are usually absent. Again, the thalami and basal ganglia tend to be fused.

At the opposite end of the spectrum is lobar holoprosencephaly, in which the appearance of the brain is more normal.[54, 63] The two hemispheres are usually well separated in this form of the disease, except in the rostral portion, where fusion usually occurs. The lateral ventricles are enlarged, although not necessarily obstructed, and frequently communicate broadly because of the absence of the septum pellucidum. However, the atria, occipital horns, and temporal horns are separate and individualized. The corpus callosum may be present, hypoplastic, or absent. The septum pellucidum, however, does not form in any type of holoprosencephaly, even the most mild lobar variety. Therefore, identification of a septum pellucidum or cavum septi pellucidi promptly excludes all forms of holoprosencephaly. However, when ventricular dilatation occurs in obstructive hydrocephalus, it is not always possible to demonstrate a septum pellucidum with confidence. The septum pellucidum is also absent in cases of complete ACC. Therefore, the inability to demonstrate a septum pellucidum does not confirm a diagnosis of lobar holoprosencephaly.

As noted above, this disorder frequently involves the face, and the facial deformations are commonly severe.[53, 55] Facial anomalies include cyclopia, ethmocephaly, cebocephaly, and median cleft lip. Cyclopia is a facial deformity characterized by median monophthalmia, synophthalmia, or anophthalmia. There is no nose or median facial bones. A proboscis is usually present and may be double (Figs. 6–34, 6–35). Hypognathia is seen in some cases. Ethmocephaly is the combination of ocular hypotelorism, usually severe, associated with a single or double proboscis. Again, the proboscis may be absent. Cebocephaly consists of ocular hypotelorism with the nose present; however, the nose demonstrates a single nostril. Less severe forms of facial dysmorphia include hypotelorism with a flat nose and median cleft lip. The more severe forms of facial dysmorphology are usually associated with alobar holoprosencephaly. Cyclopia and ethmocephaly are virtually always seen

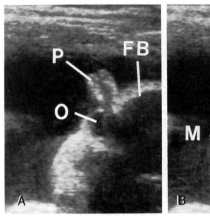
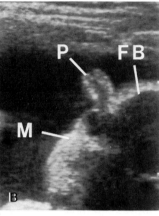

Figure 6–34. A, B, Two midsagittal sonograms of a fetus with cyclopia. FB, frontal bone; P, proboscis; O, orbit; M, absent maxillary bones.

with the alobar variety.[53] Cebocephaly and the other less severe forms of facial dysmorphology are seen in both alobar holoprosencephaly and the lesser varieties, as well. Facial anomalies, however, are not universally present, even in the severe alobar form of the disease. This has led to the dictum that *the face predicts the brain, but the brain does not always predict the face.*

The reader is referred to the excellent review of holoprosencephaly by Manelfe and Sevely upon which the following description of imaging dysmorphology in this anomaly is based.[54] The sonographer is immediately impressed by the gross malformation of the brain even upon a cursory examination of a fetus with alobar holoprosencephaly. The examiner notes that the calvarium appears to be largely filled with fluid (Figs. 6–36 to 6–38). This fluid collection represents the large monoventricular cavity in the cerebral midline that communicates posteriorly with a sac, the so-called dorsal sac (Fig. 6–36). It is prognostically not im-

portant to draw an accurate line of distinction between the monoventricular cavity and the dorsal sac, which communicate very broadly in the alobar form of this disease process. In fact, the two appear to be a single structure in most instances. The importance of visualizing the line of junction between these entities, the hippocampal ridge, is that this ridge of tissue generates one of the most characteristic and differentially diagnostic features of this process (Figs. 6–36, 6–37), a differential diagnosis that includes, most commonly, severe hydrocephalus and hydranencephaly, in addition to the lesser forms of holoprosencephaly.

The remaining cerebral tissue that surrounds the large monoventricular cavity is reduced in quantity and cephalically displaced, commonly forming a wedge of tissue anteriorly. The cephalically displaced tissue resembles a "boomerang" (Figs. 6–36, 6–37) or "horseshoe" (Fig. 6–38). No cortical mantle is seen about the dorsal cyst (Figs. 6–36 to 6–38). The basal ganglia and thalami are

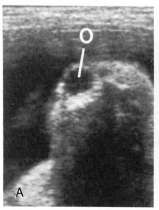
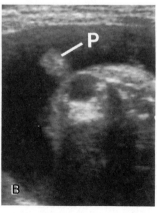

Figure 6–35. A, B, Transverse axial sonograms of the fetus in Figure 6–34. The single orbit (O) and the proboscis (P) are seen in the midline.

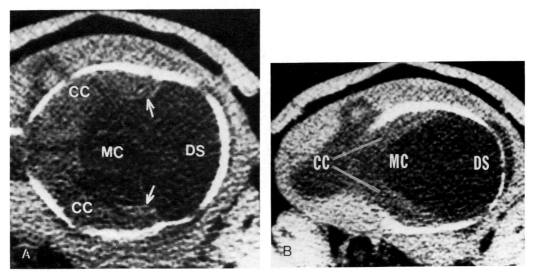

Figure 6–36. *A,* Transverse axial in utero computed tomography scan of a fetus with alobar holoprosencephaly, demonstrating the classic features of this anomaly. The monoventricle (MC) communicates with the dorsal sac (DS). The line of demarcation *(arrows)* is the hippocampal ridge. The cerebral cortex (CC) is anteriorly displaced. *B,* A more cephalic section demonstrating the "boomerang-shaped" anterior cortical mantle (CC). (*From* Filly RA, Chinn DH, Callen PW: Alobar holoprosencephaly: Ultrasonographic prenatal diagnosis. Radiology 151:455, 1984.)

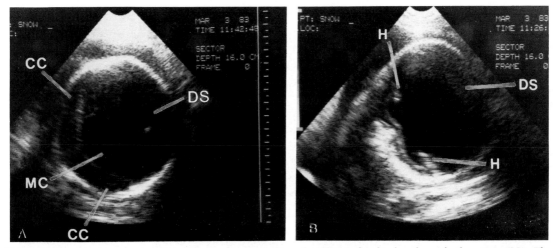

Figure 6–37. *A,* transverse axial sonogram demonstrating the anteriorly displaced cerebral cortex (CC). The monoventricular cavity (MC) communicates broadly with the dorsal sac (DS). *B,* The hippocampal ridge (H) creates a characteristic feature of alobar holoprosencephaly. (*From* Filly RA, Chinn DH, Callen PW: Alobar holoprosencephaly: Ultrasonographic prenatal diagnosis. Radiology 151:455, 1984.)

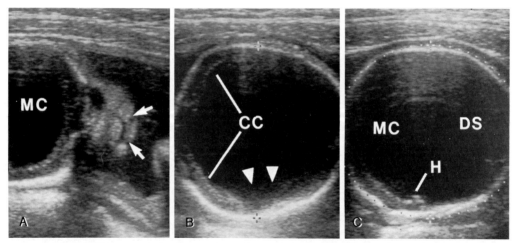

Figure 6–38. *A,* Coronal sonogram of a fetus with alobar holoprosencephaly. A central cleft of the lip *(arrows)* is seen. MC, monoventricular cavity. *B,* The hippocampal ridge is obscured by a side lobe artifact *(arrowheads),* but the symmetric, anteriorly displaced cerebral cortex (CC) is revealed, unobscured by the near calvarial reverberation. *C,* Reorientation of the transducer discloses the hippocampal ridge (H), but a near calvarial reverberation artifact now obscures the symmetry of the cerebral cortex. Differing transducer angulations are important to "bring out" specific differentially diagnostic features. The features demonstrated are now *specific* for alobar holoprosencephaly. MC, monoventricular cavity; DS, dorsal sac.

fused in the midline (Fig. 6–39). *This is an extremely important feature that immediately excludes hydrocephalus from the differential diagnosis.* In hydrocephalus, of course, the thalami should be widely separated because of the enlarged third ventricle. This leaves hydranencephaly as the most important differential diagnostic possibility. However, from a practical perspective, both

hydranencephaly and alobar holoprosencephaly have profound consequences for future mental development, and stillbirth or short survival is the rule. Pragmatic considerations aside, hydranencephaly is excluded by demonstration of either the symmetric and rostrally displaced cerebral mantle or the hippocampal ridge.

The posterior fossa is usually small, which

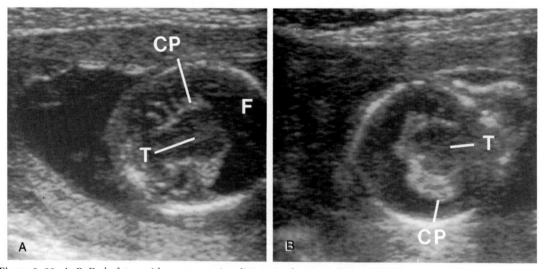

Figure 6–39. *A, B,* Early fetus with a presumptive diagnosis of a severe form of holoprosencephaly. Note the fluid-filled supratentorial compartment (F) and the fused thalami (T); the absence of a dilated third ventricle excludes hydrocephalus. Hydranencephaly remains a differential diagnostic possibility. However, both conditions have an extremely dismal prognosis. The parents elected termination by dilatation and extraction. No postmortem examination of the brain was possible. CP, choroid plexus.

Figure 6–40. *A,* Fetus with semilobar holoprosencephaly. The symmetry is obscured by a near calvarial reverberation but can be assumed to be present. Note the fused thalami (T), over which the monoventricle (M) arches. The parahippocampal gyrus (P) is in its normal position, excluding the differential diagnosis of alobar holoprosencephaly. *B,* The monoventricle extends between the hemispheres as an interhemispheric or dorsal cyst *(arrows).* The presence of fused thalami (the absence of third ventricular enlargement) excludes the diagnosis of agenesis of the corpus callosum with an interhemispheric cyst.

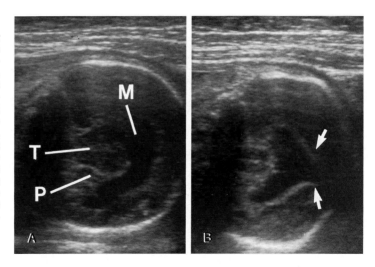

causes difficulty in ultrasonic imaging of this space. However, if visible, the posterior fossa structures are normal or only mildly hypoplastic. No falx cerebri is present. Much has been made of this feature in the diagnosis of alobar holoprosencephaly; however, a variety of artifacts may simulate the appearance of a falx when the cranium is expanded with fluid. Further, the major competing differential diagnostic possibility, hydranencephaly, frequently lacks a visible falx.

Indeed, in semilobar holoprosencephaly, the occipital lobes tend to be formed; thus, a falx and separated ventricles are seen dorsally. Fused thalami again exclude hydrocephalus, and the visible occipital brain mantle or frontal brain mantle surrounding the unseparated central ventricular cavity promptly excludes hydranencephaly (Fig. 6–40). Fetuses with complete ACC associated with a large interhemispheric cyst may closely simulate the appearance of semilobar holoprosencephaly. Segregation of these entities may be difficult. Differential diagnostic features include the presence of frontal horns and a large fluid-filled third ventricle between the thalami in ACC (Fig. 6–32), features virtually never seen in semilobar holoprosencephaly (Fig. 6–40).*

As noted elsewhere, lobar holoprosencephaly may be mimicked by ACC and by hydrocephalus with a fenestrated septum (Figs. 6–41, 6–42). Remember, demonstration of any convincing portion of the septum pellucidum excludes lobar holoprosenceph-

aly and complete ACC. However, the latter two entities should always be simultaneously considered when examining fetuses with dilated atria and occipital horns of the lateral ventricles as well as an inability to demonstrate a septum pellucidum or cavum septi pellucidi.

Fetuses with holoprosencephaly may have a head size that is normal, smaller than normal, or enlarged. The enlargement results from hydrocephalus. In addition to the ventricular malformation, there may be severe ventricular dilatation. Since the type of cases that come to light during routine obstetric scanning tend to be the more severe varieties of this disease process, the prognosis is uniformly poor, with most infants discovered in utero dying shortly after birth. Survivors usually suffer severe mental retardation. The poor prognosis is reflected in the experience of most authors who have considered this topic in the literature.[57, 63] Nonetheless, it is

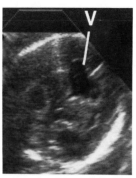

Figure 6–41. Sonogram of a fetus with ventriculomegaly (V). Note the inability to demonstrate a septum pellucidum. No definitive diagnosis was possible.

---

*Some cases of semilobar holoprosencephaly demonstrate a small third ventricle.

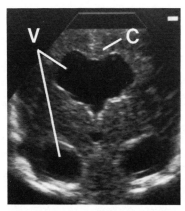

Figure 6–42. Neonatal sonogram of the fetus in Figure 6–41. Ventriculomegaly (V), the absence of a septum pellucidum, and a small corpus callosum (C) are demonstrated. Neurologic evaluation and follow-up confirmed lobar holoprosencephaly.

important to remember that the prognosis for lobar holoprosencephaly is less severe. Normal lifespan has been reported for some, but many are severely retarded. It is presumed that the uncommon individuals who may have normal mentation and a form of holoprosencephaly probably demonstrate the least structural brain disorganization and therefore the most subtle dysmorphic features. Thus, these fetuses are least likely to be detected.

All varieties of holoprosencephaly have been diagnosed in utero by sonography.[57–63] The more severe forms, as anticipated, have predominated,[57, 62] but lobar holoprosencephaly has also been recognized.[63] Obstetric management in cases of holoprosencephaly depends on the gestational age at the time of diagnosis and the severity of the abnormality.[61] If this condition is detected before 24 weeks of gestation, pregnancy termination may be elected by the parents. In the third trimester, macrocephaly due to ventricular enlargement may well prevent vaginal delivery. Thus, to avoid cesarean section in hopeless cases, cephalocentesis is usually recommended. An effective cephalocentesis should significantly reduce the size of the cranium and, in the opinion of the author, should always be considered a destructive procedure. The parents should be so counseled and the procedure treated as a destructive one. Attempts to perform a "gentle" cephalocentesis are probably ill advised.

In virtually any CNS anomaly, an analysis of the karyotype should be considered. A karyotype is clearly indicated in the case of the holoprosencephalies where a high incidence of chromosomal abnormalities has been discovered.[53, 55] Trisomy 13 is particularly common; however, other chromosomal anomalies may be detected as well.

Hydranencephaly, Porencephaly, Schizencephaly

Purists would argue that lumping these three entities together has no basis in fact. Conversely, pragmatists would see no reason to argue excessively over the incorporation of these entities into a single section of such a chapter. Hydranencephaly and porencephaly are unambiguously destructive lesions of the fetal brain.[64–71] Schizencephaly is not as unambiguously a destructive process, and many researchers consider this entity to be developmental.[72–75] Interestingly, more recent sonographic evidence supports the hypothesis that schizencephaly, like hydranencephaly and porencephaly, is the result of a destructive process.[68, 75] Probably all three represent the sequelae of in utero vascular accidents that differ only in timing and degree.[67] The timing element probably accounts for the variations in development of other CNS structures that confuse the etiologic categorization of these entities.

Hydranencephaly is the complete or nearly complete destruction of the cerebral cortex and basal ganglia (Figs. 6–43, 6–44).[64, 65] Usually, the thalami and lower brain centers are preserved although the thalami may be involved in the destructive process.[66] The choroid plexus may also be preserved; thus, although the head is often small, with functioning choroid plexus, hydrocephalus may ensue. Indeed, although evidence before the advent of diagnostic sonography seemed to indicate that normally developed brain tissue was present but then destroyed, even skeptics can no longer reasonably question this pathogenesis since complete brain destruction resulting in classic hydranencephaly has now been sonographically documented in utero.[68] It is attractive to speculate that bilateral internal carotid artery occlusion results in this abnormality, but this hypothesis is difficult to prove since these vessels are usually patent at autopsy.[64–66] Nonetheless, if one works from the premise that massive brain infarction, as may occur

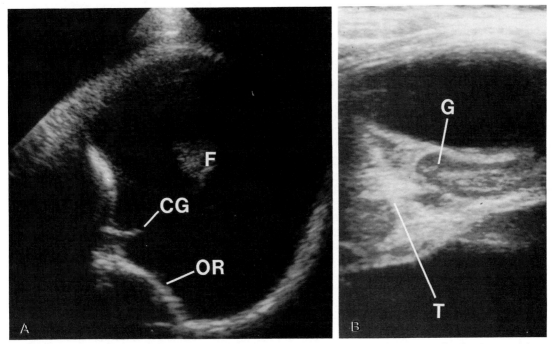

Figure 6–43. *A*, Anterior coronal scan in a fetus with hydranencephaly. No brain tissue or dural structure (falx) is seen. Only fluid (F) is present. However, the crista galli (CG) is apparent. OR, orbital roof. *B*, Posterior scan identifies a preserved gyrus of the occipital lobe. T, tentorium.

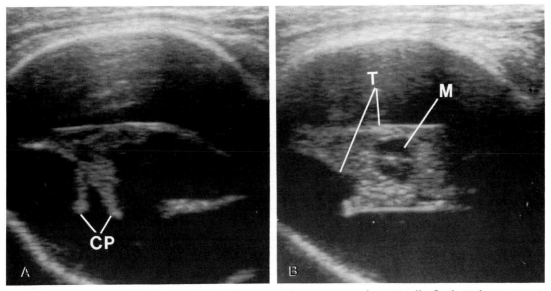

Figure 6–44. *A*, Fetus with hydranencephaly. The calvarial contents are almost totally fluid. Little structure is visible, but dangling choroid plexi (CP) are seen. *B*, Note that infratentorial structures, like the midbrain–pons (M) junction, appear entirely normal. T, tentorium.

from bilateral internal carotid artery occlusion, results in hydranencephaly, all morphologic features seen sonographically in utero can be anticipated.

It is worth recalling that severe increases in ventricular size and pressure over prolonged periods also destroy the cortical mantle. However, hydranencephaly is clearly distinct from this process, and the two can be easily separated pathologically, if not clinically, in all cases.[76] In hydranencephaly, the telencephalon is replaced by fluid-filled cavities covered only by leptomeninges. In prolonged massive hydrocephalus, a thin rim of abnormal, but identifiable, cortical brain tissue persists.

The abnormalities seen sonographically in hydranencephaly are so striking that detection is not a problem (Fig. 6–43); unfortunately, differential diagnosis is. Alternative diagnostic possibilities include massive hydrocephalus, alobar holoprosencephaly, and brain atrophy resulting in thinned but not absent cerebral hemispheres. Features that distinguish these entities have been considered in other sections; however, a few additional and important features are appropriately discussed here. First, there may be scattered preserved zones of cerebral cortical tissue in cases of hydranencephaly, although histologically the tissue is usually gliotic (Fig. 6–44). These zones occur in expected areas where tissue might be preserved by collateral arterial flow. Preserved brain tissue includes, from time to time, medial occipital lobe tissue, presumably preserved via the posterior communicating arteries, and occasionally, areas of frontal lobe tissue, presumably preserved through ophthalmic artery collaterals. The hippocampus and parahippocampal gyrus may be preserved and, when so, lie in immediate contiguity with the ambient cistern, their normal location. This position of the hippocampal tissues is quite distinct from alobar holoprosencephaly, wherein the hippocampal ridge is located peripherally. The third ventricle is present and visible but not enlarged in hydranencephaly, as opposed to severe hydrocephalus, which enlarges the third ventricle. Fusion of the thalami, as seen invariably in alobar holoprosencephaly, is never present in hydranencephaly.

Porencephaly is at the lesser end of a continuum from hydranencephaly and develops when infarction of or hemorrhage

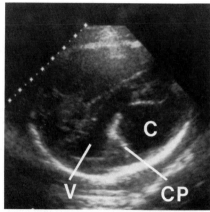

Figure 6–45. Transverse axial sonogram of a porencephalic cyst in a fetus. The large cyst (C) is located in the supply distribution of the middle cerebral artery. Despite its large size, the cyst has no mass effect. The ipsilateral ventricle (V) is enlarged. The cyst communicates with the ventricle; note that the choroid plexus (CP) hangs from the ventricle into the cyst.

into the brain parenchyma occurs. The destroyed area necroses and gradually is evacuated, usually into the adjacent ventricular lumen or subarachnoid space (Fig. 6–45). The residuum, then, is a cystic lesion that is in free communication with the ventricle or, less commonly, the subarachnoid cisterns at the external brain surface.* Since the ischemic event is often more widespread than the focal infarction that results in the porencephaly, the hemisphere tends to be small, as manifest by enlargement of the ipsilateral ventricle. The porencephalic cyst is an ex vacuo event; thus it never produces a mass effect, an important differential diagnostic point between arachnoid cysts and interhemispheric cysts as seen in ACC.

Schizencephaly, or bilateral clefts in the cerebral cortex, has been considered to be the result of bilateral middle cerebral artery infarction with subsequent development of symmetric porencephalic cysts or clefts (Fig. 6–46).† By the timing of this event (early versus late), the interruption of blood supply may also result in abnormal brain growth

---

*Areas of cystic necrosis within the brain substance that do not communicate with the subarachnoid space or the ventricular lumen are termed "false porencephalies" or cystic leukomalacia.

†More strictly, the cyst or, more appropriately, the cleft must extend from the ependyma of the ventricle to the brain surface (leptomeninges) and must be lined by gray matter. The clefts are not necessarily bilateral and may be so narrow as to contain no CSF.

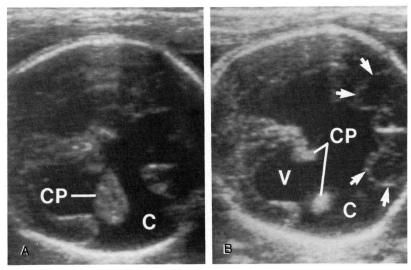

Figure 6–46. *A, B,* Schizencephaly, paired transverse axial sonograms. A large cleft (or cyst) (C) is seen in the hemisphere farther from the transducer. Choroid plexus (CP) dangles into the cyst. The ipsilateral ventricle (V) is enlarged and abnormally shaped. The lateral ventricles communicate broadly. No septum is seen; the near ventricular choroid plexus hangs down into the opposite ventricle. A near calvarial reverberation artifact obscures the symmetry of this anomaly, but careful inspection of *B (arrows)* documents that the anomaly is bilateral. (Courtesy of Laurence A Mack, MD, University of Washington, Seattle, WA.)

and development. These cysts are always lined by gray matter, a feature that speaks against the grouping of this entity with hydranencephaly and porencephaly. In any event, the dysmorphic features in "classic" cases strongly simulate the expected location of bilateral porencephalic cysts in the middle cerebral artery distribution.[72–75] The fluid collections communicate with the ventricular lumen bilaterally and extend to the calvarium. A major problem sonographically is that symmetry is difficult to demonstrate owing to the near calvarial reverberation artifact (Fig. 6–46). The unwary examiner may be contented to have observed and characterized the "down side" lesion as an isolated unilateral porencephaly.

As would be expected, the prognosis with the disorders under consideration depends on which portion of the brain has been destroyed and to what extent the other areas can compensate for the lost tissue. Hydranencephaly, of course, has a grim prognosis since nearly all of the higher brain centers have been destroyed. Interestingly, hydranencephalic newborns may appear quite normal and escape early clinical detection only to come to light after a few months.[65, 68] Early clinical detection appears to depend more on the absence of hypothalamic function than of cortical brain function. If the hypothalamus is intact, the newborn appears rel-

atively normal; however, electroencephalography shows no cortical activity, and hyperreflexia and clonus are generally present.

As a rule, in porencephaly and schizencephaly, the disability is likely to be more severe than less so, based on the observed abnormalities. More brain tissue may have been involved in the hypoxic event than can be documented sonographically. Again, experience with the later entities is small; however, extrapolation from more common CNS anomalies suggests that the more severe cases, with correspondingly poorer prognoses, tend to be detected in utero. Even so, it should be borne in mind that a poor prognosis cannot be accurately predicted in fetuses with a porencephalic cyst.

Hydrocephalus versus Nonobstructive Ventriculomegaly

The preceding sections have documented that multiple anomalies of brain development result in ventricular enlargement. The term hydrocephalus should be reserved for that dynamic process resulting in a progressive increase in ventricular volume due either to a relative or complete obstruction between sites of production and absorption of CSF or, much less commonly, to overproduction.[77, 78] Therefore, in hydrocephalus, there is necessarily an increase in relative pressure between the CSF and the intracranial venous system.

As noted, obstructive hydrocephalus is the far more common form. This type may be further subdivided into communicating or noncommunicating hydrocephalus.[78] In the former, the site of obstruction is extraventricular, most often at the arachnoid granulations, whereas in the latter, the obstruction is within the ventricular system itself. Among fetuses, communicating hydrocephalus is distinctly uncommon. Newborns and young children have a higher incidence of communicating hydrocephalus, which is most commonly seen after intraventricular hemorrhage in premature children or as a result of meningitis in older children; both conditions are rare in fetuses.

By the above definition, the term hydrocephalus ex vacuo should be dropped since the enlarged ventricles originate from a loss of surrounding brain parenchyma. Awareness of the subtleties of these definitions is, unfortunately, important. For example, in hydranencephaly there is a profound loss of brain tissues surrounding the ventricles (hydrocephalus ex vacuo). Indeed, the ventricular edge extends to the calvarial wall with no intervening brain tissue. These enlarged "ventricles" are not classified as hydrocephalus. However, in an hydranencephalic fetus, a head of normal to small size may begin to expand owing to obstruction of CSF flow (true hydrocephalus). Further, the true hydrocephlus may be either communicating or noncommunicating.

Once enlarged ventricles are noted, it is the sonographer's responsibility to make all subsequent efforts to determine whether

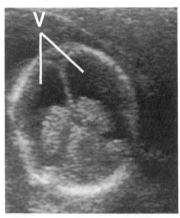

Figure 6–48. Ventriculomegaly (V) was noted at 16 weeks in a fetus with a genetic risk of Walker-Warburg syndrome. Ventriculomegaly is only one manifestation of this severe syndrome but was the only feature that could be documented. A ventricular shunt, either before or after birth, would not "cure" this fetus.

the ventricular enlargement represents true hydrocephalus or ventriculomegaly from another cause, i.e., colpocephaly or brain atrophy (Fig. 6–47). If one suspects hydrocephalus, further efforts should be made to determine whether it is isolated or associated with other anomalies of CNS or extra-CNS development, a challenge that may, in some cases, be beyond our current capabilities (Fig. 6–48). Among these, far and away, the most important are neural tube defects.[79–81] Fully one-third of all cases of hydrocephalus will be associated with myelomeningocele or encephalocele, the former being the more common. The hydrocephalus in these cases is due to the Chiari malformation. An extremely careful search of the spine by an expert examiner is warranted in all cases of ventricular enlargement.

Other causes include aqueductal stenosis (Fig. 6–49), either X-linked or idiopathic; holoprosencephaly (Fig. 6–38); hydranencephaly (Fig. 6–43); DWM (Fig. 6–26); and cloverleaf skull deformity (Fig. 6–50).[79–81] Infection and hemorrhage resulting in communicating hydrocephalus are very uncommon. The posterior fossa must be examined carefully for evidence of DWM since the supratentorial ventricular enlargement is not dependent on the size of the fourth ventricular cyst (Fig. 6–26).

There is a great temptation for the inexperienced examiner to invoke aqueductal stenosis as the cause of ventricular enlargement. There are several reasons for this.

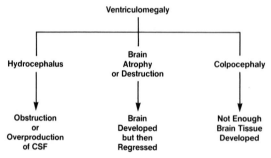

Figure 6–47. Pathologic causes of ventriculomegaly.

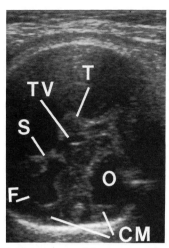

Figure 6–49. Transverse axial sonogram of a fetus who was difficult to examine. Moderately severe ventriculomegaly from the aqueductal stenosis is noted. A near calvarial reverberation artifact obscures most of the anatomy of the hemisphere closer to the transducer. Symmetry can be assumed. T, thalamus; TV, third ventricle; S, septum pellucidum; F, frontal horn; O, occipital horn; CM, cortical mantle.

First, enlargement of the lateral and third ventricles is easier to perceive than enlargement of the subarachnoid spaces (brain atrophy with large ventricles), enlargement of the fourth ventricle (communicating hydrocephalus or DWS), and spinal dysraphism (Chiari II malformation associated with myelomeningocele). Second, ventricular enlargement (with or without hydrocephalus) caused by anomalies such as ACC or lobar holoprosencephaly may require subtle observations of brain maldevelopment. Third, aqueductal stenosis is a diagnosis of exclusion even in the hands of the most sophisticated examiner. The inexperienced examiner who fails to meticulously search out these manifold possibilities often presumes their absence, inviting the erroneous conclusion that aqueductal stenosis (isolated) is the cause of the observed ventricular enlargement.

There are significant unsolved problems in managing a fetus with ventriculomegaly. We are only now beginning to understand the natural history in such cases.[82] The relationship between hydrocephalus detected in utero and that seen in neonates is only speculative. Current evidence demonstrates that the accuracy of prenatal ultrasound in discriminating true hydrocephalus from nonobstructive ventriculomegaly is less than perfect even in skilled hands.[82–88] Further,

there is a clear risk of missing associated CNS and life-threatening extra-CNS anomalies.

Pragmatically, prenatal ultrasound recognizes three patterns of ventriculomegaly.[82] These include fetuses who have *ventriculomegaly associated with severe abnormalities that would be fatal*, e.g., Meckel's syndrome. In such cases, the parents may be counseled and, if they so choose, the pregnancy terminated. The second group includes fetuses with ventriculomegaly detected serendipitously late in gestation, *associated with abnormalities that are severe but not invariably fatal*. In this circumstance, parents commonly elect vaginal delivery after cephalocentesis. Since the latter is a destructive procedure and the vaginal delivery is a further trauma to the fetus, neonatal demise is nearly always the outcome. Finally, there is the most difficult group: fetuses with isolated ventriculomegaly in whom there is *no sonographically evident associated anomaly or an anomaly that is not particularly severe*, e.g., unilateral hydronephrosis. One could include in this group of fetuses those with an anomaly such as myelomeningocele, which is not usually associated with subsequent mental retardation although it is associated with disability in most cases.

In the first two groups, a poor outcome is easily predicted. In the last group, it is not.

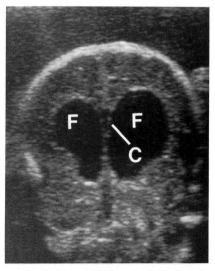

Figure 6–50. Fetus with cloverleaf skull deformity, transverse axial sonogram, frontal region. The dilated frontal horns (F) are devoid of choroid plexus. Note the compressed cavum septi pellucidi (C). This examination excludes midline anomalies.

Further, it is this group in which it is most difficult to segregate true hydrocephalus from nonobstructive ventriculomegaly and in which there is invariably a nagging suspicion that subtle, but significant, CNS or extra-CNS anomalies have been missed. This group requires an aggressive investigation that includes serial sonograms, determination of karyotype, alpha-fetoprotein analysis, and viral cultures and titers. Since it is impossible to determine intraventricular pressure safely in utero, hydrocephalus should not be diagnosed in this group unless the head is enlarged or serial sonograms document increasing ventricular and head size. Importantly, the lack of the above two features does not, however, exclude true hydrocephalus with high pressure.

The author's experience and that of others is illustrative.[82-88] In a review of 47 cases,[82] fetal ventriculomegaly was associated with other severe abnormalities in 20. In 19 of these, the family elected to terminate the pregnancy; in four cases, cephalocentesis was necessary to effect vaginal delivery, and no fetus survived. One family refused either termination or cephalocentesis and a cesarean section was performed for dystocia at term. The neonate survived for 30 minutes after delivery and was noted to have visible congenital abnormalities that had not been detected in utero.

In five cases, ventriculomegaly was detected late in pregnancy. All fetuses had associated nonlethal abnormalities, including myelomeningocele, hydronephrosis, encephalocele, and hydrops fetalis. All were delivered vaginally. Three fetuses were stillborn, and two survived less than one hour.

Twenty-two fetuses had ventriculomegaly without severe abnormalities detected in utero. In this group, ventriculomegaly remained stable throughout gestation in 19 fetuses, progressed in two, and resolved in one. Associated anomalies not detected in utero included a porencephalic cyst, an open spina bifida without an associated sac, ACC, and septo-optic dysplasia.

Until recent years, the outcome for fetuses with ventriculomegaly has been poorly delineated. Chervenak and associates reported a 72 percent mortality rate in 50 fetuses with ventriculomegaly.[84] Eighty-four percent of all fetuses had associated abnormalities. Of the 14 survivors, 13 required shunting procedures, and only six had normal intellec-

tual development. Serlo and colleagues reported similar results; of 38 fetuses with ventriculomegaly, only ten survived, six of whom were intellectually normal and four of whom were severely retarded.[85] In a study by Cochrane and coworkers, most diagnoses were made late in pregnancy (32 of 41 cases detected after 30 weeks' gestation), and pregnancy was terminated or cephalocentesis used in only four of 41 cases.[86] Still there was a high incidence of stillbirth or death shortly after delivery, with an overall mortality rate of 66 percent. Seventy-five percent of fetuses were found to have other CNS abnormalities. In a review of 40 cases, Pretorius and colleagues found an 85 percent mortality rate; only three of six survivors were intellectually normal.[87] More recently, Nyberg and associates reported 61 cases of fetal ventriculomegaly that showed a mortality rate of 66 percent.[88]

Independent of the ability of ultrasonography to discriminate nonobstructive ventricular enlargement from true hydrocephalus, it is clear that the prognosis for fetal ventriculomegaly is poor. Only about one in four fetuses with enlarged ventricles survives, as reported in the literature. The most frequent cause of death is, of course, iatrogenic: pregnancy termination, cephalocentesis. Still, the mortality rate is high even if these interventions are not employed. Moreover, only one-half of the survivors are intellectually normal. The high mortality rate is likely due to the frequent association of CNS abnormalities with anomalous development of other important organs.[82, 88] There is an 80 percent incidence of associated abnormalities. The anomalies are often severe and can affect many organ systems, including cardiovascular, gastrointestinal, and renal. Other CNS aberrations are common, as well.

As stated above, the prognosis for normal intellectual outcome is poor.[82-88] Recall that survivors tend to represent a select group that, in general, have less severe associated anomalies. Nonetheless, only about one-half have normal or near normal intelligence. Included in this group is a subset of individuals who have mild ventriculomegaly that is stable over long periods of observation and who demonstrate normal physical and mental development. Unfortunately, the degree of ventriculomegaly is not uniformly predictive of outcome.[82] Infants may have moderate to severe ventricular enlargement and demonstrate normal intellectual development after postnatal shunting. Conversely, fetuses with mild to moderate ventriculomegaly may show significantly delayed development. Rather than the degree of ventricular enlargement, it is most often the presence of other abnormalities that worsens the prognosis for the fetus.[88] It is therefore important that these anomalies be identified; however, even in the hands of highly experienced sonographers, all abnormalities may not be identified. Virtually all major series dealing with the evaluation of fetal ventricular enlargement have shown false-negative rates ranging from 20 to 39 percent.[82–88] In fetuses with abnormal ventricles, it is more likely that experienced sonographers will miss anomalies outside of the CNS than associated anomalies within the CNS.

The sonographic diagnosis of ventricular enlargement has been well described in the literature.[17, 22–25, 89] Considerable work has been done using measurements of frontal horns and lateral ventricular "widths" to define the normal limits for ventricular size in different stages of development. A set of ratio measurements, comparing the distance of the lateral wall of the lateral ventricle from the midline with the hemispheric width (LVW/HW ratio), has been proposed as a method to diagnose hydrocephalus.[89] However, the ratio measurement accuracy suffers not only from technical difficulties that alter considerably the ratio value, depending on the plane of section in which the scan is performed, but also from a very wide standard deviation that renders it insensitive to identification of early dilatation.[90] Not the least problem with this approach is the fact that the normal data are based on measurements from a linear echoing structure not actually representing the lateral ventricular wall (see the section on normal sonographic anatomy) (Figs. 6–12, 6–13).

It is preferable to determine whether ventricular enlargement is present by direct observations of the ventricle. These observations are best carried out in the region of the ventricular atrium where, in the normal fetus, the choroid plexus fills (or nearly fills) the transverse dimension of this component of the ventricular system. This is an important relationship because in early hydrocephalus, the first recognizable aberration is a relative shrinkage of the normally prominent choroid plexus within the body of the lateral ventricle. The apparent frontal horn size may seem prominent in the early second trimester, but as long as the choroid plexus can be seen filling the lateral ventricular body in its transverse dimension, hydrocephalus is not present. One should never assume that a normal head size (BPD or head circumference) excludes either ventriculomegaly or true hydrocephalus.[91, 92]

The atrial diameter is a particularly important measurement used to determine the normalcy of ventricular size. Evidence has shown that there is little, if any, change in the diameter of the lateral ventricular atrium from 15 to 35 weeks.[29] The transverse diameter of the ventricular atrium measures approximately 7 to 8 mm, with 10 mm being the upper limit of normal (Fig. 6–51). If the choroid fills the atrial lumen, no measurement is necessary. If a modest amount of fluid is seen to lie between the choroid and the ventricular wall, a measurement is advisable. If the measurement is 10 mm or less, the fetus is likely to be normal.

The lack of apparent growth in the diameter of the atrium is particularly useful to ultrasonographers (Table 6–3). The volume of the ventricle must remain relatively stable throughout the second and third trimesters, but it is dramatically reshaped by the marked growth of the adjacent brain. Apparently, the adjacent brain does not markedly reshape the atrium, accounting for the relative stability of both the atrial diameter and the ratio of choroidal width to atrial width that has been previously observed.

Recall the reverberation from the near calvarial wall often obscures the lateral ventricle lying closest to the transducer. Thus, in the vast majority of cases, the ventricles appear asymmetric when enlarged. The temptation to diagnose ventricular asymmetry should be avoided (Figs. 6–49, 6–51). Although unilateral ventricular enlargement and, indeed, unilateral ventricular hydrocephalus are a possibility, they are distinctly uncommon (Fig. 6–52).[93] One should always presume that the ventricles are symmetric unless images clearly document asymmetry.

Ventricular enlargement is easily recognized by observing the appearance of the ventricular atrium. Conversely, there is a potential to frequently overcall the presence of hydrocephalus because of the poorly ech-

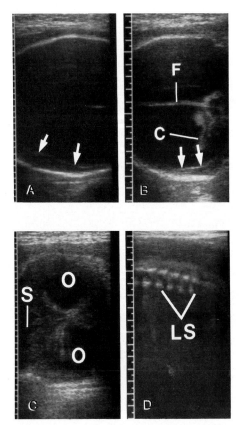

Figure 6–51. A, B, C, Fetus with massive ventriculomegaly from aqueductal stenosis, transverse axial sonograms. A near calvarial reverberation obscures the symmetry. However, the presence of uniformly distributed cortex *(arrows)* excludes the diagnoses of alobar holoprosencephaly and hydranencephaly. A small segment of septum pellucidum (S) excludes midline anomalies. O, occipital horns; F, falx; C, choroid plexus. D, The presence of a normal lumbosacral (LS) spine excludes the diagnosis of a myelomeningocele, Chiari II malformation.

ogenic adjacent brain parenchyma that may be mistakenly interpreted as cerebrospinal fluid surrounding the atrial choroid *pseudohydrocephalus)* (Fig. 6–53).[17, 94] This appearance is augmented by the technical error of applying insufficient gain when examining the brain.* Pseudohydrocephalus is easily recognized by remembering a simple fact: the *choroid plexus always rests in a gravitationally dependent position* (Fig. 6–54). Therefore, the choroid plexus *always* rests against the lateral ventricular wall unless the lateral ventricle is so large that the choroid plexus, tethered at the Monro foramen,

*When examining the head of the fetus, the ultrasonic beam passes through the attenuating calvarium. Therefore, overall gain and time-gain compensation must be increased compared with the examination of the torso.

Table 6–3. GESTATIONAL AGE VERSUS SIZE OF BRAIN STRUCTURES

Gestational Weeks		Atrium of Lateral Ventricle	Thalamus	Basal Ganglia and Insula	Temporal Operculum
15–20	Mean	5	7	6	6
	Range	(4–7)	(6–9)	(5–7)	(5–7)
	SD	0.7	0.8	0.7	0.9
21–25	Mean	6	8	7	9
	Range	(5–8)	(6–9)	(6–11)	(7–11)
	SD	0.6	0.7	1.2	1.0
26–30	Mean	7	8	9	11
	Range	(6–7)	(8–9)	(8–12)	(10–13)
	SD	0.7	0.4	1.2	0.6
31–35	Mean	7	9	11	13
	Range	(5–8)	(8–10)	(9–14)	(11–15)
	SD	0.5	0.7	1.1	0.7

(*From* Siedler DE, Filly RA: Relative growth of the higher fetal brain structures. J Ultrasound Med 6:575, 1987.)

simply is not long enough to reach the lateral wall. The choroid, a highly echogenic structure, may indeed help to obscure the lateral ventricular wall where it lies in contact with this structure (Fig. 6–55). Therefore, if the choroid plexus appears "suspended" in an "enlarged ventricle," one can immediately predict that it is a case of pseudohydrocephalus, increase the gain, and produce the appropriate images that document the error.

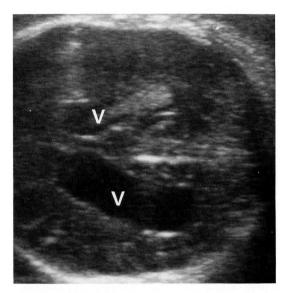

Figure 6–52. Unilateral ventriculomegaly in a fetus, transverse axial sonogram. Both lateral ventricles (V) are clearly seen. The ventricle closer to the transducer is normal in size. Choroid plexus fills the body and atrium, and the atrium measures 9 mm. Conversely, the ventricle farther from the transducer is not "filled" by the choroid (indeed, choroid plexus is not even visible in this plane of section). The atrium measures 13 mm in diameter.

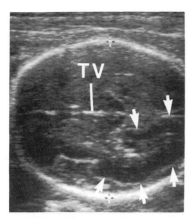

Figure 6–53. Pseudohydrocephalus, transverse axial sonogram. Lucent brain parenchyma *(arrows)* should not be mistaken for a dilated ventricle. Note the normal third ventricle (TV).

The knowledge that the choroid plexus always assumes a gravitationally dependent position also helps the sonographer to recognize true ventricular enlargement, "the dangling choroid sign" (Fig. 6–56).[95] The greater the degree of angulation of the choroid from the midline, the larger is the ventricle.

Space-Occupying Lesions: Neoplasm, Arteriovenous Malformation, Arachnoid Cyst, Choroid Plexus Cyst

Fortunately, congenital brain tumors are rare abnormalities. They account for approx-

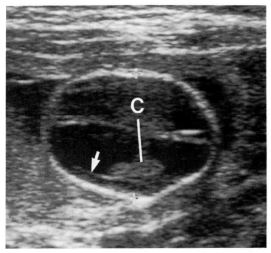

Figure 6–54. Severe ventricular enlargement, transverse axial sonogram. The gravity-dependent choroid (C) lies against the lateral wall of the lateral ventricle *(arrow)*.

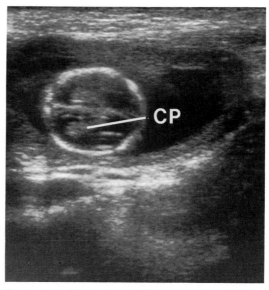

Figure 6–55. Transverse axial sonogram, normal fetal brain. Despite sonography's inability to image the lateral ventricular wall along the atrium, its position is precisely marked by the choroid plexus (CP). Using this marker, the atrial diameter can be measured (8 mm).

imately 0.3 percent of neonatal deaths in less than 28 days.[96] A variety of lesions may be found, but the most common is the teratoma, which accounts for approximately 50 percent of all congenital intracranial neoplasms.[97] This lesion may be seen at any time during life but is present most commonly in the newborn and rapidly decreases in incidence with increasing age.[98] Teratomas may be either benign or malignant although even the benign lesions tend to have devastating consequences, as will be described. Glial tumors are second in frequency and include glioblastomas, astroblastomas, and spongioblastomas. Glioblastomas predominate. Any of these lesions can produce hydrocephalus by ventricular obstruction, a common event.[98] Teratomatous lesions tend to be mixed, solid and cystic lesions, usually with a great degree of disorganization (Fig. 6–57). However, occasionally the cystic component may predominate, and there is some risk of misdiagnosing this neoplastic lesion as an arachnoid cyst. Conversely, the only reported sonographic case of glioblastoma diagnosed prenatally presented with diffusely increased echoes throughout the tumor mass.[99] The appearance was similar to that seen in a large hemorrhage or hemorrhagic infarct. Otherwise, the true nature of these abnormalities is relatively obvious.[98–101]

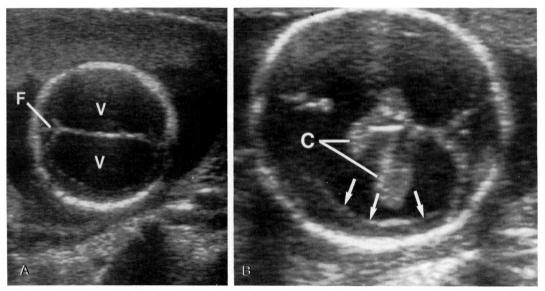

Figure 6–56. *A,* Transverse axial sonogram of a fetus with severe ventricular enlargement (V) and marked thinning of the cortex, especially medially. A large myelomeningocele was the cause. F, falx. *B,* Transverse axial sonogram taken in a more inferior plane than *A.* "Dangling choroid" (C) sign: note that the choroid of the ventricle nearer to the transducer "dangles" through the open septum into the ventricle farther from the transducer (whose choroid dangles to the limit of its length, but cannot reach the lateral ventricular wall [*arrows*]).

Dystocia may occur during vaginal delivery. This may be due both to the size of the tumor mass, which can greatly expand the calvarium, and to the secondary hydrocephalus (Fig. 6–57). Lesions are more commonly supratentorial than infratentorial, although distortion may be too great to draw this distinction. Cephalocentesis may be worthwhile if severe hydrocephalus or a large cystic component dominate the picture.[98] Unfortunately, many cases still must be delivered by cesarean section since vaginal delivery is often impossible even after cephalocentesis. Although such lesions may be small and potentially resectable,[102] thus far, only large lesions have been detected prenatally.[98–101] In each instance, the fetus has been stillborn or has died promptly in the neonatal period. For this reason, it is prudent to assume a fatal prognosis and manage cases with this outcome in mind.

At the opposite end of the spectrum is a type of mass lesion that is both common and essentially benign:[103, 104] the choroid plexus cyst (Fig. 6–58). In any modestly busy practice, it would be unusual for a month to go by without the identification of a choroid plexus cyst, if this lesion is actively sought

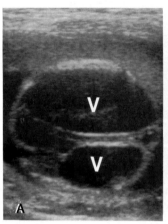

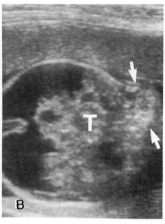

Figure 6–57. *A,* Transverse axial sonogram shows asymmetric hydrocephalus. V, ventricle. *B,* Coronal sonogram demonstrates a heterogeneous tumor mass (T) extensively involving the base of the entire supratentorial compartment and extending out of the orbit *(arrows).* The mass proved to be a teratoma.

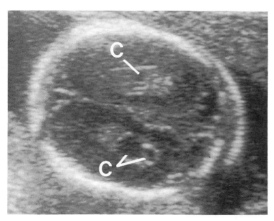

Figure 6–58. Transverse axial sonogram, bilateral choroid plexus cysts (C). The larger one is bilocular.

in all fetuses of the correct gestational age. These lesions are seen almost exclusively in fetuses between 16 and 21 weeks of gestational age and are always located in the lateral ventricle near the glomus of the choroid plexus. By the 23rd week, they are clearly regressing, and it would be distinctly unusual to see such a lesion after 25 to 26 weeks.

Because of the unique ability of ultrasound to scan large numbers of fetuses at the appropriate age range and to readily resolve even tiny cysts in the choroid plexus, these lesions, which were previously thought to be rare, are now known to be common. In fact, choroid plexus cysts are probably the most common aberration of fetal development observed sonographically

in utero. These cysts may be unilateral or bilateral; however, bilateral recognition is difficult owing to near side reverberation caused by the calvarium.

Choroid plexus cysts typically range from 0.5 to 2 cm. Commonly, they are multilocular (Fig. 6–58). Only the larger lesions expand the walls of the lateral ventricle (Fig. 6–59). The lesions themselves appear to be extraordinarily benign and transient. Unfortunately, there has been a report of an association of these cysts with chromosomal abnormalities.[105] Consideration should be given to karyotype analysis when such a cyst is seen. In the vast majority of cases, a normal karyotype is anticipated. Further, consideration should be given to interval follow-up to ensure that the cyst regresses. Again, the expectation is that virtually all will regress.

A more important, although far less common, supratentorial cyst is the arachnoid cyst.[106, 107] This lesion is the supratentorial analog of the retrocerebellar arachnoid cyst, previously described (Figs. 6–28, 6–29). However, in the larger supratentorial compartment, more variety in appearance may be anticipated. Arachnoid cysts may be either congenital or acquired;[108, 109] the acquired variety are more common. As a group of lesions seen at any time during life, they constitute only 1 percent of all intracranial masses. Thus, one may reason that the congenital variety are indeed rare. Congenital arachnoid cysts are likely to be formed by maldevelopment of the leptomeninges,

Figure 6–59. Very large choroid plexus cyst (C) seen in both axial (A) and parasagittal (B) planes. This cyst is so large it expands the ventricle (V). Polyhydramnios and other anomalies were present. Trisomy 18 was found on karyotype.

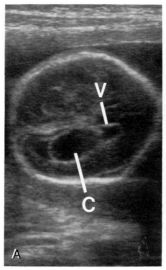
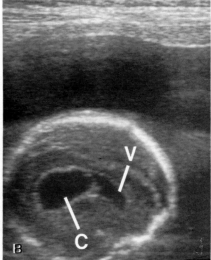

being located between the pia-arachnoid layers. The lesion originally communicates with the subarachnoid space. Acquired arachnoid cysts may follow hemorrhage or infection. Since these pathologic processes occur in utero as well as after birth, some "congenital" arachnoid cysts are likely "acquired."

Arachnoid cysts probably grow in a partially walled-off zone within the pia-arachnoid, which possesses a ball-valve communication with the subarachnoid space.[110] Thus, a fluid-filled mass is formed that may grow. Alternatively, there may be heterotopic choroid plexus–like tissue within the cyst.[111] This tissue presumably secretes CSF into a closed space, resulting in cyst formation. These lesions produce ill effects by pressure and mass effect that may result in hydrocephalus. However, they are not a cause of brain maldevelopment, and if treated before irreversible brain damage sets in, a good outcome may be anticipated.

Arachnoid cysts must be distinguished from other supratentorial cysts including choroid plexus cysts, porencephalic (schizencephalic) cysts, cystic tumors, midline cysts associated with ACC, dorsal cysts of holoprosencephaly, and arteriovenous malformations (vein of Galen aneurysms). Arachnoid cysts create a mass effect and never communicate with the lateral ventricle, while porencephalic cysts create no mass effect and most do communicate with the lateral ventricle. A cyst in the quadrigeminal plate cistern may simulate the appearance of a vein of Galen aneurysm.[107] However, no Doppler flow is seen in arachnoid cysts, whereas high-velocity signals are anticipated in a dilated vein of Galen. Choroid plexus cysts are easily identified by location. Cystic tumors (teratomas) usually have relatively large amounts of disorganized solid tissue associated with the cystic component, a feature not shared with arachnoid cysts. Distinction of arachnoid cysts from cysts seen in ACC and holoprosencephaly is based on the lack of associated brain maldevelopment invariably seen in these other disorders. The maldevelopment of the brain noted in ACC and holoprosencephaly has been discussed previously.

Already mentioned, the supratentorial arteriovenous malformation or vein of Galen aneurysm is another rare "cystic" space-occupying supratentorial mass.[112] This "cystic" lesion, unlike choroid plexus cysts or arachnoid cysts, is associated with severe cardiovascular hemodynamic abnormalities. Associated CNS disturbances are the rule. Cardiac failure, manifest in utero by hydrops fetalis (nonimmune), may be evident. The basic lesion is the arteriovenous communication that results in marked dilatation of the venous component (Galen's vein). The "cyst" is the enlarged vein. In addition to the stress placed on the heart by the arteriovenous malformation, cerebral perfusion is also compromised by diversion of blood from brain tissue directly to the venous limb ("steal" phenomenon). This results in brain infarction and the development of leukomalacia.

The features of this lesion are characteristic and easily diagnosed by prenatal sonography. The supratentorial cyst is located in or near the tentorial hiatus (the quadrigeminal plate cistern, cistern of the velum interpositum). A high-frequency turbulent Doppler signal is readily obtained from the lesion. The carotid arteries and jugular veins are enlarged and similarly show high flow signals. The heart is enlarged and hydrops fetalis may be seen. Thus, this constellation of findings enables a specific prenatal diagnosis. Unfortunately, little can be done postnatally to prevent morbidity and death; both are the rule rather than the exception.

Intracranial Hemorrhage

Intracranial hemorrhage (ICH) is an extremely common event among preterm newborns, especially those weighing less than 1500 gm and born earlier than 32 weeks.[113–114] The incidence of such hemorrhage is approximately 40 to 50 percent. The hemorrhages tend to originate in the germinal matrix, which is a highly vascular tissue located in the subependymal region of the lateral ventricles. The germinal matrix is the source of neurons migrating to the cerebral cortex.

Using computed tomography and real-time sonography, studies in premature infants show that most hemorrhages occur one to seven days after birth.[114] Although the pathophysiology of neonatal intracranial hemorrhage is unknown, the consensus is that sudden changes in blood pressure of the premature neonate may cause subependymal hemorrhages (SEH) that may subsequently rupture into the ventricular lumen (intraventricular hemorrhage [IVH]).

Hypoxic events tend to trigger such fluctuations in blood pressure, resulting in subependymal (germinal matrix) hemorrhage in preterm newborns.[113] Since fetuses have copious germinal matrix and are also susceptible to hypoxemia, one would hypothesize that such hemorrhages could also be common in fetuses. In fact and fortunately, intracranial hemorrhage in utero appears to be a peculiarly uncommon event. No series has been reported; only isolated cases appear in the literature.

Intracranial hemorrhages are most commonly categorized by the classification of Papile:[114]

Type I. Confined to the germinal matrix, i.e., subependymal hemorrhage.

Type II. Subependymal hemorrhage with rupture into the ventricle but no dilatation of the ventricle.

Type III. Same as Type II, but now the ventricle is dilated with blood.

Type IV. Extension of the hemorrhage into the brain parenchyma.

Since hypoxia is a common preceding event in the development of hemorrhages, it is important to remember that infarction and other anoxic brain injuries may be present, as well, but less readily detected by sonography.

All cases discovered in utero have been Types III or IV;[115, 116] these have the worst prognosis. In preterm newborns, Types I and II are by far the more common varieties. On the one hand, this suggests that minor grades of in utero hemorrhage go undetected on prenatal sonograms and thus are more common than the literature documents.* On the other hand, it is well known that even small hemorrhages detected sonographically remain visible for weeks after the inciting event. Thus, if intracranial hemorrhages were very common in the three to four weeks preceding birth, one would expect to find sonographic evidence of residuum frequently in the newborn. This is not the case.

A feature that is commonly seen in case reports of fetal intracranial hemorrhage is severe illness in the mother; case reports

have included evidence of severe hepatitis,[117] severe hypertension,[118] preeclampsia, seizures,[116] and acute pancreatitis.[119] However, several cases lacked significant maternal disease. In one of these, the fetus was anomalous.[120] In a second, there was a history of two stillbirths of male fetuses.[115] The fetus with ICH was also male. Nonetheless, in a few cases, the pregnancy appeared uncomplicated except for the hemorrhage.[121–123]

As in the newborn, intracranial hemorrhage, when recent, appears as a brightly echogenic focus in the fetus, either within the parenchyma of the brain or within the ventricular system. Blood in the ventricular system may show a fluid-fluid level. Intraparenchymal hemorrhage may show progressive liquefaction and excavation, resulting in a typical porencephalic cyst.

OPEN NEURAL TUBE DEFECTS

General Principles

Neural tube defects are among the most common congenital anomalies in the United States.[124–128] The incidence of these malformations has been estimated to be as high as 16 per 10,000 births in the eastern US.[124] The recurrence risk is much higher for a woman who has previously given birth to a child with a neural tube defect. In the US, the risk of recurrence after one child with a neural tube anomaly is 2 to 3 percent, and after a second abnormal child, the risk is approximately 6 percent.[126] Parents who have had a previous child with a neural tube defect may have suffered emotional as well as possible financial hardship. Such parents with an increased risk of producing another child with a neural tube defect frequently seek early prenatal testing to detect a recurrence. This has generally been accomplished with the measurement of the amniotic fluid (AF) levels of alpha-fetoprotein (AFP).

Alpha-fetoprotein is a glycoprotein that is synthesized by the normal fetal liver but is not normally produced by adult hepatocytes.[125–128] It is important to remember that AFP is *not* an abnormal "marker" protein generated by abnormally exposed neural tissues. It is a normal protein found in high concentrations in fetal serum. Serum levels are measured in milligrams per milliliter.

---

*Postnatal sonograms, obtained through the anterior fontanelle, enable resolution of much greater detail more consistently than in utero sonograms that generally require the beam to pass through the calvarium.

Under normal circumstances, some of the AFP finds its way into the amniotic fluid. The normal quantity of AFP in amniotic fluid shows a much lower level of concentration (measured in micrograms per milliliter) than fetal serum does. The mechanism by which AFP normally passes from the fetal circulation into the amniotic fluid is not fully understood, although two likely pathways are via fetal proteinuria (probably a normal event in very early pregnancy) and transudation of plasma proteins across immature fetal epithelium. The AFP found in amniotic fluid normally demonstrates a unimodal concentration curve that peaks in the early second trimester, then declines to very low levels by the end of pregnancy. Very small but measurable quantities (nanograms per milliliter) of this protein enter the maternal circulation from the amniotic fluid compartment.

If all women who had previously delivered a child with an open neural tube defect were screened by measuring amniotic fluid AFP, only 10 percent of all fetuses with a neural tube defect would be detected.[126] Ninety percent of such anomalies occur as first-time events to parents who have not previously produced a child with a neural tube defect. The only practical and safe means for large-scale screening of all pregnant women requires the measurement of maternal serum AFP levels. Measurement of AFP in amniotic fluid has been successfully employed for more than a decade to detect open neural tube defects in the fetus. Serum AFP testing is a more recent technique.

When an open neural tube defect is present, a portion of the fetus lacks its normal integumentary covering. For example, in anencephaly there is no skin covering the abnormality; instead, the cranial surface is covered by a thick angiomatous stroma. In meningocele, encephalocele, or myelomeningocele, only a membranous covering, or no covering at all, is present. This allows abnormally large quantities of AFP to "leak" into the amniotic fluid and thence into the maternal serum.

Maternal serum AFP testing has had very encouraging preliminary results.[126, 127] It seems safe to speculate that in the very near future, virtually all pregnant women in the United States will be offered AFP screening. When large numbers of women are screened, almost all sonographers doing obstetric scan-

ning will encounter cases specifically referred for "elevation of maternal serum AFP." One must be aware of the problems encountered in such testing.[128–130] Before one can understand the complexities of serum AFP testing, one must first understand the problems in amniotic fluid AFP testing. Serum AFP testing shares nearly all problems of amniotic fluid AFP testing but has a few more.

First, the maternal serum AFP may be spuriously elevated. An erroneous LNMP, a common problem, causes the measured AFP to be compared for normalcy with standards for the wrong gestational age. Twins and fetal demise also result in elevations of maternal serum AFP without a specific anomaly being present.

Second, such tests detect more abnormalities than open neural tube defects. For example, omphalocele and gastroschisis are also anomalies associated with integumentary defects and thus leak AFP into the amniotic fluid.[131, 132] Although these fetuses are abnormal, a fetus with gastroschisis has a far better prognosis than one with an encephalocele. "Knowing" by ultrasound discrimination that a fetus has one defect as opposed to the other could clearly affect a parental decision regarding subsequent management of the pregnancy, i.e., termination versus continued gestation with surgical repair of the anomaly following birth.

Third, and most important, normal living singleton fetuses may be incorrectly judged to be abnormal by either maternal serum or amniotic fluid AFP testing.[126–131] For example, fetal serum contains many thousands of times more AFP than does amniotic fluid. Thus, slight contamination of the amniotic fluid with fetal blood spuriously elevates amniotic fluid AFP levels into the abnormal zone. However, a problem that one often neglects to consider in a hospital setting must be strongly considered in a screening study. Statistically, a small percentage of normal fetuses have amniotic fluid or maternal serum AFP levels greater than two or even three standard deviations above the mean.[130] For example, two standard deviations above the mean implies that approximately 2.5 percent of normal individuals will fall above this cutoff. Even if we assume that every abnormal fetus will fall above two standard deviations, the following situation occurs in 10,000 samples tested:

2% of normals > 2 standard deviations =
200 normals

100% of abnormals > 2 standard deviations
= 16 abnormals

In this example, there would be 216 tests with an abnormal result, but only 16 of the fetuses would have a neural tube defect. A partial solution is to raise the "normal" cutoff to three, four, or even five standard deviations above the mean. However, each time one does this, the risk of "missing" an abnormal fetus increases. Unfortunately, even if one were to go as high as five standard deviations above the mean and test many thousands of women, there would still be a small but significant number of false-positive diagnoses.

What is clearly needed in such a situation is a second level of testing that discriminates the normal from the abnormal case. Sonography adequately serves as the second level of testing.[131-134] The first level of testing (AFP analysis) works with a very large group of fetuses that has a very low prevalence of disease. The second level of testing (sonography) works with a small group of fetuses with a high prevalence of disease. This statistical situation can greatly improve diagnostic accuracy with the second testing system. Additionally, the sonographer is provided with a "list" of potential abnormalities that could be identified. With this "road map," specific areas of the fetus may be preferentially examined for the presence of anomalies, a procedure that can lead to extremely accurate sonographic results.[132]

Anencephaly

This severe defect is the most common of the open neural tube defects and also the most common anomaly affecting the CNS.[125-127] It shows a clear female predominance with a female to male ratio of 4:1. An increased familial incidence has been established, as with all other neural tube defects. This probably accounts for the geographic differences in the incidence of anencephaly (for example, occurrence is greater in the United Kingdom than in the United States).

Even though anencephaly means absence of the brain, functioning neural tissue is always present.[135] The telencephalon is usually absent whereas the brainstem and portions of the mesencephalon are usually present. Absence of the cranial vault (the bones formed in membrane) is a constant finding (acrania). However, bones formed in cartilage at the base of the skull, including the orbits, are usually present.

Anencephaly results from a failure of the neural tube to close completely at its cephalic end.[9] This occurs between the second and third weeks of development, when the neural folds at the cranial end of the neural plate normally fuse to form the forebrain. The defect is covered by a thick membrane of angiomatous stroma but never bone or normal skin.

Anencephaly was the earliest fetal malformation to be recognized by sonography[136] and can be consistently detected.[131-134, 137, 138] Most often, anencephaly is discovered sonographically at the time of an attempted biparietal diameter determination for fetal age. However, more recently, it is being discovered with increasing frequency in patients referred for elevated AFP. Hopefully, in the future, virtually all cases of this universally fatal anomaly will be discovered early in pregnancy because of widespread AFP testing programs.

The finding that draws the attention of the observer to a severe abnormality is the absence of the normal cephalic outline (acrania). Though this may be recognizable toward the end of the first trimester, the calvarial bones are so small prior to the 13th week that they may go unnoticed during a routine examination. Relatively copious amounts of tissue may be present above the orbits when this anomaly is seen at an early state (Fig. 6–60). This tissue may represent either abnormally exposed brain tissue (exencephaly)[139] or buoyant angiomatous stroma. Many cases of anencephaly have been recognized as showing a typical configuration by the 16th week while a fetus examined in the 12th week with this anomaly failed to show the classic features.[140] Identification of the "head" is not sufficient to exclude anencephaly. Recall, the bony skull base and orbits are generally present and may give the impression of a cranial structure if viewed hurriedly. *Failure to identify normal bony structure and brain tissue cephalad to the bony orbits is the most reliable feature of this anomaly. Equally important, the absence of bony calvarium should be symmetric* (Fig. 6–60B, 6–61).

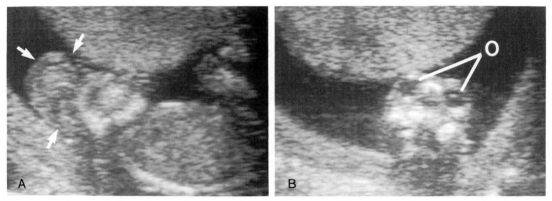

Figure 6–60. Anencephaly, early second trimester. *A,* Sagittal sonogram demonstrates a large amount of angiomatous stroma *(arrows)* cephalad to the skull base. *B,* However, coronal image of the face demonstrates the symmetric absence of calvarium above the orbits (O), thus confirming the diagnosis of anencephaly.

Common associated anomalies include spinal defects, which occur in 50 percent of anencephalic fetuses. Severe rachischisis (spina bifida) with or without myelomeningocele can often be demonstrated by sonography. Other associated anomalies may be seen, as well. However, since anencephaly is a uniformly fatal abnormality, effort should be concentrated on confirming its presence. Once a fetus has a confirmed lethal abnormality, the identification of additional anomalies is superfluous. Polyhydramnios is present in 40 to 50 percent of cases but does not usually occur until after 26 weeks of gestation. Occasionally, oligohydramnios is encountered.

A distinction should be made between anencephaly and other conditions that may be confused with it. Any similar-appearing anomaly that has caused the cranium and brain to be sufficiently small, by either abnormal growth or destruction, should be judged to carry the same fatal prognosis. However, the recurrence risk for the mother may vary considerably, ranging from no risk to 25 percent. The precise nature of the abnormality may not be detectable by ex utero examination of an abortus if dilatation and extraction was the modality employed to evacuate the uterus. Thus, the in utero sonographic examination may be the only opportunity to establish the true nature, and thus the potential recurrence risk, of the anomaly.

When severe, microcephaly may mimic the appearance of anencephaly. However,

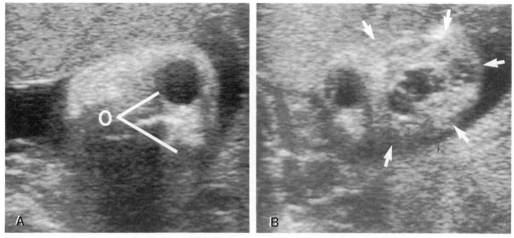

Figure 6–61. Anencephaly, middle second trimester. *A,* Coronal sonogram through the face demonstrates the "classic" appearance of anencephaly (symmetric absence of calvarium above the orbits [O]). *B,* Oblique section through the angiomatous stroma *(arrows)* overlying the skull base. The tissue is partially solid and partially cystic.

one can always identify a cranial vault when microcephaly is present (Fig. 6–62). Frequently, cortical brain tissue is identified in microcephaly, although it may be very small in quantity. If microcephaly is extremely severe, one must rely solely on identification of the cranial vault to distinguish this entity from anencephaly. In anencephaly, of course, both the cranial vault and cortical brain tissue are absent. Depending upon the etiology, i.e., autosomal recessive inheritance, microcephalic disorders may carry a 25 percent recurrence risk. Amniotic band syndrome (ABS) involving the head may present a confusing picture since this entity may destroy most of the cranial vault and brain.[141] However, ABS tends to destroy the cranium asymmetrically. Recall that in anencephaly, the absence of the cranial vault is symmetric. There is no known recurrence risk for ABS. The rare occurrence of the holoacardious "acephalic" twin can be a true anencephalic aberration. In this circumstance, the entire cranial structure may be lacking, or severe microcephaly may be present (Fig. 6–62). This condition occurs only in identical twins. The acephalic acardiac twin is a parasite on the sibling. Its blood supply comes via communications in the placenta. Since this entity occurs only in identical twins, it does not carry the recurrence risk of singleton anencephaly (there is no recurrence risk for identical twinning).[142] However, true anencephaly can occur asynchronously in twins without association of parabiotic vascular communications in the placenta. Presumably this latter situation, unlike the holoacardious identical twin, carries a recurrence risk in subsequent singleton pregnancies.

Encephalocele

This condition is the least common open neural tube defect.[131–133, 143–145] Encephalocele results from failure of the surface ectoderm to separate from the neuroectoderm.[9] This results in a mesodermal (bony calvarial) defect that allows herniation of the meninges alone (cranial meningocele) or the brain and the meninges (true encephalocele) through the bony defect. The most common site of occurrence is the occipital midline (75 percent) (Fig. 6–63) followed by the frontal midline (13 percent). Parietal lesions are noted in approximately 12 percent of cases.[146, 147] However, lesions located away from the midline are virtually always the result of the amniotic band syndrome (Fig. 6–64).

Encephaloceles are recognized as spherical, fluid- or brain-filled sacs (Fig. 6–65) extending from the bony calvarium in the occipital or frontal region.[5, 6, 143–145] Indeed, the identification of the encephalocele sac is usually not difficult. More difficult is the identification of the associated bony defect (Fig. 6–63). Importantly, acoustic shadowing may produce a spurious "defect" in the calvarium. In the suspect gestation with elevated AFP, a systematic and detailed approach should be employed to evaluate the calvarium for these defects in the typical locations described above.

Absence of brain tissue within the cranial meningocele sac is the single most favorable prognostic feature for survival.[148] Visualization of solid brain elements within the sac is usually straightforward. However, it is difficult to exclude incorporated brain tissue in sacs that appear completely fluid filled. Small amounts of incorporated brain tissue may be present toward the periphery of the sac. Associated anomalies include hy-

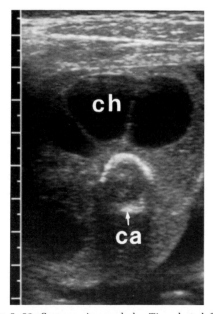

Figure 6–62. Severe microcephaly. Tiny, but definite, calvarium (ca) are detected in this severely anomalous fetus (acardiac twin at approximately 25 weeks' gestational age). The visualized calvarium excludes the possibility of anencephaly. ch, cystic hygromas.

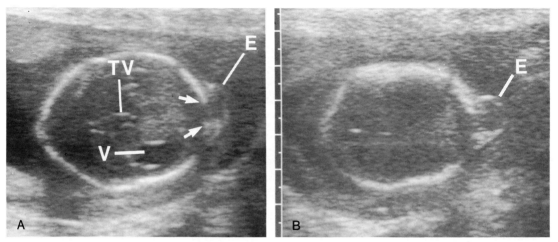

Figure 6–63. *A, B,* Small occipital encephalocele, paired transverse axial sonograms. E, encephalocele sac; V, prominent ventricle; TV, enlarged third ventricle; *arrows,* bony defect.

drocephalus (from the concomitant Chiari malformation), ACC, DWS, and Meckel's syndrome (encephalocele, microcephaly, polydactyly, cystic kidneys).

Some lesions may be mistaken for encephaloceles. The most common of these is the cystic hygroma (Fig. 6–66). Cystic hygromas have no calvarial defect (remember it is easy to create a spurious calvarial defect caused by reflective shadowing), and careful scanning confirms that the lesion is continuous with abnormal skin and subcutaneous tissues adjacent to the cystic cavity (Fig. 6–67). Nasal teratomas must be distinguished from frontal encephaloceles. The teratoma is usually more irregularly shaped and heterogeneous in its architecture. Cloverleaf skull deformity also simulates the appearance of

an encephalocele; these two entities may be distinguished by observing the presence of calvarium surrounding the three cephalic protrusions of fetuses that have the cloverleaf skull deformity.

Myelomeningocele—Spina Bifida

Myelomeningocele is the second most common open neural tube defect.[126] As with the calvarium, it is possible to have a meningocele without incorporated nerve roots or cord within it. However, isolated meningoceles are rare by comparison with the myelomeningocele. These lesions may occur anywhere along the spine but are most com-

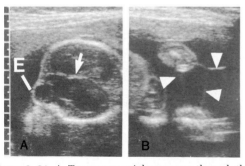

Figure 6–64. *A,* Transverse axial sonogram through the calvarium of a fetus with an encephalocele (E) that does not lie in the midline *(arrow).* This feature should suggest the amniotic band syndrome. *B,* Further search discloses numerous bands *(arrowheads)* attached to the fetus' extremities.

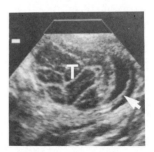

Figure 6–65. Sector real-time sonogram of a large fetal encephalocele. T, disorganized brain tissue; *Arrow,* sac margin. Avoid the temptation to call the swirled tissue in the sac "gyri and sulci." Such structures are poorly developed in young *normal fetuses;* it is unlikely that this process is more advanced in those with maldeveloped brain tissue.

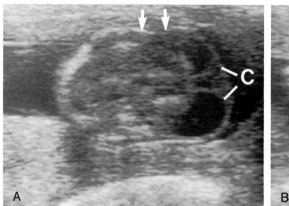
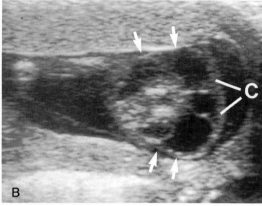

Figure 6–66. Transverse axial sonograms through the basiocciput *(A)* and neck *(B)* in a fetus with a large nuchal cystic hygroma (C). The margins of these lesions "line up" with the adjacent cutaneous tissues *(arrows)*. The adjacent subcutaneous tissues are virtually always abnormal and recognizably so.

mon in the lumbar and sacral region. The malformation results from failure of the neural tube (caudal neuropore) to close at three to four weeks, resulting in an exposed neural plate.[9] The defect is variable in size and content. Neurologic defects range from minor anesthesia to complete paraparesis and death. Prognosis is worse if the lesion is higher, larger, or associated with other anomalies.[149]

The fetal spine is easily and clearly evaluated by 16 to 17 weeks of development.[150] As discussed earlier in this chapter, the

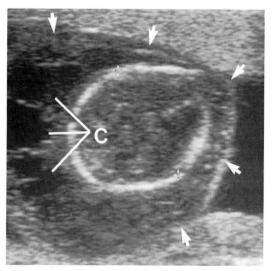

Figure 6–67. Transverse axial sonogram shows diffuse lymphangiectasia with cystic hygroma formation. The posterior cystic spaces (C) should not be misinterpreted as encephaloceles. Note that all the subcutaneous tissues *(arrows)* are abnormal.

normal POC are seen as two closely spaced parallel lines of echoes that widen normally in the cervical region. The distance between the posterior ossification centers is tantamount to the interpediculate distance (Figs. 6–21 to 6–23).[5, 6, 150] In the transverse plane of section, three ossification centers are identified, all within close proximity surrounding the spinal cord (Fig. 6–21). In spina bifida, which is the bony accompaniment to myelomeningocele, there is separation of the posterior ossification centers on the transverse and longitudinal scans (Figs. 6–68 to 6–70). Normally in transverse planes, the posterior ossification centers parallel each other or angle toward one another (Fig. 6–22). Spina bifida can be diagnosed when the posterior ossification centers splay outwardly and are farther apart than the ossification centers above or below the defect (Fig. 6–69, 6–70). The latter is noted on longitudinal images (Fig. 6–71). The cleft in the soft tissues can be seen nearly always with modern high-resolution equipment. Indeed, the cleft is more easily recognized in some cases than the bony defect itself (Fig. 6–68). Spinal defects recognized in this form are easily diagnosed if three or more vertebral segments are involved.[131, 132] If only one or two spinal segments are involved, the diagnosis becomes more difficult. Abnormal morphology of the posterior ossification centers of the spine must be used to make the diagnosis if the myelomeningocele sac is not intact or if it is flattened (Fig. 6–70). When the sac is intact and bulges into the amniotic cavity, the anomaly is then more easily recognized as a cystic extension of the posterior aspect

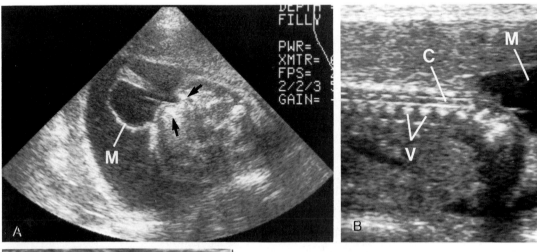

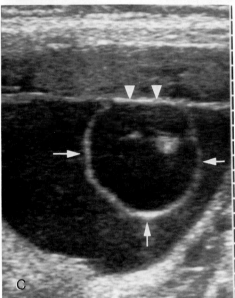

Figure 6–68. *A*, Transverse sonogram of the sacrum in a fetus with a myelomeningocele (M). Abnormal posterior ossification centers are seen *(arrows)*. *B*, Longitudinal sonogram demonstrates the myelomeningocele (M) extending from the spine. The spinal cord (C) ends at an abnormally low level (tethered cord). V, vertebral bodies. *C*, Scan oriented through the sac of the myelomeningocele. The sac margin is easily seen where it contacts amniotic fluid *(arrows)* but virtually disappears where the sac contacts the placental surface *(arrowheads)*.

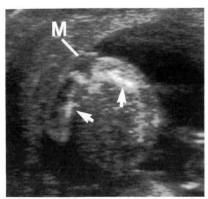

Figure 6–69. Transverse scan through the iliac wings (*arrows*) shows a small myelomeningocele (M). Note that the sac is largely obscured by contact with the myometrium.

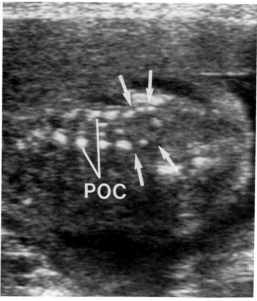

Figure 6–71. Coronal sonogram through the posterior ossification centers (POC) of the lumbosacral spine, demonstrating a small myelomeningocele. Abnormal spacing (*arrows*) of the POC is seen; this is the spina bifida lesion.

of the spine, which in real time may have a shimmering quality with fetal movement. Fetal movement, in fact, may be quite active even in the lower extremities of fetuses with myelomeningoceles although a neurologic effect on the lower extremity can be seen not uncommonly (clubfoot deformity) (Fig. 6–72).

When a specific search is made for a myelomeningocele, i.e., elevated AFP, very small lesions can be detected (Fig. 6–73A). This is especially true when a sac is present and in contact with amniotic fluid (Fig. 6–73B). When the fetal spine abuts the myometrium or placenta, the sac, even when present, may be obscured (Fig. 6–69). When the myelo-meningocele sac is obscured or absent (Fig. 6–70), one must demonstrate the bony abnormality, spina bifida, in order to suspect the presence of this anomaly. When the skin is intact over a myelomeningocele, no AFP elevation will occur. In this situation, only sonography affords an opportunity to detect the anomaly (Fig. 6–74).

As with encephaloceles, associated abnormalities are commonly present; indeed, the list includes encephalocele. Ventricular enlargement secondary to the Arnold-Chiari

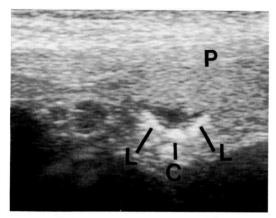

Figure 6–70. Transverse sonogram of the lumbar spine demonstrates a spina bifida lesion. This fetus with an open spinal lesion had no sac. Additionally, profound oligohydramnios was present. Thus, the only means to detect this lesion is by demonstration of the flared laminae (L), the hallmark of spina bifida. P, placenta; C, centrum.

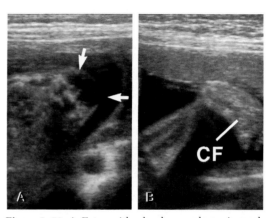

Figure 6–72. *A,* Fetus with a lumbar myelomeningocele (*arrows*). *B,* Clubfoot deformity (CF) secondary to the myelomeningocele.

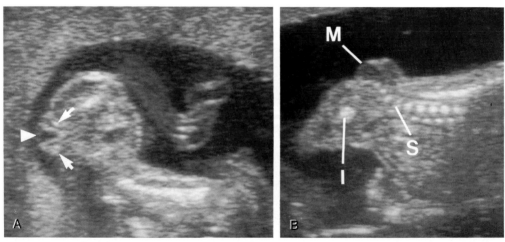

Figure 6–73. *A,* Transverse sonogram of the sacrum shows a very small myelomeningocele with the characteristic sac *(arrowhead)* and "splaying" of the posterior ossification centers *(arrows)*. *B,* Longitudinal sonogram of the same fetus. The myelomeningocele sac (M) is slightly greater than 1 cm but is very easily seen. Although smaller lesions are more difficult to detect, visualization is not strictly size dependent. I, ischial ossification center; S, sacral promontory.

(Type II) malformation is very commonly present.[149] Although not all fetuses with myelomeningocele display the Chiari (Type II) malformation, the percentage of afflicted fetuses with this malformation at the craniocervical junction is very high. Furthermore, virtually every fetus with a myelomeningocele has an abnormal posterior fossa although the abnormality may not fulfill the morphologic requirements to diagnose the Chiari (Type II) malformation.[151] As stated previously, the most common single cause of hydrocephalus in a fetus is myelomeningocele, the hydrocephalus developing secondary to the Chiari malformation. Thus, the presence of ventricular enlargement and an abnormally small or absent cisterna magna is a key observation that should always engender an extremely careful search of the spine for an open neural tube defect. However, the diagnosis of myelomeningocele should always be based on direct observation of the spinal anomaly, not on secondary signs.

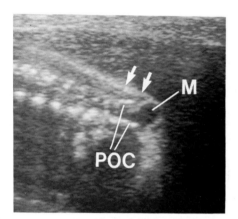

Figure 6–74. Longitudinal sonogram of the sacrum shows a very small myelomeningocele (M). This unusual myelomeningocele is skin covered *(arrows)* (compare Fig. 6–73*B*). Despite its small size (< 1 cm), it is easily seen. Note the splaying of the posterior ossification centers (POC).

DETECTION OF CNS ANOMALIES: A PRACTICAL LEVEL OF EFFORT FOR A "ROUTINE" SONOGRAM

As can be seen from the preceding discussion, sonography is an extraordinarily powerful technology that enables detection and characterization of numerous CNS malformations, some of which cause only subtle aberrations in morphology. As physicians, we must balance our desire to do the utmost for each of our patients with the practicality that performing detailed evaluations of the brain and spinal cord in every patient is simply impossible.

Fortunately, there are a few simple anatomic observations that can be made while measuring a biparietal diameter or head circumference that will exclude the vast majority of anomalies of both the brain and the spine. *The structures are three in number and are as follows: the cavum septi pellucidi, the ventricular atrium, and the cisterna magna.* These structures are easily demonstrated even by inexperienced examiners. What is substantially more difficult is understanding how demonstration of these normal structures is so effective at excluding a host of CNS malformations, especially those of the spinal cord. Importantly, this scheme helps one to recognize that an abnormality may be present, not to make specific diagnoses. *If these three structures appear well within the limits of normal, the chances that the fetus has a neutral axis anomaly of any type, including myelomeningocele, are very small, indeed.*

Open neural tube defects are the most common CNS malformations. Anencephaly, the single most common, is so severe that it is immediately detected when attempting to perform biometry of the fetal head. Not even one of the three recommended observations could possibly be made, even mistakenly, in an anencephalic fetus. Unfortunately, the second most common is myelomeningocele, the opening of which can be so subtle and difficult to detect that even the most skilled examiners fear false-negative results. As mentioned in the section on myelomeningocele, this entity is nearly always associated with the Chiari malformation. The Chiari malformation invariably effaces and most often obliterates the cisterna magna. An easily demonstrated cisterna magna with a clearly normal depth (4 to 10 mm) will be present rarely, if ever, in a fetus with a myelomeningocele. A normal-appearing cisterna magna excludes nearly all cases of myelomeningocele. The alternative method of diagnosing myelomeningoceles requires careful evaluation of every vertebral segment. With this approach, virtually 100 percent of myelomeningoceles can be detected; however, it is an approach that is entirely impractical for day to day use. Further, a normal cisterna magna excludes all but the mildest forms of DWS, cerebellar hypoplasia, and retrocerebellar arachnoid cyst.

Gross abnormalities of the supratentorial CNS (hydranencephaly, alobar holoprosencephaly, and massive hydrocephalus) are easily detected when attempting head measurements although differential diagnosis is substantially more difficult. However, less morphologically severe anomalies, such as ACC, lobar holoprosencephaly, or brain atrophy, can easily escape detection. Complete ACC and lobar holoprosencephaly are *always* associated with the absence of the septum pellucidum and, thus, the cavum septi pellucidi. Therefore, demonstration of the cavum septi pellucidi excludes nearly every subtle malformation of midline development of the brain.

Similarly, visualization of the ventricular atrium enables detection of very early ventricular enlargement, as discussed elsewhere. Importantly, enlargement of the atrium detects both obstructive hydrocephalus from any cause (communicating [rare] or noncommunicating) and nonobstructive ventricular enlargement, including developmental (colpocephaly) and destructive (brain atrophy).

The cavum septi pellucidi should be visible in the plane in which the biparietal diameter is measured. To visualize the ventricular atrium and the cisterna magna requires only minor alterations in angulation of the transducer relative to the base of the skull. Once practiced, this takes only seconds to accomplish. This brief effort to demonstrate these three structures leaves the examiner with a high level of confidence that the vast majority of lesions of CNS development, even some of the most subtle, are not present.

References

1. Carrasco CR, Stierman ED, Harnsberger HR, Lee TG: An algorithm for prenatal ultrasound diagnosis of congenital CNS abnormalities. J Ultrasound Med 4:163, 1985.
2. Goldberg BB, Isard HJ, Gershon-Cohen J, et al: Ultrasonic fetal cephalometry. Radiology 87:328, 1966.
3. Hidalgo H, Bowie J, Rosenberg ER, et al: In utero sonographic diagnosis of fetal cerebral anomalies. AJR 139:143, 1982.
4. Pasto ME, Kurtz AB: The prenatal examination of the fetal cranium, spine, and central nervous system. Semin Ultrasound, CT, and MR 5:170, 1984.
5. Fiske CE, Filly RA: Ultrasound evaluation of the normal and abnormal fetal neural axis. Rad Clin North Am 20:285, 1982.
6. Filly RA: Ultrasonography. *In* Harrison MR, Golbus MS, Filly RA (eds): The Unborn Patient: Prenatal Diagnosis and Treatment. Orlando, Grune & Stratton, 1984, pp 33–123.
7. Edwards MSD, Filly RA: Diagnosis and management of fetal disorders of the central nervous system. *In* Hoffman HJ, Epstein F (eds): Disorders of the Developing Nervous System: Diagnosis and

Treatment. Boston, Blackwell Scientific Publications, 1986, pp 55–73.

8. Clewell WH, Johnson ML, Meier PR, et al: A surgical approach to the treatment of fetal hydrocephalus. NEJM 306:1320, 1982.

9. Moore KL: The nervous system. *In* The Developing Human: Clinically Oriented Embryology, 4th Ed. Philadelphia, WB Saunders Co, 1988.

10. Day WR: Casts of foetal lateral ventricles. Brain 82:109, 1959.

11. Johnson ML, Dunne MG, Mack LA, Rashbaum CL: Evaluation of fetal intracranial anatomy by static and real-time ultrasound. J Clin Ultrasound 8:311, 1980.

12. Hadlock FP, Deter RL, Park SK: Real-time sonography: Ventricular and vascular anatomy of the fetal brain in utero. AJNR 1:507, 1980.

13. McGahan JP, Phillips HE, Ellis WG: The fetal hippocampus. Radiology 147:201, 1983.

14. Young GB: The arrow pattern: A new anatomical fetal biparietal diameter. Radiology 137:445, 1980.

15. Pilu G, DePalma L, Romero R, et al: The fetal subarachnoid cisterns: An ultrasound study with report of a case of congenital communicating hydrocephalus. J Ultrasound Med 5:365, 1986.

16. Laing FC, Stamler CE, Jeffrey RB: Ultrasonography of the fetal subarachnoid space. J Ultrasound Med 2:29, 1983.

17. Chinn DH, Callen PW, Filly RA: The lateral cerebral ventricle in early second trimester. Radiology 148:529, 1983.

18. Mahony BS, Callen PW, Filly RA, Hoddick WK: The fetal cisterna magna. Radiology 153:773, 1984.

19. Jeanty P, Chervenak FA, Romero R, et al: The sylvian fissure: A commonly mislabeled cranial landmark. J Ultrasound Med 3:15, 1984.

20. Worthen NJ, Gilbertson V, Lau C: Cortical sulcal development seen on sonography: Relationship to gestational parameters. J Ultrasound Med 5:153, 1986.

21. Reuter KL, D'Orsi CJ, Raptopoulos VD, et al: Sonographic pseudoasymetry of the prenatal cerebral hemispheres. J Ultrasound Med 1:91, 1982.

22. Denkhaus H, Winseberg F: Ultrasonic measurement of the fetal ventricular system. Radiology 131:781, 1979.

23. Jeanty P, Dramaix-Wilmet M, Delbeke D, et al: Ultrasonic evaluation of fetal ventricular growth. Neuroradiology 21:127, 1981.

24. McGahan JP, Phillips HE: Ultrasonic evaluation of the size of the trigone of the fetal ventricle. J Ultrasound Med 2:315, 1983.

25. Jorgensen C, Ingemarsson I, Svalenius E, et al: Ultrasound measurement of the fetal cerebral ventricles: A prospective, consecutive study. J Clin Ultrasound 14:185, 1986.

26. Fiske CE, Filly RA, Callen PW: The normal choroid plexus: Ultrasonographic appearance of the neonatal head. Radiology 141:467, 1981.

27. Yousefzadeh DK, Naidich TP: US anatomy of the posterior fossa in children: Correlation with brain sections. Radiology 156:353, 1985.

28. Naidich TP, Gusnard DA, Yousefzadeh DK: Sonography of the internal capsule and basal ganglia in infants: 1. Coronal sections. AJNR 6:909, 1985.

29. Seidler DE, Filly RA: Relative growth of the higher fetal brain structures. J Ultrasound Med 6:573, 1987.

30. Masdeu JC, Dobben GD, Azar-Kia B: Dandy-Walker syndrome studied by computed tomography and pneumoencephalography. Radiology 147:109, 1983.

31. Gardner E, O'Rahilly R, Prolo D: The Dandy-Walker and Arnold-Chiari malformations. Arch Neurol 23:393, 1974.

32. Goodwin L, Quisling RG: The neonatal cisterna magna: Ultrasonic evaluation. Radiology 149:691, 1983.

33. Dempsey PJ, Koch HJ: In utero diagnosis of the Dandy-Walker syndrome: Differentiation from extra-axial posterior fossa cyst. J Clin Ultrasound 9:403, 1981.

34. Lipton HL, Preiosi TJ, Moses H: Adult onset of the Dandy-Walker syndrome. Arch Neurol 35:672, 1978.

35. Lee TG, Newton BW: Posterior fossa cyst: Prenatal diagnosis by ultrasound. J Clin Ultrasound 4:29, 1976.

36. Hatjis CG, Horbar JD, Anderson GG: The in utero diagnosis of a posterior fossa intracranial cyst (Dandy-Walker cyst). Am J Obstet Gynecol 140:473, 1981.

37. Kirkinen P, Jouppila P, Valkeakari T, Saukkonen AL: Ultrasonic evaluation of the Dandy-Walker syndrome. Obstet Gynecol 59:18S, 1982.

38. Newman GC, Buschi AI, Sugg NK, et al: Dandy-Walker syndrome diagnosed in utero by ultrasonography. Neurology (NY) 32:180, 1982.

39. Depp R, Sabbagha RE, Brown T, et al: Fetal surgery for hydrocephalus: Successful in utero ventriculoamniotic shunt for Dandy-Walker syndrome. Obstet Gynecol 61:710, 1983.

40. Comstock H, Boal DB: Enlarged fetal cisterna magna: Appearance and significance. Obstet Gynecol 66:25S, 1985.

41. McCleary R, Kuhns L, Barr M: Ultrasonography of the fetal cerebellum. Radiology 151:439, 1984.

42. Archer C, Darwish H, Smith K: Enlarged cisternae magnae and posterior fossa cysts simulating Dandy-Walker syndrome on computed tomography. Radiology 127:681, 1978.

43. Kendall E: Dysgenesis of the corpus callosum. Neuroradiology 25:239, 1983.

44. Probst FP: Congenital defects of the corpus callosum: Morphology and encephalographic appearances. Acta Radiol [Diagn] 331:1S, 1973.

45. Harwood-Nash DC: Absence of the corpus callosum. *In* Harwood-Nash DC (ed): Neuroradiology in Infants and Children, Vol 3. St Louis, CV Mosby Co, 1976, p 1019.

46. Rakic P, Yakovlev PI: Development of the corpus callosum and cavum septi in man. J Comp Neurol 132:45, 1968.

47. Comstock CH, Culp D, Gonzalez J, Boal DB: Agenesis of the corpus callosum in the fetus: Its evolution and significance. J Ultrasound Med 4:613, 1985.

48. Gebarski SS, Gebarski KS, Bowerman RA, Silver TM: Agenesis of the corpus callosum: Sonographic features. Radiology 151:443, 1984.

49. Mok PM, Gunn TR: The diagnosis of absence of the corpus callosum by ultrasound. Australas Radiol 26:121, 1982.

50. Skeffington F: Agenesis of the corpus callosum: Neonatal ultrasound appearance. Arch Dis Child 57:713, 1982.

51. Skidmore MB, Dolfin T, Becker LE, et al: The sonographic diagnosis of agenesis of the corpus callosum. J Ultrasound Med 2:55, 1983.

52. Babcock DS: The normal, absent and abnormal corpus callosum: Sonographic findings. Radiology 151:449, 1984.

53. Cohen MM, Jirasek JE, Guzman RT, et al: Holoprosencephaly and facial dysmorphia: Nosology, etiology and pathogenesis. Birth Defects: Original Article Series 7:125, 1971.

54. Manelfe C, Sevely A: Neuroradiologic study of holoprosencephalies. J Neuroradiol 9:15, 1982.

55. Warkang J, Lemire R, Cohen M: Holoprosencephaly: Cyclopia series. In Mental Retardation and Congenital Malformations of the Central Nervous System. Chicago, Year Book Medical Publishers, 1981, pp 176–190.

56. Cohen MM: An update on the holoprosencephalic disorders. J Pediatr 101:865, 1982.

57. Filly RA, Chinn DH, Callen PW: Alobar holoprosencephaly: Ultrasonographic prenatal diagnosis. Radiology 151:455, 1984.

58. Chervenak FA, Isaacson G, Hobbins JC, et al: Diagnosis and management of fetal holoprosencephaly. Obstet Gynecol 66:322, 1985.

59. Greene MF, Benacerraf BR, Frigoletto FD: Reliable criteria for the prenatal sonographic diagnosis of alobar holoprosencephaly. Am J Obstet Gynecol 156:687, 1987.

60. Toth Z, Csecsei K, Szeifert G, et al: Early prenatal diagnosis of cyclopia associated with holoprosencephaly. J Clin Ultrasound 14:550, 1986.

61. Chervenak FA, Isaacson G, Mahoney MJ, et al: The obstetric significance of holoprosencephaly. Obstet Gynecol 63:115, 1984.

62. Cayea PD, Balcar I, Alberti O, Jones TB: Prenatal diagnosis of semilobar holoprosencephaly. AJR 142:401, 1984.

63. Hoffman-Tretin JC, Horoupian DS, Koenigsberg M, et al: Lobar holoprosencephaly with hydrocephalus: Antenatal demonstration and differential diagnosis. J Ultrasound Med 5:691, 1986.

64. Muir CS: Hydranencephaly and allied disorders. Am J Dis Child 34:231, 1959.

65. Lemire RJ, Loeser JD, Leech RW, Alvord EC: Normal and Abnormal Development of the Human Nervous System. Hagerstown, MD, Harper & Row, 1975, p 251.

66. Friede RL: Developmental Neuropathology. New York, Springer Verlag, 1975, p 109.

67. Jung JH, Graham JM, Schultz N, Smith DW: Congenital hydranencephaly/porencephaly due to vascular disruption in monozygotic twins. Pediatr 73:467, 1984.

68. Green MF, Benacerraf B, Crawford JM: Hydranencephaly: US appearance during in utero evolution. Radiology 156:779, 1985.

69. Straus S, Bouzouki M, Goldfarb A, et al: Antenatal ultrasound diagnosis of an unusual case of hydranencephaly. J Clin Ultrasound 12:420, 1984.

70. Fleischer A, Brown M: Hydramnios associated with fetal hydranencephaly. J Clin Ultrasound 5:41, 1977.

71. Lee TG, Warren BH: Antenatal diagnosis of hydranencephaly by ultrasound: Correlation with ventriculography and computed tomography. J Clin Ultrasound 5:271, 1977.

72. Page LK, Brown SB, Gargano FP, Shortz RW: Schizencephaly: A clinical study and review. Childs Brain 1:348, 1975.

73. Miller GM, Stears JC, Guggenheim MA, Wilkening GF: Schizencephaly: A clinical and CT study. Neurology 34:997, 1984.

74. Williams JP, Blalock CP, Dunaway CL, Chalhub EG: Schizencephaly. J Comput Assist Tomogr 7:135, 1983.

75. Klingensmith WC, Cioffi-Ragan DT: Schizencephaly: Diagnosis and progression in utero. Radiology 159:617, 1986.

76. Sutton LN, Bruce DA, Schut L: Hydranencephaly versus maximal hydrocephalus: An important clinical distinction. Neurosurg 6:35, 1980.

77. Chuang S: Perinatal and neonatal hydrocephalus. Perinatology Sept–Oct:8, 1986.

78. Harwood-Nash F: Neuroradiology in Infants and Children, Vol 2. St. Louis, CV Mosby Co, 1976, pp 609–677.

79. McElroy DB: Hydrocephalus in children. Nurs Clin North Am 15:23, 1980.

80. Shannon MW, Nadler HL: X-linked hydrocephalus. J Med Genet 5:326, 1968.

81. Carter LO: Clues to the etiology of neural tube malformations. Dev Med Child Neurol 16(suppl):3, 1976.

82. Hudgins RJ, Edwards MJB, Goldstein R, et al: Natural history of fetal ventriculomegaly. Pediatrics, in press.

83. Glick PL, Harrison MR, Nakayama DK, et al: Management of ventriculomegaly in the fetus. J Pediatr 105:97, 1984.

84. Chervenak FA, Berkowitz RL, Tortura M, Hobbins JL: The management of fetal hydrocephalus. Am J Obstet Gynecol 151:933, 1985.

85. Serlo W, Kirkinen P, Jouppila P, Herva R: Prognostic signs in fetal hydrocephalus. Childs Nerv Syst 2:93, 1986.

86. Cochrane DD, Miles ST, Nimrod C, et al: Intrauterine hydrocephalus and ventriculomegaly: Associated anomalies and fetal outcome. Canad J Neurol Sci 12:51, 1984.

87. Pretorius DH, Davis K, Manco-Johnson ML, et al: Clinical course of fetal hydrocephalus: 40 cases. AJR 144:827, 1985.

88. Nyberg DA, Mack LA, Hirsch J, et al: Fetal hydrocephalus: Sonographic detection and clinical significance of associated anomalies. Radiology 163:187, 1987.

89. Pretorius DH, Drose JA, Manco-Johnson ML: Fetal lateral ventricular ratio determination during the second trimester. J Ultrasound Med 5:121, 1986.

90. Fiske CE, Filly RA, Callen PW: Sonographic measurement of lateral ventricular width in early ventricular dilatation. J Clin Ultrasound 9:303, 1981.

91. Gillieson MS, Hickey NM: Prenatal diagnosis of fetal hydrocephalus with a normal biparietal diameter. J Ultrasound Med 3:227, 1984.

92. Callen PW, Chooljian D: The effect of ventricular dilatation upon biometry of the fetal head. J Ultrasound Med 5:17, 1986.

93. Hartung RW, Yiu-Chiu V: Demonstration of unilateral hydrocephalus in utero. J Ultrasound Med 2:369, 1983.

94. Case KJ, Hirsch J, Case MJ: Simulation of significant pathology by normal hypoechoic white matter in cranial ultrasound. J Clin Ultrasound 11:281, 1983.

95. Cardoza J, Filly RA, Podrasky AE: Exclusion of pseudohydrocephalus by a simple observation: The dangling choroid sign. AJR, in press.
96. Fraumeni JR, Miller RW: Cancer deaths in the newborn. Am J Dis Child 127:186, 1969.
97. Koos WT, Miller MH: Intracranial Tumors of Infants and Children. St Louis, CV Mosby, 1971, pp 12–14.
98. Lipman SP, Pretorius DH, Rumack CM, Manco-Johnson ML: Fetal intracranial teratoma: US diagnosis of three cases and a review of the literature. Radiology 157:491, 1985.
99. Riboni G, DeSimoni M, Leopardi O, Molla R: Ultrasound appearance of a glioblastoma in a 33 week fetus in utero. J Clin Ultrasound 13:345, 1985.
100. Hoff NR, Mackay IM: Prenatal ultrasound diagnosis of intracranial teratoma. J Clin Ultrasound 8:247, 1980.
101. Shawker TH, Schwartz RM: Ultrasound appearance of a malignant fetal brain tumor. J Clin Ultrasound 11:35, 1983.
102. Whittle IR, Simpson DA: Surgical treatment of neonatal intracranial teratoma. Surg Neurol 15:268, 1981.
103. Chudleigh P, Pearce JM, Campbell S: The prenatal diagnosis of transient cysts of the fetal choroid plexus. Prenat Diag 4:135, 1984.
104. Ostlere SJ, Irving HC, Lilford RJ: Choroid plexus cysts in the fetus. Lancet 1:1491, 1987.
105. Ricketts NEM, Lowe EM, Patel NB: Prenatal diagnosis of choroid plexus cysts. Lancet 1:213, 1987.
106. Diakoumakis EE, Weinberg B, Mollin J: Prenatal sonographic diagnosis of a suprasellar arachnoid cyst. J Ultrasound Med 5:529, 1986.
107. Mack LA, Rumack CM, Johnson ML: Ultrasound evaluation of cystic intracranial lesions in the neonate. Radiology 137:451, 1980.
108. Oliver LC: Primary arachnoid cysts. Br Med J 1:1147, 1958.
109. Starkman SP, Brown TC, Linell EA: Cerebral arachnoid cysts. J Neuropath Exp Neurol 17:484, 1958.
110. Williams B, Guthkelch DL: Why do central arachnoid pouches expand? J Neurol Neurosurg Psychol 37:1085, 1974.
111. Koto A, Horoupian DS, Shulman K: Choroidal epithelial cyst. J Neurosurg 47:955, 1977.
112. Reiter AA, Huhta JC, Carpenter JR, et al: Prenatal diagnosis of arteriovenous malformation of the vein of Galen. J Clin Ultrasound 14:623, 1986.
113. Morales WJ: Effect of intraventricular hemorrhage on the one-year mental and neurologic handicaps of the very low birthweight infant. Obstet Gynecol 70:111, 1987.
114. Papile T, Burstein J, Burstein R, et al: Incidence and evolution of subependymal and intraventricular hemorrhage: A study of infants with birth weights less than 1500 grams. J Pediatr 92:529, 1978.
115. Lustig-Gillman I, Young BK, Silverman F, et al: Fetal intraventricular hemorrhage: Sonographic diagnosis in clinical implications. J Clin Ultrasound 11:277, 1983.
116. Minkoff H, Schaffer RM, Delke I, Grunebaum AN: Diagnosis of intracranial hemorrhage in utero after a maternal seizure. Obstet Gynecol 65(suppl):22, 1985.
117. Chinn DH, Filly RA: Extensive intracranial hemorrhage in utero. J Ultrasound Med 2:285, 1983.
118. Bondurant S, Boehm FH, Fleischer AC, Machin JE: Antepartum diagnosis of fetal intracranial hemorrhage by ultrasound. Obstet Gynecol 63(suppl):255, 1984.
119. Kim MS, Elyaderani MK: Sonographic diagnosis of cerebral ventricular hemorrhage in utero. Radiology 142:479, 1982.
120. Mintz MC, Argerleman BG: In utero sonographic diagnosis of intracerebral hemorrhage. J Ultrasound Med 4:375, 1985.
121. Donn SM, DiPietro MA, Faix RG, Bowerman RA: The sonographic appearance of old intraventricular hemorrhage present at birth. J Ultrasound Med 2:283, 1983.
122. Donn SM, Barr M, McLeary RD: Massive intracerebral hemorrhage in utero: Sonographic appearance and pathologic correlation. Obstet Gynecol 63(suppl):28, 1984.
123. McGahan JP, Haesslein HC, Meyers M, Ford KB: Sonographic recognition of in utero intraventricular hemorrhage. AJR 142:171, 1984.
124. Greenberg F, James LM, Oakley GP: Estimates of birth prevalence rates of spina bifida in the United States from computer-generated maps. Am J Obstet Gynecol 145:570, 1983.
125. Kimball ME, Milunsky A, Alpert E: Prenatal diagnosis of neural tube defects. III. A reevaluation of alpha-fetoprotein assay. Obstet Gynecol 49:532, 1977.
126. Main DM, Mennuti MT: Neural tube defects: Issues in prenatal diagnosis and counseling. Obstet Gynecol 67:1, 1986.
127. U.K. collaborative study on alpha-fetoprotein in relation to neural tube defects. Maternal serum alpha-fetoprotein measurement in antenatal screening for anencephaly and spina bifida in early pregnancy. Lancet 1:1323, 1977.
128. Milunsky A, Alpert E: Prenatal diagnosis of neural tube defects. I. Problems and pitfalls: Analysis of 2495 cases using the alpha-fetoprotein assay. Obstet Gynecol 48:1, 1976.
129. Milunsky A, Alpert E: Prenatal diagnosis of neural tube defects. II. Analysis of false positive and false negative alpha-fetoprotein results. Obstet Gynecol 48:6, 1976.
130. Goldberg MF, Oakley GP: Interpreting elevated amniotic fluid alpha-fetoprotein levels in clinical practice: Use of the predictive value positive concept. Am J Obstet Gynecol 133:126, 1979.
131. Slotnick N, Filly RA, Callen PW, et al: Sonography as a procedure complementary to alpha-fetoprotein testing for neural tube defects. J Ultrasound Med 1:319, 1982.
132. Hashimoto BE, Mahony BS, Filly RA, et al: Sonography, a complementary examination to alpha-fetoprotein testing for neural tube defects. J Ultrasound Med 4:307, 1985.
133. Linkfors KK, McGahan JP, Tennant FP, et al: Midtrimester screening for open neural tube defects: Correlation of sonography with amniocentesis results. AJR 149:141, 1987.
134. Roberts CJ, Evans KT, Hibbard BM, et al: Diagnostic effectiveness of ultrasound in detection of neural tube defect. Lancet 2:1068, 1983.
135. Warkany J: Anencephaly. In Congenital Malformations: Notes and Comments. Year Book, 1971, pp 189–200.

136. Sunden B: On the diagnostic value of ultrasound in obstetrics and gynecology. Acta Obstet Gynecol Scand 43(suppl):1, 1964.

137. Campbell S, Johnstone FD: Anencephaly: Early ultrasonic diagnosis and active management. Lancet 2:1226, 1972.

138. Johnson A, Losure TA, Weiner S: Early diagnosis of fetal anencephaly. J Clin Ultrasound 13:503, 1985.

139. Cox GG, Rosenthal SJ, Holsapple JW: Exencephaly: Sonographic findings and radiologic–pathologic correlation. Radiology 155:755, 1985.

140. Goldstein RB, Filly RA, Callen PW: Sonography of anencephaly: Pitfalls in early diagnosis. JCU, in press.

141. Mahony BS, Filly RA, Callen PW, Golbus MS: The amniotic band syndrome: Antenatal sonographic diagnosis and potential pitfalls. Am J Obstet Gynecol 152:63, 1985.

142. Mahony BS, Filly RA, Callen PW: Amnionicity and chorionicity in twin pregnancy: Prediction using ultrasound. Radiology 155:205, 1985.

143. Graham D, Johnson TRB, Winn K, Sanders RC: The role of sonography in the prenatal diagnosis and management of encephalocele. J Ultrasound Med 1:111, 1982.

144. Chervenak FA, Isaacson G, Mahoney MJ, et al: Diagnosis and management of fetal cephalocele. Obstet Gynecol 64:86, 1984.

145. Chatterjee MJ, Bondoc B, Adhate A: Prenatal diagnosis of occipital encephalocele. Obstet Gynecol 153:646, 1985.

146. Ingraham FD, Swah H: Spina bifida and cranium bifidum: A survey of 546 cases. NEJM 228:559, 1943.

147. Suwanwela C, Suwanwela N: A morphological classification of sincipital encephalomeningoceles. Neurosurg 36:201, 1972.

148. Mealey J, Ozenitis AJ, Hockley AA: The prognosis of encephaloceles. J Neurosurg 32:209, 1970.

149. Lorber J: Results of treatment of myelomeningocele: An analysis of 524 unselected cases, with special reference to possible selection for treatment. Dev Med Child Neurol 13:279, 1971.

150. Filly RA, Simpson GF, Linkowski GD: Fetal spine morphology and maturation during the second trimester. J Ultrasound Med 6:631, 1987.

151. Naidich TP: Personal communication.

7

THE FETAL MUSCULOSKELETAL SYSTEM

Barry S. Mahony, M.D.

Shortly after the turn of the century, radiographic studies began to provide insights regarding fetal bone lengths, as well as the timing and sequence of ossification. These observations led to atlases of fetal growth still in use today.[1] Then, during the 1950s, Gray and associates published an elegant series of articles that documented normal embryogenesis of the fetal appendicular musculoskeletal system.[2-7] They recognized that the proximal and cephalad structures of the appendicular skeleton developed slightly before the distal and caudad structures. These studies, as well as those by Garn and colleagues, documented that by ten menstrual weeks of pregnancy (eight weeks after conception), the bones, joints, and musculature have differentiated into structures with form and relative positions identical to those of an adult (Fig. 7–1).[8, 9] The remainder of gestation and postnatal development involves increasing size and complexity of structures already present by the end of the first trimester of pregnancy.

The advent of ultrasonography, especially high-resolution real-time ultrasound, opened exciting opportunities to evaluate fetal growth and development dynamically in utero. The flexibility and rapid frame rate of real-time ultrasound permit a survey of the fetal axial and appendicular skeleton and

provide direct visualization of fetal movements. Furthermore, antenatal ultrasound does not suffer the inherent problems of fetal radiography, i.e., ionizing radiation, variable magnification, and obscuration from underlying maternal structures. The absence of ionizing radiation enables the sonographer to obtain numerous images of the fetus in various planes of section in an attempt to minimize the number of structures not well visualized because of overlying maternal or fetal parts. When contained within the focal zone of the ultrasound transducer, an object is imaged free of distortion. Currently, antenatal sonography displays more fetal abnormalities than does radiography and has become the most accurate image modality for the diagnosis of skeletal dysplasias.[10]

The extremely high subject contrast between the ossified portions of the fetus and adjacent soft tissue structures enables sonographic visualization of the fetal skeleton shortly after ossification begins. Justifiably, therefore, much of the sonographic literature concerns the evaluation of osseous structures. Of probable equal importance, however, are the nonossified structures of the cartilages, musculature, joints, and vasculature. Future attention to these structures, as well as to the dynamics of fetal movement, undoubtedly will provide helpful informa-

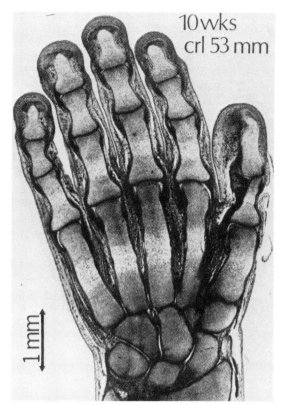

Figure 7–1. Histologic section of the fetal hand at approximately 12 menstrual weeks (ten weeks post conception) shows adult proportions. By ten menstrual weeks the musculoskeletal system has differentiated into structures with adult form and proportions. (From Garn SM: Contributions of the radiographic image to our knowledge of human growth. AJR 137:231, 1981. Copyright: American Roentgen Ray Society.)

tion regarding fetal development and malformation.

NORMAL PRENATAL DEVELOPMENT

Osteogenesis of the skeleton begins toward the end of the embryonic period when endochondral ossification commences in the midshaft of long bones, where a cartilaginous model converts into bone. In the flat bones of the skull, maxilla, mandible, zygoma, and squamous portion of the temporal bone, the mesoderm differentiates into osteoblasts to form intramembranous ossification centers. Sonography first images the primary ossification centers simultaneously with or shortly after their inception, often before the end of the first trimester. At later stages of development, the most central and oldest cells of the cartilaginous epiphyses at the ends of the long bones convert into the secondary ossification centers, which, in turn, become visible sonographically. In most instances, this process does not occur until postnatal life, when the secondary ossification center expands from the center centrifugally until the cartilaginous epiphysis becomes completely ossified.

Primary ossification of the clavicle and mandible begins at eight menstrual weeks. By the end of the first trimester of pregnancy, the appendicular long bones, phalanges, scapula, ilium, base and inferior portions of the skull, and spine (centrum and vertebral arches of each vertebra) have begun to ossify. During the fourth month of gestation, the ischium, metacarpals, and metatarsals ossify. By the end of the fourth month (16 menstrual weeks), the flat bones of the calvarium have ossified rostrally to reach the top of the head but remain separated by the sutures and fontanelles. During the fifth and sixth months, the pubis, the tarsal calcaneus, and talus ossify. Ossification of the remaining tarsals and all of the carpal bones does not occur until after birth. Only the secondary ossification centers within the epiphyseal cartilages of the distal femur, proximal tibia, and, occasionally, the proximal humerus appear prenatally. The remaining secondary epiphyseal ossification centers do not appear until after birth.

Structures of the limb joints also develop from mesoderm during the embryonic period and increase in size and complexity during fetal development. All large joints possess complete joint cavities by the end of the embryonic period. During subsequent stages of fetal growth, the synovial cavities develop their characteristic bursae and recesses. Synovial villi grow during the third month of gestation, and articular fat pads develop at four to five months of gestation. Articular cartilage appears during fetal development but at birth is only slightly more fibrous than the adjacent epiphyseal cartilage.

Limb musculature differentiates in situ from mesenchyme surrounding the developing bones. Muscular activity begins in the second month of gestation when the joints start to form. Shortly thereafter, real-time ultrasound, especially with the increased resolution capabilities of transvaginal probes, begins to visualize definite and discrete embryonic movements of the extremities and spine. Since ultimate joint structure depends upon joint movement during the initial stages of joint formation, failure of joint motion during the early stages of pregnancy, either from mechanical inhibition or from neuromuscular maldevelopment, may result in club foot, arthrogryposis, or other congenital joint problems and postural deformities.[11, 12]

Although the high subject contrast produced by the very echogenic skeletal ossification may dominate the ultrasound image, echopenic epiphyseal cartilage and musculature are readily apparent sonographically and, therefore, may provide helpful information regarding subsequent limb function. The fetal ultrasound delineates the major individual muscles and muscle groups quite well, as well as the echogenic fascial planes coursing within muscle groups. Major blood vessels (femoral and popliteal arteries) can occasionally be identified pulsating within the soft tissues of the limb. Fetal joint spaces, with the exception of the knee and shoulder, are not well seen sonographically; however, echogenic material, presumably synovium, fat, and microvasculature, permits visualization of the knee and shoulder joints.

NORMAL SONOGRAPHY

Observation and documentation of each fetal bone is neither practical nor necessary in the vast majority of obstetric sonograms. Numerous structures of the fetal musculoskeletal system, however, can be seen as early as the beginning of the second trimester of pregnancy when they are typically bathed in adequate amounts of amniotic fluid in the focal zone of the transducer and are not shadowed by other fetal parts or obscured by extreme maternal obesity. Subsequently, the amount of amniotic fluid and fetal positioning occasionally dictate which portions of the fetal musculoskeletal system may be well imaged sonographically. For example, oligohydramnios may limit fetal motion such that in no plane of section can sonography evaluate a certain structure because of obscuration by other overlying and adjacent parts. In cases with extreme polyhydramnios, on the other hand, the frequent and rapid fetal movements, as well as increased distance from the transducer surface, render detailed survey difficult and time consuming. Nevertheless, when a specific indication exists, persistence, patience, and practice usually allow adequate visualization to anticipate the presence or absence of many abnormalities affecting growth and development.

The Skull and Axial Skeleton

Even before intramembranous ossification of the flat calvarial bones has reached the top of the head, measurements of the biparietal diameter (BPD) provide an accurate

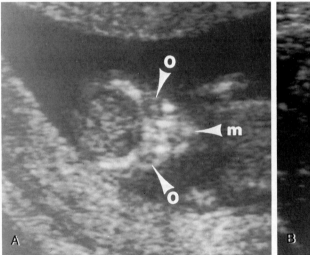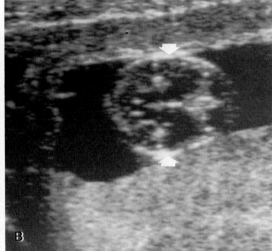

Figure 7–2. Coronal (A) and axial (B) scans of the fetal head at 12 menstrual weeks demonstrate that calvarial ossification has not reached the top of the head (A) but that ossification extends rostrally enough to permit accurate biparietal diameter measurement (*small arrows*). O, orbits; m, mandible.

assessment of the menstrual age near the beginning of the second trimester of pregnancy (Fig. 7–2).[13] By about 16 menstrual weeks, the calvarium has become ossified, except where sutures or fontanelles persist. At the base of the skull, the greater wing of the sphenoid and petrous ridge define the anterior, middle, and posterior cranial fossae. With proper transducer angulation, the orbits can be quite well seen as early as the beginning of the second trimester. Intraocular distances correlate with other biometric parameters and may predict hyper- or hy-

potelorism.[14] Maxillary and mandibular ossification assists in the visualization of the facial anatomy. Depending upon fetal positioning, antenatal sonography may detect facial clefts and other facial abnormalities, especially when these are suspected on the basis of other sonographic findings, i.e., holoprosencephaly (Fig. 7–3).[15] Ossification of the skull base and maxilla obscures almost all cleft palates.

The ribs become visible sonographically early in the second trimester and serve as excellent landmarks for the thorax. Although

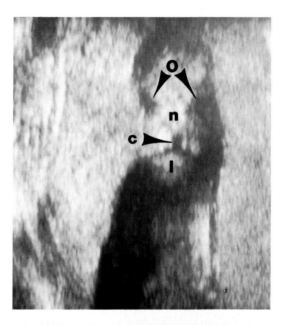

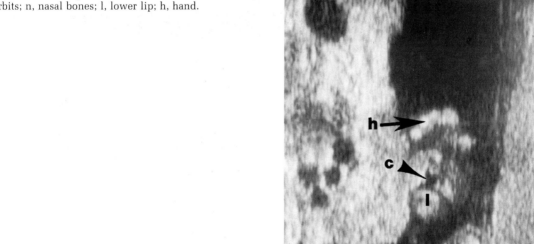

Figure 7–3. Coronal scans of the face at 17 menstrual weeks clearly show a cleft upper lip (c). This was an incidental finding in an otherwise normal fetus. O, orbits; n, nasal bones; l, lower lip; h, hand.

the three ossification centers (the centrum and two vertebral arches) of each vertebral body first appear early in the second trimester, they attain adequate definition to permit reliable diagnostic information regarding the spine only during the second half of the mid-trimester. Optimal visualization of fetal anatomic detail occurs at approximately 18 to 22 menstrual weeks (Fig. 7–4). With meticulous technique, most, but not all, cases of fetal spinal dysraphism manifest sonographically at this time with the characteristic findings of splaying of the two posterior ossification centers.[16] Planes of section transverse to the long axis of the spine best display this finding. The two posterior elements, corresponding approximately to the junction between the lamina and pedicles bilaterally, characteristically converge at all spinal levels. Because of the extreme importance of the spine in fetal diagnosis, the sonographer should examine carefully each spinal level from the base of the calvarium through the level of the ischial ossification centers. The renal hilus serves as a landmark for localization of approximately the first lumbar vertebra.

Care must be taken so that during fetal flexion, one does not image the sacrum obliquely. In such circumstances, one may confuse the normally divergent pedicles of the sacrum with the lamina, thereby leading to the false diagnosis of spinal dysraphism (Fig. 7–5).[17] Occasionally, longitudinal planes of section provide helpful information regarding the spine. Most sonographers, however, consider longitudinal scans less reliable for the detection of dysraphism because of the extreme subtlety of findings. Normal longitudinal scans show a smooth lumbosacral lordosis and thoracic kyphosis, with slight flaring of the paired posterior elements in the cervical and lumbar regions and tapering in the sacrum. Longitudinal scans show multiple vertebral body segmentation abnormalities of the spine better than transverse planes of section and permit measurements of spinal length, a feature that may prove useful in delineation of some dwarf syndromes or other pathologic conditions.[18, 19]

The Appendicular Skeleton[20]

The primary ossification centers of the shoulder and pelvis provide excellent anatomic landmarks to orient imaging of the appendicular skeleton. Imaging of the scapula in the long axis coronally produces an unmistakable Y-configuration with the supraspinatus, infraspinatus, and subscapularis muscles in their respective fossae. The scapula manifests a triangular configuration when imaged posteriorly (Fig. 7–6). When not obscured by the flexed fetal head, the clavicle can be quite well seen. It grows in a linear fashion at approximately 1 mm per

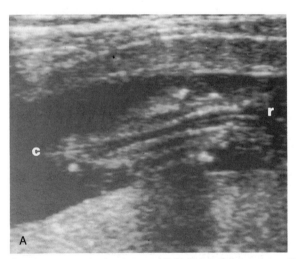 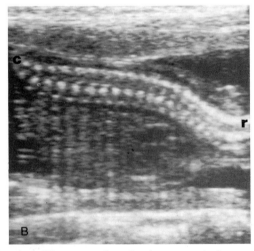

Figure 7–4. Longitudinal scans of the normal spine at 12 (A) and 20 (B) menstrual weeks show smooth thoracic kyphosis and lumbosacral lordosis with slight flaring of the paired posterior elements in the cervical and lumbar regions. Although the spinal elements have begun to ossify by 12 weeks, optimal visualization occurs at approximately 18 to 22 weeks when ultrasound can clearly define individual vertebrae. r, rostral; c, caudal.

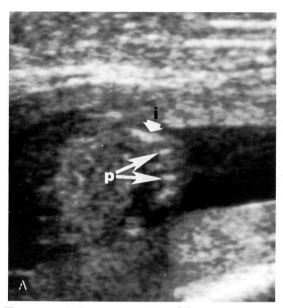
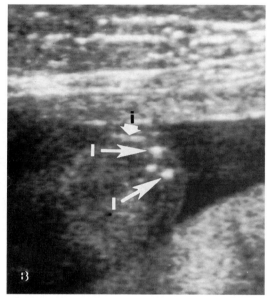

Figure 7–5. A, Transverse section of the sacrum at 15 menstrual weeks shows apparent splaying of the posterior elements. This scan was taken slightly obliquely through the vertebra and shows the normally divergent pedicles; B, A scan obtained in a true cross-section shows the normally convergent laminae. i, iliac wing; p, pedicles, l, laminae.

week, such that at 20 menstrual weeks, it measures roughly 20 mm and at 40 weeks, its length is approximately 40 mm.[21] Visualization of the iliac wings, ischium, and pubis assists in the localization of pelvic structures such as the urinary bladder and the caudal end of the spine.

Throughout the course of the examination, the fetus often flexes, extends, abducts, and adducts the extremities. Since the fetus often holds the humerus adducted against the fetal thorax and the femur flexed at approximately 90 degrees to the long axis of the spine, use of the shoulder and hip landmarks permits the excellent and rapid visualization and measurement of these long bones.

The epiphyseal cartilage of the humeral head resides between the primary ossification centers of the distal clavicle, scapula, and humerus. Late in gestation, the fetal shoulder typically localizes immediately deep to the myometrium, within several centimeters of the transducer surface. This enables detection of the developing secondary ossification center of the proximal humeral epiphysis within the center of the echopenic epiphyseal cartilage (Fig. 7–7).[22] Occasionally, an echogenic rim, probably synovium or microvasculature within the joint space and biceps tendon sheath, surrounds the superolateral margin of the humeral head.

The deltoid and triceps muscles are readily apparent.

Upper extremity flexion may render the elbow difficult to image. In many cases, however, the nonossified coronoid fossa delineates the medial and lateral humeral epi-

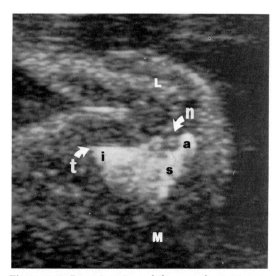

Figure 7–6. Posterior view of the scapula at 19 menstrual weeks demonstrates the scapular tip (t), inferior angle (i), spine (s), notch (n), and acromion (a). M, medial; L, lateral.

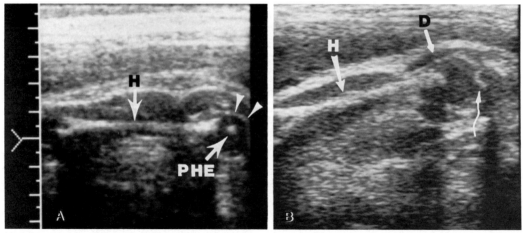

Figure 7–7. *A,* Longitudinal scan of the humerus shows the proximal humeral epiphyseal ossification center (PHE) within the center of the epiphyseal cartilage *(arrowheads).* This provides strong evidence for concomitant lung maturity. *B,* In this fetus, the PHE is not yet visible. The echogenic focus *(curved arrow)* probably represents the biceps tendon groove, not the PHE. H, humerus; D, deltoid. *(From* Mahony BS, Bowie JD, Killam AP, et al: Epiphyseal ossification centers in the assessment of fetal maturity: Sonographic correlation with the amniocentesis lung profile. Radiology 159:521, 1986. Copyright: Radiological Society of North America.)

condyles and creates a distinctive appearance (Fig. 7–7). With the arm held in extension, the echopenic cartilage of the distal humerus and of the proximal radius and ulna can be identified. Although sonography does not delineate the elbow joint capsule well, real-time scanning frequently confirms appropriate motion, including supination and pronation. The more proximal extent of the ulna at the elbow distinguishes the ulna from the radius, but at the wrist, the ossified diaphyses of the ulna and radius end at the same level (Fig. 7–8). Demonstration of this relationship effectively excludes many paraxial limb reduction anomalies that characteristically foreshorten the distal radius.

Antenatally, the carpals produce a conglomerate zone of midrange gray echoes, since they do not ossify until after birth. The ossified metacarpals and phalanges, however, produce high-amplitude echoes that are quite readily imaged by the middle of the second trimester of pregnancy, especially if the fetus extends the hand.

Perhaps because the fetus tends to move

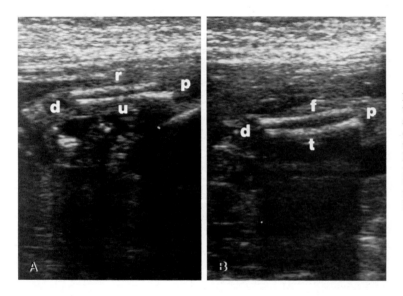

Figure 7–8. Longitudinal scans of the forearm *(A)* and lower leg *(B)* show that the radius and ulna end distally at the same level, as do the tibia and fibula. At the elbow, however, the ulna extends more proximally, whereas the tibia and fibula begin at the same level at the knee. r, radius; u, ulna; f, fibula; t, tibia; p, proximal; d, distal.

the lower extremities less than the upper ones, antenatal sonography often defines details of the lower limbs better than those of the upper limbs. The echopenic epiphyseal cartilage of the femoral head localizes between the primary ossification centers of the ischium and of the femoral diaphysis. The cartilages of the acetabulum, femoral neck, and greater trochanter abut the highly echogenic primary ossification centers of the ischium and femoral diaphysis.

The fetus tends to maintain the knee flexed at approximately 90 degrees (unlike the elbow, which the fetus often holds at greater angles of flexion). The knee may be well visualized in nearly all third trimester pregnancies. Furthermore, highly echogenic material in the fetal knee clearly delineates its anatomy in many cases. The echogenic material in and about the knee, presumably synovial tissues, fat, and microvasculature, clearly define the echopenic cartilage of the distal femur, patella, and proximal tibia and fibula, as well as the quadriceps tendon, patellar ligament, and intercondylar notch between the cartilaginous medial and lateral femoral condyles.[20] In the third trimester of pregnancy, the secondary epiphyseal ossifi-

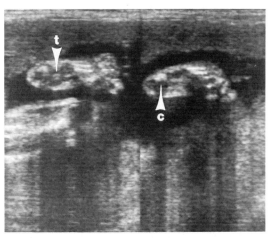

Figure 7–10. Scans of the foot show the talar and calcaneal ossification centers, which first appear at approximately 22 to 24 menstrual weeks. t, talus; c, calcaneus.

cation centers of the distal femur and proximal tibia become visible, centrally positioned within their respective cartilages. Awareness of the secondary ossification centers' central location within the cartilage obviates confusion with the echogenic synovium or microvasculature within the intercondylar notch (Fig. 7–9).

The tibia and fibula end at the same level proximally as well as distally (Fig. 7–8). The distal tibial and fibular primary ossification centers join their echopenic epiphyseal cartilages at the ankle. The talus and calcaneus ossify at approximately 22 to 24 menstrual weeks (Fig. 7–10). Prior to that time, the discrete echopenic cartilages of the calcaneus, talus, cuboid, and navicular may be seen. Metatarsal and phalangeal ossification enables their enumeration in the early second trimester. The echopenic gaps between the ossified diaphyses result from the cartilaginous ends of the bones.

Measurements of the Fetal Extremities[13]

The landmarks of the pelvis and shoulder, coupled with the predominant fetal posture and tone, render localization and measurement of the femur and humerus relatively simple. Presumably because the fetus displays greater freedom of motion of the humerus than of the femur, most biometric charts concern measurement of femoral

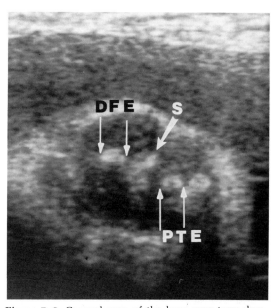

Figure 7–9. Coronal scan of the knee near term demonstrates the echogenic distal femoral (DFE) and proximal tibial (PTE) epiphyseal ossification centers within their respective hypoechoic epiphyseal cartilages. The echogenic synovium (S) within the intercondylar notch should not be confused with an epiphyseal ossification center.

length and its correlation with menstrual age (Table 7–1). Most biometric studies making such a correlation yield consistent results, which, however, may be influenced by technical factors. Unfortunately, few studies report the lengths of other limb bones, and none of these studies list demographic data or assess measurement error. Because of these limitations, one must consider the relationship between menstrual age and limb bone lengths (other than femoral length) not well defined at this time.[13] Table 7–2 provides data that may be helpful as guidelines of approximate expected limb bone lengths.[23]

One should use only charts that relate extremity length to menstrual age when predicting menstrual age on the basis of femoral

Table 7–1. FEMUR LENGTH GROWTH AND DATING CURVES*

	Growth Curve				Dating Curve		
		Femur Length				Menstrual Age	
Menstrual Age (wk)	Lower Limit‡ (cm)	Predicted Value† (cm)	Upper Limit§ (cm)	Femur Length (cm)	Lower Limit** (wk)	Predicted Value‖ (wk)	Upper Limit†† (wk)
12	0.6	0.7	0.8	1.0	11.9	13.2	14.6
13	0.9	1.0	1.1	1.2	12.4	13.7	15.2
14	1.1	1.3	1.5	1.4	12.9	14.4	15.9
15	1.4	1.6	1.8	1.6	13.5	14.9	16.6
16	1.7	2.0	2.3	1.8	14.0	15.6	17.3
17	2.0	2.3	2.6	2.0	14.6	16.2	18.0
18	2.2	2.6	3.0	2.2	15.2	16.9	18.7
19	2.5	2.9	3.3	2.4	15.8	17.5	19.4
20	2.7	3.1	3.5	2.6	16.4	18.2	20.2
21	2.9	3.4	3.9	2.8	17.1	18.9	21.0
22	3.2	3.7	4.2	3.0	17.7	19.7	21.8
23	3.4	4.0	4.6	3.2	18.4	20.4	22.6
24	3.6	4.2	4.8	3.4	19.1	21.1	23.4
25	3.9	4.5	5.1	3.6	19.8	21.9	24.3
26	4.0	4.7	5.4	3.8	20.5	22.7	25.1
27	4.2	4.9	5.6	4.0	21.2	23.5	26.0
28	4.5	5.2	5.9	4.2	21.9	24.3	26.9
29	4.6	5.4	6.2	4.4	22.6	25.1	27.8
30	4.8	5.6	6.4	4.6	23.4	25.9	28.7
31	5.0	5.8	6.6	4.8	24.1	26.7	29.6
32	5.2	6.0	6.8	5.0	24.9	27.6	30.6
33	5.3	6.2	7.1	5.2	25.7	28.4	31.5
34	5.5	6.4	7.3	5.4	26.4	29.3	32.5
35	5.7	6.6	7.5	5.6	27.2	30.2	33.4
36	5.8	6.8	7.8	5.8	28.0	31.0	34.4
37	5.9	6.9	7.9	6.0	28.8	31.9	35.4
38	6.1	7.1	8.1	6.2	29.6	32.8	36.4
39	6.3	7.3	8.3	6.4	30.4	33.7	37.3
40	6.4	7.4	8.4	6.6	31.2	34.6	38.4
				6.8	32.0	35.5	39.3
				7.0	32.8	36.4	40.3
				7.2	33.6	37.3	41.3
				7.4	34.4	38.1	42.3
				7.6	35.2	39.0	43.3
				7.8	36.0	39.9	44.2
				8.0	36.8	40.8	45.2

*Use the dating curve to predict menstrual age for a given femur length and the growth curve to determine if the femur is too short for a given menstrual age.

†Femur length = − 3.8929 + 0.42062 (menstrual age) − 0.0034513 (menstrual age)^2.

‡Lower limit = predicted value − 0.14 (predicted value).

§Upper limit = predicted value + 0.14 (predicted value).

‖Menstrual age = antilog [log menstrual age = 2.35301 + 0.231815 (femur length) − 0.007804 (femur length)^2].

**Lower limit = antilog (predicted log menstrual age − 0.103).

††Upper limit = antilog (predicted log menstrual age + 0.103).

From Warda AH, Deter RL, Rossavik IK, et al: Fetal femur length: A critical reevaluation of the relationship to menstrual age. Obstet Gynecol 66:69, 1985. Copyright: The American College of Obstetricians and Gynecologists.

Table 7–2. APPROXIMATE EXPECTED EXTREMITY BONE LENGTHS (IN MILLIMETERS) AT DIFFERENT MENSTRUAL AGES

Menstrual Week	Humerus			Ulna			Radius			Tibia			Fibula			Menstrual Week
	Percentile			Percentile			Percentile			Percentile			Percentile			
	5th	50th	95th	5th	50th	95th	5th	50th	95th	5th	50th	95th	5th	50th	95th	
12	–	9	–	–	7	–	–	7	–	–	7	–	–	6	–	12
13	6	11	16	5	10	15	6	10	14	–	10	–	–	9	–	13
14	9	14	19	8	13	18	8	13	17	7	12	17	6	12	19	14
15	12	17	22	11	16	21	11	15	20	9	15	20	9	15	21	15
16	15	20	25	13	18	23	13	18	22	12	17	22	13	18	23	16
17	18	22	27	16	21	26	14	20	26	15	20	25	13	21	28	17
18	20	25	30	19	24	29	15	22	29	17	22	27	15	23	31	18
19	23	28	33	21	26	31	20	24	29	20	25	30	19	26	33	19
20	25	30	35	24	29	34	22	27	32	22	27	33	21	28	36	20
21	28	33	38	26	31	36	24	29	33	25	30	35	24	31	37	21
22	30	35	40	28	33	38	27	31	34	27	32	38	27	33	39	22
23	33	38	42	31	36	41	26	32	39	30	35	40	28	35	42	23
24	35	40	45	33	38	43	26	34	42	32	37	42	29	37	45	24
25	37	42	47	35	40	45	31	36	41	34	40	45	34	40	45	25
26	39	44	49	37	42	47	32	37	43	37	42	47	36	42	47	26
27	41	46	51	39	44	49	33	39	45	39	44	49	37	44	50	27
28	43	48	53	41	46	51	33	40	48	41	46	51	38	45	53	28
29	45	50	55	43	48	53	36	42	47	43	48	53	41	47	54	29
30	47	51	56	44	49	54	36	43	49	45	50	55	43	49	56	30
31	48	53	58	46	51	56	38	44	50	47	52	57	42	51	59	31
32	50	55	60	48	53	58	37	45	53	48	54	59	42	52	63	32
33	51	56	61	49	54	59	41	46	51	50	55	60	46	54	62	33
34	53	58	63	51	56	61	40	47	53	52	57	62	46	55	65	34
35	54	59	64	52	57	62	41	48	54	53	58	64	51	57	62	35
36	56	61	65	53	58	63	39	48	57	55	60	65	54	58	63	36
37	57	62	67	55	60	65	45	49	53	56	61	67	54	59	65	37
38	59	63	68	56	61	66	45	49	54	58	63	68	56	61	65	38
39	60	65	70	57	62	67	45	50	54	59	64	69	56	62	67	39
40	61	66	71	58	63	68	46	50	55	61	66	71	59	63	67	40

Modified from: Jeanty P: Letter to the editor. Radiology 147:602, 1983.
Copyright: Radiologic Society of North America.

length. On the other hand, one should employ charts that correlate extremity length with other parameters of gestational age assessment (BPD, head circumference, and similar measurements) in detecting whether or not a fetus suffers from a short-limb dysplasia. To utilize either set of charts effectively, one must understand that published measurements of the fetal long bones correspond to measurements only of the ossified diaphyses. Epiphyseal cartilages, although visible sonographically at the ends of the long bones, have not been included in charts regarding fetal bone measurements. Furthermore, presumably because of the wide biologic variability in fetal size as gestation progresses, skeletal measurements obtained from an initial sonogram during the third trimester of pregnancy are of limited value in the assessment of menstrual age.

Attention to technical detail in fetal bone measurement will maximize reproducibility and minimize error. The sonographer should obtain several scans in the long axis of the bone to ensure optimal long bone measurement. Since the primary ossification center may be factitiously foreshortened when scanned obliquely through the bone, the longest diaphyseal measurement characteristically is most accurate. Conversely, measurement of the femoral length only on views that include the epiphyseal cartilages at either end of the ossified diaphysis will avoid overestimation of the femoral length (Fig. 7–11).[24] The specular echo from the edge of the epiphyseal cartilage should not be included in diaphyseal measurement.[24]

The ends of the femoral ossified diaphysis flare slightly to join the larger epiphyses, giving the femur a slightly bowed appearance especially apparent in the medial aspect of the femur.[25] Shadowing by the diaphyseal ossification obscures the details of the extremity deep to the surface of the bone and yields a false impression that the diaphysis is too thin for the width of the epiphyseal cartilage; therefore, the true diaphyseal width is extrapolated from that of the epiphyseal cartilages.[20]

As previously mentioned, the most central cells of the cartilage in the epiphyses of the distal femur (DFE) and the proximal tibia (PTE) begin to ossify during the third trimester of pregnancy (Figs. 7–7, 7–9). In some fetuses, the epiphyseal ossification center of the proximal humerus (PHE) also begins to

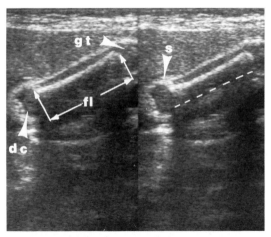

Figure 7–11. The recommended view for femur length (fl) measurement shows the epiphyseal cartilages at either end of the ossified diaphysis. The specular echo (s) from the edge of the epiphyseal cartilage at the knee should not be included in femur length measurement. The width of the epiphyseal cartilage is only slightly greater than the width of the diaphysis. gt, cartilaginous greater trochanter; dc, cartilaginous distal femoral epiphysis; *dotted line,* approximate location of the medial border of the diaphysis.

ossify near term. Although these epiphyseal ossification centers appear and enlarge at variable rates, they do so in a predictable sequence: the DFE at approximately 28 to 35 menstrual weeks, followed two to three weeks later by the PTE, which precedes the appearance of the PHE.[22, 26, 27] The secondary epiphyseal ossification centers enlarge centrifugally as gestation progresses such that if the DFE measures $\geq$ 7 mm in diameter, the fetus is most likely $\geq$ 37 menstrual weeks. This may be a helpful feature in the prediction of menstrual age when the patient only presents for her initial sonogram in the third trimester. Furthermore, a fetus without a visible DFE is most likely $\leq$ 37 menstrual weeks. The PTE grows more rapidly than does the DFE so that the size of the PTE approaches that of the DFE near term.

Antenatal sonography reliably identifies and measures the secondary ossification centers, and their size correlates well with the amniotic fluid's lecithin/sphingomyelin ratio.[22] In 1986, the author studied the epiphyseal ossification centers in 50 fetuses and correlated their features with the amniocentesis lung profile.[22] In this study, all fetuses with a visible PHE had a mature amniocentesis, as well as those whose DFE and PTE were large (> 11 mm in combined diameters) and similar in size (DFE $\leq$ 1 mm larger than the PTE). Identification and measurement of the secondary ossification centers, therefore, may provide valuable information regarding menstrual age and fetal maturation.

FETAL MUSCULOSKELETAL ABNORMALITIES

Fetal musculoskeletal abnormalities are neither rare nor esoteric.[28] Furthermore, the sonographer now plays a central and crucial role in the antenatal diagnosis and consequent obstetric management of an affected pregnancy. Cases of fetal musculoskeletal abnormalities undergo initial sonographic examination for one of several reasons:

1. If one performs the ultrasound because of a specific genetic risk for an inheritable musculoskeletal abnormality, documentation of a similar fetal anomaly provides convincing evidence for the recurrence of the specific syndrome. Pedigree analysis, therefore, assists in the prenatal detection of and distinction among the various inheritable syndromes involving the musculoskeletal system. Most inheritable musculoskeletal abnormalities exhibit an autosomal inheritance pattern with either recessive or dominant transmission. Table 7–3 briefly reviews the risks for recurrence of autosomally inherited entities, both for a couple who have had a prior affected pregnancy and for a couple at least one of whom manifests the syndrome. Variation in penetrance and expressivity alter these idealized statistics.

2. In the absence of a positive familial history for dysplasia or other musculoskeletal abnormalities, serendipitous discovery of a limb anomaly on a sonogram performed for obstetric indications mandates a careful search for other characteristic features that, when present, may permit confident antenatal diagnosis of a specific syndrome. For example, Pretorius and colleagues correctly identified the specific type of skeletal dysplasia in utero in seven of 13 patients on the basis of associated sonographic findings, only one of whom had a familial risk.[29] In their series, the most helpful features to evaluate, when attempting to diagnose the specific type of dysplasia after detection of shortened limbs, included spinal appearance, thoracic shape, associated hydrops, and polyhydramnios.

3. Detection of other abnormalities may occasionally lead the sonographer to suspect and discover subtle musculoskeletal abnormalities that might otherwise go unnoticed. For this reason, when one detects a fetal abnormality on the sonographic examination, one should evaluate the limbs for possible dwarfism or other musculoskeletal abnormalities.[29]

Whereas detailed extremity examination is neither warranted nor feasible in the vast majority of pregnancies, detection of other fetal structural abnormalities or of polyhydramnios mandates careful evaluation of the fetal musculoskeletal system. Fortunately, associated risk factors (polyhydramnios, other structural abnormalities, or familial risk) characteristically occur with most extremity malformations, especially those not evident on the basis of femoral measurement

Table 7–3. INHERITANCE PATTERNS AND RECURRENCE RISKS

	Recurrence Risk	
Mode of Transmission	***Sibling of Proband (Prior Pregnancy with Affected Child)***	***Child of Affected Parent***
Autosomal recessive (AR)	1. 25% for each offspring	3. Not increased unless: (both rare) a. Mate is carrier: 50% recurrence b. Mate is homozygote: 100% recurrence
Autosomal dominant (AD)	2. If one parent affected: 50% for each offspring If both parents affected: 75% affected offspring (50% heterozygotes, 25% homozygotes)	4. Same as 2.

alone. Nevertheless, the relatively simple maneuver of measuring the fetal femur will lead to the accurate identification of most fetal skeletal abnormalities between 19 and 33 menstrual weeks, especially the lethal syndromes, as well as to the serendipitous detection of such entities as focal femoral shortening and the mermaid syndrome.[30–32] For many reasons, therefore, measurement of the femoral length must be a routine, documented, and integral part of the obstetric sonographic examination.[33]

Fetal Dwarf Syndromes

Discordance of the fetal femoral length with the gestational age, as determined by correlation with calvarial size, menstrual dates, or previous examination, permits detection of many short-limbed bone dysplasias before 22 menstrual weeks, sometimes as early as 12 to 13 menstrual weeks when one can first measure the femoral length reliably.[29] A fetus whose bones measure greater than two standard deviations below the mean for a known menstrual age must be suspected of dwarfism. Although some bone dysplasias (especially heterozygous achondroplasia) do not exhibit definitively shortened bone length early in gestation, a shortened femoral length confirms the presence of dwarfism.[10]

Following the detection of dwarfism, the sonographer's role is to characterize the abnormality and to search for associated anomalies in an attempt to determine a specific diagnosis antenatally, thereby providing essential prognostic information necessary to obstetric management and subsequent genetic counseling. Radiographs only occasionally clarify confusing cases in which the sonographic features do not enable a definitive diagnosis of a specific dwarf syndrome antenatally. Prenatal radiographs often suffer from limitations caused by overlapping structures, fetal motion, and variable magnification. In the absence of characteristic sonographic features, however, third trimester radiographs may provide helpful information leading to the diagnosis of a specific dwarf syndrome.[29]

Fortunately, a finite list of recognizable dwarf syndromes manifest antenatally or at birth.[34, 35] One need not memorize the names and specific features of all the dysplasias

detectable antenatally, but awareness of several principles and familiarity with specific features to search for facilitate diagnosis and appropriate management. The following discussion presents a diagnostic approach to these syndromes for the sonographer and amalgamates pertinent information from textbooks of human malformation syndromes.[36–38]

Lethal Dwarf Syndromes

The most crucial dwarf syndromes for the sonographer to identify and characterize antenatally include those in which the fetus has little or no chance of survival (Table 7–4). The proper prognosis will obviate heroic in utero intervention to save a fetus with a lethal syndrome. Unfortunately, all lethal short-limbed dwarf syndromes (except homozygous achondroplasia) occur in a sporadic or autosomal recessive pattern. Antenatal sonography, therefore, most often serendipitously discovers cases with these lethal syndromes. On the other hand, however, all lethal short-limbed dwarf syndromes typically manifest on the antenatal sonogram with striking micromelia or other characteristic features that often permit distinction from nonlethal dwarfisms. Using antenatal sonography, the probable diagnosis of lethal short-limbed dwarfism can be made in approximately 85 percent of cases.[29] The lethal short-limbed dwarfisms that manifest antenatally include (1) achondrogenesis, (2) homozygous recessive osteogenesis imperfecta (Type II), (3) severe hypophosphatasia, (4) thanatophoric dysplasia, (5) homozygous dominant achondroplasia, (6) camptomelic dysplasia, (7) short-rib polydactyly syndrome, and (8) chondrodysplasia punctata (rhizomelic type). The former three entities, each inherited in an autosomal recessive manner, characterize themselves by features secondary to hypomineralization of bone. The latter five processes produce severe manifestations or characteristic features that most often permit distinction from the entities that carry a less dire prognosis.

FOCAL HYPOMINERALIZATION: ACHONDROGENESIS.[39, 40] Achondrogenesis, characterized histologically by disorganization of cartilage and absence of normal bony architecture, causes death in utero or shortly after birth. Profound limb length reduction typically involves all extremity tubular bones. Two

Table 7–4. LETHAL SHORT-LIMBED OSTEOCHONDRODYSPLASIAS

Dysplasia	Inheritance Pattern	Characteristic or Distinctive Sonographic Features	Comments
A. Focal hypomineralization 1. Achondrogenesis	AR*	Decreased/absent ossification of vertebral bodies and sacrum	Ossified calvarium distinguishes from severe hypophosphatasia
B. Diffuse hypomineralization 2. Osteogenesis imperfecta (type II)	AR	Multiple fractures, "thick" bones	
3. Severe hypophosphatasia	AR	Thin, delicate bones; ± absence of entire bones	Very decreased/absent alkaline phosphatase in amniocytes
C. Others 4. Thanatophoric dysplasia	Sporadic ?AR if cloverleaf skull	14% have cloverleaf skull	Severe micromelia and cloverleaf skull without affected parents = thanatophoric, platyspondylisis
5. Homozygous dominant achondroplasia	AD†	± Cloverleaf skull	Both parents achondroplastic dwarfs
6. Camptomelic dysplasia	?AR	Anterior bowing of tibia and fibula; scoliosis	Diaphyses bent but of overall normal length (distinguishes from other dysplasias with bent bones)
7. Short-rib polydactyly	?AR	Polydactyly; small thorax; ± cleft lip, short tibia, renal cysts	Micromelia more severe than chondroectodermal dysplasia or asphyxiating thoracic dystrophy
8. Chondrodysplasia punctata (rhizomelic type)	AR	Severe shortening of humeri and femora, multiple contractures	Characteristic dorsal and ventral vertebral body ossification

*AR, autosomal recessive.
†AD, autosomal dominant.

types and three subtypes of achondrogenesis have been described. Ossification of the vertebral bodies and sacrum, normally clearly seen by the beginning of the second trimester of pregnancy, is virtually absent in all types of achondrogenesis, except in one subtype in which the vertebral bodies and sacrum may be only underdeveloped. The absent vertebral body ossification manifests best sonographically on transverse views of the spine that show less than three ossification centers per spinal segment. In contrast to the striking lack of vertebral body ossification, the calvarium is normally ossified in all fetuses with achondrogenesis, except those with Type I. Although not present in all fetuses with achondrogenesis, the combination of severe limb reduction, absent vertebral body ossification, and normal calvarial ossification serves to differentiate achondrogenesis from all other lethal short-limbed dysplasias. On the basis of these sonographic features, a specific antenatal diagnosis of achondrogenesis has been made in the absence of familial risk (Fig. 7–12).

DIFFUSE HYPOMINERALIZATION: OSTEOGENESIS IMPERFECTA (TYPE II)[41, 42] AND SEVERE HYPOPHOSPHATASIA.[43] Direct evidence for diffuse hypomineralization may be quite subtle but includes (1) an easily compressible calvarium with abnormally clear visualization of brain anatomy, and (2) irregular visualization of the ribs, spine, and long bones that may produce less than normal posterior shadowing (Fig. 7–13).[41] The lack of calvarial ossification may lead to sonographic artifacts, increased through transmission and absence of reverberation, as the sound beam penetrates the fetal head. This often permits clear visualization of the peripheral sulci and gyri of the brain in the near field. One must exercise caution in the exclusion of a diffuse hypomineralization syndrome, however, since the extent of calcification necessary to produce a sonographically normal-appearing bone is undetermined.

Sonographic distinction between congenital hypophosphatasia and homozygous recessive osteogenesis imperfecta may be dif-

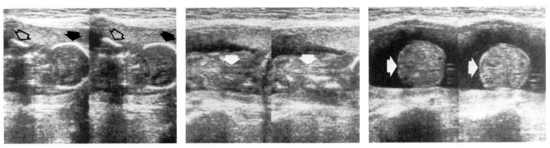

Figure 7–12. Documentation of severe limb reduction, absent vertebral ossification, and normal calvarial ossification permitted antenatal diagnosis of achondrogenesis in this case of approximately 19 menstrual weeks. *Open arrows,* shortened humerus; *closed black arrows,* normal calvarial ossification; *closed white arrows,* absent vertebral ossification that permits visualization of the spinal cord. (Courtesy of Roy A Filly, MD, University of California, San Francisco, CA.)

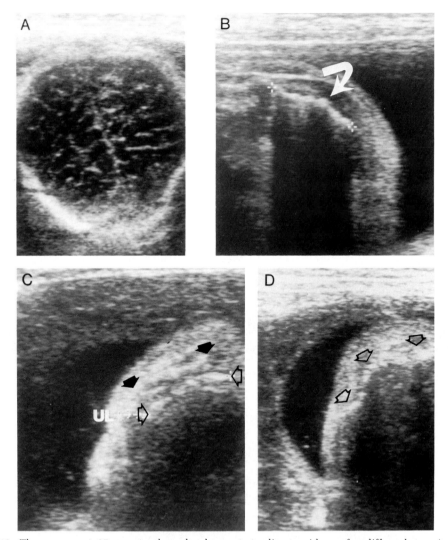

Figure 7–13. These scans at 35 menstrual weeks demonstrate direct evidence for diffuse hypomineralization associated with osteogenesis imperfecta (Type II). *A,* Peripheral sulci and gyri of the brain can be seen through the poorly ossified calvarium. *B,* The femur *(curved arrow)* is shortened, with multiple fractures. *C,* The ulna (UL; *open arrows)* and radius *(closed arrows)* are also shortened and deformed, with multiple fractures and a dot-dash appearance indicative of poor ossification. *D,* A rib *(open arrows)* also shows fracture deformity and a dot-dash appearance.

ficult, since both syndromes exhibit a generalized pattern of poor ossification, including the calvarium. Nevertheless, demonstration of numerous fractures in a fetus with shortened, thickened, and acutely angulated or bowed limb bones provides strong evidence for homozygous recessive osteogenesis imperfecta (Type II) (Fig. 7–14). Rib fractures also strongly suggest the diagnosis, especially when accompanied by the previously mentioned sonographic features of hypomineralization.[29]

The apparent thickening of the limb bones probably results from the exuberant callus typical of osteogenesis imperfecta as well as from the hypomineralization that may not shadow the width of the bone deep to the near field diaphyseal surface. Probably because of the exuberant callus, one rarely visualizes the fracture lines of the multiply fractured bones.

When manifest antenatally, severe hypophosphatasia exhibits as moderate micromelia and diffuse hypomineralization, the degree of which is similar to that in osteogenesis imperfecta (Type II) but without the multiple fractures. However, in severe hypophosphatasia, the tubular bones are delicate or may even be absent, in contrast to the thickened bones of osteogenesis imperfecta (Type II). Transmission occurs in an autosomal recessive manner, probably with more than one allele. Antenatal diagnosis can be made on the basis of a combination of sonographic findings and biochemical evaluation. The amniocytes of an affected homozygote in utero have marked diminution of alkaline phosphatase. Approximately 60 percent of carriers have increased urine and plasma levels of phosphoethanolamine.

OTHER LETHAL DWARF SYNDROMES

THANATOPHORIC DYSPLASIA[44, 45] AND HOMOZYGOUS DOMINANT ACHONDROPLASIA.[46] Thanatophoric ("death-seeking") dwarfism probably represents the most common lethal skeletal dysplasia manifest antentally. It occurs sporadically and is characterized by striking rhizomelic shortening, bowed limbs, polyhydramnios, a narrow thorax, and markedly flattened vertebral bodies. At present, the platyspondylisis may be occasionally detectable sonographically, and provides a distinctive radiographic feature that can confirm the diagnosis of thanatophoric dwarfism antenatally.[29]

Approximately 14 percent of thanatophoric dwarfs have the cloverleaf skull deformity, a severely enlarged and trilobed head readily apparent on the antenatal sonogram (Fig. 7–15). Even though the cloverleaf skull malformation may occur in a variety of syndromes, it manifests only in short-limbed dwarfs who have either thanatophoric dysplasia or homozygous achondro-

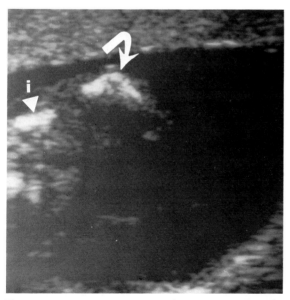 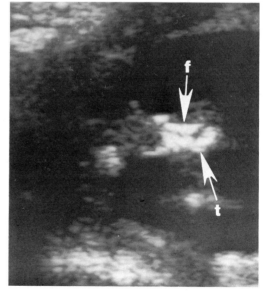

Figure 7–14. Even at approximately 14 menstrual weeks, acute angulation of the femur and tibia may indicate fractures of recurrent homozygous recessive osteogenesis imperfecta (Type II). *Curved arrow*, femur; t, tibia; f, fibula; i, iliac wing.

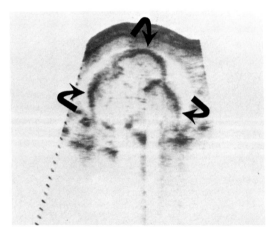

Figure 7–15. Identification of the trilobed appearance of the skull (*arrows*), characteristic of the cloverleaf skull deformity in this fetus with severe micromelia and no familial risk, permitted the correct and specific antenatal diagnosis of thanatophoric dwarfism. Polyhydramnios is present. (*From* Mahony BS, Filly RA, Callen PW, Golbus MS: Thanatophoric dwarfism with the cloverleaf skull: A specific antenatal sonographic diagnosis. J Ultrasound Med 4:151, 1985. Copyright: American Institute of Ultrasound in Medicine.)

plasia. Since the parents of thanatophoric dwarfs are of normal stature, whereas the parents of a fetus with homozygous achondroplasia will be readily recognizable as achondroplastic dwarfs, no confusion should exist between these two lethal short-limbed dwarf syndromes. Sonographic detection of a short-limbed dwarf with the cloverleaf skull deformity whose parents are of normal stature, therefore, permits the confident antenatal diagnosis of thanatophoric dysplasia when no familial risk for short-limbed dwarfism exists. A specific diagnosis of thanatophoric dysplasia has been made on the basis of these sonographic features alone. This diagnosis is important since isolated thanatophoric dwarfism occurs sporadically, whereas the association of thanatophoric dwarfism and cloverleaf skull may be transmitted in an autosomal recessive manner and therefore have a 25 percent recurrence risk.

CAMPTOMELIC DYSPLASIA.[47] Most authors now believe that camptomelic ("bent-limbed"; alternatively spelled campomelic) dysplasia represents a distinct entity typified by characteristic anterior bowing of the lower extremity tubular bones (especially the femurs and tibia), anomalies of the cervical and thoracic spine with scoliosis, and hypoplastic or absent scapulae. Although numerous dysplasias can cause bent bones, this syndrome may be diagnosed antenatally by sonographic detection of the characteristic anterior bowing of the extremity tubular bones in conjunction with scoliosis. Unlike other lethal dwarfisms that exhibit diaphyseal shortening, in camptomelic dysplasia, the diaphyseal length is often quite normal. The limb shortening results from the anterior bowing and distinguishes camptomelic dysplasia from other causes of bent bones.

SHORT-RIB POLYLDACTYLY SYNDROME[48] AND CHONDRODYSPLASIA PUNCTATA (RHIZOMELIC TYPE). These dysplasias, which have an extremely poor prognosis, exhibit some features that resemble dysplasias with better prognoses. However, the severity of limb shortening and selected features often serve to differentiate them from their less severe counterparts.

The short-rib polydactyly syndromes show striking micromelia, the degree of which distinguishes them from chondroectodermal dysplasia (Ellis-van Creveld syndrome) and asphyxiating thoracic dystrophy (ATD). The shortened thorax with a small circumference associated with the short-rib polydactyly syndromes may be so striking as to be unmistakable. Careful search for polydactyly, renal cysts, and disproportionate tibial shortening may lend corroborative evidence for a short-rib polydactyly syndrome but often does not help distinguish it from chondroectodermal dysplasia and ATD.

The rhizomelic type of chondrodysplasia punctata results in either neonatal death or severe mental retardation with death in early childhood. It exhibits severe micromelia of the humeri and femora, with multiple joint contractures. The vertebral bodies have characteristic dorsal and ventral ossification centers, separated by a bar of cartilage that might be detectable sonographically and permit a specific antenatal diagnosis. Furthermore, attention to the epiphyses might reveal the characteristic calcific stippling of the humeral and femoral epiphyses in this autosomal recessive disorder. In any case, the severe and symmetric rhizomelic shortening should distinguish this entity with a very poor prognosis from others that result in a less severe rhizomelia (heterogzygous achondroplasia and ATD) and that have a variable prognosis.

Osteochondrodysplasias with a Variable or Good Prognosis

As delineated above, the lethal osteochondrodysplasias characteristically present with severe findings or pathognomonic features that often enable the sonographer to make an accurate diagnosis and prognosis. On the other hand, antenatal sonography may detect numerous defects of tubular growth that have a good or variable prognosis but one which is certainly not uniformly lethal in early infancy. For example, diastrophic dysplasia causes increased infant mortality, but those who survive infancy can expect normal intellectual development and a normal lifespan if progressive kyphoscoliosis does not compromise their pulmonary and cardiac function. Unfortunately, many osteochondrodysplasias occur in an autosomal recessive pattern or sporadically, such that the sonographer is the first to recognize a problem. In addition, the dysplasias often do not exhibit adequately distinguishable features to permit the confident antenatal

diagnosis of a specific syndrome, except in the presence of a familial risk.

Tables 7–5 and 7–6 present the characteristic features of the osteochondrodysplasias manifest at birth, with a variable or good prognosis. Note that not all persons with these osteochondrodysplasias are short-limbed dwarfs (Table 7–6). These reference tables represent a condensation of information from several sources and delineate features that might be detectable on an antenatal sonogram.[35–38] Distinctive features or patterns, if present, may assist the sonographer in specifying the type of dysplasia present once an abnormality has been identified. A characteristic tail-like appendage overlying the sacrum of a fetus with moderate limb shortening, for example, may suggest metatrophic dysplasia. Absent ossification of the DFE, PTE, calcaneus, and talus late in the third trimester in a fetus with relatively short limbs, on the other hand, may suggest spondyloepiphyseal dysplasia congenita. Several bone fractures in a fetus with bone lengths that are normal, or near

Table 7–5. NONLETHAL SHORT-LIMBED OSTEOCHONDRODYSPLASIAS

Dysplasia	Inheritance Pattern	Characteristic or Distinctive Sonographic Features	Comments
A. Variable prognosis			
1. Chondroectodermal dysplasia (Ellis-van Creveld)	AR,* variable expressivity	Postaxial hexadactyly, 50% have large ASD	Very frequent in one Amish group
2. Asphyxiating thoracic dystrophy	AR	Narrow thorax; ± rhizomelic shortening; ± polydactyly, renal cysts	Almost always Caucasian, may be very similar to 1
3. Metatrophic dysplasia	Heterogeneous	Narrow thorax, kyphoscoliosis, relatively long trunk	± Characteristic tail-like appendage over sacrum
4. Roberts syndrome, pseudothalidomide syndrome	AR, variable expressivity	Tetraphocomelia, midline facial clefts	Pseudothalidomide syndrome, much less severe manifestations
5. Diastrophic dysplasia	AR	Multiple contractures, "hitchhiker" thumb	More muscle mass than arthrogryposis
B. Good prognosis			
1. Heterozygous achondroplasia	AD†, over 80% spontaneous mutation	Rhizomelic micromelia	Characteristic fetal growth curve, narrow interpedicular distance of lumbar spine (subtle)
2. Spondyloepiphyseal dysplasia congenita	AD, variable expressivity	Short, bowed femora; short spine and trunk	Delayed ossification of epiphyseal centers, calcaneous, and talus
3. Kniest's dysplasia	Probably AD	Kyphoscoliosis, short trunk, broad thorax	
4. Mesomelic and acromesomelic dysplasia	AR or AD (depends on type)	Micromelia of middle or distal segments	Distribution of shortening distinguishes from lethal syndromes

*AR, autosomal recessive.
†AR, autosomal dominant.

Table 7–6. OSTEOCHONDRODYSPLASIAS WITH NORMAL BODY PROPORTIONS

Dysplasia	Inheritance Pattern	Prognosis	Characteristic or Distinctive Sonographic Features	Comments
Osteogenesis imperfecta (types I, III, IV)	AD* or sporadic	Variable	± Several fractures with normal or near normal bone lengths	
Cleidocranial dysplasia	AD; wide expressivity, high penetrance	Good	Clavicular hypoplasia/ aplasia, brachycephaly	⅓ occur by spontaneous mutation
Otopalatodigital syndrome	AD in males	Mild mental retardation	Hypoplasia of proximal radius, short thumbs	Not manifest at birth in females
Larsen's syndrome	Sporadic	Good	Talipes, hypertelorism, multiple dislocations, ± kyphoscoliosis	
Osteopetrosis congenita	AR†	Variable	Hepatosplenomegaly	Probably requires x-ray diagnosis

*AD, autosomal dominant.
†AR, autosomal recessive.

normal, imply osteogenesis imperfecta (Type I or III) (Fig. 7–16). Distribution of limb foreshortening may also provide a helpful diagnostic feature in distinguishing the mesomelic or acromesomelic dysplasias from other syndromes.

One must make special note of heterozygous achondroplasia because of its high incidence and good prognosis. A spontaneous mutation leads to heterozygous achondroplasia in over 80 percent of cases; the remaining cases have been transmitted in an autosomal dominant manner. Retardation of endochondral bone formation typically produces rhizomelic shortening of the limbs. In heterozygous achondroplasia, the length of the fetal femora shows a characteristic growth curve, which distinguishes this entity from other osteochondrodysplasias (Fig. 7–17).[10, 49] Until approximately 20 menstrual weeks, the femora are normal in length but then fall away from the normal curve and pass below the 99 percent prediction interval by approximately 27 menstrual weeks. Even without a known familial genetic predisposition, fetuses that demonstrate this typical femoral growth curve should be suspected of being heterozygous achondroplastic dwarfs. Unfortunately, other skeletal dysplasias may produce similar degrees of femoral shortening late in gestation, such that the antenatal sonographic diagnosis of heterozygous achondroplasia requires sequential scans over an extended period commencing early in gestation. One cannot exclude heterozygous achondroplasia on the basis of a normal femoral length before 27 menstrual weeks. On the other hand, when the sonographer first examines a woman in the third trimester and detects limb shortening with a predominant rhizomelic pattern but without other distinguishing features, heterozygous achondroplasia should be a prime diagnostic consideration. Since narrowing of the interpedicular distance of the lower lumbar spine has been reported to be specific for this syndrome, attention to this region on transverse views of the spine might be useful in the future, although this may be an extremely subtle sign.

As a general rule, the osteochondrodysplasias with a variable or good prognosis tend to manifest with less severe features than do the lethal syndromes. The degree of micromelia in lethal syndromes often is so striking that the fetal limbs remain positioned at approximately 90 degrees from the trunk. Shortened limb bones associated with the nonlethal syndromes, on the other hand, tend to acquire an adequate overall length that permits a more normal relationship with the trunk. Some of these nonlethal syndromes exhibit variable expressivity of phenotype with the result that some patients manifest a phenotype more severely than do others with the same syndrome. As an example, severe manifestations of Roberts syndrome include striking limb shortening from marked tetraphocomelia, as well as microcephaly and bilateral cleft lip and palate. Prenatal or perinatal death occurs almost uniformly when Roberts syndrome mani-

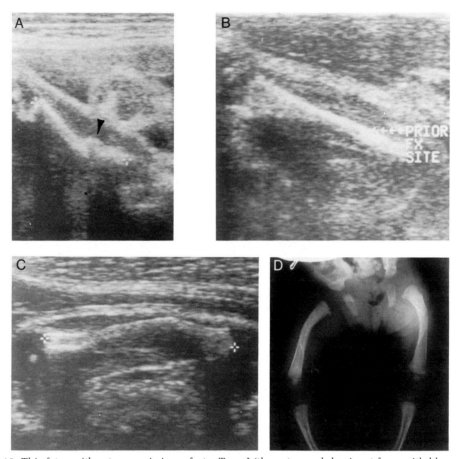

Figure 7–16. This fetus with osteogenesis imperfecta, Type I (the autosomal dominant form with blue sclera) has normal extremity bone lengths. At 29 menstrual weeks, however, a left tibial fracture *(A)* with some callus formation is evident *(arrowhead)*. Nineteen days later, the left tibial fracture has healed *(B)*, but the femur angulates *(C)* at the junction of its proximal and middle thirds, indicative of fracture deformity. A postnatal radiograph *(D)* confirms the antenatal findings.

Figure 7–17. Plot of femur length versus biparietal diameter (BPD) in seven cases of heterozygous achondroplasia shows that the femur length falls below the 99 percent confidence limit at a BPD of 57 to 65 mm in five cases *(dashed lines)* and at a BPD of 51 to 69 mm in two cases *(solid lines)*. This is the characteristic growth curve for heterozygous achondroplasia. *(From Kurtz AB, Filly RA, Wapner RJ, et al: In utero analysis of heterozygous achondroplasia: Variable time of onset as detected by femur length measurements. J Ultrasound Med 5:137, 1986. Copyright: American Institute of Ultrasound in Medicine.)*

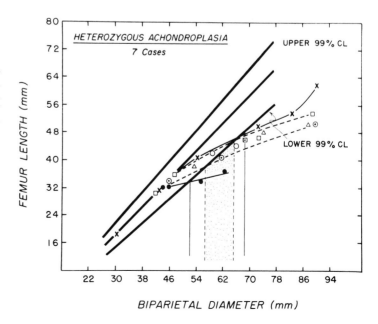

fests severely. Many authors, therefore, categorize Roberts syndrome as a lethal dwarfism. However, the severe phenotype of Roberts syndrome and a significantly less severe and nonlethal phenotype, termed the pseudothalidomide syndrome, may occur in the same family. Survivors with the pseudothalidomide syndrome have limb lengths that may approach normal. Despite the confusing features created by the variable expressivity in this example, the general rule holds that extreme manifestations of limb shortening signify a dire prognosis.

Asphyxiating thoracic dystrophy (ATD, Jeune's syndrome) also occurs in an autosomal recessive manner, but the phenotype manifests with variable expressivity. The clinical manifestations range widely from prenatal or perinatal death to latent phenotypes without respiratory symptomatology. In patients with a positive family history for ATD, the 25 percent recurrence risk alerts the sonographer to search diligently for specific features indicative of recurrence. Several reports document the correct antenatal sonographic diagnosis of ATD in families with a prior affected pregnancy.[50, 51] The antenatal sonographic features of recurrent ATD include rhizomelic dwarfism in association with a fetal thorax that is unmistakably small. Unfortunately, the normal sonographic relationship between thoracic size and menstrual age is not adequately defined. Furthermore, since many of the osteochondrodysplasias (and all of the lethal skeletal dysplasias reported by Pretorius and colleagues) result in a small thorax; this feature alone does not help distinguish ATD from other syndromes.[29] When unmistakably severe, however, a small thorax helps to predict a poor prognosis (Fig. 7–18).

Miscellaneous Abnormalities

Focal Limb Abnormalities

For a fetus with a genetic risk of a focal limb reduction abnormality, detailed sonographic examination may identify an aplasia or a hypoplasia of the major long bones. Table 7–7 presents the nomenclature for these focal limb reduction anomalies.

Documentation that the radius does not end at the same level distally as the ulna, in conjunction with sharp radial angulation of the hand at the wrist, confirms the presence of radial hypoplasia or aplasia (Fig. 7–19). A variety of heritable syndromes produce radial aplasia or hypoplasia, including Fanconi's anemia, the Holt-Oram syndrome, and the thrombocytopenia-absent radius syndrome. If specifically sought, other major limb reduction abnormalities should be detected by antenatal sonography. In addition, a fetus of a diabetic mother may rarely exhibit proximal focal femoral deficiency that presents as asymmetric femoral shortening, a feature one would only detect by measuring both femora. The yield for antenatal detection of each of these rare anomalies would be expected to be low but accurate.

Even in the absence of a genetic or biochemical risk, the detection of a limb reduction deformity may lead to the correct antenatal diagnosis of a specific entity. The amniotic band syndrome, for example, is a common but nonheritable cause of various fetal malformations involving the limbs, craniofacial region, and trunk.[52] It occurs in approximately one in 1200 live births. Rupture of the amnion leads to entrapment of fetal parts by fibrous mesodermic bands that emanate from the chorionic side of the amnion. Entrapment or entanglement of fetal parts by the bands may cause amputation or slash defects in nonembryologic distributions. Depending upon the degree of fetal entanglement and the orientation and location of the bands that slash across the developing fetus, deformities occur ranging from subtle amputation or lymphedema to amputation of large portions of the fetus (Figs. 7–20, 7–21). Although extremity amputations may result from genetic or teratogenic causes, in such cases the amputations tend to be bilaterally symmetric, unlike the asymmetric amputations of the amniotic band syndrome. Even when the aberrant bands of tissue are not visualized sonographically, documentation of characteristic fetal deformities provides evidence strongly suggestive of the amniotic band syndrome. These deformities include multiple clefts in bizarre and nonembryologic distributions, large gastropleural schisis with exteriorization of the liver, and encephalocele occurring in a location other than midline. The limb–body wall complex represents a similar but very severe and lethal set of fetal malformations, probably resulting from early rupture of the amnion between the third and fifth week of embryogenesis.[53] Severe sco-

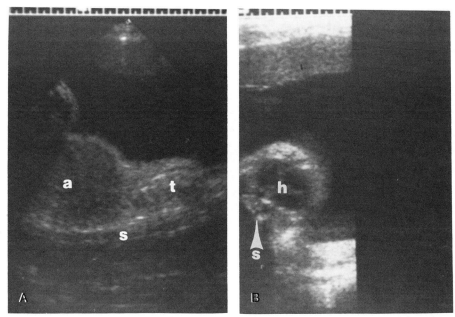

Figure 7–18. Sagittal scan of the fetal trunk (A) and transverse scan of the thorax (B) demonstrate an unmistakably small thorax in this fetus with asphyxiating thoracic dystrophy. The normal-sized heart practically fills the thorax. Polyhydramnios is present. t, thorax; a, abdomen; s, spine; h, heart.

Table 7–7. NOMENCLATURE FOR LIMB ANOMALIES

Achiria	Absence of hands
Achiropody	Absence of hands and feet
Acromelia	Shortening of distal segments (hands, feet)
Adactyly (ectrodactyly)	Absence of fingers or toes
Amelia (ectromelia)	Absence of extremity
Apodia	Absence of feet
Camptomelia (campomelia)	Bent limb
Diastrophic	Distorted
Equinus	Extension of foot
Hemimelia	Absence (complete or incomplete) of limb below knee or elbow
Mesomelia	Shortening of middle segments (forearm, lower leg)
Micromelia	Shortened limbs; dwarfism
Paraxial	Beside axis of limb
Phocomelia	Deficient development of middle portions of limb with preservation of proximal and distal segments
Polydactyly	Extra digits
Postaxial	Posterior to axis of limb, i.e., postaxial hexadactyly = 6 digits with extra digit along dorsal aspect of hand or foot
Rhizomelia	Shortening of proximal segment (femur, humerus)
Symbrachydactyly	Short fused digits
Talipes	Clubfoot
Thanatophoric	Death seeking
Varus	Bent inward

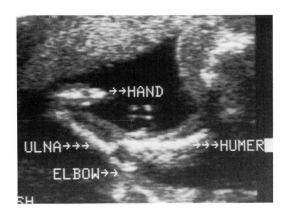

Figure 7–19. This fetus has radial aplasia with absence of visualization of the radius and sharp radial angulation of the hand at the wrist. humer, humerus. (Courtesy of Jack H Hirsch, MD, Swedish Hospital Medical Center, Seattle, WA.)

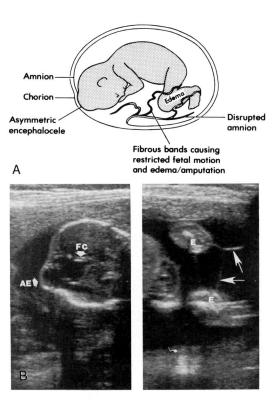

Figure 7–20. *A,* In the amniotic band syndrome, rupture of the amnion causes variable malformations ranging from subtle to severe. The bands may create bizarre slash defects across the face, cause gastropleural schisis, or entangle the extremities, causing edema or amputation. Adherence of the fetus to the chorion may cause asymmetric encephalocele. *B,* This fetus has an asymmetric encephalocele (AE) and numerous bands *(arrows)* attached to the extremities (E). FC, falx cerebri. (*From* Mahony BS, Filly RA, Callen PW, Golbus MS: The amniotic band syndrome: Antenatal sonographic diagnosis and potential pitfalls. Am J Obstet Gynecol 152:63, 1985.)

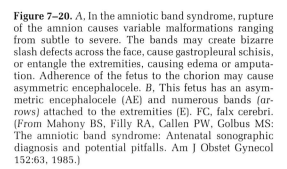

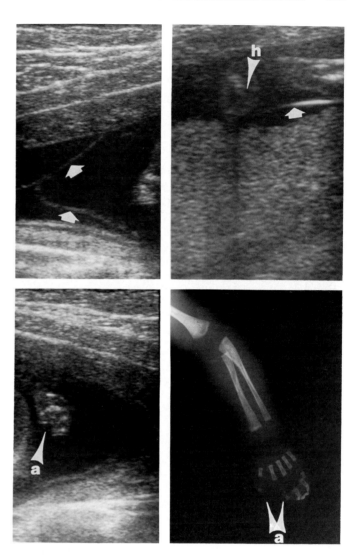

Figure 7–21. This pregnancy demonstrated numerous bands *(arrows)* attached to the fetal extremities (h, hand) and subtle amputations (a), indicative of the amniotic band syndrome.

liosis with resultant postural deformity is present in the majority of these cases (Fig. 7–22).

Postural Deformities

Attention to fetal positioning and limb motion should permit detection of several abnormalities characterized sonographically by anomalous posture. Detection of these anomalies often occurs in the setting of a familial risk of recurrence or of other severe anomalies.

Talipes (clubfoot), for example, frequently occurs in conjunction with oligohydramnios, neuromuscular abnormalities, or a genetic syndrome. Oligohydramnios, presumably leading to in utero crowding, should be readily apparent, as are many of the neuromuscular abnormalities, including meningomyelocele or arthrogryposis. On the other hand, talipes may be the major or only sonographic manifestation of other neuromuscular abnormalities or genetic syndromes, such as muscular dystrophies, Trisomy 13, and Trisomy 18. Serendipitous discovery of talipes, therefore, should alert the sonographer to search diligently for other abnormalities and to consider genetic amniocentesis.[54]

Most sonographic reports of talipes describe talipes equinovarus (Fig. 7–23).[54, 56] This deformity is characterized sonographically by constant visualization of the long axis of the foot on the same plane of section as, but at right angles to, the tibia and fibula. One must exercise caution in making the

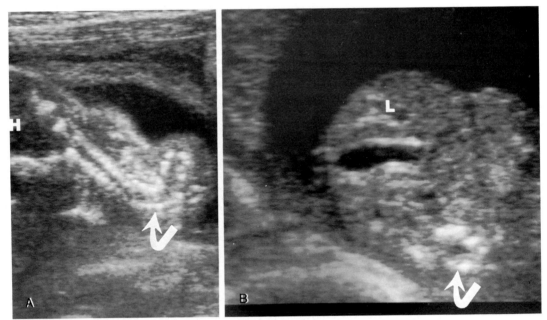

Figure 7–22. Limb–body wall complex probably results from early amnion rupture and produces very severe and lethal malformations, including severe scoliosis (A) and gastropleural schisis (B). H, head; *arrows*, spine; L, liver exteriorized through gastropleural schisis. (Case courtesy of Jack H Hirsch, MD, Swedish Hospital Medical Center, Seattle, WA.)

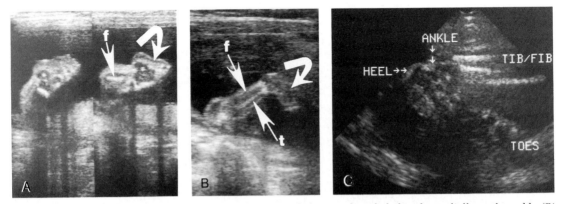

Figure 7–23. In talipes equinovarus, the foot remains extended (A) and angled sharply medially at the ankle (B) such that the long axis of the foot and lower leg are in the same plane of section. t, tibia; f, fibula; *curved arrow*, foot. The fetus in C, however, held the foot in equinovarus position throughout the course of the examination but did not have talipes at birth. tib/fib, tibia and fibula.

definitive diagnosis of talipes, since the fetus may hold the feet in a position strongly suggestive of talipes in the absence of neonatal deformity.[55]

Arthrogryposis multiplex represents a heterogeneous group of conditions typified by decreased or absent movement of multiple joints, often associated with contractures (Fig. 7–24).[36, 57] Some syndromes (myotonic dystrophy, diastrophic dwarfism, bilateral renal agenesis, and Trisomy 18) may cause the features of arthrogryposis multiplex, in which cases the sonogram or amniocentesis may yield the correct cause. In many cases, however, arthrogryposis multiplex does not occur as part of a recognizable syndrome. First, arthrogryposis multiplex with primary limb involvement may occur sporadically and produce fixed symmetric involvement with extended limbs at the knees and elbows, internal rotation of the shoulders, flexion of the hands and wrists, and equinovarus of the feet. Survivors have normal intelligence. Second, the limitation of joint movement in conjunction with scoliosis often results in uniformly flexed limbs; mild mental retardation may be present. Up to one-third of such persons have a familial history of this condition. And third, the limitation of joint motion associated with a severe central nervous system disturbance causes persistently flexed limbs and severe mental retardation, often with microcephaly.

Pterygium syndromes may produce multiple flexion contractures from webs extending across limb joints.[37] In general, these syndromes do not impair overall health. For example, popliteal pterygium syndrome, which recurs in an autosomal dominant manner but with variable expressivity and incomplete penetrance, usually produces bilateral webs extending from the ischial tuberosities to the heels. Multiple pterygium syndrome, on the other hand, occurs in an autosomal recessive fashion and causes webbing of variable severity and distribution, involving the neck, axilla, elbow, knee, and digits. Other defects, especially cleft lip and anomalies of the external genitalia, frequently accompany these syndromes. X-linked dominant and autosomal dominant pterygium multiplex syndromes have also been described.

Subtle Hand and Foot Deformities

Meticulous sonographic examinations now may enable antenatal detection of a wide variety of hand and foot deformities, including polydactyly, symbrachydactyly, and clinodactyly.[56] These anomalies usually occur in conjunction with other severe anomalies. Prenatal diagnosis may facilitate diagnosis of a lethal trisomy syndrome or permit proper parental counseling and early neonatal treatment of many of these anom-

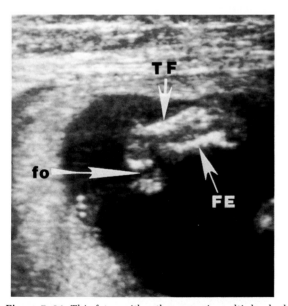 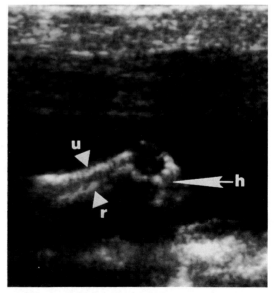

Figure 7–24. This fetus with arthrogryposis multiplex had multiple joint contractures. It remained motionless and contorted during the examination. FE, femur; TF, tibia and fibula; fo, foot; r, radius; u, ulna; h, hand.

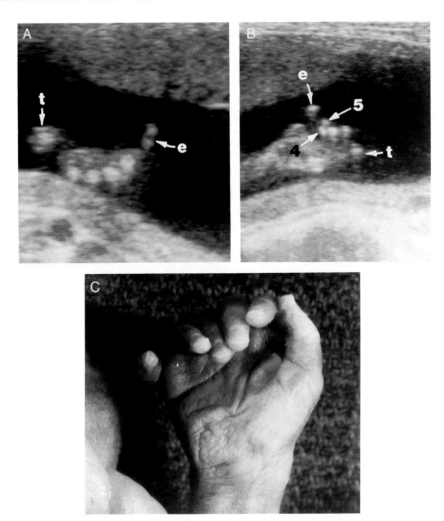

Figure 7–25. Transverse scan *(A)* through the hand, at the level of the metacarpals, demonstrates a supernumerary digit. This antenatal sonogram *(B)* and corresponding postnatal radiograph *(C)* show polydactyly and overlapping of the fifth (5) over the fourth (4) digit. On this basis, given the presence of holoprosencephaly, the correct antenatal sonographic diagnosis of Trisomy 13 was made. t, thumb; e, supernumerary digit.

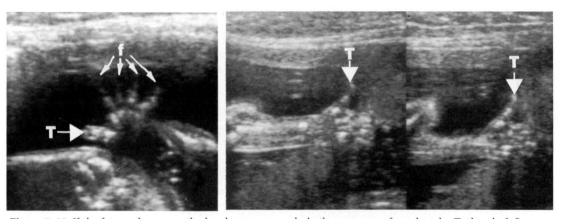

Figure 7–26. If the fetus splays open the hand, one may exclude the presence of syndactyly. T, thumb; f, fingers.

alies.[58] Detection of polydactyly, for example, in conjunction with other features of an osteochondrodysplasia such as chondroectodermal dysplasia or asphyxiating thoracic dystrophy, may imply the specific diagnosis. A persistently fisted hand with overlapping of the digits suggests Trisomy 13 (Fig. 7–25). Subtle hypoplasias or syndactyly, however, may be extremely difficult to detect. One may exclude the presence of syndactyly of the hand only if the fetus clasps the hands together and interdigitates or splays open the fingers (Fig. 7–26).

Antenatal sonography accurately depicts the fetal musculoskeletal system. Measurement of the fetal long bones permits detection of many skeletal dysplasias, even in the absence of familial risks. Observation of the characteristic features may enable differentiation among many of the syndromes, so that the sonographer may render an accurate antenatal diagnosis and prognosis. Detailed examination may detect focal musculoskeletal abnormalities and postural changes that will alert the parents, obstetrician, and pediatrician to potential perinatal problems and facilitate optimal management.

References

1. Todd TW: The reliability of measurements based upon subcutaneous bony points. Am J Phys Anthropol 18:275, 1925.
2. Gray DJ, Gardner E: Prenatal development of the human knee and superior tibiofibular joints. Am J Anat 86:235, 1950.
3. Gardner E, Gray DJ: Prenatal development of the human hip joint. Am J Anat 87:163, 1950.
4. Gray DJ, Gardner E: Prenatal development of the human elbow joint. Am J Anat 88:429, 1951.
5. Gardner E, Gray DJ: Prenatal development of the human shoulder and acromioclavicular joints. Am J Anat 92:219, 1953.
6. Gray DJ, Gardner E, O'Rahilly R: The prenatal development of the skeleton and joints of the human hand. Am J Anat 101:169, 1957.
7. Gardner E, Gray DJ, O'Rahilly R: The prenatal development of the skeleton and joints of the human foot. J Bone Surg Am 41-A:847, 1959.
8. Garn SM, Burdi AR, Babler WJ, et al: Early prenatal attainment of adult metacarpal-phalangeal rankings and proportions. Am J Phys Anthropol 43:327, 1975.
9. Garn SM: Contributions of the radiographic image to our knowledge of human growth. AJR 137:231, 1981.
10. Kurtz AB, Filly RA, Wapner RJ, et al: In utero analysis of heterozygous achondroplasia: Variable time of onset as detected by femur length measurements. J Ultrasound Med 5:137, 1986.
11. Drackman DB, Coulombre AJ: Experimental clubfoot and arthrogryposis multiplex congenita. Lancet 2:523, 1962.
12. Drackman DB, Sokoloff L: The role of movement in embryonic joint development. Dev Biol 14:401, 1966.
13. Deter RL: Evaluation of studies of normal growth. In Deter RL, Harrist RB, Birnholz JC, Hadlock FP (eds): Quantitative Obstetrical Ultrasonography. New York, John Wiley & Sons, 1986, pp 65–111.
14. Jeanty P, Cantraine F, Cousaert E, et al: The binocular distance: A new way to estimate fetal age. J Ultrasound Med 3:241, 1984.
15. Hegge FN, Prescott GH, Watson PT: Fetal facial abnormalities identified during obstetric sonography. J Ultrasound Med 5:679, 1986.
16. Hashimoto BE, Mahony BS, Filly RA, et al: Sonography, a complementary examination to alpha-fetoprotein testing for fetal neural tube defects. J Ultrasound Med 4:307, 1985.
17. Dennis MA, Drose JA, Pretorius DH, Manco-Johnson ML: Normal fetal sacrum simulating spina bifida: "Pseudodysraphism." Radiology 155:751, 1985.
18. Birnholz JC: Fetal lumbar spine: Measuring axial growth with US. Radiology 158:805, 1986.
19. Abrams SL, Filly RA: Congenital vertebral malformations: Prenatal diagnosis using ultrasonography. Radiology 155:762, 1985.
20. Mahony BS, Filly RA: High-resolution sonographic assessment of the fetal extremities. J Ultrasound Med 3:489, 1984.
21. Yarkoni S, Schmidt W, Jeanty P, et al: Clavicular measurement: A new biometric parameter for fetal evaluation. J Ultrasound Med 4:467, 1985.
22. Mahony BS, Bowie JD, Killam AP, et al: Epiphyseal ossification centers in the assessment of fetal maturity: Sonographic correlation with the amniocentesis lung profile. Radiology 159:521, 1986.
23. Jeanty P: Letter to the editor. Radiology 147:602, 1983.
24. Goldstein RB, Filly RA, Simpson G: Pitfalls in femur length measurements. J Ultrasound Med 6:203, 1987.
25. Abrams SL, Filly RA: Curvature of the fetal femur: A normal sonographic finding. Radiology 156:490, 1985.
26. Chinn DH, Bolding DB, Callen PW, et al: Ultrasonographic identification of fetal lower extremity epiphyseal ossification centers. Radiology 147:815, 1983.
27. Mahony BS, Callen PW, Filly RA: The distal femoral epiphyseal ossification center in the assessment of third-trimester menstrual age: Sonographic identification and measurement. Radiology 155:201, 1985.
28. Poznanski AK: Bone dysplasias: Not so rare, definitely important. AJR 142:427, 1984.
29. Pretorius DH, Rumack CM, Manco-Johnson ML, et al: Specific skeletal dysplasias in utero: Sonographic diagnosis. Radiology 159:237, 1986.
30. Hegge FN, Prescott GH, Watson PT: Utility of a screening examination of the fetal extremities during obstetrical sonography. J Ultrasound Med 5:639, 1986.
31. Graham M: Congenital short femur: Prenatal sonographic diagnosis. J Ultrasound Med 4:361, 1985.
32. Raabe RD, Harnsberger HR, Lee TG, Mukuno DH: Ultrasonographic antenatal diagnosis of "mermaid

syndrome": Fusion of fetal lower extremities. J Ultrasound Med 2:463, 1983.

33. American Institute of Ultrasound in Medicine: Official Guidelines and Statements on Obstetrical Ultrasound, October 1985.

34. Special Report: International Nomenclature of Constitutional Diseases of Bone. AJR 131:352, 1978.

35. Sillence DO, Rimoin DL, Lachman R: Neonatal dwarfism. Ped Clin North Am 25:453, 1978.

36. Bergsma D (ed): Birth Defects Compendium, 2nd Ed. New York, Liss, 1979.

37. Taybi H: Radiology of Syndromes and Metabolic Disorders, 2nd Ed. Chicago, Year Book, 1983.

38. Spranger JW, Langer LO, Wiedemann HR: Bone Dysplasias: An Atlas of Constitutional Disorders of Skeletal Development. Philadelphia, WB Saunders, 1974.

39. Whitley DB, Gorlin RJ: Achondrogenesis: New nosology with evidence of genetic heterogeneity. Radiology 148:693, 1983.

40. Mahony BS, Filly RA, Cooperberg PL: Antenatal sonographic diagnosis of achondrogenesis. J Ultrasound Med 3:333, 1984.

41. Brown BS: The prenatal ultrasonographic diagnosis of osteogenesis imperfecta lethalis. J Can Assoc Radiol 35:63, 1984.

42. Merz E, Goldhofer W: Sonographic diagnosis of lethal osteogenesis imperfecta in the second trimester: Case report and review. JCU 14:380, 1986.

43. Kousseff BG, Mulivor RA: Prenatal diagnosis of hypophosphatasia. Obstet Gynecol 57:9S, 1981.

44. Fink IJ, Filly RA, Gallen PW, Fiske CC: Sonographic diagnosis of thanatophoric dwarfism in utero. J Ultrasound Med 1:337, 1982.

45. Mahony BS, Filly RA, Callen PW, Golbus MS: Thanatophoric dwarfism with the cloverleaf skull: A specific antenatal sonographic diagnosis. J Ultrasound Med 4:151, 1985.

46. Filly RA, Golbus MS: Ultrasonography of the normal and pathologic fetal skeleton. Radiol Clin North Am 20:311, 1982.

47. Balcar I, Bieber FR: Sonographic and radiographic findings in campomelic dysplasia. AJR 141:481, 1983.

48. Meizner I, Bar-Ziv J: Prenatal ultrasonic diagnosis of short-rib polydactyly syndrome (SRPS) type III: A case report and a proposed approach to the diagnosis of SRPS and related conditions. JCU 13:284, 1985.

49. Filly RA, Golbus MS, Carey JC, et al: Short-limbed dwarfism: Ultrasonic diagnosis by mensuration of fetal femur length. Radiology 138:653, 1981.

50. Schinzel A, Savoldelli G, Briner J, et al: Prenatal sonographic diagnosis of Jeune syndrome. Radiology 154:777, 1985.

51. Skiptunas S, Weiner S: Early prenatal diagnosis of asphyxiating thoracic dysplasia (Jeune's syndrome): Value of fetal thoracic measurement. J Ultrasound Med 6:41, 1987.

52. Mahony BS, Filly RA, Callen PW, Golbus MS: The amniotic band syndrome: Antenatal sonographic diagnosis and potential pitfalls. Am J Obstet Gynecol 152:63, 1985.

53. Patten RM, Van Allen, M, Mack LA, et al: Limb–body wall complex: In utero sonographic diagnosis of a complicated fetal malformation. AJR 146:1019, 1986.

54. Benacerraf BR, Frigoletto FD: Prenatal ultrasound diagnosis of clubfoot. Radiology 155:211, 1985.

55. Hashimoto BE, Filly RA, Callen PW: Sonographic diagnosis of clubfoot in utero. J Ultrasound Med 5:81, 1986.

56. Jeanty P, Romero R, d'Alton M, et al: In utero sonographic detection of hand and foot deformities. J Ultrasound Med 4:595, 1985.

57. Miskin M, Rothberg R, Rudd NL, et al: Arthrogryposis multiplex congenita—prenatal assessment with diagnostic ultrasound and fetoscopy. J Pediatr 95:463, 1979.

58. Benacerraf BR, Frigoletto FD, Greene MF: Abnormal facial features and extremities in human trisomy syndromes: Prenatal US appearance. Radiology 159:243, 1986.

EVALUATION OF THE FETAL HEART BY ULTRASOUND

Klaus G. Schmidt, M.D.
Norman H. Silverman, M.D.

Because of the technologic advances complemented by the increasing ability of ultrasonographers to recognize normal and abnormal fetal anatomy, the use of ultrasonography as a diagnostic obstetric tool continues to expand. Although structural abnormalities of the heart and great vessels are fairly common congenital abnormalities, occurring in approximately eight of 1000 live newborns,[1, 2] fetal cardiac ultrasonography, or fetal echocardiography, has only recently attracted more attention. Because the fetal heart is small and beats rapidly, it could be imaged reliably only after high-resolution real-time ultrasound scanners became available. Since the advent of cross-sectional scanners, which provide real-time directed M-mode and pulsed Doppler echocardiography and color-coded Doppler flow mapping, the ultrasonographer is able to recognize congenital heart defects,[3–11] arrhythmias,[12–17] or disturbed cardiac function in utero.[18–20] The information from fetal echocardiography has augmented genetic counseling, has permitted sophisticated monitoring of cardiac arrhythmias during transplacental treatment, and may help determine a site and route of delivery when a serious cardiac abnormality has been recognized. In the future, acquisition of such information may allow decisions about cardiac surgery in utero.[21, 22]

CLINICAL INDICATIONS

Indications for fetal echocardiography include the previous occurrence of congenital heart disease in siblings or parents; a maternal disease known to affect the fetus, such as diabetes mellitus or connective tissue disease; and the maternal use of drugs that might cause cardiac abnormalities in the fetus, such as lithium, alcohol, or progesterones.[23] Obstetric examinations indicating abnormal cardiac findings due to chromosomal abnormalities, diaphragmatic hernia, exomphalos, hydrops, excessive or very little amniotic fluid volume, or the presence of a very fast or slow fetal heart rate are other reasons for referral. The most common indication is a family history of congenital heart disease (Table 8–1). Although in the authors' experience—and in that of others[24]—the rate of recurrence is low when there is one previously affected child, this rate might be considerably higher when there is more than one previously affected child or when the mother has congenital heart disease.[24–26] Most of those women, who are referred be-

Table 8–1. INDICATIONS FOR ECHOCARDIOGRAPHY AND INCIDENCE OF STRUCTURAL CARDIAC ABNORMALITIES IN 561 FETUSES

Family history of CHD	246	
Siblings (n = 222) and recurrence		5 (2.2%)*
Mother (n = 24) and recurrence		3 (12.5%)†
Maternal disease affecting the fetus	37	
Diabetes (n = 25) and fetal CHD		2 (8%)
Maternal ingestion of teratogens	24	
Lithium (n = 14) and fetal CHD		1 (7%)
Alcohol (n = 6) and fetal CHD		2 (33%)
Extracardiac fetal abnormalities	53	
Chromosomal defects (n = 10) and fetal CHD		5 (50%)
Diaphragmatic hernia, exomphalos, cystic hygroma, and similar defects (n = 43) and fetal CHD		10 (23%)
Nonimmune fetal hydrops	48	
Fetal CHD		18 (38%)
Abnormal amniotic fluid volume	8	
Fetal CHD		2 (25%)
Fetal arrhythmias	145	
Heart block (n = 15) and fetal CHD		8 (53%)
Heart block (n = 15) and maternal connective tissue disease		6 (40%)
Tachyarrhythmia (n = 15) and fetal CHD		0
PAC (n = 76) or PVC (n = 2) and fetal CHD		1 (1.3%)

*3 cardiomyopathies (previous sibs: cardiomyopathy), 1 pulmonary stenosis (previous sib: cardiomyopathy), 1 atrioventricular septal defect (previous sib: ventricular septal defect, coarctation).

†1 Ebstein's anomaly (mother: Ebstein's), 1 pulmonary stenosis (mother: pulmonary stenosis), 1 atrioventricular septal defect (mother: primum atrial septal defect).

CHD, congenital heart disease; PAC, premature atrial contractions; PVC, premature ventricular contractions.

cause their disease is considered to be a risk to fetal cardiac development, have diabetes mellitus. Euglycemic control in diabetics at the time of conception and in early pregnancy may diminish the risk, and the authors have not found cardiac abnormalities in the offspring of such diabetic women. Structural cardiac defects are encountered more frequently when other fetal abnormalities have been detected previously on obstetric ultrasound examination, especially when there is nonimmune hydrops, exomphalos, or diaphragmatic hernia.

In the presence of a very slow fetal heart rate (< 80 beats/min), the fetus is at high risk of associated heart disease; fetal echocardiography should be performed not only to evaluate the arrhythmia but also to rule out the presence of a structural cardiac defect. The association of complete heart block with structural cardiac defects appears to have an extremely poor prognosis, presumably because of their adverse interaction and the atrioventricular valve regurgitation that frequently complicates the condition. In fetuses with complete heart block but without structural cardiac defect, the mother frequently suffers from a connective tissue disorder.[27, 28] Other arrhythmias have, in the authors' experience, no association with any structural abnormality of the heart. All incidences found reflect a trend, but the individual numbers are too small to extrapolate a true incidence of fetal cardiac disease. Although these clues have been useful, continuously expanding experience makes hard and fast indications difficult to articulate.

The authors prefer to perform the initial study between 18 and 22 weeks of gestation because the valves are well developed, the size of the heart is adequate for study, and the fetal size and position usually allow best access to the heart. If necessary, however, it is possible to display the fetal cardiac anatomy and to analyze cardiac rhythm and function from 16 weeks to term.

EQUIPMENT

The cornerstone of fetal echocardiography is high-resolution imaging with cross-sectional (two-dimensional) echocardiography. When studying the fetal heart, it is also desirable to use ultrasound systems equipped with M-mode, pulsed Doppler, and continuous wave Doppler ultrasound. The authors have gained additional information using color Doppler flow mapping. The transducer frequency for cardiac imaging should be as high as possible; the authors prefer 7.5 or 5 MHz transducers but have also used transducers with a 3 MHz frequency. Both linear array and sector scanners may be used to image the fetal heart. The authors prefer the sector scanner because it provides easier access to the fetal heart. Since this format has commonly been used in cardiology, the additional modalities of ultrasound, such as M-mode, conventional Doppler, or color Doppler flow mapping, are usually available. Image magnification and cineloop facilities that allow one to image the beating heart in real time or in slow motion have augmented our diagnostic ability. Recording the studies on videotape for later playback and analysis is very valuable. The video recorder used for replay of the study should have slow motion, forward and reverse playing, and single frame advance capabilities. This facilitates analysis, especially when studies are recorded and interpreted subsequently by different people. The authors have also used an offline computer-assisted analysis system with cineloop and full measurement facilities.

M-mode echocardiography can be most easily understood as a true display of information under the single cursor or scan line. This provides an "ice pick" view of the heart, but because the sample rate runs at between 1000 and 2000 Hz (cycles per second), accurate measurements of the dimensions of walls, cavities, and vessels can easily be made. It also provides exquisite detail of structural motion that is too fast to be perceived by sector scanning, which has a frame rate of 20 to 60 Hz. For example, the rapid motion of valve opening and closure, the fine flutter of valve leaflets, the small motion of atrial contraction, and the rates of change in muscle thickening or cavity size diminution are clearly displayed.

Pulsed Doppler ultrasound demonstrates the direction and characteristics of the blood flow within the fetal heart and the great vessels and allows the qualitative and quantitative definition of flow disturbances such as those that occur with valvar stenotic or regurgitant lesions. As is the authors' practice after birth, pulsed Doppler ultrasound can also be used as a form of flow mapping or "intracardiac stethoscope." Doppler ultrasound uses the change in frequency (the so-called "Doppler shift") of sound waves reflected from the red blood cells within the cardiovascular system. If the red cells are traveling toward the transducer, the pitch increases, and if the cells are traveling away from the transducer, the pitch is lowered. These Doppler signals are displayed above or below the baseline, respectively. By timing the receiving period, it is possible to "listen" at a specific distance from the transducer (range gating). This is displayed by a small line or box (the so-called "sample volume") on the cursor, which can be steered through any sector line or depth of the image. The size of the sample volume

may vary from 1.5 to 9 mm in axial depth. Lateral resolution varies depending on the focal length of the transducer. The angle between the blood flow and the path of the Doppler sound is called the angle of insonance (angle θ). The more perpendicular the sound wave is to the blood flow, the less is the frequency (or velocity) change. The ideal approach for sampling, then, is axial to the blood flow. For practical purposes of measurement, it is desirable to keep the angle θ to less than 25°. The Doppler carrier frequency used is 3 or 5 MHz, preferably the higher frequency to ensure lower ultrasound exposure of the fetus. Current state of the art pulsed Doppler employing fast Fourier analysis has become accepted as standard. Currently, most ultrasound systems convert the frequency shift into a velocity display automatically through the formula:

$$v = (f_d \times c)/(2f_o \times \cos \theta)$$

where v is the velocity (m/sec), f_d is the frequency shift (Hz), c is the conducting velocity of sound in water (1560 m/sec), f_o is the carrier frequency of the transducer (e.g., 3 or 5 MHz), and θ is the angle of insonance. One problem with pulsed Doppler ultrasound is that high-velocity flow cannot be determined accurately because of the finite sampling rate. The frequency shift from range gating techniques can only be sampled at a rate that depends on the number of pulses of sound emitted by the transducer. If the frequency shift of the red blood cell targets exceeds the sampling frequency, aliasing of the signal occurs. This is analogous to observing a wagon wheel apparently spinning backward as it is moving forward, which relates to the optic sampling frequency (27 cycles/sec for the human eye) being exceeded. To measure high velocities of flow, two alternatives are available: high pulse repetition frequency or continuous wave Doppler ultrasound. High pulse repetition frequency Doppler has an advantage in the fetus because the beam and the sample volume can be guided through the sector image to define the origin of the flow disturbance. With the systems the authors have used, continuous wave Doppler cannot be directed through the image and therefore is of limited value in the fetus. In other systems, the problem is eliminated with continuous wave Doppler that is steerable through the sector image. Nevertheless, with high-velocity signals, a blind aligning of the transducer at the site of the flow disturbance may be an efficacious way of determining the peak velocity.

Doppler ultrasound exposes the fetus to higher levels of ultrasonic energy than M-mode or cross-sectional imaging. Although echocardiography, to date, has not been reported to have harmful effects on the developing fetus, Doppler ultrasonic energy should be kept at or below a 100 mW/cm² spatial peak-temporal average, and Doppler interrogation should be limited to as short a time as possible.* On the other hand, Doppler ultrasound provides information unavailable with other techniques in the fetus and, despite the concern as to its bioeffects, remains a most valuable technique.

Color-coded Doppler flow mapping may aid in detecting flow disturbance and flow direction (see Figs. 8–26, 8–46) and should be used when appropriate. Color Doppler flow mapping is a new technology that provides some information about flow direction and the extent of flow disturbance. Flow mapping is a multigate Doppler technique in which sampling along all the scan lines and depths in the field occurs simultaneously. No hard and fast standard of color Doppler display is in use; however, flow toward the transducer is commonly depicted as warm colors (orange and red), and flow away from the transducer is depicted as cold colors (blue). Disturbed flow signals are depicted by adding the color green. As these colors are displayed across the cross-sectional image in real time, not only can the direction of blood flow be mapped in time but the direction and magnitude of flow disturbances resulting from leaks and stenoses can also be assessed. This technique has been valuable for the assessment of congenital heart disease in utero. Unfortunately, the energy levels of this ultrasound method are higher than those of older established methods and have led to certain manufacturers recommending that this technique should not be used in the fetus.

The authors do limit color Doppler examination to brief periods of time and consider the information it provides an important addition to ultrasound in general. Some have suggested that the use of this Doppler technique may allow more rapid identification of a pathologic condition, thereby limiting the time of examination and the exposure of the fetus to further ultrasound examination. Some have also suggested that, because of the experimental nature of this technique, informed consent from the parents should be obtained.

TECHNIQUE

Cross-Sectional Imaging

In order to define the cardiac position and situs, it is necessary to orient the cross-sectional image to the fetal body by noting the position of the head, body, and limbs. It is also important to estimate fetal age using biparietal diameter or femoral length measurements, because cardiac dimensions relate to gestational age and fetal weight.[5, 29–31] The best access to the heart is through the fetal abdomen, but imaging is also possible through the rib cage and from the back, because the fetal lungs are filled with fluid and are not a barrier to the passage of ultrasound, as they are postnatally. In later gestation, however, when the fetal back may be very close to the maternal abdominal wall, much of the ultrasonic energy is absorbed by the vertebral bodies, scapulae, and ribs, which have become ossified, resulting in poorer imaging potential from this direction. To improve imaging, it may be necessary to turn the mother onto one or another side, or to elevate her chest or pelvis. The authors have often found it helpful to have the mother walk around or empty her bladder, or to delay the examination for hours or even days. In the presence of polyhydramnios, the fetus may lie at some distance from the transducer when the mother is recumbent. The fetus can be brought closer to the transducer by having the mother rest on her knees and elbows.

Once the fetal heart is located, only slight movements of the transducer are needed to display the cardiac structures because, with the fetal heart being at some distance from the transducer, small movements subtend great angle changes. The authors consider a complete cardiac examination to encompass scanning of the fetal heart from side to side

*For more details on the bioeffects of ultrasound, see NIH Publication 84-667: Diagnostic Ultrasound Imaging In Pregnancy. US Department of Health and Human Services, 1984.

and from top to bottom. Reference planes similar to those obtained postnatally are gathered, namely four-chamber, long- and short-axis views (Fig. 8–1). It should be noted that these terms are derived from traditional cardiac reference planes established postnatally.

Although the four-chamber view (Fig. 8–1A) is very valuable for defining the comparative sizes of the chambers, it allows the display of only the atrioventricular connections. It does not pass through a plane that allows recognition of the aorta and pulmonary arteries and therefore will not define the complexes of transposition of the great arteries, tetralogy of Fallot, truncus arteriosus, or a double-outlet right ventricle. It also does not pass through the outlet part of the ventricular septum and will not define outlet ventricular septal defects and aortic override

as found in tetralogy of Fallot, truncus arteriosus, or a double-outlet right ventricle. It may not pass through a plane where most ventricular septal defects lie. The arterial valve anatomy is not defined in the four-chamber view, so aortic and pulmonic stenosis cannot be detected from this plane. Abnormalities of the aortic arch, such as interruption and coarctation, will not be identified either. The authors therefore recommend that the mere display of a four-chamber view is not adequate for a fetal cardiac examination. It should be appreciated that when the four-chamber view is obtained from a subcostal equivalent view, simply rotating the transducer along its axis by approximately 90° brings the great veins and great arteries into view, allowing one to establish the venoatrial, atrioventricular, and ventriculoarterial connections.

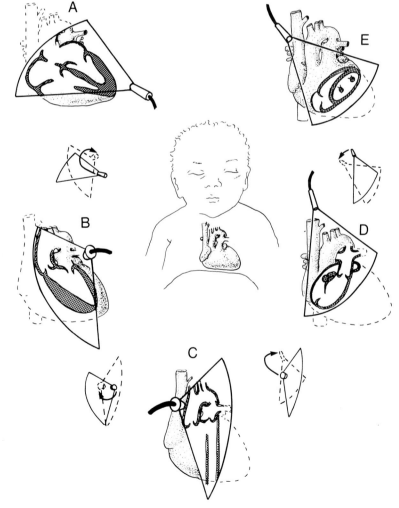

Figure 8–1. Schematic representation of the different views and approaches used to image the fetal heart and great vessels. The fetal heart has a more horizontal axis compared with its postnatal lie in the chest *(center)*. Note that all the views are shown as being obtained from the chest or the abdominal wall; however, it is also possible to achieve all these imaging planes from the back. *A,* Four-chamber view showing both atria and the foramen ovale within the atrial septum, both ventricles, and the atrioventricular valves. *B,* After slight clockwise rotation and tilt of the transducer toward the fetal left shoulder, the long axis comes into view. *C,* Further clockwise rotation and tilt of the transducer results in sagittally oriented planes, which are valuable for depicting the aortic arch and the "ductus–arch." *D,* Perpendicular to the long axis, the short axis views are obtained. At the base of the heart, the aorta lies centrally and is surrounded by the structures of the right ventricle and the pulmonary artery, as postnatally. *E,* Further toward the apex, the left ventricular structure with two papillary muscles can be seen.

The cardiac segments should be assessed sequentially in a manner similar to that performed postnatally.[32] In utero, the left and right sides of the body must be established to define the cardiac position within the chest. Inappropriate identification or the assumption of levocardia and situs solitus can lead to basic errors. Although the echocardiographic views might be obtained from unusual transducer planes, the reference to cardiac position and situs (atrial arrangement) is facilitated by noting that the left atrium lies closer to the vertebral column and the right ventricle lies closer to the anterior chest wall (Fig. 8–2). Furthermore, in situs solitus, the fluid-filled stomach is left-sided, whereas the hepatic veins and the inferior vena cava, as well as the superior vena cava, drain into the right-sided atrium (Fig. 8–3). Magnifying the image considerably aids the recognition of anatomic details (Fig. 8–4B).

The definition of the atrial situs requires the identification of the venous connections and atrial structures. Usually the venous connections can be distinguished in utero (Fig. 8–3). Sometimes even the specific structures of the atrial appendages may be visible, thus substantiating the atrial situs (Fig. 8–3). More often, however, the atrial structures are identified indirectly by the presence of the valve of the inferior vena cava (eustachian valve) within the right atrium and by the demonstration of the flap valve of the foramen ovale, which is the septum primum, within the left atrium (Fig. 8–5). When the situs is ambiguous, these atrial structures may be absent or vestigial. In these situations, one has to rely on additional scanning of the abdomen for the relative positions of the aorta and the azygos, hemiazygos, or inferior caval veins to define the nature of any ambiguous situs, as has been reported after birth.[33, 34] In situs solitus (the usual atrial arrangement), the aorta is more posterior and leftward, whereas the inferior vena cava is more anterior and on the right of the spine (Fig. 8–6). The identification of these vessels can be complemented by interrogation with pulsed Doppler ultrasound. In situs inversus there is a mirror image arrangement of these vessels, with the aorta posterior and to the right, the inferior vena cava anterior and to the left, and the stomach on the right. When the situs is ambiguous, there is either left atrial isomerism (polysplenia syndrome or double left-sidedness) or right atrial isomerism (asplenia syndrome or double right-sidedness). In left atrial isomerism, the inferior vena cava is usually interrupted above the renal veins, and lower body venous drainage is achieved by means of azygos or hemiazygos veins. These veins are identified posterior to the aorta, either on the same or on the opposite side of the spine. Doppler interrogation allows the rapid differentiation of arterial and venous structures (Fig. 8–7). In right atrial isomerism, there is almost invariably juxtaposition of the abdominal aorta and the inferior vena cava on the same side of the spine, either side by side or in an anteroposterior relationship, the posterior vessel being the aorta. Again, in this situation it has been extremely valuable to confirm which vascular structure is which by pulsed Doppler interrogation of these vessels.

Having established the situs, the atrioventricular and ventriculoarterial connections are determined using a variety of examining planes. The four-chamber view (Fig. 8–1A) is easily obtained by tracing the inferior vena cava to the right atrium and then angling the transducer slightly cranially until the four chambers are visualized (Fig. 8–8). The relatively large fetal liver and the noninflated

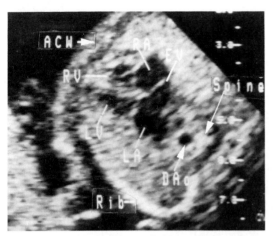

Figure 8–2. Magnified horizontal section through the fetal heart (four-chamber view) and thorax. The right ventricle (RV) is seen close to the anterior chest wall (ACW), wheres the left atrium (LA) lies more posteriorly in front of the descending aorta (DAo) and the spine. The eustachian valve (EV) is noted within the right atrium (RA). LV, left ventricle. In this and most subsequent echocardiographic images, a centimeter-scale marker is included on the right of the figure.

Figure 8–3. Series of magnified parasagittal views in the fetus, representing a sweep from the left to the right side. *A*, The fluid-filled stomach (St) is seen inferior to the left ventricle (LV). The right ventricle (RV) lies anteriorly and is in continuation with the main pulmonary artery (MPA), which gives rise to the left pulmonary artery (LPA). A part of the aortic arch (AoA) can be seen above the pulmonary "arch." The left atrium (LA) lies between the left pulmonary artery and the left ventricle. *B*, In a sagittal view obtained to the right of the previous section, the inferior vena cava (IVC) and a hepatic vein (HV) draining into the right atrium (RA) are demonstrated. The eustachian valve (EV) separates the inferior vena cava from the rest of the right atrium and is pointing towards the atrial septum. Note the narrow-based, finger-like left atrial appendage (LAA) lying behind the aortic root (Ao). The descending aorta (DAo) is seen lying between the left atrium (LA) and the spine. *C*, This section was obtained by directing the transducer further to the fetal right side in a sagittal orientation demonstrating the entry of the inferior (IVC) and superior (SVC) vena cava into the right atrium (RA). The right atrium is characterized by the presence of the eustachian valve (EV) and of a broad-based right atrial appendage (RAA). The right pulmonary artery (RPA) is visible in cross section, posterior to the superior vena cava.

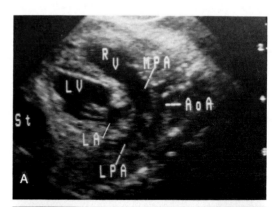

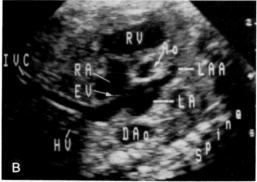

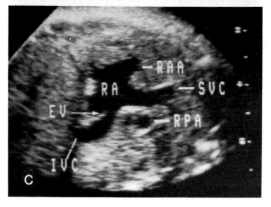

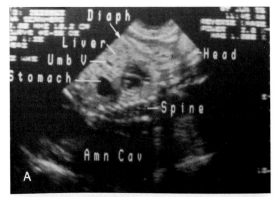

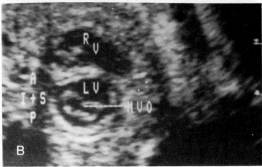

Figure 8–4. Short-axis view of a fetal heart at 22 weeks' gestation. A, This frame shows the position of the head, spine, and abdominal organs (stomach, liver), indicating the superior, inferior, anterior, and posterior directions. Amn Cav, amniotic cavity; Diaph, diaphragm; Umb V, umbilical vein. The depth in the panel is up to 11 cm. B, After magnification (3×), this frame shows the heart, which lies between 2.5 and 4.5 cm away from the transducer. The cardiac structures are better demonstrated than in A; the left ventricle (LV), the mitral valve orifice (MVO), and the right ventricle (RV) can be identified. A, anterior; I, inferior; P, posterior; S, superior.

Figure 8–5. Magnified fetal sagittal view at the site of entry of the inferior vena cava (IVC) into the right atrium with its broad-based right atrial appendage (RAA). The eustachian valve (EV) is seen within the right atrium, and the flap valve of the foramen ovale or septum primum (1) is seen within the left atrium (LA). The asterisks indicate the boundaries of the foramen ovale. AO, aorta; PA, pulmonary artery; A, anterior; I, inferior; P, posterior; S, superior.

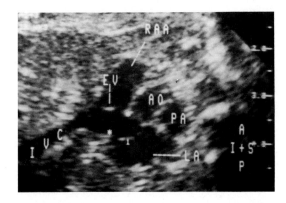

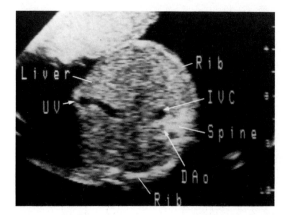

Figure 8–6. Horizontal section at the umbilical level in a fetus of 22 weeks' gestation demonstrating normal situs. The liver and umbilical vein (UV) lie anterior; the spine lies posterior. Note the inferior vena cava (IVC) more anterior and to the right of the spine, whereas the descending aorta (DAo) can be seen more posterior and to the left of the spine.

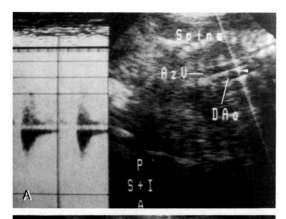

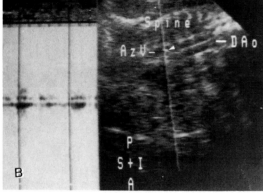

Figure 8–7. Abdominal sagittal view in a fetus of 23 weeks' gestation with left atrial isomerism (polysplenia syndrome) and complete heart block. *A,* In the right panel, two parallel vessels are recognized on the same side of the spine. The Doppler sample volume is placed in the anterior vessel *(arrowhead).* The Doppler display *(left)* shows an arterial flow signal at a rate of 57 beats/min, thus identifying the descending aorta (DAo). *B,* In the right panel, the Doppler sample volume is now seen in the posterior vessel *(arrowhead).* The Doppler display *(left)* demonstrates a low-velocity venous flow signal, thus indicating an azygous vein (AzV). This finding strongly suggests the presence of an interrupted inferior vena cava with azygous continuation of the lower body veins. A, anterior; I, inferior; P, posterior; S, superior.

lungs keep the diaphragm at a higher level within the chest, making the heart lie more horizontal than it does after birth. The four-chamber view usually allows identification of the prominent eustachian valve within the right atrium and the flap valve of the foramen ovale (septum primum) within the left atrium. In real time, the septum primum moves forward to the left atrial cavity and back toward the atrial septum twice during each cardiac cycle. The phasic movement of this interatrial valve appears to mirror the interatrial flow dynamics in the fetus. Both atrioventricular valves may be seen in the

normal heart, and the tricuspid valve lies closer to the cardiac apex than the mitral valve does. The right ventricle often shows the septal attachment of the tricuspid valve leaflets, the moderator band, or the associated large anterior papillary muscle. The right ventricle may also appear slightly larger than the left ventricle.[5]

The four-chamber view allows the definition of atrioventricular connections, the evaluation of atrioventricular valve malformations, the comparative assessment of chamber size, and the identification of some positions of ventricular septal defects. Furthermore, scanning more cranially toward the outflow tracts in the four-chamber view may display the ventriculoarterial connections (Fig. 8–9), but this is not always possible, and other planes should also be used to define these connections.

By rotating the transducer clockwise from the four-chamber view and tilting it slightly toward the fetal left shoulder, the scan plane is oriented in the long axis of the heart, similar to that of long-axis views observed postnatally (Fig. 8–1B). These views allow a better definition of venoatrial, atrioventricular, and ventriculoarterial connections. The crossing of the right and the left ventricular outflow tracts, as well as the perpendicular relationship of the aorta (posterior) and the pulmonary artery (anterior), can be defined (Fig. 8–10). This crossing of the great arteries will be absent when they are transposed. Furthermore, long-axis planes demonstrate

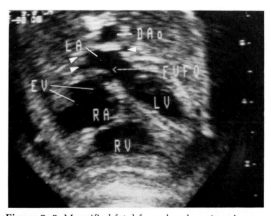

Figure 8–8. Magnified fetal four-chamber view demonstrating the eustachian valve (EV) within the right atrium (RA) and the flap valve of the foramen ovale (FVFO), i.e., the septum primum, within the left atrium (LA). The *arrowheads* indicate pulmonary veins entering the left atrium. DAo, descending aorta; LV, left ventricle; RV = right ventricle.

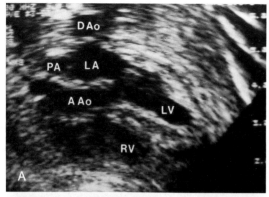

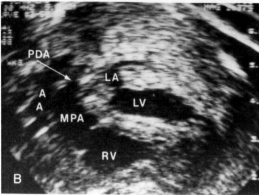

Figure 8–9. From the fetal four-chamber view, with anterior angulation of the transducer, the ventriculoarterial connections are imaged. *A,* The ascending aorta (AAo) is seen arising from the left ventricle (LV). The circular pulmonary artery (PA) lies above the left atrium (LA) and behind the ascending aorta. DAo, descending aorta; RV, right ventricle. *B,* With even further anterior angulation of the ultrasonic beam, the main pulmonary artery (MPA) is displayed arising from the right ventricle (RV), as it lies below the aortic arch (AA). The ductus arteriosus (PDA) is seen arising from the distal end of the main pulmonary artery.

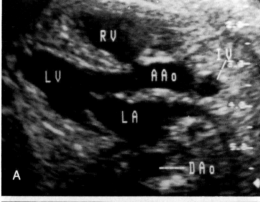

Figure 8–10. Magnified fetal long-axis view demonstrating the left atrioventricular and both ventriculoarterial connections. *A,* The left atrium (LA) drains into the left ventricle (LV) via the mitral valve. The ascending aorta (AAo) arises from the left ventricle. The innominate vein (IV) is seen coursing anterior to the aorta. The descending aorta (DAo), running posterior to the left atrium, is imaged in cross section. *B,* With slight angulation of the scan plane to the fetal left side, the pulmonary artery (PA) is seen arising from the right ventricle (RV) and running below the aortic arch (AA).

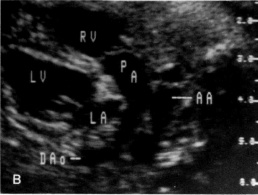

the left-sided structures of the heart just as they would postnatally (Fig. 8–10A). With slight motion of the scan plane toward the fetal left side, the right ventricular outflow tract, pulmonary valve, main pulmonary artery, and descending aorta can also be demonstrated (Fig. 8–10B). From the long axis, slight clockwise rotation allows one to display the aortic root and the entire aortic arch (Fig. 8–1C), including the origin of the head and neck arteries, the aortic isthmus, the innominate vein, and the right pulmonary artery (Fig. 8–11). This plane is important because the origin of the head and neck vessels may help to identify the side of the

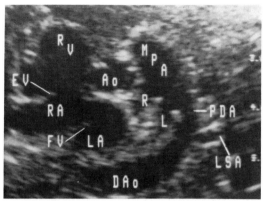

Figure 8–12. Magnified fetal sagittal view at 36 weeks of gestation, demonstrating the continuation of the main pulmonary artery (MPA), ductus arteriosus (PDA), and descending aorta (DAo), the so-called "ductus-arch." The ascending aorta (Ao) is seen in cross section; the main pulmonary artery gives rise to the right (R) and left (L) branch pulmonary arteries. The ductus begins after the branch pulmonary arteries are given off and ends where the left subclavian artery (LSA) arises from the descending aorta. Note that the ductus at this stage of gestation appears to be narrower than the pulmonary artery or the descending aorta. The other structures identified in this view are the eustachian valve (EV) within the right atrium (RA), the flap valve of the foramen ovale (FV) within the left atrium (LA), and the right ventricle (RV).

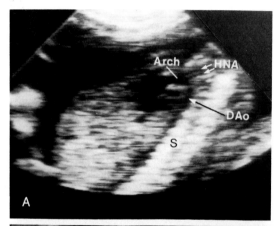

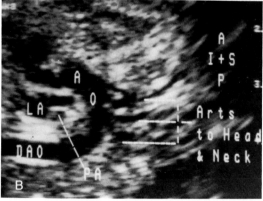

Figure 8–11. Fetal sagittal view of the entire aortic arch in an 18 week fetus. A, The arch, with the head and neck arteries (HNA), can be seen; the descending aorta (DAo) lies in front of the spine (S). B, This magnified view, obtained from a different fetus, shows three arteries (Arts) to the head and neck, arising from the aortic arch (AO). These arteries are the innominate, the left carotid, and the left subclavian. In the concavity of this arch, the left atrium (LA) and the right pulmonary artery (PA) are seen. Note that the "ductus-arch" cannot be seen in this plane. A, anterior; I, inferior; P, posterior; S, superior.

aortic arch. Moving the plane slightly farther leftward shows the main pulmonary artery and its continuation into the descending aorta, where the ductus arteriosus is defined as that vessel connecting the pulmonary trunk, at the site of the origin of its branches, to the descending aorta (the "ductus-arch," Fig. 8–12). Aortic isthmus narrowing is a normal feature in utero (Fig. 8–13) but may be distinguished from coarctation.

From these classic long-axis planes, views in the short axis, similar to those obtained postnatally, can be acquired (Fig. 8–1D,E). The short axis here refers to images obtained perpendicular to the long axis of the heart. Because of the horizontal lie of the fetal heart, the long- and short-axis views are often at right angles to or parallel to the fetal spine, respectively. The short-axis views allow the visualization of the fetal heart from the level of the cardiac apex through the level of the ventricles (where the papillary muscle architecture in the left ventricle is best displayed) and more cranially (where the mitral valve morphology is characteristic [Fig. 8–4B]) up to the level of the great arteries (where the right ventricular outflow

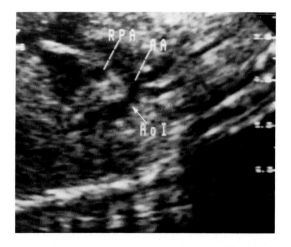

Figure 8–13. Magnified fetal sagittal view of the aortic arch (AA), demonstrating the normal aortic isthmus (AoI), which is relatively narrow. RPA, right pulmonary artery.

tract, the pulmonary trunk with its bifurcation into the branch pulmonary arteries [Fig. 8–14], and the ductus arteriosus can be seen). In this plane, obstructive lesions of the right ventricular outflow tract and of both semilunar valves can be displayed, and the size and position of the great arteries assessed. With high-resolution equipment, even the proximal coronary arteries may be displayed in this plane, thus helping to define the aortic vessel (Fig. 8–15).

M-Mode Echocardiography

Real-time directed M-mode echocardiography is a useful addition to cross-sectional imaging in the evaluation of fetal ventricular cavity dimension and wall thickness or valve and wall motion, as well as cardiac arrhythmias.[12, 15, 18, 29–31, 35, 36] Both long- and short-axis views at the level of the atrioventricular valves allow the assessment of ventricular size (Fig. 8–16). Previous studies have provided percentiles of ventricular sizes and arterial diameters from which comparisons can readily be made (Figs. 8–17, 8–18). At the base of the heart, the movement of both semilunar valves can be seen, and the diameter of the great arteries measured (Fig. 8–19). Pericardial effusions, especially when small, are best substantiated by M-mode display, which demonstrates the separation of the parietal and visceral pericardium, better distinguishing a pericardial effusion from a pleural effusion in the hydropic fetus (Fig. 8–20). For the exploration of fetal arrhythmias, M-mode recordings can be obtained from any plane, which allows the simultaneous display of movements of an atrial and a ventricular wall or of a semilunar and an atrioventricular valve.

Text continued on page 181

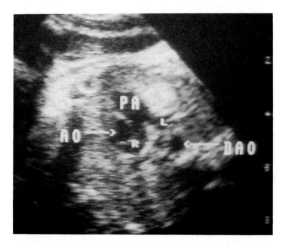

Figure 8–14. Fetal short-axis view at the level of the aortic root (AO), depicting the pulmonary artery (PA) and its bifurcation into the right (R) and left (L) pulmonary arteries. The descending aorta (DAO) is seen in cross section behind the bifurcating pulmonary branches.

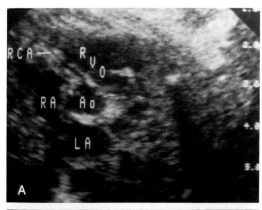

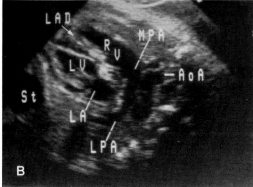

Figure 8–15. *A,* A magnified fetal short-axis view displays the right coronary artery (RCA), which arises from the aortic root (Ao). RVO, right ventricular outflow tract; LA, left atrium; RA, right atrium. *B,* A long-axis view of the right ventricular (RV) outflow tract shows the left anterior descending coronary artery (LAD) running on the ventricular septum. AoA, aortic arch; LA, left atrium; LPA, left pulmonary artery; LV, left ventricle; MPA, main pulmonary artery; St, stomach.

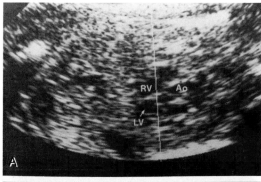

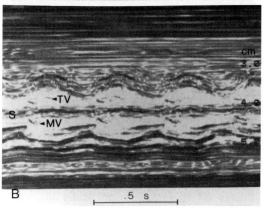

Figure 8–16. Real-time directed M-mode echocardiography at ventricular level in the fetus. *A,* In this cross-sectional image, the M-mode cursor line crosses the right (RV) and left (LV) ventricles, seen in long axis. Ao, aorta. *B,* The M-mode recording shows normal contractions and thickening of both ventricular walls in systole. The movement of the tips of the tricuspid (TV) and mitral (MV) valves is seen. The ventricular septum (S) and both ventricular free walls have about the same thickness.

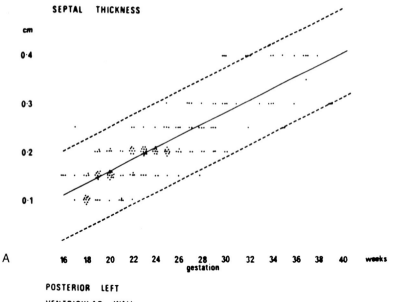

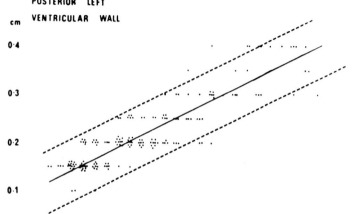

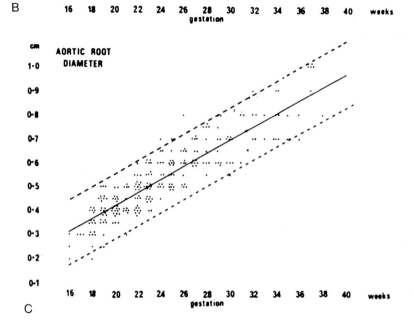

Figure 8–17. Graphic display of normal M-mode measurements of septal thickness *(A)*, posterior left ventricular wall thickness *(B)*, and aortic root diameters *(C)* in fetuses from 16 weeks to term. Values in centimeters (y-axis) are plotted against gestational age (x-axis); the *dotted lines* represent twice the standard error of the mean *(straight line)*. (From Allan LD, Joseph MC, Boyd EGC, et al: M-mode echocardiography in the developing human fetus. Br Heart J 47:573, 1982.)

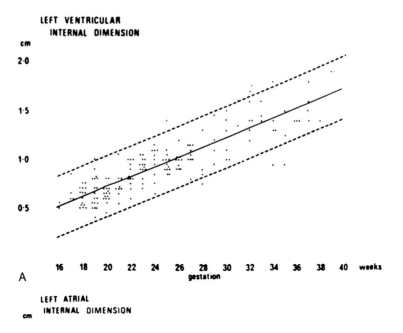

**LEFT VENTRICULAR
INTERNAL DIMENSION**

A

**LEFT ATRIAL
INTERNAL DIMENSION**

Figure 8–18. Graphic display of normal M-mode measurements of left ventricular *(A)*, left atrial *(B)*, and right ventricular *(C)* internal diameters in fetuses from 16 weeks to term. (*From* Allan LD, Joseph MC, Boyd EGC, et al: M-mode echocardiography in the developing human fetus. Br Heart J 47:573, 1982.)

B

**RIGHT VENTRICULAR
INTERNAL DIMENSION**

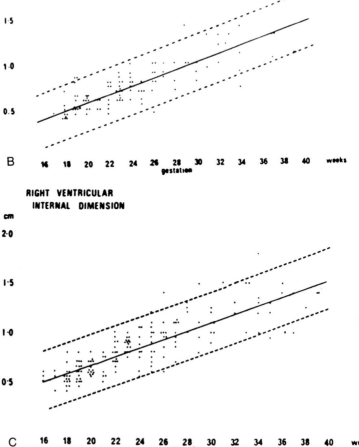

C

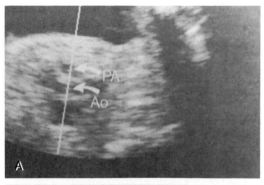

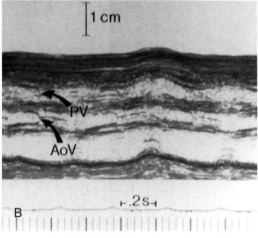

Figure 8–19. M-mode echocardiogram at the level of both great arteries. *A,* At the base of the heart, the M-mode reference line crosses the pulmonary artery (PA) and the aortic root (Ao). *B,* The typical systolic motion of both semilunar valves as open boxes is demonstrated. The *black arrows* indicate the closure of the pulmonary valve (PV) and of the aortic valve (AoV). The diameters of both great vessels can easily be measured from this M-mode recording.

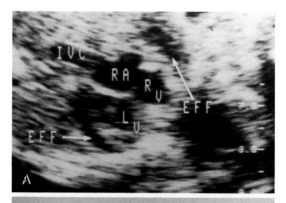

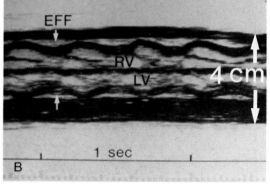

Figure 8–20. *A,* Magnified cross-sectional image of the heart at 22 weeks' gestation in a fetus with nonimmune hydrops. Although the pericardial effusion (EFF, *arrows*) may be seen, it can better be substantiated from the M-mode recording in the same fetus *(B).* The dense echoes of the pericardium and the rhythmically contracting ventricular myocardium are separated by the echo-free area of the effusion. IVC, inferior vena cava; LV, left ventricle; RA, right atrium; RV, right ventricle.

The start of an atrial contraction is defined either by the onset of contraction of the atrial wall or by the F-point of an atrioventricular valve motion (Fig. 8–21). The start of a ventricular contraction is defined by the onset of ventricular wall motion, by the closure of an atrioventricular valve (C-point), or by the opening of a semilunar valve (Fig. 8–21). Since the electromechanical delay differs between these points, one should consistently use the same markers in each study.

Imaging of the atrial wall motion may be difficult because of its small amplitude, but this technique is most valuable because the direct result of atrial contraction can be seen in most cases by careful examination (Fig. 8–22). If the M-mode recordings are obtained from the posterior fetal aspect, their display is inverted with respect to conventional M-mode display. The M-mode tracings can be read more easily by inverting the recording and viewing it through a mirror (Fig. 8–23). These two maneuvers allow an orientation and pattern recognition similar to that achieved postnatally.

When structural abnormalities of the heart are coupled with an arrhythmia, such as with complete heart block[13, 15, 16] or, less frequently, with a tachyarrhythmia,[37] M-mode echocardiography is especially valuable. Even with direction of the cursor through the cardiac image, the variable fetal position may not allow a standardized beam orientation such as is possible postnatally, which makes the quantitative interpretation of M-mode echocardiography more difficult.

Doppler Echocardiography

Pulsed Doppler echocardiography is obtained by guiding the sample volume through the cross-sectional reference image. Doppler interrogation within vascular structures, either at the level of the umbilical cord or within the fetal body, identifies arterial or venous flow (Figs. 8–8, 8–24), assisting the ultrasonographer to distinguish arteries and veins and to evaluate the direction of blood flow in complex cardiovascular malformations. Normal flow velocity profiles across both the atrioventricular and the semilunar valves have been defined in the fetus (Fig. 8–25);[38–41] normal values for peak and

Figure 8–21. Schematic representation depicting the motion of cardiac structures as visualized by M-mode echocardiography, and ladder diagrams from these recordings. *A,* The ultrasound beam passes through a ventricle and an atrioventricular valve within it. The atrioventricular valve leaflets can be seen opening in early diastole (D-E portion), moving toward each other in mid-diastole (E-F), and moving away from each other again in late diastole during atrial contraction (F-A). The beginning of this second opening (F-point) indicates the onset of atrial contraction. The closure of the valve leaflets (C-point) or the beginning of the forward motion of the posterior ventricular wall (PW) indicates the onset of the ventricular contraction. The ladder diagram *(below)* marks these events; the delay between atrial and ventricular activation is the atrioventricular (AV) conduction time. *B,* The ultrasound beam passes through the root of a great artery (A) and the semilunar valve within it, then through an atrium behind that vessel. The M-mode recording shows the onset of the forward motion of the atrial wall (AW, *open arrow*) that defines the beginning of atrial contraction. The opening of the semilunar valve (SV, *black arrow*) defines beginning of the ventricular contraction. The ladder diagram *(below)* demonstrates these events as in the top panel.

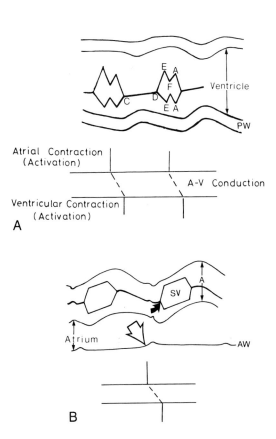

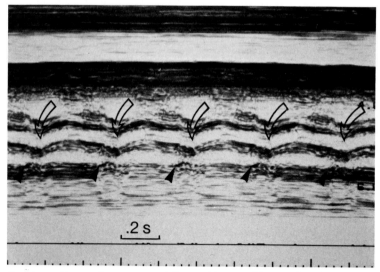

Figure 8–22. M-mode echocardiogram from a 24 week fetus with normal heart. The ultrasound beam passes through the right atrioventricular junction, the aortic root, and the left atrium. Atrial contraction *(arrowheads)* can be seen preceding ventricular contraction, which is indicated by aortic valve opening *(open arrows)* in this example.

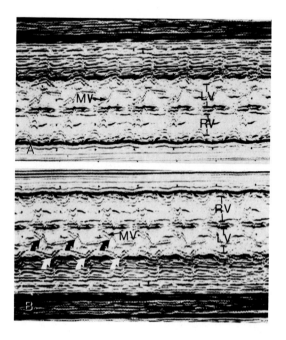

Figure 8–23. Fetal M-mode recording at ventricular level; the fetus is lying with its back toward the ultrasound transducer. *A,* The original display appears inverted compared with conventional M-mode display. Pattern recognition, therefore, becomes difficult. The M-mode recording shows the left ventricle (LV) on top and runs from right to left. *B,* Inverting the recording and viewing it in a mirror allows an orientation as seen postnatally. The same effect was achieved in this example by turning the negative of the original photograph backward, to display the appropriate lateral inversion, and printing it upside down. The onset of atrial contraction *(black arrows)* and of ventricular contraction *(white arrows)* can now easily be defined in the correct temporal sequence. MV, mitral valve; RV, right ventricle.

Figure 8–24. Pulsed Doppler interrogation at the site of the umbilical cord. *A,* The Doppler sample volume lies within the umbilical artery (UA, *arrow*). In the lower panel, a characteristic umbilical arterial signal is displayed above the baseline, demonstrating flow toward the transducer. *B,* The Doppler sample volume is now seen within the umbilical vein (UV, *arrow*); the fetal body and head are also shown. In the lower panel, a venous flow signal of fairly uniform low velocity throughout systole and diastole is demonstrated below the baseline; this flow is directed away from the transducer and toward the fetal body. Because the wall filter was set at 400 Hz, compared with 50 Hz in *A,* the origin of the spectral signals is blanked out.

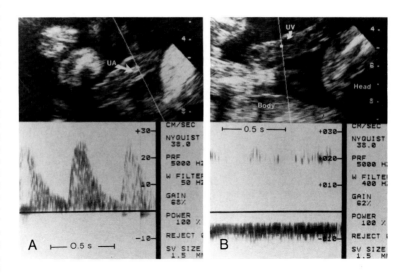

mean temporal flow velocities, as well as for volume flow across these valves, have been established (Table 8–2). The flow velocity curve across a fetal atrioventricular valve is normally characterized by a v-component (due to venous filling), which is followed by a higher a-component (due to atrial contraction) (Fig. 8–25A). This pattern is different from that observed postnatally and in the adult where the v-component is higher than the a-component; this difference may relate to the fetal ventricular size or to diminished ventricular compliance. Because the flow through the atrioventricular orifice relates to filling in that portion of diastole, the high a-component in the fetus suggests that a substantial amount of filling occurs as a result of atrial contraction. This may explain why fetal tachycardia is so poorly tolerated in the fetus and may lead to the development of fetal hydrops.

The highest velocity in the fetal heart is

Figure 8–25. Normal fetal Doppler flow profiles across an atrioventricular and a semilunar valve are shown. *A,* In a four-chamber view *(top),* the left atrium (LA), the right atrium (RA), the left ventricle (LV), and the right ventricle (RV) are seen. The sample volume lies below the tricuspid valve. The Doppler display *(bottom)* shows the diastolic inflow into the right ventricle above the baseline, indicating its direction toward the transducer. A biphasic signal is seen with a smaller v-component resulting from rapid venous filling, followed by a larger a-component *(black arrowheads)* resulting from atrial contraction. This pattern with predominant a-waves is typical for the fetus. The mirrorlike display below the baseline is an artifact caused by too high a gain setting. *B,* In a fetal short-axis

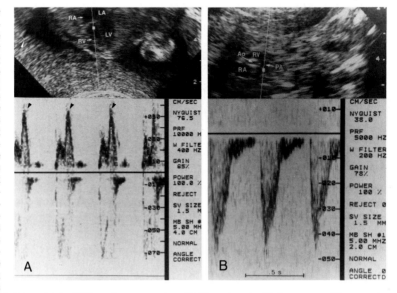

view *(top),* the right atrium (RA), right ventricle (RV), pulmonary artery (PA), and aorta (Ao) are seen. The sample volume lies distal to the pulmonary valve within the pulmonary artery. The Doppler flow signal below the baseline is directed away from the transducer *(bottom).*

Table 8–2. FLOW MEASUREMENT IN THE NORMAL FETAL HEART

	Peak Velocity (cm/sec)	Mean Temporal Velocity (cm/sec)
Tricuspid valve*	51 ± 9.1	11.8 ± 3.1
Mitral valve*	47 ± 8.3	11.2 ± 2.3
Pulmonary valve*	60 ± 12.9	16 ± 4.1
Aortic valve*	70 ± 12.2	18 ± 3.3
Right ventricular output†		307 ± 127 ml/kg/min
Left ventricular output†		232 ± 106 ml/kg/min

*Angle-corrected maximal and mean temporal flow velocities across the cardiac valves are expressed as mean ± SD.

†Cardiac output derived from tricuspid and mitral valve area and mean velocities (mean ± SD).

Adapted from Reed KL, Meijboom EJ, Sahn DJ, et al: Cardiac Doppler flow velocities in human fetuses. Circulation 73:41, 1986.

recorded within the ductus arteriosus;[42] color-coded Doppler flow mapping demonstrates aliased and disturbed flow in the fetal ductus (Fig. 8–26). By using Doppler inter-

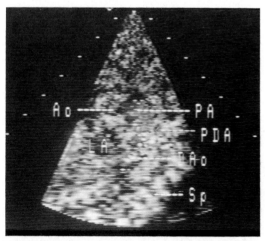

Figure 8–26. Color* Doppler flow map taken in a short-axis view in a fetus of 34 weeks' gestation, with complete heart block and a structurally normal heart. The red and blue color bars indicate flow directed toward and away from the transducer, respectively. Normal flow directed away from the transducer is seen in the pulmonary artery (PA) indicated by blue color, but a change in color occurs in the ductus arteriosus (PDA) and in the descending aorta (DAo). This color change into yellow and turquoise represents a phenomenon called aliasing. Aliasing occurs when the velocity of the blood flow exceeds the equipment's ability to recognize the velocity accurately. In this case, the acceleration of the flow velocity is related to the narrowing of the ductus arteriosus that occurs as the fetus matures. Ao, aorta; LA, left atrium; Sp, spine.

*See color plate, p xvi.

rogation in a direction where the velocity of blood flow is axial to the sample volume, one may obtain high-velocity profiles across stenotic or regurgitant atrioventricular and semilunar valves, which permits estimation of the pressure difference across these valves (Fig. 8–27). For this purpose, the modified Bernoulli equation is used, which states that the pressure drop (measured in mm Hg) across an orifice is proportional to four times the squared peak velocity (measured in m/sec) across that valve:

$$P = 4 V_d^2$$

where V_d is the high velocity in the stenotic area or just distal to it.[43, 44]

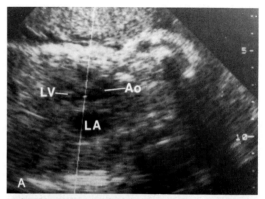

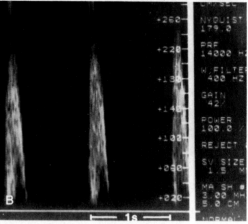

Figure 8–27. *A,* Long-axis view of a fetal heart at 32 weeks' gestation, with mild subaortic obstruction and complete heart block. The Doppler sample volume lies just above the aortic valve in the ascending aorta (Ao). The left atrium (LA) and left ventricle (LV) are also seen. *B,* Although the angle at the site of Doppler interrogation is more than 25°, thus underestimating the flow velocity, high pulse repetition frequency Doppler demonstrates a jet velocity of 2.5 m/sec. Some of this increase in velocity is related to the increased stroke volume associated with complete heart block.

Doppler ultrasound also aids in the analysis of cardiac rhythm disturbances. Sampling in any arterial vessel provides a measurement of heart rate, and sampling within the region of an atrioventricular valve provides information about valve opening and closure. By increasing the size of the sample volume, it is possible to obtain signals from two chambers or vessels simultaneously, for example, from both the descending aorta and left atrial wall in complete heart block, demonstrating the asynchronous contraction of atria and ventricles (Fig. 8–28). The characteristics of the pulse in the umbilical artery have been used to demonstrate altered flow dynamics in growth-retarded fetuses. The ratio of the peak systolic velocity divided by the minimal diastolic velocity is called the S/D or A/B ratio; it changes normally during gestation.[45, 46] Higher ratios suggest a decreased flow to the placenta that may be due to a higher resistance of the placental vascular bed such as seems to occur in growth-retarded fetuses.[47] With ratios, the measurements may be less dependent on the angle of insonance. In the authors' experience,

Doppler ultrasound was an essential technique that enabled them to demonstrate stenotic and regurgitant lesions[48] and to diagnose arrthythmias in a fetus with congenital heart disease. The use of this modality allows the detection of cardiac lesions, for example, mitral regurgitation in cardiomyopathy, not possible by other methods.

INTERPRETATION

Detection of Structural Defects

Among 561 fetuses the authors have studied for an indication mentioned above, a structural cardiac abnormality was found in 9 percent (Table 8–3). Normal cardiac anatomy with a cardiac rhythm disturbance was present in 18 percent. The remaining studies were within normal limits. The diagnosis of the structural cardiac defect was confirmed postnatally in all except two fetuses.

The most common structural abnormality in the authors' experience was an atrioventricular septal defect (Fig. 8–29). Often this

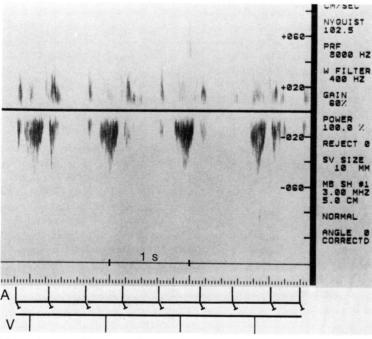

Figure 8–28. Pulsed Doppler recording from a fetus with complete heart block. Note in the right-hand side of the figure that the sample volume (SV) size has been increased to 10 mm. It has been placed astride the descending aorta and the left atrium in such a way as to allow simultaneous sampling of aortic flow and left atrial wall motion. The aortic flow is seen as the broader signal below the baseline. The smaller signals above and below the baseline indicate the wall "knock" of the left atrial contractions. The ladder diagram *(below)* demonstrates a ventricular rate of 65 beats/min but an atrial rate of about 130 beats/min; both chambers beat independently of each other.

Table 8–3. STRUCTURAL ABNORMALITIES IN 561 FETUSES

	N	Survivors
Atrioventricular septal defect (including 4 with L-ISO and CHB)	11	2
Ventricular septal defect (VSD) (including 1 with L-ISO and CHB)	7	4
Cardiomyopathy (CMP) (including 3 with familial CMP)	7	2
Univentricular atrioventricular connection (3 left-sided, 1 right-sided)	4	0
Pulmonary atresia/stenosis without VSD	4	1
Ebstein's anomaly	3	0
Double-outlet right ventricle (including 1 with pulmonary stenosis)	3	0
Aortopulmonary transposition with VSD	2	0
Aortic atresia	2	0
Absent pulmonary valve complex	1	0
Truncus arteriosus	1	0
Multiple rhabdomyoma	1	0
Other	5	2

CHB, complete heart block; L-ISO, left atrial isomerism.

defect was part of a complex cardiac lesion including left atrial isomerism, complete heart block, and nonimmune hydrops. Three of these pregnancies were terminated because of a fetal chromosomal defect. Seventy-five percent of the remaining fetuses with atrioventricular septal defect died either in utero or during the neonatal period.

Ventricular septal defects were also found frequently (Fig. 8–30). Occasionally the spontaneous closure of ventricular septal defects was observed on subsequent fetal examinations when there was no additional lesion. Seven cases of cardiomyopathy were encountered, more often the congestive form with a dilated, poorly contracting ventricle and atrioventricular valve regurgitation associated with fetal hydrops (Figs. 8–31, 8–32). One fetus presented with a hypertrophic cardiomyopathy (Fig. 8–33) and was clini-

cally identified to have Noonan's syndrome at birth. Two fetuses appeared to have normal cardiac function at 20 weeks' gestational age but, shortly after birth, were recognized to have congestive cardiomyopathy, suggesting that it may not always be possible to detect this abnormality prenatally and that myocardial dysfunction may occur either after examination in utero or after birth.

Complex forms of cardiac defects were diagnosed, such as univentricular atrioventricular connection in four fetuses, presenting in one as an absent right-sided atrioventricular connection with ventriculoarterial discordance (Figs. 8–34, 8–35), and in three as an absent left-sided atrioventricular connection, a double-outlet right ventricle, and a hypoplastic or an interrupted aortic arch (Figs. 8–36, 8–37). Ebstein's anomaly was detected in three fetuses (Figs. 8–38, 8–39);

Text continued on page 191

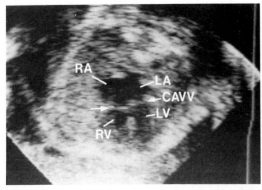

Figure 8–29. Fetal four-chamber view at 32 weeks' gestation. An atrioventricular (canal) septal defect is demonstrated. The common atrioventricular valve (CAVV, *white arrows*) straddles a common atrioventricular orifice dividing the large defect seen in this view into an atrial and a ventricular component. LA, left atrium; LV, left ventricle; RA, right atrium; RV, right ventricle.

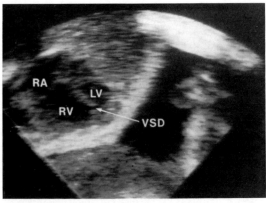

Figure 8–30. Fetal four-chamber view in a 32 week fetus. An isolated ventricular septal defect (VSD) is depicted in the apical muscular part of the ventricular septum. LV, left ventricle; RA, right atrium; RV, right ventricle.

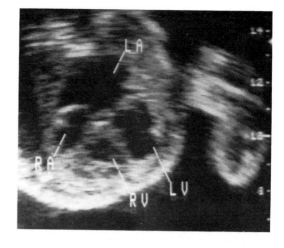

Figure 8–31. Magnified four-chamber view in a 31 week fetus with cardiomyopathy, severe mitral regurgitation, and hydrops. In this end-systolic frame, the left atrium (LA) and the left ventricle (LV) are considerably dilated, whereas the right atrium (RA) and the right ventricle (RV) appear to be of normal size.

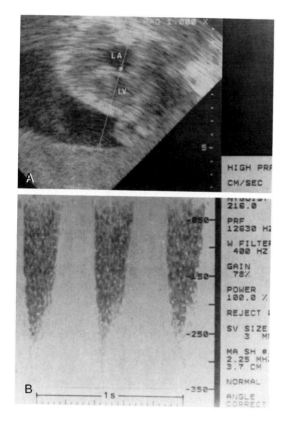

Figure 8–32. *A,* In a four-chamber view of a 28 week fetus with cardiomyopathy, the Doppler sample volume is above the mitral valve within the left atrium, which is considerably dilated. A turbulent jet of high velocity, directed away from the transducer, is displayed on high pulse repetition frequency Doppler in systole *(B),* indicating mitral insufficiency.

Figure 8–33. Long-axis view in a fetus with hypertrophic cardiomyopathy. This fetus was examined because of polyhydramnios. The ventricular septum (VS) and the right ventricular (RV) and the left ventricular (LV) free wall are thickened, and both ventricular cavities are diminutive. AAo, ascending aorta; Amn Cav, amniotic cavity; LA, left atrium.

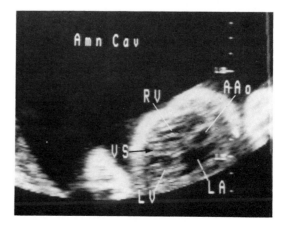

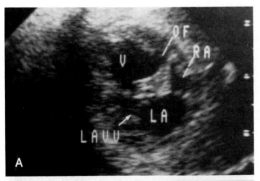

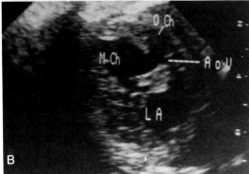

Figure 8–34. Long-axis orientation in a fetus of 38 weeks, with a univentricular heart and absent right-sided atrioventricular connection ("tricuspid atresia"). *A,* Instead of a right atrioventricular valve, there is echodense tissue between the right atrium (RA) and the dilated ventricle (V). The left atrium (LA) is enlarged and drains via a left atrioventricular valve (LAVV) into the ventricle. An outlet foramen (OF) is displayed anteriorly, leading into an outlet chamber, which can better be appreciated in *B. B,* This frame demonstrates a semilunar valve connected to the outlet chamber (OCh). Since the aorta arises anteriorly from that outlet chamber (see Fig. 8–35), this is the aortic valve (AoV). The single atrioventricular valve is demonstrated lying between the left atrium (LA) and main chamber (MCh) or ventricle.

Figure 8–35. *A,* In a long-axis view of the same fetus as in Figure 8–34, the aorta (Ao) and the pulmonary artery (PA) are seen exiting the heart in parallel, indicating transposition. The aorta, which arises from the outlet chamber and runs anterior to the pulmonary artery, can easily be defined as such because it gives rise to an innominate artery (IA). The pulmonary artery can be seen to arise from the main ventricular chamber (V) posteriorly. *B,* In this view obtained by tilting the transducer slightly to the fetus' right side, the pulmonary artery (PA), which arises posteriorly from the ventricle (V) and branches into the right (RPA) and left (LPA) pulmonary arteries, is seen. *C,* In a short-axis view at the base of the heart, both tricuspid semilunar valves are seen. LA, left atrium; OF, outlet foramen; OCh, outlet chamber.

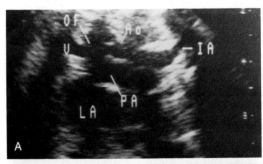

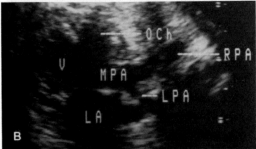

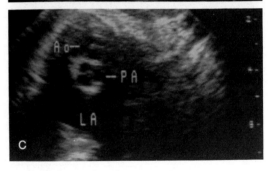

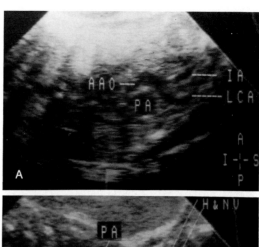

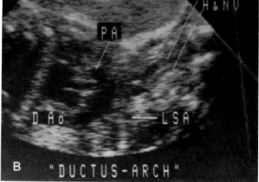

Figure 8–36. Sagittal view in a fetus of 34 weeks' gestation with absent left-sided atrioventricular connection, double-outlet right ventricle, and interrupted aortic arch. *A,* The ascending aorta (AAo) and the proximal arch, which runs on top of the right pulmonary artery (PA), are seen giving rise to the innominate artery (IA) and to the left carotid artery (LCA). A, anterior; I, inferior; P, posterior; S, superior. *B,* After slight angulation of the transducer to the fetus' left side, the dilated pulmonary artery (PA) and its continuation via the ductus arteriosus into the descending aorta (DAo) come into view (the so-called "ductus-arch"). The left subclavian artery (LSA) can be seen arising from the descending aorta, which is separated from the arch and the head and neck vessels (H&NV).

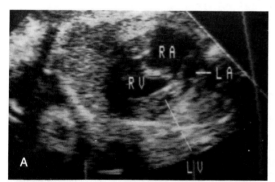

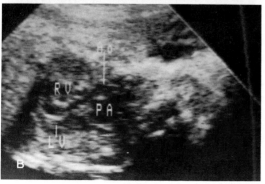

Figure 8–37. Four-chamber view in the same fetus as in Figure 8–36. *A,* The dilated right-sided structures and the hypoplastic left-sided structures of the heart are demonstrated: LA, left atrium; LV, left ventricle; RA, right atrium; RV, right ventricle. *B,* In a long-axis view, the aorta (Ao) and the pulmonary artery (PA) are seen to arise from the large right ventricle (RV); no vessel arises from the hypoplastic left ventricle (LV).

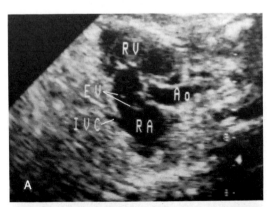

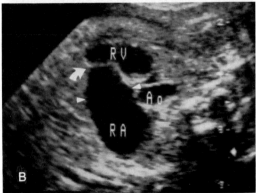

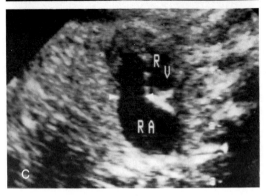

Figure 8–38. Magnified sagittal views in a fetus of 20 weeks' gestation with Ebstein's anomaly. *A*, The inferior vena cava (IVC) drains into the dilated right atrium (RA); the eustachian valve (EV) can be seen marking the approximate position of the atrioventricular groove. The right ventricle (RV) and aorta (Ao) are also seen. *B*, The displacement of the valve leaflets, especially of the posteroinferior leaflet *(thick arrow)*, is demonstrated during systole when the leaflets are apposed. The tricuspid valve ring, which is part of the atrioventriclar groove, is marked by *small arrowheads*. *C*, In a diastolic frame, the displaced posteroinferior leaflet is shown tethered to the diaphragmatic surface of the right ventricular wall.

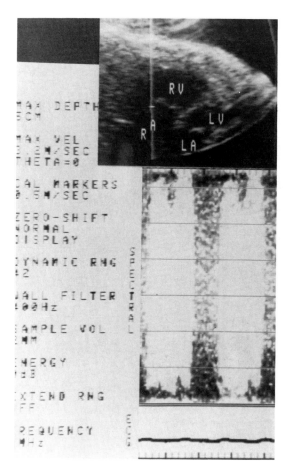

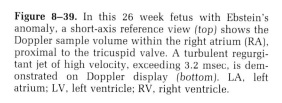

Figure 8–39. In this 26 week fetus with Ebstein's anomaly, a short-axis reference view *(top)* shows the Doppler sample volume within the right atrium (RA), proximal to the tricuspid valve. A turbulent regurgitant jet of high velocity, exceeding 3.2 msec, is demonstrated on Doppler display *(bottom)*. LA, left atrium; LV, left ventricle; RV, right ventricle.

one of them died in utero with severe hydrops, and the other two died during the first week of life. One of these fetuses was the product of a mother who had the same lesion; another one was born to a mother who had taken high doses of lithium, a known cardiac teratogen,[23, 49] during early pregnancy.

Two fetuses were found to have transposition of the great arteries with a ventricular septal defect; one also had pulmonary atresia (Fig. 8–40). In a thoracopagus twin detected as early as 16 weeks, the authors noted the hearts to be fused with shared atria and shared ventricles, one common atrioventricular valve, and only one dilated great artery in each body (pulmonary atresia in one, aortic hypoplasia with interrupted arch in the other) (Fig. 8–41). Several other lesions were encountered once, including absent pulmonary valve complex (Figs. 8–42, 8–43), persistent truncus arteriosus (Fig. 8–44), and multiple intracardiac rhabdomyoma due to tuberous sclerosis (Fig. 8–45).

Using pulsed Doppler ultrasound, the authors detected severe atrioventricular valve regurgitation in ten fetuses (Figs. 8–32, 8–39). All of these presented with fetal hydrops but with different cardiac defects, such as Ebstein's anomaly, aortic or pulmonary atresia, atrioventricular septal defect, cardiomyopathy, or double-outlet right ventricle with atretic left-sided atrioventricular valve. Doppler echocardiography also aided the detection of pulmonary regurgitation in one fetus (Fig. 8–43) and disturbed flow in both left and right ventricular outflow tract obstructions in three fetuses (Fig. 8–27). Display of an abnormal flow pattern indicating valvar stenosis and regurgitation were augmented in five cases using color-coded Doppler flow mapping (Fig. 8–46). Color Doppler studies did not always reproduce the results obtained by pulsed or high pulse repetition frequency Doppler, especially when the fetal lie was unfavorable or when the fetus was situated at a distance greater than 10 cm from the maternal abdominal wall. Instru-

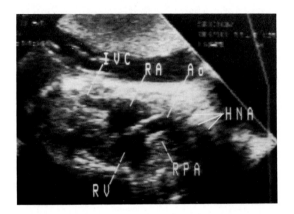

Figure 8–40. Sagittal view in a fetus presenting with the back lying anteriorly. This 32 week fetus had transposition of the great arteries, with ventricular septal defect and pulmonary atresia. The inferior vena cava (IVC) is seen draining into the right atrium (RA), which is connected to the right ventricle (RV). The aorta (Ao) arises anteriorly from the right ventricle and gives rise to the head and neck arteries (HNA). The right pulmonary artery (RPA) is diminutive, indicating severe obstruction of the pulmonary outflow tract.

Figure 8–41. Thoracopagus twins at 24 weeks. Both bodies are visualized; the fused hearts share the atria (A, A) and the ventricles (B, V). Only one common atrioventricular valve (CAVV), shared between the two hearts, can be seen.

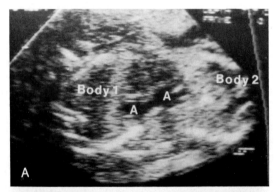

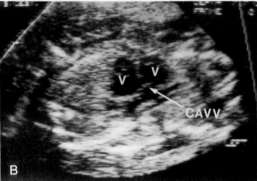

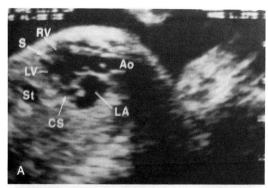

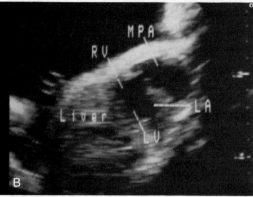

Figure 8–42. Sagittal views in a fetus of 31 weeks' gestation, with absent pulmonary valve complex and tetralogy of Fallot. *A,* The ascending aorta (Ao) is seen overriding a large ventricular septal defect. CS, coronary sinus; LA, left atrium; LV, left ventricle; RV, right ventricle; S, ventricular septum; St, stomach. *B,* With the scan plane directed more to the left, the dysplastic pulmonary valve and the markedly dilated main pulmonary artery (MPA) are demonstrated. *C,* More to the right, the aortic arch is shown. Note the discrepancy between the size of the aortic arch and the right pulmonary artery (RPA), which lies underneath it.

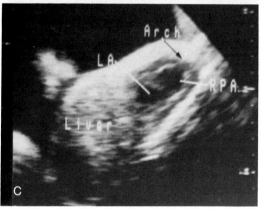

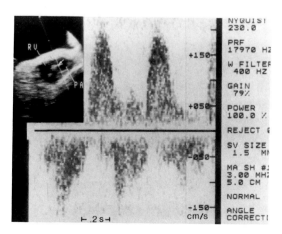

Figure 8–43. Pulsed Doppler ultrasound examination in the same fetus as in Figure 8–42. In the *top left* reference image, the Doppler sample volume lies in the pulmonary artery (PA), distal to the dysplastic pulmonary valve *(arrow)*; the right ventricle (RV) is also seen. The spectral Doppler display is not corrected for angle. A diastolic signal of disturbed flow at a high velocity is demonstrated above the baseline (directed toward the transducer) and reflects pulmonary regurgitation, whereas the systolic signal below the baseline (directed away from the transducer) indicates pulmonary stenosis.

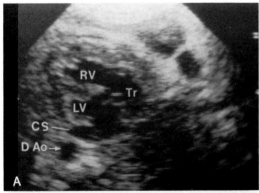

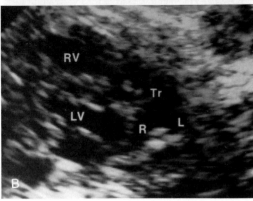

Figure 8–44. Long-axis orientation in a fetus of 32 weeks' gestation with truncus arteriosus. *A,* The single truncal vessel (Tr) is seen overriding a ventricular septal defect. The coronary sinus (CS) is dilated because of a left superior vena cava connection. DAo, descending aorta; LV, left ventricle; RV, right ventricle. *B,* After magnification and slight movement of the transducer to the fetal left side, the common origin of a pulmonary artery from the truncus and its division into right and left pulmonary branches (R, L) can be seen.

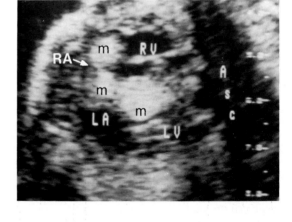

Figure 8–45. Magnified four-chamber view in a 29 week fetus presenting with nonimmune hydrops. A considerable amount of ascites (Asc) is demonstrated. Echodense masses (m) are depicted in the ventricular septum between the right ventricle (RV) and the left ventricle (LV), but can also be seen at the right atrial (RA) level. These masses are multiple rhabdomyoma due to tuberous sclerosis. LA, left atrium.

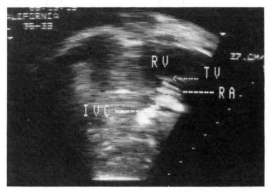

Figure 8–46. Color* Doppler flow map taken in a short-axis view of a 29 week fetus with tricuspid regurgitation due to a structural cardiac defect (univentricular atrioventricular connection, aortic arch hypoplasia). In this systolic frame, the tricuspid valve (TV) can be seen between the right ventricle (RV) and the right atrium (RA). A regurgitant jet, refluxing all the way back into the inferior vena cava (IVC), is depicted in red and yellow colors, indicating its direction toward the transducer.

*See color plate, p xvi.

ments with greater sensitivity than those the authors used initially may obviate this problem.

Although Doppler ultrasound readily defines stenotic and regurgitant lesions, there are pitfalls of which one has to be aware. Because of beam divergence, ambiguity in the position of the sample volume may occur in closely situated structures; for example, sampling within the right atrium close to the aorta may lead to the misinterpretation of tricuspid regurgitation because, in fact, the signal of a normal flow in the ascending aorta was sampled. This becomes particularly important when short-focused high-frequency transducers are used. Unfavorable fetal position or great distance from the transducer, such as in cases of polyhydramnios, may limit the Doppler technique in certain cases. Attempts have been made to calculate the fetal cardiac output from blood flow velocity profiles,[38, 39, 41] but unfortunately, this calculation requires accurate measurement of valve or vessel diameters; inaccuracy of even 1 mm may yield an unacceptable high error in the calculation of fetal cardiac output, particularly when the flow vessel diameter is small. Color-coded flow mapping may facilitate the Doppler display, thereby shortening the study time, but in the fetus, color flow mapping also appears to have significant technical limitations due to aliasing and depth resolution. Off-axis signals may also not be well defined by color flow mapping.

Diagnostic Errors

It is important to recognize that, in spite of the increased experience with fetal echocardiography, errors in interpretation are still possible. The authors have made a false-negative diagnosis of a structurally normal heart in four fetuses of their series. One had a ventricular septal defect, one had aortic coarctation coupled with double-orifice mitral valve, one had mild pulmonary stenosis, and one had situs inversus (mirror image dextrocardia). The last error should not be made if the correct position of the heart within the chest is determined first. In complex cardiac defects, the main lesion may be recognizable, but secondary lesions may be missed unless careful attention is paid to the entire examination. In general, experience suggests that prenatal findings in complex congenital defects tend to underestimate the severity of the spectrum of abnormalities.

Both false-negative and false-positive findings have been reported previously.[7, 8, 11, 50] When evaluating the cause of errors, the authors found that most of the serious ones had been made using older equipment that had poor resolution and no magnification or Doppler facilities. Other errors unrelated to equipment are beyond the ultrasonographer's control, including technical factors such as suboptimal imaging, which may occur with maternal obesity, polyhydramnios, or fetal lie. Because the resolution of echocardiographic imaging is limited to distances of 1 to 1.5 mm, structural abnormalities such as relatively small ventricular septal defects may be technically impossible to image. Mild aortic or pulmonic stenosis may be difficult to detect because valve morphology may not be distorted, and blood flow velocity may be lower than after birth owing to low ventricular pressures present in fetal life. Other defects, such as mild aortic coarctation or a secundum atrial septal defect, may be indistinguishable from similar conditions in the normal fetus. Furthermore, cardiac lesions may develop or worsen later in pregnancy, as the authors have observed in cases of cardiomyopathy, and may require serial studies during the second and third trimesters. On the other hand, some lesions may disappear on subsequent studies, such as ventricular septal defects closing spontaneously.

Outcome of Fetuses with Structural Cardiac Defects

Reports that the overall outcome of a fetus with a structural cardiac abnormality is unfavorable[10, 48, 50, 51] were confirmed in the authors' series (Table 8–3). Six pregnancies were electively terminated: two because of severe fetal cardiac defects, the others because of chromosomal abnormalities. There were 33 fetal or neonatal deaths, and only 12 children (24 percent) were alive at the end of the neonatal period. Five of these 12 infants underwent cardiac surgery within the first months of life, including one who had cardiac transplantation. The incidence of death in those fetuses presenting with nonimmune hydrops and cardiac defects was high (16 of 18 cases). In ten of these, there was severe atrioventricular regurgitation, and all of them died either before birth or within the first week of life. Cardiac defects coupled with complete atrioventricular block were present in eight fetuses; in this group, there were seven prenatal or

Table 8–4. FETAL ARRHYTHMIAS DETECTED BY ULTRASOUND

	N	Therapy	Neonatal Survivors
Premature atrial contractions	76	–	76
Premature ventricular contractions	2	–	2
Supraventricular tachycardia	12	11*	10
Atrial flutter	3	3†	3
Complete heart block	15	–	8

*Effective treatment: digoxin alone in 7, digoxin and verapamil in 1, digoxin and procainamide in 1. In 1 fetus, severe bradycardia occurred after administration of digoxin and verapamil, leading to emergency cesarean section; this arrhythmia was controlled after birth. In 1 fetus, digoxin, verapamil, propranolol, procainamide, and amiodarone failed to convert the cardiac rhythm; this fetus died. One fetus was not treated because of severe additional abnormalities and died subsequently.
†Effective treatment with digoxin alone in all of them.

neonatal deaths. The prognosis for fetal survival appears to be poor in the presence of structural abnormalities coupled with atrioventricular valve regurgitation, complete heart block, or fetal hydrops. It is important to note that because the technique is in its early stages, those defects most likely to be symptomatic are more likely to be recognized.

Fetal Cardiac Arrhythmias

Analysis and comprehension of fetal cardiac arrhythmias using M-mode or Doppler ultrasound is facilitated by the construction of ladder diagrams (Fig. 8–21). Ladder diagrams allow the definition of the sequence of atrial and ventricular events and are used in electrophysiology for delineating arrhythmias. The horizontal lines indicate the division between the atria, the atrioventricular node, and the ventricles. With normal conduction, atrial (sinus) activity precedes atrioventricular nodal activity, which precedes ventricular activity (Fig. 8–22). It is important to recognize that echocardiography cannot identify the electrical events but only the mechanical events that succeed them. Mechanical events are less precise and less easy to define, underscoring the limitations of the technique. Despite these limitations, fetal echocardiography is the most practical method currently available for analyzing fetal arrhythmias and has proved to be remarkably valuable.

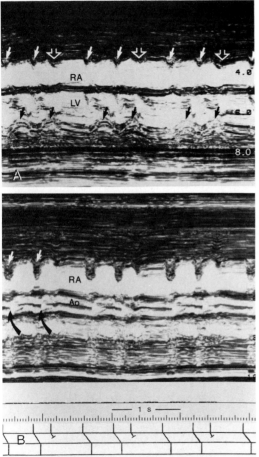

Figure 8–47. M-mode recording from a fetus with premature atrial contractions. *A,* The ultrasound beam passes through the right atrium (RA), the atrioventricular junction, and the left ventricle (LV). After two regular atrial beats *(white arrows),* there is an ectopic beat *(open arrows).* This premature atrial contraction is not conducted, since it is not followed by a ventricular contraction *(black arrows).* The compensatory pause is 720 msec; it is an incomplete compensatory pause, because a complete one would last twice the atrial interval (900 msec). *B,* In the same patient, the ultrasound beam now passes through the right atrium (RA) and the aortic root (Ao). The *white arrows* indicate atrial contraction, and the *black arrows* mark the opening of the aortic valve, indicating the effect of ventricular contraction. Two ventricular beats are followed by an incomplete compensatory pause due to premature atrial beats.

Most frequently, an irregular fetal heart rate results from isolated premature atrial contractions (Fig. 8–47, Table 8–4). These are characterized by a compensatory pause that is almost invariably an incomplete one. Compensatory pauses are the same phenomenon seen in electrocardiography after birth; if they are complete, they account for two intervals of regular heartbeats. Isolated premature atrial contractions are fairly common, accounting for about two-thirds of fetal arrhythmias noted in the authors' series; they are benign and usually transient, and they do not require any treatment.[12–16] The authors do, however, recommend abstaining from smoking and ingesting caffeine-containing products. This rhythm disturbance should be followed by the primary physician, because supraventricular tachycardia may develop on rare occasion; however, it does not require further routine echocardi-

ographic examination. Isolated premature ventricular contractions are characterized by a compensatory pause that is usually complete (Fig. 8–48); they are, in the authors' experience, much rarer than premature atrial contractions, but others have noted a higher incidence.[17] Premature ventricular beats are also benign and do not require treatment.

Tachyarrhythmias were present in 15 percent of the authors' cases with a fetal cardiac rhythm disturbance. Most common is a supraventricular tachycardia (Fig. 8–49), which may lead to fetal cardiac failure, hydrops, and death. Doppler echocardiography demonstrates the reduction of stroke volume during runs of supraventricular tachycardia (Fig. 8–50). On rarer occasions, fetal tachyarrhythmia is caused by atrial flutter (Fig. 8–51), usually presenting with variable degrees of atrioventricular block. Atrial flutter may also lead to fetal cardiac failure and

Figure 8–48. Fetal premature contractions that are more likely to be premature junctional or ventricular contractions. *A,* In this M-mode display, the movements of the mitral valve (M) and of the left ventricular posterior wall (PW) can be seen. The irregularity in the rhythm is caused by a premature fifth beat. Whereas all other beats are preceded by an atrial kick, seen on the mitral valve echo *(arrows),* the premature beat is not. Furthermore, the compensatory pause is complete, because two intervals of regular beats also last approximately 1020 msec, as seen in the ladder diagram below. This favors the diagnosis of a premature junctional or ventricular contraction. *B,* Pulsed Doppler sampling within the umbilical artery in a different fetus reveals a similar pattern of irregularity. The premature beat *(open arrow)* is followed by a complete compensatory pause and, therefore, is more likely to be of ventricular origin.

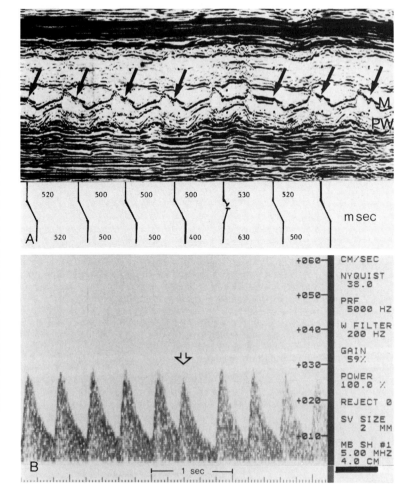

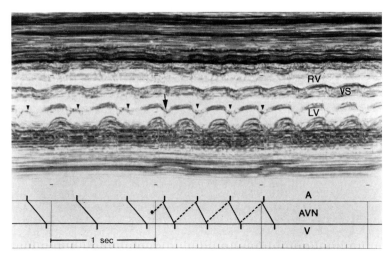

Figure 8–49. M-mode recording of a 30 week fetus with a supraventricular tachycardia. This example demonstrates the atrioventricular re-entry mechanism at the onset of the tachycardia. To the left of the recording, there is a normal sinus rhythm; note that the atrial click *(black arrowheads)* on the mitral valve echo, indicating atrial contraction, is fairly separated from the preceding valve movement during early diastolic filling. After three regular beats, a premature atrioventricular nodal depolarization causes retrograde atrial and antegrade ventricular activation, thus starting a re-entry cycle. The first atrial click on the mitral valve echo appears at the same time as the early diastolic filling deflection *(black arrow)*; during the tachycardia, it then can be seen in a different position, closer to the early filling wave than during the sinus rhythm. A, atrial contraction; AVN, atrioventricular node activation; LV, left ventricle; RV, right ventricle; V, ventricular contraction; VS, ventricular septum.

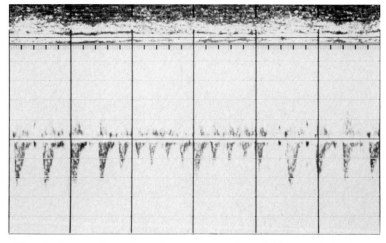

Figure 8–50. Pulsed Doppler interrogation within the pulmonary artery of a fetus with short runs of supraventricular tachycardia. Note the reduction in stroke volume at the onset of tachycardia, after the first four regular beats. Ten beats in tachycardia are followed by a pause and resumption of the normal sinus rhythm. Horizontal lines are markers of frequency shift (1 kHz or 0.25 m/sec); vertical lines are time markers (1 sec).

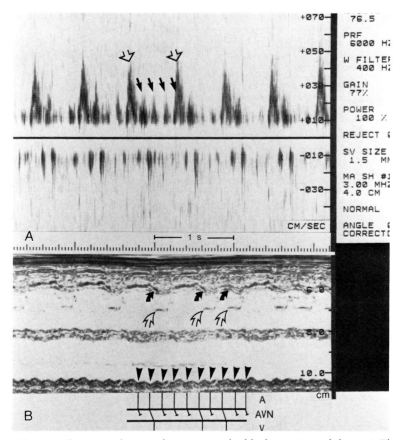

Figure 8–51. Atrial flutter with varying degrees of atrioventricular block in a 36 week fetus. *A,* The sample volume is placed across the descending aorta and the left atrial wall. Pulsed Doppler interrogation demonstrates atrial contractions (smaller flow signals, *black arrows*) and ventricular contractions (bigger flow signals, *open arrows*). In this recording, there is constantly a 4:1 atrioventricular block. This results in an apparently regular heart rate of about 100 beats/min. *B,* M-mode recording from the same fetus. The ultrasound beam passes through the right ventricle anteriorly and the left atrium posteriorly. At the back of the heart, rapid atrial contractions at about 400 beats/min can be seen *(black arrowheads).* Ventricular activation is inferred from either the tricuspid valve closure *(open arrows)* or the onset of ventricular wall motion *(black arrows).* The ladder diagram demonstrates the presence of a 4:1 atrioventricular block on the left side, with one following beat showing a 2:1 block. These varying degrees of atrioventricular block result in an irregular heart rate. A, atrium; AVN, atrioventricular node; V, ventricle.

hydrops. When the survival of the fetus would be compromised by early delivery, intrauterine treatment by administering medications to the mother should be used, as it has been successful on numerous occasions.[12, 13, 19, 52, 53] It is now established practice to use the transplacental route for antiarrhythmic drug administration. Since supraventricular tachycardia is most likely the result of atrioventricular re-entry (see Fig. 8–49), as experience with this arrhythmia in infancy suggests, digoxin is the drug of first choice.[12, 13, 19, 52–54] If it fails to convert the fetal heart rate to sinus rhythm, the authors also administer verapamil, propranolol, procainamide, or quinidine, in that order (Table 8–5).

The authors' dosage schedule for these drugs is based on loading doses for the conversion of cardiac arrhythmias in adults (Table 8–5). Except for digoxin, which may be given orally, other antiarrhythmic drugs carry some risk, and most are administered intravenously in a delivery set-up room. The mother remains in a position where rapid obstetric intervention is possible. Direct echocardiographic monitoring of the fetal heart should be performed during such cardioversion. Enteral absorption of digoxin may be limited during pregnancy, and additional administration of other drugs, such as verapamil, may decrease its clearance.[52] Therefore, the maintenance therapy should be monitored by maternal serum concentra-

Table 8–5. DOSAGE SCHEDULE FOR ANTIARRHYTHMIC TRANSPLACENTAL TREATMENT

	Loading		Maintenance			Plasma Level	
Drug	*Dose*	*Route*	*Dose*	*Route*	*Interval*	*Therapeutic*	*Toxic*
Digoxin	0.5 mg (initially) + 0.25 mg q 6 hr (total: 1.25– 1.5 mg)	iv					
	or 1.5–2 mg (in 24–48 hr)	po	0.25–0.75 mg	po	24 hr	1–2 ng/ml	>2.5 ng/ml
Verapamil†	0.1–0.2 mg/kg	iv (1–2 min)	80–120 mg	po	6–8 hr	80–300 ng/ml	>300 ng/ml
Propranolol*	0.1–0.2 mg/kg	iv	10–40 mg	po	8–6 hr	50–100 ng/ml	
Procainamide	15 mg/kg, max: 1 gm	iv‡	0.5–1 gm	po	4 hr	3–6 µg/ml	>8 µg/ml
Quinidine- Sulfate	—§	—§	0.3–0.4 gm	po	6–8† hr	2–6 µg/ml	>8 µg/ml

*Do not use verapamil and propranolol at the same time!

†Atropine (0.5–1 mg) should be on hand for managing the side effect of maternal or fetal bradycardia due to atrioventricular block.

‡As infusion, about 50 mg/min.

§Start with maintenance; po only. Decrease digoxin, and check serum levels if used simultaneously.[67]

tions. Besides the authors' own experience of antiarrhythmic medication administration, other drugs, such as amiodarone, have also been reported to be successful for converting supraventricular tachycardia.[54] Newer antiarrhythmic agents, such as mex- iletine, tocainide, encainide, and flecainide, have not yet been used in fetal tachyarrhythmias. The authors would like to stress that, except for digoxin, other agents are best administered in a tertiary care facility by a team consisting of pediatric cardiologists,

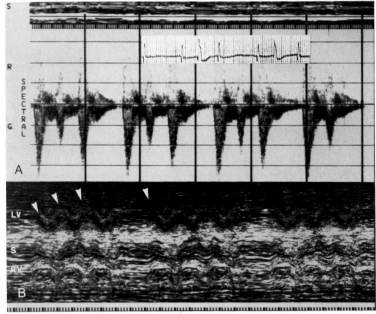

Figure 8–52. Group beating in a 38 week fetus with bradycardia and junctional or ventricular escape beats, demonstrated by pulsed Doppler *(A)* and M-mode echocardiography *(B)*. A, The pulsed Doppler interrogation (paper speed: 50 mm/sec) in the descending aorta demonstrates a less effective stroke volume from the second beat when compared with the first and the third beat of each group. Whereas group beating with three beats followed by a pause is usually noted with second degree atrioventricular block (Wenckebach-type), the less effective second beat strongly suggests that this is due to premature contractions rather than to atrioventricular block. The inset shows a scalp electrode electrocardiogram (paper speed: 25 mm/sec) obtained after a rupture of the membranes had occurred. Premature junctional escape beats are seen, confirming the echocardiographic diagnosis. B, The M-mode tracing (paper speed: 75 mm/sec), obtained from the same fetus, demonstrates the motion of the left ventricular (LV) wall, ventricular septum (S), and right ventricular (RV) wall. The same group-beating phenomenon is seen *(arrowheads)*, but the less effective nature of the premature beat cannot be noted.

electrophysiologists, obstetricians, anesthesiologists, and support personnel, as these antiarrhythmic drugs may have serious side effects to the mother and fetus.

Prolonged fetal bradyarrhythmia may result from several mechanisms, including the frequent occurrence of nonconducted premature atrial contractions, group beating, or complete heart block. Group beating may occur because of different electrophysiologic mechanisms, the most common of which is Wenckebach's phenomenon (usually second degree atrioventricular block). The authors have also observed group beating with bradycardia and junctional or ventricular escape beats (Fig. 8–52). Doppler ultrasound is valuable for distinguishing these different conditions (Figs. 8–52, 8–53).

Bradyarrhythmia due to complete heart block was present in 15 percent of the authors' cases of fetal arrhythmia (Figs. 8–28, 8–54). Complete heart block may occur coupled with structural cardiac defects—affected fetuses often present with nonimmune hydrops—but it may also be an isolated finding. In fetuses without structural defects, the mother often suffers from connective tissue disease. These women almost always have antibodies to soluble tissue ribonucleoprotein antigens (Ro[SS-A] and La[SS-B]) that may pass the placental barrier and may be found in the affected newborn.[28, 55] No therapeutic approach is presently available for the sick fetus with heart block. Attempted direct fetal cardiac pacing has failed to prevent death.[56] The authors have attempted transabdominal stimulation with an extracardiac pacemaker applied to the maternal abdominal wall, with the same outcome. The prognosis of complete heart block in the fetus is especially poor when structural heart disease or hydrops is also present. However, most fetuses with complete heart block survive when this is an isolated phenomenon, regardless of any association with maternal connective tissue disease.

It is a useful rule of thumb that in fetal arrhythmias, rapid (> 200 beats/min) and slow (< 80 beats/min) heart rates require further evaluation, whereas isolated irregular beats are of little concern. Should irregularities of fetal rhythm be associated with runs of tachycardia or bradycardia, they are of more concern. Isolated irregularities of fetal cardiac rhythm do not, in the authors'

experience, occur together with specific structural cardiac abnormalities; only complete heart block has this association.

COMMENTS

Incidence

The spectrum of abnormalities the authors found does not reflect the common incidence of the different types of congenital cardiac defects.[1, 2, 57, 58] On the contrary, rarer and more complex forms of congenital cardiac defects are detected, presumably because they are more likely to be symptomatic. Both the frequent diagnosis of complex lesions and the high incidence of structural cardiac defects may relate to the criteria the authors set for evaluating the population for the development of congenital heart defects. The risk of developing congenital heart disease has been thought to increase when there is a family history of either congenital heart defects or extracardiac malformations.[24–26, 59, 60] Maternal congenital heart disease appears to carry a risk factor as great as 10 to 15 percent for subsequent pregnancies, whereas the recurrence of congenital heart disease with one affected sibling is about 2 percent.

Impact of Fetal Echocardiography on Obstetric Management

Decisions on the further obstetric management of the pregnancy may be influenced by fetal echocardiography. Because of its potential for prenatal distinction of simple and complex structural abnormalities of the heart, this information has been made available for genetic counseling, aiding the decision for elective termination of the pregnancy, as in four of the authors' cases in which chromosomal defects were present. Elective termination of pregnancy based purely on the morphologic information of fetal echocardiography was performed in only two fetuses, but the detection of serious cardiac defects may become a much more frequent reason for terminating pregnancy when the technique becomes more generally applied. The role of fetal echocardiography

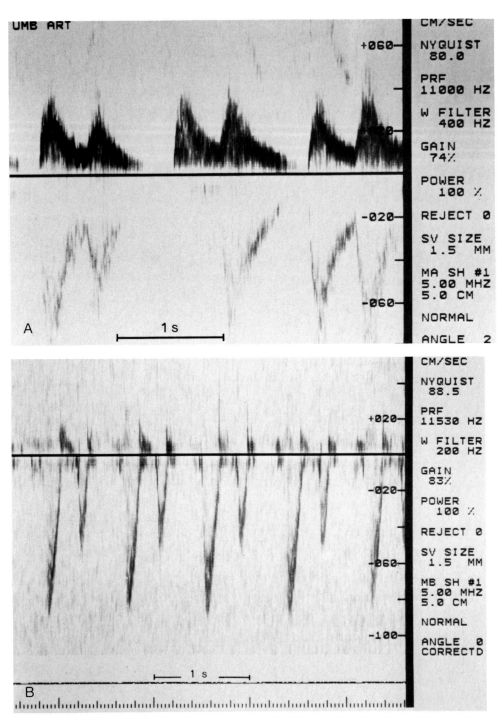

Figure 8–53. Doppler ultrasound recording showing group beating (bigeminal rhythm) in two fetuses with premature contractions. *A,* In this example taken from the umbilical artery (umb art), the mother had received digoxin because supraventricular tachycardia occurred in the fetus. Therefore, fetal group beating may well be related to fetal digitalis intoxication (either because of digoxin-induced atrioventricular block of the Wenckebach type or because of bigeminal premature ventricular contractions), but may result from nonconducted premature atrial contractions as well. Although the Doppler interrogation did not allow the distinction between these possible causes, the M-mode recording obtained from the same fetus (see Fig. 8–47) clearly showed nonconducted premature atrial contractions as being the cause of this bigeminal rhythm and indicated a satisfactory therapeutic response to the digoxin therapy. *B,* In this example taken from another fetus' pulmonary artery, the less effective ejection of every second beat is likely to result from premature contractions. Since this rhythm was so persistent that no sequence of regular beats could be recorded, it was not possible to distinguish between an atrial and a ventricular origin of the premature contractions. Postnatal follow-up demonstrated a normal sinus rhythm.

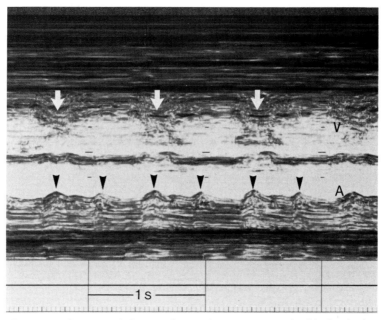

Figure 8–54. M-mode tracing of a 32 week fetus with complete atrioventricular block. The beam passes through the right ventricle (V) and the left atrium (A). Ventricular contractions *(white arrows)* at a rate of 68 beats/min are seen occurring independently of atrial contractions *(black arrowheads)*; the atrial rate is 142 beats/min.

in detecting severe structural abnormalities is therefore comparable with that of amniocentesis or fetal blood sampling, which is used as a diagnostic tool for the assessment of severe chromosomal or inborn metabolic disorders. When terminating the pregnancy is not an alternative, fetal echocardiography plays an important role in determining the course of appropriate management.[61, 62] If immediate neonatal support is contemplated, the delivery can also be planned at a center with facilities for medical and surgical cardiac treatment of these neonates. The detection of cardiac defects may also influence the route of delivery; for example, when prolonged labor may cause myocardial ischemia, cesarean section might be contemplated.[62]

In the authors' series, most fetuses with major cardiac defects had a prior examination by an obstetric ultrasonographer who recognized some cardiac disturbance. The impact of fetal echocardiography will be greater when it becomes an accepted and familiar technique for primary care ultrasonographers. Since it appears that fetal echocardiography is considerably more complex than obtaining a fairly "normal-looking" four-chamber view, obstetric ultrasonographers will require further training in the

recognition of structural abnormalities of the fetal heart. When cardiac examination of the fetus becomes a routine part of the primary ultrasonographic examination, it is conceivable that an entirely new perspective may emerge on congenital heart disease, including diagnosis and physiology, which may shift the emphasis for early treatment to the prenatal period.

Outlook

New therapeutic strategies may develop because of fetal echocardiography. Prenatal surgery, already an established treatment for hydrocephalus or hydronephrosis, may become an alternative approach to the treatment of congenital heart defects. Experimental data indicate the potential of performing certain forms of fetal cardiovascular surgery to palliate or remove severe right heart obstructive lesions,[21, 22] which may allow better development of these malformed hearts. For the same reason, interventional catheterization in the fetus has been proposed as a possible therapeutic approach in the future.[51] Fetal echocardiography is the only technique currently available as a prenatal test for congenital heart defects. Although magnetic resonance imaging has been used to demonstrate fetal cardiac anatomy,[63] there are obviously limitations to its applicability and safety.

Monitoring of the fetal cardiovascular function by echocardiography during treatment of arrhythmias or congestive heart failure with medication administered by both a maternal[12–15, 18–20, 52–54, 64] and a direct fetal route[64, 65] may be expanded considerably in the future. Moreover, fetal echocardiography may allow the detection of undesired side effects of drugs taken for maternal indications, such as the constriction of the ductus arteriosus after indomethacin therapy in the mother.[42]

Fetal echocardiography provides new information about the development of the heart in the presence of structural or functional disease;[37, 48, 51, 66] this knowledge will contribute to a better understanding of the natural history of congenital heart disease.

Acknowledgment: We are indebted to Dr. Melvin Scheinman (Division of Cardiology) for his advice concerning antiarrhythmic therapy and to many of our obstetric colleagues, especially Drs. Mitchell Golbus and Robert Anderson (Division of Genetic Counseling and Prenatal Diagnosis) and Drs. Roy Filly and Peter Callen (Division of Radiology), for their help, advice, and support. We wish to thank Mrs. Heather Silverman for editorial assistance with this manuscript and Mrs. Mary Helen Briscoe for artwork.

References

1. Mitchell SC, Korones SB, Berendes HW: Congenital heart disease in 56,109 births. Incidence and natural history. Circulation 43:323, 1971.
2. Hoffman JIE, Christianson R: Congenital heart disease in a cohort of 19,502 births with long-term follow-up. Am J Cardiol 42:641, 1978.
3. Allan LD, Tynan MJ, Campbell S, et al: Echocardiographic and anatomical correlates in the fetus. Br Heart J 44:444, 1980.
4. Lange LW, Sahn DJ, Allen HD, et al: Qualitative real-time corss-sectional echocardiographic imaging of the human fetus during the second half of pregnancy. Circulation 62:799, 1980.
5. Sahn DJ, Lange LW, Allen HD, et al: Quantitative real-time cross-sectional echocardiography in the developing normal human fetus and newborn. Circulation 62:588, 1980.
6. Huhta JC, Hagler DJ, Hill LM: Two-dimensional echocardiographic assessment of normal fetal cardiac anatomy. J Reprod Med 29:162, 1984.
7. Allan LD, Crawford DC, Anderson RH, Tynan MJ: Echocardiographic and anatomical correlations in fetal congenital heart disease. Br Heart J 52:542, 1984.
8. Silverman NH, Golbus MS: Echocardiographic techniques for assessing normal and abnormal fetal cardiac anatomy. J Am Coll Cardiol (suppl) 5:20S, 1985.
9. Fermont L, deGeeter B, Aubry MC, et al: A close collaboration between obstetricians and pediatric cardiologists allows antenatal detection of severe cardiac malformations by two-dimensional echocardiography. In Doyle EF, Engle MA, Gersony WM, et al (eds): Pediatric Cardiology, Proceedings of the Second World Congress. New York, Springer, 1986, pp 34–37.
10. Allan LD, Crawford DC, Anderson RH, Tynan M: Spectrum of congenital heart disease detected echocardiographically in prenatal life. Br Heart J 54:523, 1985.
11. Sandor GGS, Farquarson D, Wittmann B, et al: Fetal echocardiography: Results in high-risk patients. Obstet Gynecol 67:358, 1986.
12. Kleinman CS, Donnerstein RL, Jaffe CC, et al: Fetal echocardiography. A tool for evaluation of in utero cardiac arrhythmias and monitoring of in utero therapy: Analysis of 71 patients. Am J Cardiol 51:237, 1983.
13. Allan LD, Anderson RH, Sullivan ID, et al: Evaluation of fetal arrhythmias by echocardiography. Br Heart J 50:240, 1983.
14. DeVore GR, Siassi B, Platt LD: Fetal echocardiography. III. The diagnosis of cardiac arrhythmias using real-time-directed M-mode ultrasound. Am J Obstet Gynecol 146:792, 1983.
15. Silverman NH, Enderlein MA, Stanger P, et al: Recognition of fetal arrhythmias by echocardiography. J Clin Ultrasound 13:255, 1985.
16. Strasburger JF, Huhta JC, Carpenter RJ, et al: Doppler echocardiography in the diagnosis and management of persistent fetal arrhythmias. J Am Coll Cardiol 7:1386, 1986.
17. Steinfeld L, Rappaport HL, Rossbach HC, Martinez E: Diagnosis of fetal arrhythmias using echocardiographic and Doppler techniques. J Am Coll Cardiol 8:1425, 1986.
18. Kleinman CS, Donnerstein RL, DeVore GR, et al: Fetal echocardiography for evaluation of in utero congestive heart failure. N Engl J Med 306:568, 1982.
19. Wiggins JW, Bowes W, Clewell W, et al: Echocardiographic diagnosis and intravenous digoxin management of fetal tachyarrhythmias and congestive heart failure. Am J Dis Child 140:202, 1986.
20. Simpson PC, Trudinger BJ, Walker A, Baird PJ: The intrauterine treatment of fetal cardiac failure in a twin pregnancy with an acardiac, acephalic monster. Am J Obstet Gynecol 147:842, 1983.
21. Turley K, Vlahakes GJ, Harrison MR, et al: Intrauterine cardiothoracic surgery: The fetal lamb model. Ann Thorac Surg 34:422, 1982.
22. Slate RK, Stevens MB, Verrier ED, et al: Intrauterine repair of pulmonary stenosis in fetal sheep. Surg Forum 36:246, 1985.
23. Zierler S: Maternal drugs and congenital heart disease. Obstet Gynecol 65:155, 1985.
24. Allan LD, Crawford DC, Chita SK, et al: Familial recurrence of congenital heart disease in a prospective series of mothers referred for fetal echocardiography. Am J Cardiol 58:334, 1986.
25. Whittemore R, Hobbins JC, Engle MA: Pregnancy and its outcome in women with and without surgical treatment of congenital heart disease. Am J Cardiol 50:641, 1982.

26. Nora JJ, Nora AH: Maternal transmission of congenital heart diseases: New recurrence risk figures and the questions of cytoplasmic inheritance and vulnerability to teratogens. Am J Cardiol 59:459, 1987.

27. McCue CM, Mantakas ME, Tingelstad JB, Ruddy S: Congenital heart block in newborns of mothers with connective tissue disease. Circulation 56:82, 1977.

28. Scott JS, Maddison PJ, Taylor PV, et al: Connective-tissue disease, antibodies to ribonucleoprotein, and congenital heart block. N Engl J Med 309:209, 1983.

29. Allan LD, Joseph MC, Boyd EGC, et al: M-Mode echocardiography in the developing human fetus. Br Heart J 47:573, 1982.

30. St John Sutton MG, Gewitz MH, Shah B, et al: Quantitative assessment of growth and function of the cardiac chambers in the normal human fetus: A prospective longitudinal echocardiographic study. Circulation 69:645, 1984.

31. DeVore GR, Siassi B, Platt LD: Fetal echocardiography. IV. M-mode assessment of ventricular size and contractility during the second and third trimesters of pregnancy in the normal fetus. Am J Obstet Gynecol 150:981, 1984.

32. Anderson RH, Becker AE, Freedom RM, et al: Sequential segmental analysis of congenital heart disease. Pediatr Cardiol 5:281, 1984.

33. Silverman NH, de Araujo LML: An echocardiographic method for the diagnosis of cardiac situs and malpositions. Echocardiography 4:35, 1987.

34. De Araujo LML, Silverman NH, Filly RA, et al: Prenatal detection of left atrial isomerism by ultrasound. J Ultrasound Med, 6:667, 1987.

35. Stewart PA, Tonge HM, Wladimiroff JW: Arrhythmia and structural abnormalities of the fetal heart. Br Heart J 50:550, 1983.

36. Kleinman CS, Donnerstein RL: Ultrasonic assessment of cardiac function in the intact human fetus. J Am Coll Cardiol (suppl) 5:84S, 1985.

37. Birnbaum SE, McGahan JP, Janos GG, Meyers M: Fetal tachycardia and intramyocardial tumors. J Am Coll Cardiol 6:1358, 1985.

38. Reed KL, Meijboom EJ, Sahn DJ, et al: Cardiac Doppler flow velocities in human fetuses. Circulation 73:41, 1986.

39. Huhta JC, Strasburger JF, Carpenter RJ, et al: Pulsed Doppler fetal echocardiography. J Clin Ultrasound 13:247, 1985.

40. Reed KL, Sahn DJ, Scagnelli S, et al: Doppler echocardiographic studies of diastolic function in the human fetal heart: Changes during gestation. J Am Coll Cardiol 8:391, 1986.

41. Maulik D, Nanda NC, Saini VD: Fetal Doppler echocardiography: Methods and characterization of normal and abnormal hemodynamics. Am J Cardiol 53:572, 1984.

42. Huhta JC, Moise KJ, Fisher DJ, et al: Detection and quantitation of constriction of the fetal ductus arteriosus by Doppler echocardiography. Circulation 75:406, 1987.

43. Hatle L, Brubakk A, Tromsdal A, Angelsen B: Noninvasive assessment of pressure drop in mitral stenosis by Doppler ultrasound. Br Heart J 40:131, 1978.

44. Hatle L, Angelsen BA, Tromsdal A: Non-invasive assessment of aortic stenosis by Doppler ultrasound. Br Heart J 43:284, 1980.

45. Stuart B, Drumm J, FitzGerald DE, Duignan NM: Fetal blood velocity waveforms in normal pregnancy. Br J Obstet Gynaecol 87:780, 1980.

46. Schulman H, Fleischer A, Stern W, et al: Umbilical velocity wave ratios in human pregnancy. Am J Obstet Gynecol 148:985, 1984.

47. Trudinger BJ, Giles WB, Cook CM, et al: Fetal umbilical artery flow velocity waveforms and placental resistance: Clinical significance. Br J Obstet Gynaecol 92:23, 1985.

48. Silverman NH, Kleinman CS, Rudolph AM, et al: Fetal atrioventricular valve insufficiency associated with nonimmune hydrops: A two-dimensional echocardiographic and pulsed Doppler ultrasound study. Circulation 72:825, 1985.

49. Weinstein MR, Goldfield MD: Cardiovascular malformations with lithium use during pregnancy. Am J Psychiatry 132:529, 1975.

50. Huhta JC, Strasburger JF, Carpenter RJ, Reiter A: Fetal echocardiography: Accuracy and limitations in the diagnosis of cardiac disease. (Abstr.) J Am Coll Cardiol 5:387, 1985.

51. Allan LD, Crawford DC, Tynan MJ: Pulmonary atresia in prenatal life. J Am Coll Cardiol 8:1131, 1986.

52. Kleinman CS, Copel JA, Weinstein EM, et al: Treatment of fetal supraventricular tachyarrhythmias. J Clin Ultrasound 13:265, 1985.

53. Dumesic DA, Silverman NH, Tobias S, Golbus MS: Transplacental cardioversion of fetal supraventricular tachycardia with procainamide. N Engl J Med 307:1128, 1982.

54. Arnoux P, Seyral P, Llurens M, et al: Amiodarone and digoxin for refractory fetal tachycardia. Am J Cardiol 59:166, 1987.

55. Taylor PV, Scott JS, Gerlis LM, et al: Maternal antibodies against fetal cardiac antigens in congenital complete heart block. N Engl J Med 315:667, 1986.

56. Carpenter RJ, Strasburger JF, Garson A, et al: Fetal ventricular pacing for hydrops secondary to complete atrioventricular block. J Am Coll Cardiol 8:1434, 1986.

57. Scott DJ, Rigby ML, Miller GAH, Shinebourne EA: The presentation of symptomatic heart disease in infancy based on 10 years' experience (1973–82). Br Heart J 52:248, 1984.

58. Fyler DC, Buckley JP, Hellenbrand WE, et al: Report of the New England Regional Infant Cardiac Program. Pediatrics (suppl) 65:375, 1980.

59. Copel JA, Pilu G, Kleinman CS: Congenital heart disease and extracardiac anomalies: Associations and indications for fetal echocardiography. Am J Obstet Gynecol 154:1121, 1986.

60. Nora JJ, Nora AH: The evolution of specific genetic and environmental counseling in congenital heart diseases. Circulation 57:205, 1978.

61. Sanders SP, Chin AJ, Parness IA, et al: Prenatal diagnosis of congenital heart defects in thoracoabdominally conjoined twins. N Engl J Med 313:370, 1985.

62. Huhta JC, Carpenter RJ, Moise KJ, et al: Prenatal diagnosis and postnatal management of critical aortic stenosis. Circulation 75:573, 1987.

63. Lowe TW, Weinreb J, Santos-Ramos R, Cunningham FG: Magnetic resonance imaging in human pregnancy. Obstet Gynecol 66:629, 1985.

64. Redel DA, Hansmann M: Prenatal diagnosis and

treatment of heart disease. *In* Dellenbach P (ed): 1. Symposium International d'Echocardiologie Foetale. Strasbourg, Milupa Dietetique, 1982, pp 127–134.

65. Hansmann M, Redel DA: Prenatal symptoms and clinical management of heart disease. *In* Dellenbach P (ed): 1. Symposium International d'Echocardiologie Foetale. Strasbourg, Milupa Dietetique, 1982, pp 137–149.

66. Allan LD, Crawford DC, Tynan M: Evolution of coarctation of the aorta in intrauterine life. Br Heart J 52:471, 1984.

67. Spinnato JA, Shaver DC, Flinn GS, et al: Fetal supraventricular tachycardia: In utero therapy with digoxin and quinidine. Obstet Gynecol 64:730, 1984.

ULTRASOUND EVALUATION OF THE FETAL THORAX AND ABDOMEN

Ruth B. Goldstein, M.D.
Peter W. Callen, M.D.

With the advent of high-resolution real-time sonography, there has been a dramatic improvement in the ability both to diagnose congenital anomalies prenatally and to confirm the presence of normal fetal morphology prenatally. Along with anomalies of the central nervous and skeletal systems, anomalies of the thorax and abdomen constitute a major group of fetal abnormalities currently detectable with prenatal sonography. While many of these anomalies can be diagnosed by direct visualization of the abnormal morphologic features (i.e., in gastroschisis, loops of bowel floating freely in amniotic fluid), in some cases, suspicion of an abnormality will first be raised merely by the abnormal relationships of chest or abdominal structures (i.e., in congenital diaphragmatic hernia, fluid-filled ectopic stomach in the chest).

THE FETAL THORAX

The Normal Chest

By the second and third trimesters of pregnancy, the pleural, pericardial, and perito-neal cavities are morphologically distinct,[1] and the contents of these spaces, as well as their relationships, can be studied during real-time sonography. During routine survey of the fetal chest, coronal, axial, and sagittal views may be useful in confirming the normal intrathoracic relationships. The position of the fetus is usually flexed, and transverse scanning through the fetal chest may require stepwise correction in the transducer's angulation relative to the skin surface. Despite this technical difficulty, it is still helpful to begin the fetal thoracic examination by scanning transversely through the fetal thorax at right angles to the fetal spine, from the pulmonary apices down to the diaphragm. At the level of the pulmonary apices, the clavicles are a distinguishing landmark, just as the diaphragm is a caudal one (Fig. 9–1). The fetal diaphragm appears as a smooth hypoechoic muscular margin between the fetal lungs and the liver or spleen (Fig. 9–2). Using routine transverse scanning of the chest in this way, much useful information can be quickly obtained regarding chest shape, size, and symmetry; cardiac size and morphology; and pulmonary echotexture. With coronal or parasagittal imaging, the

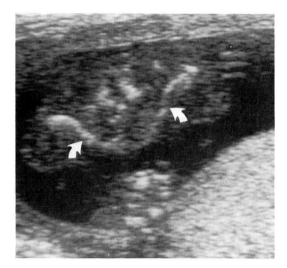

Figure 9–1. The clavicles *(arrows)* are sufficiently mineralized to provide a reliable anatomic marker in the fetus.

Figure 9–2. The fetal diaphragm *(arrows)* is a smooth, hypoechoic band of tissue separating the thoracic and abdominal cavities. C, heart.

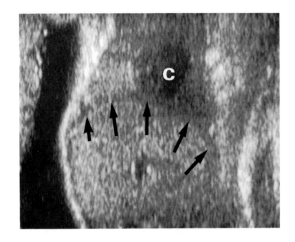

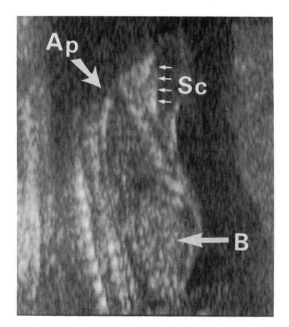

Figure 9–3. Parasagittal image. The polarity of the bell-shaped thorax is helpful in determining the fetal lie. Ap, thoracic apex; Sc, scapula; B, collapsed bowel.

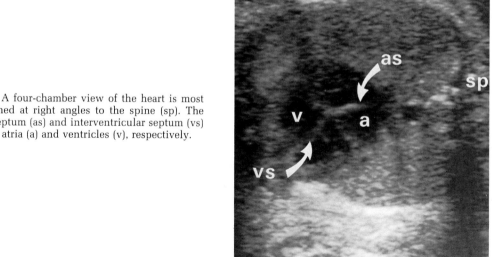

Figure 9–4. A four-chamber view of the heart is most easily obtained at right angles to the spine (sp). The interatrial septum (as) and interventricular septum (vs) separate the atria (a) and ventricles (v), respectively.

typical bell shape of the thorax becomes apparent, the apex of which is helpful in determining the fetal presentation (Fig. 9–3).

The mediastinum is centrally positioned in the chest, and the majority of the cardiac volume positioned to the left of the midline (Fig. 9–4). A simple four-chamber view of the heart (visualized in all fetuses in the second and third trimesters) should be a part of routine obstetric scanning and is most easily obtained with a transverse scanning plane through the lower fetal thorax, at right angles to the spine (Fig. 9–4). The ventricular chambers are assessed for symmetry and to exclude the rare occurrence of a cardiac mass, e.g., rhabdomyoma in tuberous sclerosis (Fig. 9–5). The right and left ventricles are most easily distinguished by virtue of their position in the anteroposterior plane

in the chest; the most anterior ventricular chamber is the right ventricle, and the most posterior ventricular chamber, the left ventricle. The superior and inferior venae cavae are seen as anechoic tubular structures that may be followed to their confluence in the right atrium. Blood flow from the right to the left atrium results in regular opening and closing of the foramen ovale, which may occasionally be seen during real-time scanning. Using currently available high-resolution equipment, some investigators believe that a small amount of pericardial fluid in some fetuses is a normal finding.[2, 3] Mediastinal structures, such as the aortic arch, ductus arteriosus, and great vessels, can be visualized with regularity (Fig. 9–6). With effort, even small structures, such as the fetal trachea, esophagus, and thyroid gland, may currently be reported with sonography.[5]

Figure 9–5. Fetus at risk for tuberous sclerosis. *A*, Oblique scan through the fetal chest and heart (c). An echogenic cardiac mass (m) is a rhabdomyoma. *B*, Oblique coronal image through the abdomen and chest of the same fetus. The echogenic cardiac rhabdomyoma (m) extends to the diaphragmatic surface of the heart. The hypoechoic diaphragm (d) and liver (L) are indicated by *arrows*.

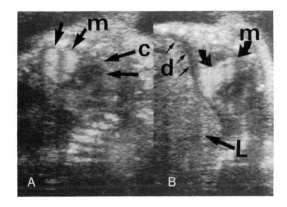

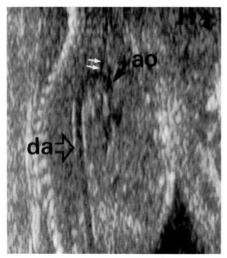

Figure 9–6. Aortic arch. The ascending aorta (ao) and descending aorta (da) are readily visualized. The origin of the great vessels is marked by *small arrows*. H, fetal head.

More cephalad, the oropharynx, tongue, and mandible (with tooth buds) are often distinguished (Fig. 9–7).

The Lung

The fetal lungs appear homogeneous and of moderate echogenicity. Early in gestation, the pulmonary parenchyma appears similar to or slightly less echogenic than the liver, and as gestation progresses, there is a trend toward increased pulmonary echogenicity relative to the liver. Although some have attempted to reliably correlate increasing pulmonary echogenicity, coarsening of the lung echotexture, and increasing through-sound transmission with pulmonary maturity, these attempts have largely been unsuccessful.[6, 7] Some have even suggested pulmonary maturity might be assessed through visual cues, i.e., pulmonary "squishiness," suggesting developing lung compliance.[8] Despite the work of many qualified investigators, at this time amniocentesis, accompanied by the analysis of lecithin/sphingomyelin ratios and phosphotidylglycerol, remains the most reliable method for the important determination of fetal lung maturity (see Chap. 14).

Pulmonary hypoplasia is most closely correlated with and inversely related to gestational age. In the presence of oligohydramnios, however, the degree to which the fetal lungs are underdeveloped or hypoplastic may be more severe than predicted by gestational age. Although sonographic features ("small" lungs, echogenic lungs, and similar findings) in the fetal chest alone cannot accurately predict pulmonary function, a correlation between pulmonary hypoplasia and a small chest circumference has been noted.[9, 10] This notion is supported by nomograms constructed for normal chest and heart circumferences that demonstrate that these measures increase linearly during gestation between 24 gestational weeks and term (Fig. 9–8).[9, 11] Interestingly, Chitkara and associates, in a study of normal fetuses, found the ratio of chest to abdomen circumference to be virtually constant throughout gestation after 16 weeks.[11] The chest and

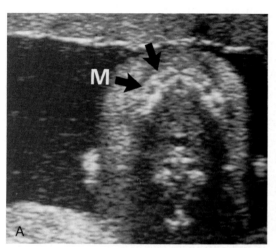

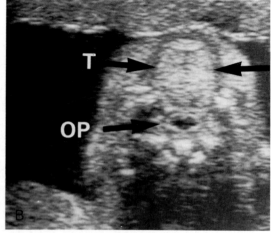

Figure 9–7. *A,* Transverse axial view of the fetal mandible (M), in mid-pregnancy. Hypoechoic toothbuds may be seen. *B,* The same fetus cephalad to the image in *A.* The tongue (T) and oropharynx (OP) are indicated by *arrows.*

Gestational age (wk)	No.	Predictive percentiles								
		2.5	5	10	25	50	75	90	95	97.5
16	6	5.9	6.4	7.0	8.0	9.1	10.3	11.3	11.9	12.4
17	22	6.8	7.3	7.9	8.9	10.0	11.2	12.2	12.8	13.3
18	31	7.7	8.2	8.8	9.8	11.0	12.1	13.1	13.7	14.2
19	21	8.6	9.1	9.7	10.7	11.9	13.0	14.0	14.6	15.1
20	20	9.5	10.0	10.6	11.7	12.8	13.9	15.0	15.5	16.0
21	30	10.4	11.0	11.6	12.6	13.7	14.8	15.8	16.4	16.9
22	18	11.3	11.9	12.5	13.5	14.6	15.7	16.7	17.3	17.8
23	21	12.2	12.8	13.4	14.4	15.5	16.6	17.6	18.2	18.8
24	27	13.2	13.7	14.3	15.3	16.4	17.5	18.5	19.1	19.7
25	20	14.1	14.6	15.2	16.2	17.3	18.4	19.4	20.0	20.6
26	25	15.0	15.5	16.1	17.1	18.2	19.3	20.3	21.0	21.5
27	24	15.9	16.4	17.0	18.0	19.1	20.2	21.3	21.9	22.4
28	24	16.8	17.3	17.9	18.9	20.0	21.2	22.2	22.8	23.3
29	24	17.7	18.2	18.8	19.8	21.0	22.1	23.1	23.7	24.2
30	27	18.6	19.1	19.7	20.7	21.9	23.0	24.0	24.6	25.1
31	24	19.5	20.0	20.6	21.6	22.8	23.9	24.9	25.5	26.0
32	28	20.4	20.9	21.5	22.6	23.7	24.8	25.8	26.4	26.9
33	27	21.3	21.8	22.5	23.5	24.6	25.7	26.7	27.3	27.8
34	25	22.2	22.8	23.4	24.4	25.5	26.6	27.6	28.2	28.7
35	20	23.1	23.7	24.3	25.3	26.4	27.5	28.5	29.1	29.6
36	23	24.0	24.6	25.2	26.2	27.3	28.4	29.4	30.0	30.6
37	22	24.9	25.5	26.1	27.1	28.2	29.3	30.3	30.9	31.5
38	21	25.9	26.4	27.0	28.0	29.1	30.2	31.2	31.9	32.4
39	7	26.8	27.3	27.9	28.9	30.0	31.1	32.2	32.8	33.3
40	6	27.7	28.2	28.8	29.8	30.9	32.1	33.1	33.7	34.2

*Measurements in centimeters.

Figure 9–8. Fetal thoracic circumference measurements. (*From:* Chitkara U, Rosenberg J, Chervenak FA, et al: Prenatal sonographic assessment of the fetal thorax: Normal values. Am J Obstet Gynecol 156:1069, 1987.)

cardiac circumference may be measured on cross-sectional views of the fetal thorax, obtained at right angles to the fetal spine at the level of the atrioventricular valves in diastole. In their study, Nimrod and coworkers found a small chest circumference to be suggestive of pulmonary hypoplasia. When the fetal chest is evaluated in this way, however, false-negative diagnoses for pulmonary hypoplasia arise when space-occupying pulmonary masses or pleural effusions are present.[12] Under these circumstances, the chest circumference may be normal or enlarged despite the presence of severe pulmonary hypoplasia; thus, the chest circumference is unreliable in predicting pulmonary hypoplasia.

Unlike small effusions that may occur in the pericardial space of normal fetuses, fluid accumulations in the pleural space are not seen in normal fetuses, and thus fetal pleural fluid should always be interpreted as abnormal.

Intrathoracic Abnormalities

Chest masses in the fetus may appear echogenic and solid or cystic and should be considered life threatening. In general, by the time they are large enough to identify sonographically, they exert mass effect, with lung compression and deviation of the mediastinum and heart. The differential diagnosis of a fetal chest mass includes congenital diaphragmatic hernia (CDH), congenital cystic adenomatoid malformation (CCAM), pulmonary sequestration, bronchogenic or neurenteric cyst, congenital lobar emphysema, or bronchial atresia. The sonographic appearance of these entities may be very similar, and thus differentiation may be difficult. As a general rule, however, regardless of the precise identity of a fetal chest mass, poor fetal prognosis is predicted when this abnormality is accompanied by fetal hydrops and maternal polyhydramnios. Although many investigators believe nonimmune fetal hydrops results from the mass effect of these abnormalities (associated with compression of the stomach, heart, and great vessels), this has not been proven. Because each of these entities may be associated with other congenital and chromosomal abnormalities, careful survey of the fetus for other anomalies, as well as chromosomal analysis of the fetus, is warranted when a lesion of this nature is suspected.

Congenital Diaphragmatic Hernia

During embryologic development, the muscular diaphragm forms between the sixth and 14th menstrual weeks as a result of a complicated chain of events involving the fusion of four structures: the septum transversum (future central tendon), pleuroperitoneal membranes, dorsal mesentery of the esophagus (future crura), and body wall. The most posterior aspect of the diaphragm, derived from the body wall, forms last.[1]

A failure of fusion during this period results in a CDH, the most common developmental abnormality of the diaphragm, which occurs in approximately one in 2000 to 5000 live births.[1, 13] The defect is usually unilateral (97 percent), on the left (75 to 90 percent), with the herniated bowel located posteriorly in the chest.[13] The reported incidence of associated morphologic anomalies varies from few to 56 percent, and these include cardiac, renal, central nervous system (CNS), and chromosomal abnormalities.[14, 15]

Patients carrying a fetus with a CDH are often first referred for sonography because the fundus is clinically judged to be too large for the menstrual dates and polyhydramnios is suspected. The definitive sonographic diagnosis of fetal CDH relies on the visualization of abdominal organs in the chest, and the sonographic hallmark of a CDH is a fluid-filled mass just behind the left atrium and ventricle in the lower thorax as seen on a transverse view (Fig. 9–9). Even if a specific viscus is not identified, other sonographic features should raise strong suspicion of a CDH. These include absence of the normally placed stomach (seen in virtually all normal fetuses after 15 weeks),[16] shift of the mediastinum, small fetal abdominal circumference, and polyhydramnios (Fig. 9–10). In the more common left-sided lesion, stomach, small and large bowel, and the left lobe of liver may herniate into the chest. With real-time sonography, peristalsis of the bowel in the fetal chest may even be detected. The detection of liver in the chest may be more difficult.

Occasionally an oblique section through a normal fetal chest may result in an image that may be confused with a CDH. This occurs because infradiaphragmatic structures such as bowel and liver are included

in the same image as the lower thorax (Fig. 9–11). As a general rule, however, no bowel should be identified in the chest on the same image as the four-chamber view of the heart (Fig. 9–4).[17] Thus, whenever this confusion arises, the four-chamber view of the heart, as well as the appropriate parasagittal or coronal views of the chest that include the fetal diaphragm and the infradiaphragmatic abdominal anatomy, should be sought to exclude or confirm the presence of a CDH. Fortunately, whenever a large CDH is present, there is usually sufficient shift of the heart and mediastinum (and possibly a pleural effusion) to confirm the sonographer's suspicion.

The herniation of bowel through the defect may occur as an intermittent event, and thus the size and contents of the hernia may change from one examination to another. This phenomenon may explain why small hernias may not be diagnosed until late in gestation despite the fact that the diaphragmatic defect occurred much earlier.

In *right-sided* hernias, which occur less commonly, the right lobe of the liver alone may herniate. Although this type of hernia may be associated with other suggestive findings, such as hydrothorax and ascites,[18] right-sided lesions may be more difficult to identify owing to the similar echotexture of the liver and lungs. Identification of the

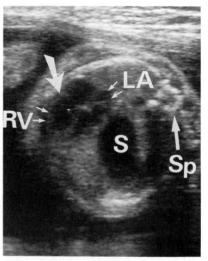

Figure 9–9. Congenital diaphragmatic hernia (CDH). Transverse view of the thorax. The stomach (S) has herniated into the chest, behind the four-chamber heart *(large arrow)*. RV, right ventricle; LA, left atrium, Sp, spine.

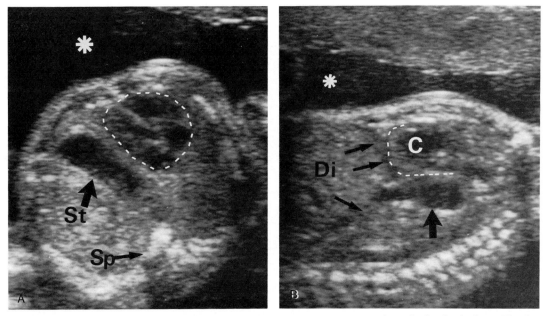

Figure 9–10. Congenital diaphragmatic hernia (CDH). *A*, Transverse image through the fetal chest. The heart *(dashed circumference)* has been displaced to the right by a fluid-filled stomach (St) behind the left heart. Sp, spine. *B*, Sagittal image demonstrating the herniated stomach *(large arrow)* through the diaphragm (Di), behind the heart *(dashed line)*. Also note the presence of polyhydramnios *(asterisk)*.

gallbladder in the chest may be a useful ancillary finding confirming the diagnosis in these cases.

The mortality associated with CDH is extremely high (50 to 80 percent).[14, 19] Polyhydramnios, which is commonly associated with this defect, is an especially poor prognostic indicator. In one reported series, the survival of those infants with CDH and associated polyhydramnios was 11 percent,

compared with a survival rate of 55 percent in the group without polyhydramnios.[19] The chief cause of perinatal mortality in these infants is pulmonary insufficiency secondary to pulmonary hypoplasia (both ipsilateral and contralateral to the side of the hernia) or persistent fetal circulation.[19, 20] Both pulmonary hypoplasia and persistent fetal circulation are presumed to result from persistent and severe lung compression in

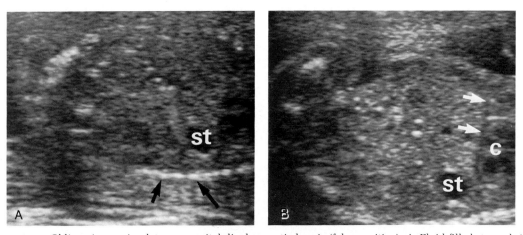

Figure 9–11. Oblique image simulates congenital diaphragmatic hernia (false positive). *A*, Fluid-filled stomach (st) is imaged in an area surrounded by ribs *(arrows)*, simulating the location of the stomach in the fetal thorax. *B*, A more direct coronal image demonstates normal relationships: intact hypoechoic diaphragm *(arrows)*, stomach (st) below the diaphragm, and heart (c) in the fetal thorax.

intrauterine life. Despite the most valiant efforts at surgical correction postnatally, prognosis appears to be most closely related to the volume of herniated bowel contents and the timing of the herniation. Thus larger hernias and those that occur earliest in gestation carry the worst prognoses.[17, 19] Unfortunately, the degree of pulmonary hypoplasia currently cannot be established by the antepartum sonographic appearance of lung volume or compression.

Sonographically, CDH may be confused with other intrathoracic fetal abnormalities, such as CCAM, bronchogenic cysts, or extralobar sequestration. However, normal upper fetal abdominal anatomy would be expected in the other lesions.

Congenital Cystic Adenomatoid Malformation

Congenital cystic adenomatoid malformation is a rare pulmonary lesion that can be diagnosed by ultrasound antenatally.[21–27] Like CDH, it may be associated with fetal hydrops, maternal polyhydramnios, and pulmonary hypoplasia. The prenatal diagnosis can be helpful in planning both the site of delivery and the immediate postnatal care and in counseling the parents about the outcome.

Congenital cystic adenomatoid malformation is a hamartomatous pulmonary lesion.[28–31] It is typically unilateral and usually involves one lobe or segment. Stocker and associates described the pathologic appearance of lesions as macrocystic, medium-sized cystic, and solid.[28] Some forms, particularly the medium-sized cystic lesions, have been associated with chromosomal and other congenital anomalies. Therefore, chromosomal analysis as well as careful fetal survey should always be performed when this lesion is suspected. Relatively few cases have been described antenatally. The sonographic appearance has ranged from a multicystic mass to a solid pulmonary lesion with mass effect and mediastinal shift (Figs. 9–12, 9–13). The antenatal sonographic findings and outcome were described in 12 cases by Adzick and colleagues.[22] Among these cases, two general categories of lesions emerged: those that appeared microcystic and those that appeared macrocystic on sonography. The distinction between these groups, although somewhat different from the pathologic descriptions, seemed to be useful in separating those fetuses who had poor outcomes (those with solid-appearing lesions and hydrops) from those who did well (those with macrocystic lesions and no hydrops). The lesions that appeared sonographically solid were histologically found to contain many small cysts, and were thought to appear solid secondary to the numerous reflections from interfaces of the myriad tiny cysts (similar to infantile polycystic kidney disease). As with all space-occupying chest lesions, the prognosis of a fetus with CCAM appears to be adversely affected by fetal hydrops, polyhydramnios, a solid-appearing or microcystic lesion, and lesions of large volume.[22] Although associ-

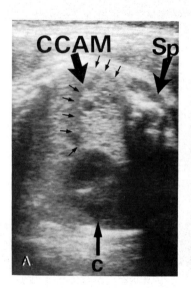
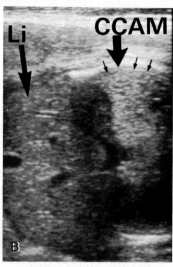

Figure 9–12. Congenital cyst adenomatoid malformation (CCAM). *A, B,* Echogenic mass lesion with scattered cysts in the right fetal chest (CCAM), with displacement of the heart (c) to the left. Sp, spine; Li, liver.

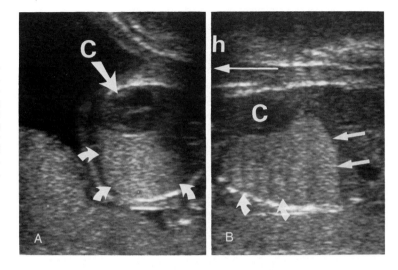

Figure 9–13. Congenital cyst adenomatoid malformation (CCAM). A, Transverse image demonstrating homogeneous, solid-appearing pulmonary lesion *(curved arrows)* displacing the heart (C) to the right. B, Oblique coronal view demonstrating mass effect of CCAM *(curved arrows)*, with bowing of the diaphragm *(straight arrows)*. C, heart; h, head.

ated fetal hydrops carries a poor prognosis in these fetuses, it is interesting to note that the majority of patients with isolated CCAM who survive after delivery will be asymptomatic during the neonatal period. In these cases, the lesions are amenable to surgical correction, and the infant stands a good chance of survival.[30]

Pulmonary Sequestration

While the exact etiology of these abnormalities is unknown, pulmonary sequestrations probably represent bronchopulmonary foregut abnormalities.[31] The lesions have been divided into extralobar and intralobar forms, and the former (the one most commonly found in infants and neonates) is the only form that has been described antenatally.[26, 32–34] The extralobar lesion consists of a mass of ectopic pulmonary tissue that is enveloped by its own pleura outside of the normal visceral pleura. This tissue does not communicate with the tracheobronchial tree and receives its arterial supply ectopically from the thoracic aorta, and its venous drainage is to systemic (inferior vena cava, azygous, or portal veins) rather than pulmonary veins.[35, 36] Sequestrations occur most commonly on the left (90 percent) in the posterior and basal segments. The extralobar form is associated with other anomalies, including foregut abnormalities and CDH (an associated finding in 30 percent of the cases).[31, 37]

Sonographically, a pulmonary sequestration appears as an echogenic mass in the fetal thorax.[26, 32–34] Like CCAM and CDH, they too have been associated with fetal hydrops and maternal polyhydramnios that is presumed to be secondary to mass effect and compression of the fetal esophagus or mediastinum and heart. Although these lesions may be similar to CDH, they may be distinguished from it by virtue of the normal intra-abdominal anatomy associated with pulmonary sequestration.

Bronchogenic cysts are uncommon congenital anomalies that result from an abnormal development in the budding or branching of the tracheobronchial tree, probably between the 26th and 40th day of fetal life, when the most active tracheobronchial development is occurring.[38] They also represent foregut abnormalities and result from abnormal budding of the ventral diverticulum of the foregut.[31, 38] Recall that the respiratory tract and the esophagus are derived from the primitive foregut: the esophagus from the posterior aspect and the tracheobronchial tree from the anterior aspect. Therefore, posterior mediastinal neurenteric cysts occur as an anomaly of the posterior (dorsal) aspect of the foregut and notochord and, as expected, are associated with spinal anomalies. Abnormal development in the *middle* of the foregut is felt to result in esophageal duplications, and abnormal budding of the anterior diverticulum of the foregut results in bronchial cysts, most of which occur in the mediastinum, with a minority occurring in the pulmonary parenchyma.[31] Bronchogenic cysts are not usually associated with other congenital anomalies.[31, 39] They may enlarge in infancy and

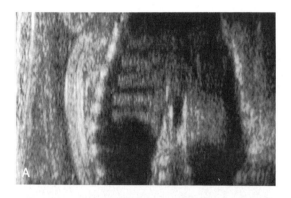

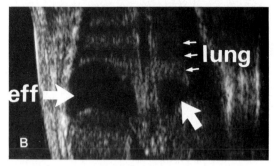

Figure 9–14. Fetal pleural effusions *(eff)*. *A, B,* The fluid may conform to the normal chest contour, with slight compression of the lung parenchyma. This appearance is not reliable for predicting future pulmonary function.

cause respiratory distress. Very few cases have been detected antenatally, but those that have have appeared as unilocular or multilocular cystic masses in the fetal chest.[26]

Congenital bronchial atresia is another unusual pulmonary anomaly that rarely has been described on antenatal sonography as an echogenic pulmonary mass lesion.[40] The cause is unknown, but the *focal* obliteration of a segment of the bronchial lumen results and occurs most commonly in the left upper lobe. Other relatively common sites are the right upper middle lobes. This lesion rarely occurs in the lower lobe,[31] and in this way might be distinguished from extralobar pulmonary sequestration or CDH.

Pleural Effusion

Fluid in the pleural space of the fetus is abnormal at any gestational age. Pleural effusions may occur in the fetus as an isolated abnormality or in association with more se-

rious conditions, such as immune or nonimmune hydrops or posterior urethral valves associated with urinary ascites. In cases of nonimmune hydrops fetalis (NIHF), prognosis is usually poor,[41–43] and these serous effusions represent only a single manifestation of a more serious underlying dysfunction (cardiac anomaly, lymphangiectasia, intrauterine infection, Turner's syndrome, chromosomal anomaly, and similar defects). In the case of immune hydrops fetalis, current therapy is directed toward intrauterine transfusion or prompt delivery, depending on the gestational age.[44]

Sonographically, pleural effusions appear as anechoic fluid collections in the fetal chest that usually conform to the normal chest and diaphragmatic contour (Fig. 9–14) but, when large enough, may be associated with bulging of the chest and flattening or inversion of the diaphragm (Figs. 9–15, 9–16).[43] An isolated fetal pleural effusion (hydrothorax), without other associated anomalies, may be chylous in nature. Although chylous effusions in the feeding infant or adult typically appear whitish and have been described as "milky," chylous effusions in the fetus do not contain chylomicrons, are not "milky" in appearance (the fetus is "fasting"), and are indistinguishable sonographically from the serous effusions of

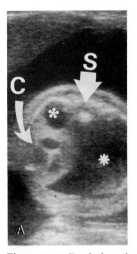

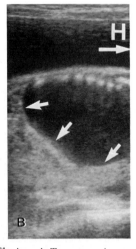

Figure 9–15. Fetal pleural effusion. *A,* Transverse image of the fetal thorax. Largely unilateral effusion *(asterisk).* The heart (C) is shifted. S, spine. *B,* The diaphragm was bowed by the mass effect of this large fetal effusion *(arrows).* This effusion was drained and redrained following catheter failure in utero at 30 and 32 menstrual weeks. The fetus was born approximately two weeks later and did not require ventilatory assistance. H, head.

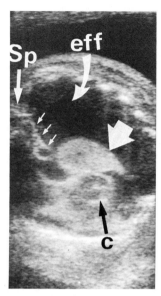

Figure 9–16. Fetal pleural effusion. Transverse image of the fetal thorax demonstrates bowing of the mediastinum. Sp, spine; eff, effusions; c, heart; *large arrow,* lung.

hydrops fetalis. Aspiration of the fluid, which appears "golden" or "straw-colored" prenatally, for analysis or the development of a "milky" color in the fluid postpartum after the infant has begun feeding[45–49] is the only way to confirm the chylous origin. Sonographic features suggestive of fetal chylothorax include the following: (1) the pleural effusion occurs as an isolated finding; (2) the size of the effusion is disproportionately large compared with other findings and other effusions; and (3) the effusion occurs first as an isolated finding and is later followed by the development of other features associated with hydrops fetalis, such as ascites and integumentary edema.

Interestingly, chylothorax is the most frequent cause of isolated pleural effusion leading to respiratory distress in the newborn.[46, 47] The importance of this diagnosis is underscored by the fact that respiratory distress of the newborn associated with pleural effusions carries a 15 to 25 percent mortality rate.[48, 49] The etiology is unknown.[46–50] It is more common in males and is usually unilateral, although a small fraction will be bilateral.[47] Prenatal sonographic findings have been reported in a limited number of cases.[45, 59, 51] In the most severe cases, these effusions have been associated with mediastinal shift, fetal hydrops, and maternal po-

lyhydramnios.[44, 48] In some cases, drainage of large effusions in utero have been performed in an attempt either to relieve mediastinal shift thought to be the cause of hydrops or to allow for better lung expansion and growth in utero.[45, 48] In some instances, in utero thoracentesis has been performed just before delivery for the purposes of improving ventilation in the immediate postpartum period.[51] Postnatally, these effusions are treated with chest tube drainage for days to weeks, and in a series of cases diagnosed at birth, the condition eventually resolved with normal outcome in almost all.[46, 50]

Cystic Hygromas

Cystic hygromas (CH) are multiseptate cystic masses that are often bilateral and located posterolaterally along the neck, occasionally extending into the upper thorax. The incidence is said to be one in 6000 pregnancies.[52, 53] They are felt to represent dilated obstructed jugular lymph sacs, and thus CH is considered under the general category of lymphangiomas.[54, 55] Although pediatricians may be asked to evaluate children with cystic hygromas, the sonographer often detects this condition in utero in association with generalized lymphedema, an invariably lethal condition. The likely explanation for this dichotomy is that if the lymph sacs and their draining veins connect and drain in utero, the edema may resolve before birth.[54] In some of these cases, webbing of the neck may result.

Cystic hygromas most commonly occur in association with Turner's syndrome. They may also be seen in otherwise normal healthy individuals and fetuses with Noonan's syndrome, fetal alcohol syndrome, familial pterygium coli, and the trisomy syndromes.[54–56] Focal cystic hygromas or lymphangiomas occasionally occur in locations other than the nuchal area. This subset of lesions may not be associated with other anomalies or chromosomal abnormalities.[57]

The differential diagnosis of a cystic neck mass would include encephalocele (bony defect often associated with ventricular dilatation), branchial cleft cyst (usually anterolateral), thyroglossal duct cyst (midline), and teratoma (solid elements). On ultrasound, a thick midline septation that separates the cystic masses is often seen in pa-

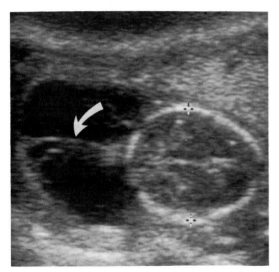

Figure 9–17. Cystic hygroma. A thick midline septation *(arrow)* is characteristic.

tients with cystic hygroma (Fig. 9–17). This probably represents the nuchal ligament; the remaining septations are likely due to fluid dissecting in the connective tissue.

THE FETAL ABDOMEN

By the second trimester, most of the fetal abdominal organs are large enough to have attained their normal adult position and structure. Viscera, including the liver, gall-bladder, spleen, stomach, and kidneys, may be easily identified using ultrasound. The fetal abdomen, however, differs from that of the adult in several ways:

1. The umbilical arteries and veins are patent and provide important anatomic landmarks for fetal abdominal anatomy and measurements.

2. The ductus venosus is patent and, unlike in the adult liver, may be visualized sonographically in that of the fetus as the conduit between portal veins and systemic veins.

3. The proportions of the fetal body differ from those of the adult in that the relative size of the abdomen compared with body length is larger in the fetus and the liver occupies a larger volume relative to the abdomen.[58]

4. The fetal pelvic cavity is small, and thus structures, such as the urinary bladder, ovaries, and uterus, that lie within the pelvis

in the adult tend to lie almost completely in the abdominal cavity in the fetus. Thus the filled bladder in the fetus is not confined to the pelvis, and ovarian cysts, for example, may be visualized in the fetal abdominal cavity or flanks.

5. The apron of the greater omentum is relatively small, contains relatively little fat, and remains unfused in the fetus. The incomplete fusion of the omentum may account for the observation that ascitic fluid may accumulate between omental sheets in the fetus, a distinctly unusual finding in the adult (Fig. 9–18).[59]

The Abdomen in the Embryo: The First Trimester

The *yolk sac* is often the first sonographically identified structure within the gestational sac in intrauterine pregnancies. It is connected to the primitive gut by a focal constriction known as the yolk stalk or omphalomesenteric duct. The dorsal part of the yolk sac is incorporated into the primitive gut, and the remaining yolk sac and stalk detach from the developing midgut loop by the end of the eighth menstrual week.[60]

The yolk sac becomes visible on transabdominal sonography by five to six menstrual weeks (when it is presumed to still be attached to the midgut) as a tiny anechoic round structure with an echogenic rim

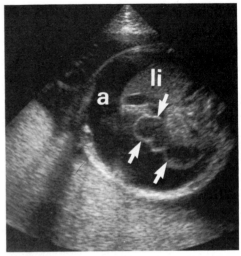

Figure 9–18. Fetal ascites. Fluid has accumulated between the unfused omental sheets *(arrows)*. a, ascites; li, liver.

("bull's eye") (see Chap. 3). It lies within the chorionic cavity between the amniotic membrane and chorion and is surrounded by fluid. After the eighth menstrual week, the yolk sac gradually involutes but may remain visible on sonograms until approximately 14 to 15 menstrual weeks, at which time the chorioamniotic membranes fuse and obliterate the distinct "chorionic" cavity that houses the yolk sac.[61] On occasion, remnants of the intra-abdominal yolk stalk or omphalomesenteric duct persist and result in a diverticulum near the terminal ileum, the so-called "Meckel's diverticulum" (present in approximately 2 percent of adults).[62] Meckel's diverticulum has not been described on antenatal sonography.

The *allantois* is a small structure in the human fetus, and although it is not identified on antenatal sonography, it gives rise to other anatomic structures, abnormalities of which may be identified on antenatal sonography. The allantois forms as a caudal outpouching of the yolk sac at day 16 (approximately four menstrual weeks).[60] Its function is quite limited in human fetuses, but primitive blood formation occurs in its wall in early embryonic development, and the vessels of the allantois become the umbilical arteries and veins. The extraembryonic portion of the allantois degenerates during the second fetal month. Remnants of this structure result in detectable allantoic cysts that usually occur between umbilical vessels and most commonly in the proximal umbilical cord, near its insertion in the ventral abdominal wall. Sonographically, they appear as thin-walled anechoic structures within the cord and may be quite large (Fig. 9–19). The remaining intraembryonic allantois connects the apex of the fetal bladder to the umbilicus. As the bladder enlarges, the allantois involutes and gives rise to the urachus, a midline structure located between the umbilical arteries. The urachus in turn involutes during fetal development, giving rise to the median umbilical ligament, a fibrous cord of tissue between the bladder apex and umbilicus. Patent areas along this remnant result in urachal cysts or sinuses. Although these nonoccluded segments along the former urachus are commonly found in autopsy specimens, they usually are not clinically discovered unless they become infected in the adult.[63] Patencies of the urachus (urachal sinuses or diverticula) have been described

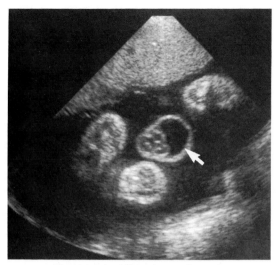

Figure 9–19. Allantoic cyst *(arrow)*.

in fetuses with bladder outlet obstruction and prune-belly syndrome.[64, 65]

The *umbilical cord* forms during the first five weeks of gestation (seven menstrual weeks) as a fusion of the omphalomesenteric (yolk stalk) and allantoic ducts. The umbilical cord acquires its epithelial lining as a result of the enlargement of the amniotic cavity and the resultant enveloping of the amniotic membrane (Fig. 9–20).[60]

The intestines, growing at a faster rate than the abdomen, herniate into the proximal umbilical cord at approximately nine menstrual weeks and remain there until approximately the middle of the 12th menstrual week.[66, 67] This physiologic cord herniation may be visualized as a bulge or thickening of the cord near the fetus on sonography (Fig. 9–21).[68] While in the base of the umbilical cord, the midgut loop grows and rotates 90° on the axis of the superior mesenteric artery. When the loops of bowel return to the fetal abdomen, they rotate another 180° in a counterclockwise direction, completing the normal rotation of the bowel.[66] The site of the cord insertion at the junction with the ventral abdominal wall is an important anatomic landmark in the developing fetus, and this area is routinely investigated to exclude a ventral abdominal wall defect such as gastroschisis or omphalocele (see Chap. 10). To avoid falsely positive diagnoses because of this physiologic umbilical cord herniation (between the ninth and 12th menstrual weeks), it has been

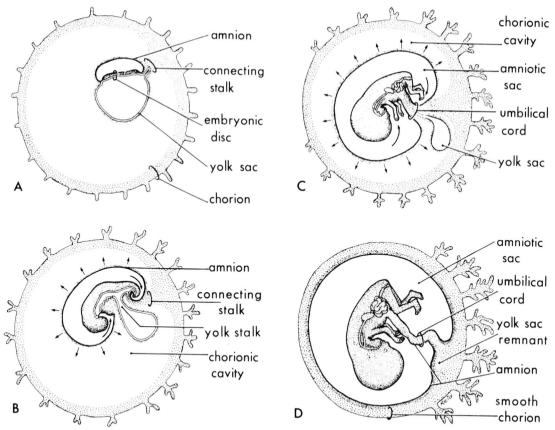

Figure 9–20. Development of the umbilical cord. As the amniotic cavity enlarges, its membrane envelops the cord, forming the epithelial lining of the cord. (*From* Moore, KL: The Developing Human: Clinically Oriented Embryology, 4th Ed. Philadelphia, WB Saunders Co, 1988.)

suggested that the diagnosis of ventral abdominal wall defects should not be made before 14 weeks, after which the normal migration of midgut back into the abdomen

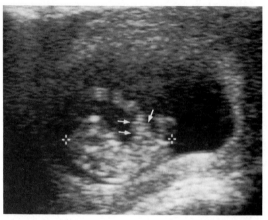

Figure 9–21. Physiologic umbilical hernia. A bulge in the cord at the insertion site (*arrows*) is a normal finding before 13 menstrual weeks. The crown-rump length measurement is indicated by *cursors.*

has occurred.[68, 69] Likewise, the normal cord floating in amniotic fluid may appear quite prominent in close proximity to the ventral abdominal wall and should not be confused for bowel that has herniated through a ventral abdominal wall defect, such as a gastroschisis.

The vessels of the umbilical cord may be followed using sonography as they enter the abdomen and travel toward the liver and iliac arteries. The single thin-walled *umbilical vein* (UV) may be followed cephalad from the cord insertion to the left portal vein (Fig. 9–22). The UV has no branches to the liver; therefore, if branching structures are identified associated with a vein near the ligamentum teres, it is the left portal vein (possibly the umbilical portion of the left portal vein), not the UV (Fig. 9–23). In certain cases of fetal compromise (chorioangiomas or immune hydrops fetalis), the UV may appear quite prominent (Fig. 9–24). Although some researchers have suggested

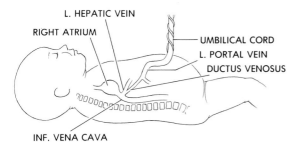

Figure 9–22. Schematic representation of the course of the umbilical vein.

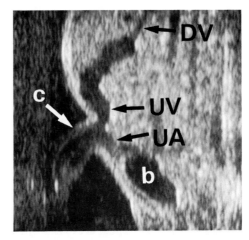

Figure 9–24. Fetus with placental chorioangioma. The umbilical vein appears prominent. c, umbilical cord; b, bladder; UV, umbilical vein; UA, umbilical artery; DV, ductus venosus.

that increasing UV diameter correlates with increasing fetal distress, the authors and others have not found this to be a reliable indicator to either confirm or exclude fetal compromise.[70, 71] From the left portal vein, blood flows either through the ductus venosus to systemic veins (inferior vena cava or left hepatic vein) bypassing the liver, or medially from the left portal vein and portal sinus to the right portal vein, perfusing the fetal liver (Fig. 9–25). The ductus venosus, which has the structure of a muscular vein,[58] in this way forms the conduit between the portal system and systemic veins. Sonographically, the ductus venosus is a thin intrahepatic channel with echogenic walls. It lies within the two layers of the lesser omentum (hepatogastric ligament), in a groove between the left lobe and the caudate lobe (fissure for the ligamentum venosum), and thus becomes an anatomic landmark for both the hepatogastric ligament and caudate lobe of the liver (Fig. 9–26). Although 40 to 60 percent of umbilical venous flow passes

into the liver through the portal veins, the remainder passes directly to the cava via this fetal conduit.[72] The ductus venosus is patent during fetal life and remains so until shortly after birth, when transformation of the ductus into the *ligamentum venosum* occurs (beginning in the second week after birth).[58]

The two *umbilical arteries* may be followed caudad from the cord insertion, in their normal path adjacent to the fetal bladder, to the internal iliac arteries (Fig. 9–27).

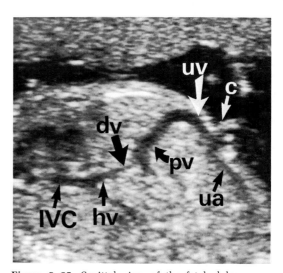

Figure 9–25. Sagittal view of the fetal abdomen. c, umbilical cord insertion; ua, umbilical artery. The umbilical vein (uv) courses cephalad to the left portal vein (pv). The ductus venosus (dv) is a narrow channel that connects the left portal vein to the left hepatic vein (hv) or inferior vena cava (IVC).

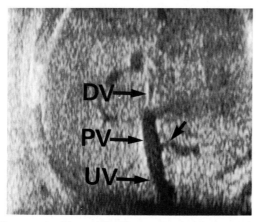

Figure 9–23. The umbilical vein (UV) as it becomes the left portal vein (PV). The branch vessel *(arrow)* distinguishes this vessel (PV) from the umbilical vein. DV, ductus venosus.

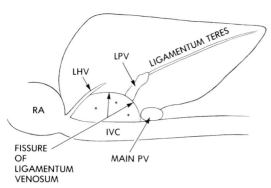

Figure 9–26. Schematic diagram of the sagittal hepatic venous anatomy, through the plane of the left hepatic vein. From the left portal vein (LPV), the ductus venosus travels in the fissure of the ligamentum venosum to the left hepatic vein (LHV) or inferior vena cava (IVC). In this plane, the liver dorsal to the fissure is the caudate lobe (*asterisk*). RA, right atrium.

Post partum, most of the intra-abdominal umbilical arteries become the medial umbilical ligaments, and proximally they become the superior vesical arteries in the adult.[58]

The Abdomen in the Fetus in the Second and Third Trimesters

An enormous amount of information about the normal fetal abdomen may be gleaned during the routine survey with currently available real-time equipment. The liver, gallbladder, and spleen are detected as distinct structures in most fetuses after midpregnancy and may be evaluated for size, echotexture, and normal morphology. Information regarding the hollow gastrointestinal (GI) tract, as well as the urinary tract and filled bladder, may also be readily obtained.

The Hepatobiliary System and Spleen

The *liver* is a relatively large organ in the fetus, accounting for approximately 10 percent of the total weight of the fetus at 11 menstrual weeks and 5 percent of the total weight at term. It is the site of most hematopoiesis in the fetus between the eighth and 14th menstrual weeks, and bile formation by hepatic cells begins at the end of the first trimester (approximately 14 menstrual weeks).[73]

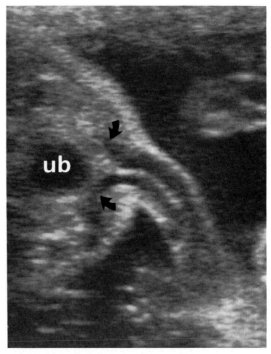

Figure 9–27. The umbilical cord insertion demonstrates the proximity of the distal umbilical arteries (*arrows*) to the wall of the urinary bladder (ub).

Many of the adult anatomic relationships of the liver and its lobes may be depicted even in the small fetus. The hepatic veins can often be traced to their confluence at the intrahepatic inferior vena cava (Fig. 9–28).

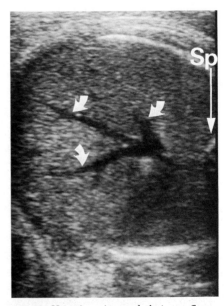

Figure 9–28. Hepatic veins and their confluence. *Arrows*, right, middle, and left hepatic veins; Sp, spine.

The right and left hepatic lobes are distinguished by the separating landmarks of the main lobar fissure, middle hepatic vein, and gallbladder. The left hepatic lobe and caudate lobe are separated by the hepatogastric ligament, in which courses the ductus venosus.

Few abnormalities of the liver have been described on antenatal sonography; these include hepatic calcifications and space-occupying lesions. Diffuse and branching calcifications in the fetal liver have been observed in association with ischemic hepatic infarcts, although the mechanism is unknown.[74] Calcification within the hepatic parenchyma in the fetus may be seen in the setting of intrauterine infection with such organisms as Toxoplasma and herpes simplex virus. Other considerations for fetal hepatic calcifications might include calcified portal vein thromboemboli;[75, 76] these findings have been described in the neonate but not in the fetus.

Fetal hepatic neoplasms, also uncommon, include hepatic teratoma, hepatoblastoma, hemangioma, and hamartoma and should be considered in the differential diagnosis of a focal hepatic space-occupying mass.[77, 78] Few have been diagnosed antenatally, but hepatic hemangioma is thought to be the most common benign liver tumor in infants.[79]

Rarely is a cyst visualized in the fetal liver. The two major categories of cystic disease of the liver seen in infancy and childhood are nonparasitic hepatic cysts and mesenchymal hamartomas.[80] Both of these entities are felt to represent developmental abnormalities, and both have been diagnosed in the fetus with sonography. The prenatal diagnosis of a solitary nonparasitic cyst, lined by biliary epithelium of the liver, was reported by Chung.[81] Most of these solitary cysts probably result from a focal developmental interruption of the biliary tree.[82] Likewise, a large multilocular cystic hepatic mass was discovered in a fetus at 25 weeks' gestational age and was confirmed at autopsy to be a mesenchymal hamartoma.[83] Hamartomas of this nature, however, are usually discovered in the first year of life, and fatalities have been attributed to treatment complications or other causes, rather than to the lesion itself. The relationship between infant death and the hepatic lesion in this case was unknown.

Diffuse cystic diseases of the liver may occur in association with cysts of other organs, including the kidneys, pancreas, and lungs, and although these have not been reported antenatally, Davies and associates reported a case of an infant in whom saccular dilation of intrahepatic bile ducts was associated with infantile polycystic kidneys and was detected within the first three days of life. This cystic liver disease was presumed to have been present prenatally[84] and was therefore a potentially detectable abnormality in the fetus. Hepatic hemangioma, although generally not included under hepatic cystic disease, may appear quite cystic on sonograms and might appropriately be considered in the differential diagnosis. Hepatoblastoma, the most common malignant neonatal hepatic neoplasm, rarely appears cystic.[85]

The *gallbladder* forms as a caudal part of the hepatic diverticulum at approximately seven menstrual weeks.[73] In the authors' experience, the gallbladder is sonographically visible in almost all fetuses after midpregnancy (20 weeks). Despite its small size, it is readily detected by virtue of the intrinsic contrast between it and the surrounding liver parenchyma. Both the gallbladder and portal-umbilical vein appear as oblong fluid-filled structures on the transverse view of the fetal abdomen through the liver. The gallbladder, however, should be distinguished by its location to the right of the portal-umbilical vein and usually may be identified as an oblong, more oval structure, whereas the umbilical vein appears as a more anechoic "channel" (Fig. 9–29). It has been suggested that the gallbladder plays a passive role in fetal life as it is most commonly observed filled after 20 weeks' gestational age and has not been demonstrated to contract in response to a fatty meal.[86]

Abnormalities of the fetal biliary tree that have been detected using sonography include choledochal cysts and fetal cholelithiasis.[87–90] Choledochal cysts are uncommon abnormalities and clinically present most often in the second and third decades of life.[91] Although several morphologic forms occur, the most common is Type I, or a cystic dilatation of the common bile duct. The abnormality has been detected uncommonly on antenatal sonography, seen as early as 25 menstrual weeks, but in most cases, prenatal diagnoses have been made in the third trimester.[87] Because choledochal

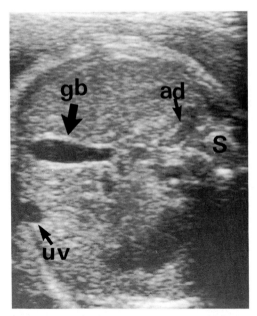

Figure 9–29. Fetal gallbladder (gb); umbilical vein (uv). The fetal adrenal gland (ad) and spine (S) are also visualized.

cysts may be associated with intermittent biliary obstruction and severe biliary cirrhosis, early diagnosis is important, and surgical resection is considered optimal therapy.

On prenatal sonography, a choledochal cyst appears in the right upper quadrant. Differential diagnosis includes dilated bowel, hepatic or omental cyst, cyst of renal origin, or dilated loop of bowel, such as might be seen in the setting of duodenal atresia. The likelihood of the presence of a choledochal cyst is greater if the location is subhepatic and intraperitoneal, if the morphology does not change with observed peristalsis of the fetal bowel, and lastly, if tubular (ductal) structures are identified entering and leaving the cyst.[87, 88]

Cholelithiasis is uncommon in children and extremely rare in utero. Beretsky and Lankin described its diagnosis in the fetus at 36 weeks' gestational age.[89] Cholelithiasis was confirmed on an immediate postnatal sonographic examination, but the stones disappeared on follow-up sonograms in approximately one month. The etiology of fetal gallstone formation is unknown, just as the cause of their disappearance was unknown in this case, and whether they dissolve or are passed, fetal and neonatal gallstones do not persist, as a general rule.

Biliary atresia, a sclerosing process of both intra- and extra-hepatic bile ducts, is a life-threatening abnormality in the neonate. Although this process is often associated with nonvisualization of the gallbladder on neonatal sonography, this disease has not been detected prenatally. The etiology of biliary atresia (congenital versus acquired) remains unknown and controversial, but many researchers believe this to be an acquired disease, possibly related to viral infection.[92–96] It has not been described in stillborns, and it is unlikely that it will be detected on prenatal sonography.

The *spleen* can be identified in virtually all fetuses between 18 and 40 menstrual weeks (Fig. 9–30).[97] It increases in size during gestation.[98, 99] In the fetus, the spleen is of similar echotexture to the kidney and slightly less echogenic than the liver.[100] Nomograms for splenic size have been published,[97] and splenic enlargement has been associated with Rhesus (Rh) immunization disease, premature rupture of the membranes (PROM), and cytomegalovirus infections.[101]

The *kidneys* may be identified in the expected location in the flanks and will be sonographically visible in 90 percent of patients at 17 to 22 weeks' gestational age.[102] The flanks are relatively shallow in the fetus, and thus the anterior surface of the kidneys project more anteriorly in the fetus than in the adult (see Chap. 11).

The fetal *adrenal glands* are relatively large in the third trimester and at birth are 20 times their relative adult size.[103, 104] Because of their large size and typical sonographic morphology, they are readily visualized in the third trimester of pregnancy. It is estimated that at least one gland may be

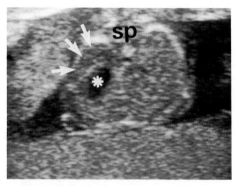

Figure 9–30. The fetal spleen is indicated by the *arrows* and is located behind the fluid-filled stomach *(asterisk).* sp, spine.

identified in 90 percent of fetuses greater than 27 gestational weeks of age.[105] The relatively thick outer zone of the fetal adrenal is hypoechoic and presumed to represent a combination of the inner fetal zone of the adrenal cortex (from which neonatal adrenal hemorrhages originate) and an outer thin "permanent" cortex. The fetal zone comprises approximately 80 percent of the bulk of the fetal adrenal gland before birth[105] but atrophies and disappears within three to 12 postnatal months.[104] The echogenic inner zone of the fetal adrenal gland is presumed to represent the fetal adrenal medulla (Fig. 9–31). The adrenal glands are so prominent in the fetus that they have been confused for renal parenchyma in cases in which one or both kidneys are absent, i.e., renal aplasia, or ectopically located. Interestingly, unlike the situation in the adult, the left adrenal is usually imaged superior to the upper pole of the left kidney in fetal life and apparently moves to its normal position (more anterior and medial to the left kidney) in early childhood.[106] Abnormalities in the fetal adrenal gland are rarely discovered, but adrenal neuroblastoma has been described on antenatal sonograms.[107] Human chorionic gonadotropin (hCG) contributes to adrenal growth in the first half of pregnancy; thereafter, adrenocorticotropic hormone (ACTH) controls the

fetal adrenal. This may, in part, explain the smaller adrenals sometimes noted in anencephalics who lack a well-developed hypothalamic-pituitary axis.[105, 108]

It is unusual to visualize the fetal *pancreas* by virtue of its morphology alone because of the paucity of retroperitoneal fat in the fetal abdomen and the similar echotexture compared with surrounding structures. Visualization of the fetal pancreas may be accomplished, however, with special care and attention to the associated anatomic landmarks of the superior mesenteric artery and vein in the fetus. The head of the pancreas is relatively larger than its body in the neonates, as compared with the adult.[58]

The Hollow GI Tract in the Fetus

The esophagus, trachea, and stomach originate from the foregut. The esophagus becomes anatomically separate from the trachea in the sixth and seventh menstrual weeks. The stomach assumes its adult shape and position at approximately nine to ten menstrual weeks.[109, 110] The fetus begins to swallow early in the second trimester (16 to 18 menstrual weeks), and the volume of amniotic fluid swallowed increases dramatically with age (from 7 ml per day at 16 menstrual weeks to approximately 400 to 750 ml per day at term), resulting in increased volumes of fluid delivered to the stomach, small bowel, and colon during development.[58, 60, 111–113] Distally in the GI tract, as a result of developmental changes as well as the increasing volume of fluid delivered to the bowel, the appearance of small bowel and colon changes in a fairly predictable pattern during gestation, and Zilianti and Fernández have correlated these changing patterns with gestational age.[114]

The normal fetal esophagus is collapsed and not usually visualized sonographically. The fluid-filled *stomach*, however, may be identified in virtually all normal second and third trimester pregnancies. Sonographically, the stomach "bubble" appears as an anechoic crescent-shaped structure in the left abdominal cavity (Fig. 9–31) and is usually visualized in the same axial image in which the abdominal circumference is measured. Movement of the gastric musculature begins in approximately the fourth to fifth

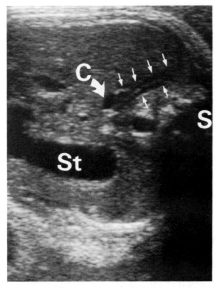

Figure 9–31. The fetal adrenal gland is indicated by the *small arrows*. Note that it "kisses" the inferior vena cava (C), a useful anatomic relationship. S, spine; St, stomach.

month of gestation, and in mid-gestation, this, in combination with increased swallowing, results in the delivery of increasing amniotic fluid volume distally into the small bowel and colon where fluid and nutrients are reabsorbed.[16]

After the 15th to 16th menstrual week, meconium begins to accumulate in the distal part of the small intestine as a combination of desquamated cells, bile pigments, and mucoproteins.[115] Early in the second trimester, the meconium-filled small bowel appears quite echogenic, mimicking echogenic fetal abdominal masses, the so-called fetal abdominal "pseudomasses" (Fig. 9–32).[110, 116, 117] At this stage, the small bowel most likely assumes this appearance because the bowel lumen is not yet distended and the opposed walls (possibly in combination with undiluted meconium) appear echogenic. As more amniotic fluid is swallowed, however, and as this fluid enters the intestines, these echogenic areas give rise to more typical and readily identifiable sonolucent fluid-filled loops of small bowel (Fig. 9–33).[116, 117] Active small bowel peristalsis, which first occurs early in the second trimester,[110] is commonly noted in these fluid-filled loops during real-time sonography after 26 to 30 menstrual weeks.[118]

Sonographically, the *colon* is first identi-

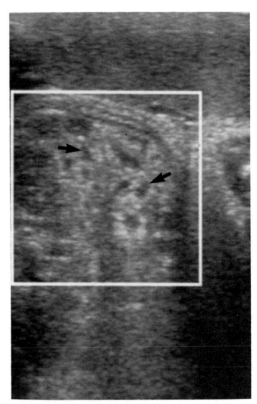

Figure 9–33. Normal fluid-filled small bowel *(arrows)* becomes visible later in gestation as more swallowed amniotic fluid is delivered distally.

fied at the end of the second trimester and is visualized in virtually all fetuses after 28 menstrual weeks.[114, 118] The colon appears as a long tubular hypoechoic structure with well-defined walls, located in the flanks and upper abdomen (Fig. 9–34). Unlike the small

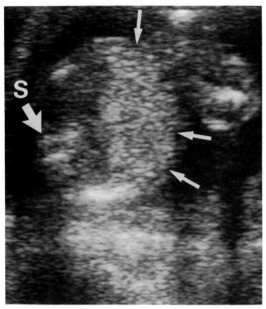

Figure 9–32. Early in gestation, collapsed fetal small bowel may appear as an echogenic mass (pseudomass), indicated by the *arrows*. S, spine.

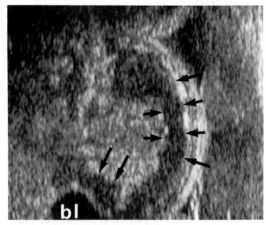

Figure 9–34. Normal fetal colon *(arrows)*. Low-level echoes (meconium) are seen within this tubular structure, in the flanks and pelvis. bl, urinary bladder.

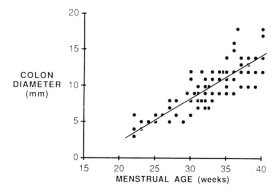

Figure 9–35. Maximum colon diameter compared with gestational age. (*From* Nyberg DA, Mack LA, Patten RM, Cyr DR: Fetal bowel: Normal sonographic findings. J Ultrasound Med 6:3, 1987.)

bowel, the colon does not usually exhibit active peristalsis that is sonographically detectable in the fetus but acts as a reservoir for the meconium that is propelled to the colon by the small bowel.[118] As a result, the normal colonic diameter increases linearly during gestation (Fig. 9–35). On occasion, the tubular fluid-filled nature of the colon may simulate a dilated ureter. More commonly, low-level echoes, probably secondary to meconium, are detected (Fig. 9–36).

Sonographically Detectable Abnormalities in the Fetal Abdomen

Stomach

GASTRIC PSEUDOMASSES. Although the fetal stomach is readily visualized as a fluid-

filled structure in the left upper quadrant, occasionally, a discrete echogenic area is imaged within it (Figs. 9–37, 9–38). Unlike abnormalities of the distal small bowel, these findings have not been associated with meconium ileus or peritonitis and are considered to be benign. Fakhry and coworkers reported this finding in seven of 624 prenatal sonograms,[119] six of which were performed in the middle of the second trimester. Repeat sonography in five of these seven fetuses demonstrated the disappearance of this intraluminal gastric mass in three to five weeks. One fetus was presumed to be afflicted by a recessive genetic disorder, and the patient suffered a miscarriage at 24 weeks. The last fetus had evidence of meconium peritonitis on pre- and postnatal studies but was otherwise normal, without evidence of cystic fibrosis. Thus, while the etiology of these gastric pseudomasses is

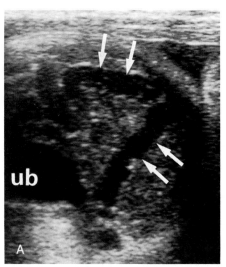
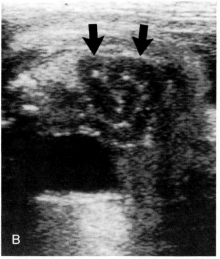

Figure 9–36. *A,* Later in gestation, tubular structures in the flanks are presumed to be colon (*white arrows*). Low-level echoes seen within the bowel are probably secondary to meconium. ub, urinary bladder. *B,* Similar tubular structures are most likely ileum (*black arrows*). In some instances, ileal loops appear similar to colon.

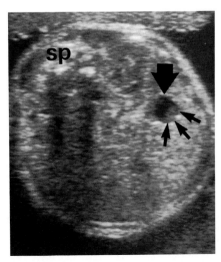

Figure 9–37. Gastric pseudomass. A transaxial view of the fetal abdomen demonstrates that the stomach *(large arrow)* is fluid-filled and contains a small mass of medium echoes *(small arrows)* presumed to represent swallowed "debris." sp, spine.

unknown, they are presumed to result from aggregates of swallowed cells and debris, before coordinated and active gastric peristalsis has developed. They have not been reported late in gestation.

ABSENT STOMACH. The stomach can be

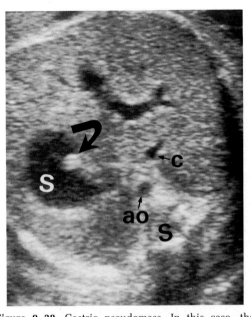

Figure 9–38. Gastric pseudomass. In this case, the echogenic focus *(curved arrow)* along the lesser curvature of the fetal stomach may represent swallowed debris or the incisura angularis. S *(white)*, stomach; ao, aorta; c, inferior vena cava; S *(black)*, spine.

visualized in virtually all second and third trimester pregnancies.[16] In cases in which it is not visualized, the examiner should consider anomalies such as esophageal atresia, CDH, or oligohydramnios as the cause.

Esophageal atresia occurs in one in 2500 live births.[120] The causative insult is unknown but probably occurs at approximately six menstrual weeks. Sonographically, esophageal atresia is suspected when the fluid-filled stomach is absent. Associated polyhydramnios is the rule and is thought to result from impaired fetal swallowing.[16, 121] Therefore, the combination of polyhydramnios and absent stomach should raise suspicion of this anomaly.[121–123] Sonographic visualization of the proximal esophageal pouch has been described.[124] Fetal anomalies are commonly associated with tracheoesophageal (TE) fistula, including vertebral, anal, cardiac, renal, and limb anomalies (VACTERL). Thus if TE fistula is suspected sonographically, a careful survey should be performed in search of other fetal abnormalities.

In the most common forms of esophageal atresia (greater than 90 percent), there is an associated distal communication between the respiratory and the GI tracts. Therefore, fluid enters the stomach through the fistula, and thus it is possible that a fluid-containing stomach might be visualized even when esophageal atresia is present. The true accuracy of the sonographic diagnosis of this more common form of tracheoesophageal fistula (communicating) is unknown, but it is likely that some cases may be overlooked on prenatal sonograms by virtue of the presence of fluid identified within the fetal stomach. Despite the presence of a fistula, however, the distal passage of fluid is impeded sufficiently in some cases to result in a poorly-filled fetal stomach on prenatal sonograms, thus conforming to the expected findings of atresia without fistula.

Congenital diaphragmatic hernia, because it most commonly occurs on the left, with stomach herniated into the chest, also results in a nondetectable fluid-filled stomach in the expected location in the fetal abdomen. This may be distinguished from esophageal atresia by virtue of the accompanying intrathoracic abnormalities associated with CDH, in contradistinction to the usual normal-appearing thorax in most cases of esophageal atresia.

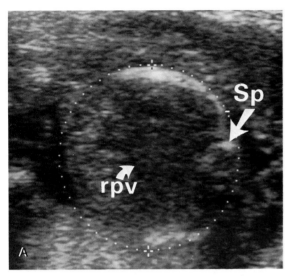

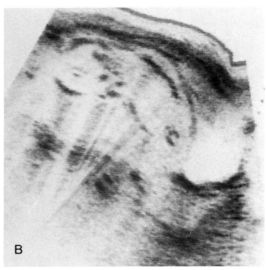

Figure 9–39. Absent or poorly visualized stomach in association with oligohydramnios. *A*, Transverse view of the fetal abdomen. The fluid-filled stomach is poorly visualized. Sp, spine; rpv, right portal vein. *B*, Longitudinal image of the same fetus. Profound oligohydramnios.

In the authors' practice, the most common setting in which the fluid-filled stomach is poorly visualized or appears collapsed is in the presence of *oligohydramnios* (Fig. 9–39). The authors believe this most likely results from paucity of amniotic fluid available for swallowing. This is in contradistinction to the situation in which esophageal atresia without fistula is present, where polyhydramnios would be the likely accompaniment. We have also noticed a poorly filled stomach in some cases in which the fetus is severely distressed, as in nonimmune hydrops. In these cases, polyhydramnios may also be present.

DILATED STOMACH AND DUODENUM: THE "DOUBLE BUBBLE." *Duodenal atresia* is the most common type of fetal small bowel atresia, occurring in one in 10,000 live births.[125] Most investigators currently believe that the atresia results from the failure of recanalization of the duodenum, which normally occurs at about ten menstrual weeks.[126] It may be detected prenatally with sonography by the presence of a dilated fluid-filled stomach and proximal duodenum,[127–130] the sonographic equivalent of the "double bubble" (Figs. 9–40, 9–41). Its greatest significance is its association with other congenital anomalies in 48 percent of cases: 30 percent Trisomy 21, 22 percent gut malrotations, and 20 percent congenital heart disease, and less commonly, tracheoesophageal fistulas, renal malformations, and hepatobiliary and pancreatic duct anomalies.[127, 131–133] It is associated with polyhydramnios in 45 percent of cases[125] and symmetric growth retardation in 50 percent.[134]

Duodenal atresia is not the only cause of the "double bubble," however. Duodenal stenosis, annular pancreas, and peritoneal bands may also result in this sonographic

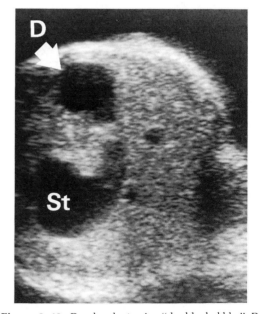

Figure 9–40. Duodenal atresia: "double bubble." D, duodenum; St, stomach.

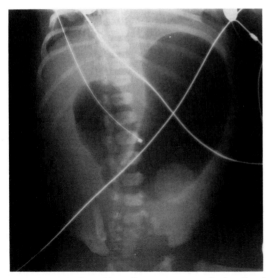

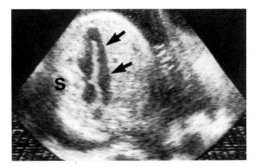

Figure 9–42. Midgut volvulus. The overall appearance of these "isolated" fluid-filled proximal bowel loops (*arrows*) did not change configuration during real-time imaging. S, spine.

Figure 9–41. Plain film of a neonate with duodenal atresia: "double bubble."

appearance and should also be considered in the differential diagnosis. Duodenal atresia, however, has the most significant association with chromosomal and other anomalies. It usually involves the descending or second portion of the duodenum (distal to the ampulla), whereas duodenal stenosis usually involves the horizontal (third) or ascending (fourth) parts of the duodenum.[126] Nevertheless, it is unlikely that the distinction between atresia and stenosis can be made on antenatal sonography. Unfortunately, no case of duodenal atresia has been diagnosed prior to 26 menstrual weeks.[125, 135] In the absence of other life-threatening anomalies, infants with duodenal stenosis or atresia do well if provided prompt neonatal surgical correction.[128]

When a greater number of echo-free areas are present in the upper fetal abdomen than would be expected with a mid-duodenal obstruction, and these bowel loops do not change in configuration over time, it can be presumed that the site of obstruction is more distal in the small bowel (Figs. 9–42, 9–43). In this instance, etiologies, including volvulus, malrotation, or peritoneal bands, should be considered. These "high" obstructions in the small bowel are also often accompanied by polyhydramnios. In fact, obstruction of the small bowel as far distally as the terminal ileum has been associated with polyhydramnios, whereas obstructions of the colon are generally not associated with excessive amniotic fluid volume.

Midgut Abnormalities

SMALL BOWEL DILATATIONS. Sonographically, the fetal small and large bowel are distinguished largely on the basis of type-specific morphology and location in the ab-

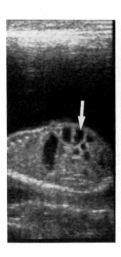

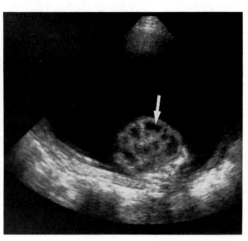

Figure 9–43. Distal jejunal atresia. Abnormal fluid-filled bowel loops. More loops are visualized than are expected with duodenal atresia. Marked polyhydramnios was also present.

domen. Small bowel is characteristically located more centrally in the fetal abdomen and, after mid-pregnancy, appears as a cluster of fluid-filled structures with discernible walls that may demonstrate active peristalsis during real-time imaging. The colon is a tubular hypoechoic structure larger in caliber, containing low-level echoes, and located along the periphery of the fetal abdomen. Because there is such variability in the appearance of normal fetal bowel, sonographers often feel uncertain in making the diagnosis of bowel obstruction. It has been suggested that measurements of bowel loops may be of some help. For example, in their study, Nyberg and colleagues found that small bowel loops never exceeded 7 mm in diameter and colonic diameter increased linearly with gestational age after 22 weeks, reaching up to 18 mm at term.[118] Crelin, on the other hand, suggests that the sigmoid colon can normally reach a diameter of 2 to 3 cm at birth.[58] Regardless, although measurements of small and large bowel may be useful in some instances to confirm the sonographer's impressions of fetal bowel obstruction, other features in the fetal abdomen may be more helpful in initially alerting the sonographer to bowel obstruction during a routine examination. These include:

1. Polyhydramnios associated with "high" small bowel obstructions (jejunal and duodenal).

2. Disproportionate dilatation of proximal small bowel relative to distal small bowel.

3. Failure to detect normal colon late in gestation.

4. Abdominal circumference disproportionately large for dates.

5. Fetal ascites or peritoneal calcifications.

6. Diminished or absent peristalsis in dilated small bowel loops.

Dilated loops of bowel cannot always be identified as small bowel with certainty because the typical sonographic appearance attributed to small bowel may be lost when a distal obstruction is present. For example, the authors misinterpreted dilated meconium-filled ileum as dilated colon because the loops were dilated, assumed an appearance typical for colon, were located in a position typical for colon, and did not exhibit peristalsis (Fig. 9–44). After birth, the diagnosis of meconium ileus, microcolon, and cystic fibrosis was confirmed. Interestingly, in this case, the collapsed nonvisualized microcolon had been displaced by a large, distended, immobile, meconium-filled ileum with features indistinguishable from those of colon.[136]

A rare form of fetal bowel dysfunction, *congenital chloridorrhea* (CCD), may be detected prenatally through the abnormal appearance of fetal bowel. It is inherited as an autosomal recessive trait and results from impaired active transport of chloride from the distal ileum and colon, resulting in profuse chloride diarrhea in the infant.[137, 138] The diagnosis has been suggested on prenatal sonography by virtue of an enlarged abdominal circumference associated with dilated fluid-filled loops of bowel with active peristalsis in a fetus at risk of the dis-

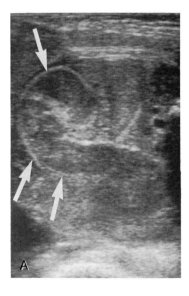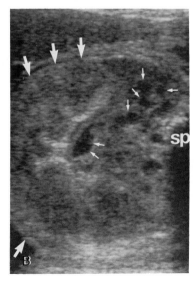

Figure 9–44. Meconium ileus in association with cystic fibrosis. The appearance of the dilated ileum was misinterpreted as colon. Post partum, the infant was shown to have a microcolon. *A,* Dilated loop of small bowel, low in the anterior abdomen, appeared similar to the sigmoid colon *(large arrows). B,* Dilated meconium-filled loop of bowel in the anterior midabdomen simulates the appearance of the transverse colon *(larger arrows),* in contrast to the smaller fluid-filled loops in the central abdomen, more typical of small bowel *(small arrows).* sp, spine.

ease.[137, 138] Of all causes of small bowel obstruction or dilation, however, CCD is one of the rarest and should really be seriously considered only in a fetus at risk of the disease.

The true function of the *colon* in utero is unknown. Histologically, there are some features present in the fetal colon that suggest the colon may be involved in processes such as water absorption or secretion,[110] but from an imaging perspective, the colon merely acts as a reservoir for the storage of meconium in the fetus. Meconium normally does not pass the rectal folds or anal sphincter in fetal life unless the fetus is distressed late in gestation, during which time meconium may be passed through the rectum, resulting in meconium staining of the amniotic fluid. Although some investigators have related this to cord compression[139] or fetal hypoxia,[140] others have even suggested that the passage of meconium may be a normal physiologic event, reflecting increasing fetal maturity.[141] Regardless, meconium staining appears to occur exclusively in more mature fetuses. Matthews and Warshaw correlated meconium staining of the amniotic fluid with gestational age. They found that over 98 percent of the infants born with evidence of meconium-stained amniotic fluid were at least 37 menstrual weeks old, and no infant who had meconium-stained amniotic fluid was less than 34 weeks. Because the innervation of the intestine develops in a craniocaudal direction, these authors suggested that perhaps more premature infants have less developed and possibly less reactive colonic gastrointestinal motility.[142]

Because the colon largely serves as a reservoir in the fetus, it seems unlikely that low colonic obstructions involving the sigmoid or rectum would result in a colonic appearance that differs significantly from normal (when associated with normal amniotic fluid volume). Nevertheless, some authors have suggested that anorectal atresia or low bowel obstructions may, in fact, be visualized on sonograms prenatally. Harris and coworkers reviewed prenatal sonographic findings in 11 proven cases of anorectal atresia and found evidence of a peculiar focal bowel dilatation in the pelvis or lower abdomen suggestive of low colonic obstruction in four of the 11 cases (36 percent).[143] Although the numbers are small, it appears that features suggestive of colonic

obstruction may be present on prenatal sonograms. The sensitivity of ultrasound for colonic obstruction appears to be directly related to gestational age, and in their cases, the distal colonic obstructions were more obvious as the fetuses approached term.[143] Why a low large bowel atresia would manifest as colonic dilatation is not explained. The prenatal diagnosis of anal atresia is important, however, both for early antenatal surgical correction and for alerting the sonographer and perinatologist to the potential presence of commonly associated defects, such as vertebral, cardiovascular, tracheoesophageal fistulae, renal, and limb anomalies (VACTERL). Other causes of distal bowel obstruction to be considered are the meconium plug syndrome and Hirschsprung's disease.[118, 144]

ASCITES. True ascites in the fetal abdomen is always abnormal. Intraperitoneal fluid is most readily identified in the peritoneal recesses of the subhepatic space, the flanks, and the lower abdominal cavity or pelvis. Unlike in adults, in fetuses, because of the small size of the pelvis, large fluid collections are rarely noted in the rectovesical recess. Occasionally, ascites is visualized as a fluid collection between the two leaves of unfused omentum (Fig. 9–18).[59]

Fetal ascites may be associated with hydrops fetalis, in which case intraperitoneal fluid will be associated with pleural effusions, possibly pericardial effusion, and often integumentary edema. In cases of nonimmune hydrops, the prognosis is poor. The ascites may also occur as an isolated finding, and in these cases, bowel perforation (atresias, volvulus, stenoses) or urinary ascites, secondary to bladder outlet obstruction associated with bladder or fornical rupture, should be considered. The prognosis in cases of bowel obstruction may be quite good, but in the authors' experience, those associated with bladder rupture have had a poor outcome.[145]

When isolated fetal ascites is found on prenatal sonography, a search for the etiology of the ascites should be made. Identifiable features that may be helpful include peritoneal calcifications, intra-abdominal cysts (meconium pseudocysts), dilated urinary bladder or hydronephrosis, and bowel dilatation as evidence of obstruction.

Ascites is always abnormal in the fetus, and thus the implications for fetal prognosis and intervention may be quite significant for both the mother and fetus. Familiarity with a potential pitfall, "*pseudoascites*," may be helpful in avoiding the falsely positive diagnosis of fetal ascites. When the fetal abdomen is examined, a thin rim of lucent tissue is often observed along the anterior surface of the fetal abdominal cavity just beneath the skin; this may appear quite similar to ascites. This appearance, referred to as pseudoascites, is thought to represent the hypoechoic anterior abdominal musculature (internal oblique, external oblique, and transverse muscles) in the fetus (Fig. 9–45).[146] It is distinguished from true ascites through the following observations:

1. Owing to the insertion of the oblique muscles into the ribs, this lucent rim "fades" posterolaterally and is not visualized between the dorsal ribs and liver.

2. True ascites generally insinuates itself between the bony rib cage and viscera (both liver and spleen) and can be confirmed by its presence in the peritoneal recesses of the fetal subhepatic space, flanks, or pelvis, whereas pseudoascites cannot.

3. True ascites surrounds bowel loops in the abdomen, whereas pseudoascites does not.

4. Although ascites frequently outlines the falciform ligament and umbilical vein, pseudoascites does not.

CALCIFICATION IN THE ABDOMEN. Calcification in the fetal abdomen appears as a bright reflector with shadowing on sonograms. When these calcifications are localized to peritoneal recesses (subhepatic areas, pelvis or flanks, or scrotal sacs) and are unaccompanied by solid lesions, the vast majority of cases are secondary to meconium peritonitis.

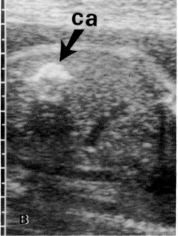

Figure 9–45. "Pseudoascites." The hypoechoic abdominal musculature *(arrows)* "fades" along the interface with the ribs *(open arrow)*. Also note that the hypoechoic pseudoascites does not outline the umbilical vein (uv).

If calcifications are parenchymal or are associated with a solid mass, then neuroblastoma, fetal teratoma, hamartoma, and prior viral infection (i.e., toxoplasmosis, rubella, cytomegalovirus, and herpes simplex [TORCH]) should be considered.[74-76] Occasionally, echogenic foci with shadowing may be associated with bladder outlet obstruction and bladder rupture (see Chap. 11).

MECONIUM PERITONITIS. Meconium peritonitis is a sterile chemical peritonitis that results from intrauterine perforation of the small bowel with spillage of sterile meconium into the peritoneal cavity. Secondary peritoneal inflammation and calcification occur (Fig. 9–46). The bowel perforations are thought to occur after the onset of gastric

Figure 9–46. Calcification in association with meconium peritonitis. *A*, Transverse image of the fetal abdomen demonstrates ascites (a) and peritoneal calcifications (ca). S, spine. *B*, Sagittal image of the same fetus. Calcification (ca) with shadowing secondary to meconium peritonitis.

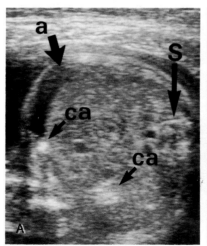

movement and bowel peristalsis, and in some instances have occurred as early as 24 weeks of life (the mean menstrual age at diagnosis is 29.5 weeks).[147] Meconium peritonitis is commonly accompanied by fetal ascites and polyhydramnios.[147] It may be associated with obstructive bowel lesions and malformations such as atresias, volvulus, malrotations, and less commonly, meconium ileus and cystic fibrosis. In many cases the perforation heals spontaneously, leaving behind small foci of calcification scattered about the peritoneal lining as the only evidence of prior perforation in the neonate. In only 50 percent of the cases of meconium peritonitis can the cause be demonstrated post partum, the most common being volvulus, atresia, and intussusception.[148] In male fetuses, because of the patent processus vaginalis, these calcifications may extend into the scrotal sac.[149] Alternatively, the meconium and fibrinous peritoneal reaction may become encysted, resulting in a meconium pseudocyst, which may attain quite a large size and appear as a calcified soft tissue mass in the fetal abdomen on sonography.[150] It has been noted that the calcifications of meconium peritonitis are not seen until at least 10 days after the peritoneal spillage, and thus, if the fetus is scanned after perforation but before this interval, ascites may be the only finding.[151]

Importantly, although cystic fibrosis (CF) is a concern, in most cases in which the antenatal sonographic features of meconium peritonitis are described in the literature (calcification and pseudocyst formation), the fetuses were not afflicted with CF. On the contrary, most cases of bona fide meconium ileus diagnosed in infancy are associated with CF. Nevertheless, because 15 percent of children with CF show associated meconium peritonitis and 10 to 25 percent of children with CF have associated intestinal atresia, CF should be considered in the differential diagnosis whenever peritoneal calcifications are detected in the fetus.[152]

ABDOMINAL CYSTS. Cysts are occasionally discovered in the fetal abdomen during routine prenatal sonography and are almost always benign. The largest fetal abdominal cysts encountered in the authors' practice have originated from the urinary system and represent dilated renal pelves or perinephric urinomas. Although the authors attempt to determine the site of origin of all abdominal cysts, this is not always possible; one rule that has been helpful and reliable is that if the cyst touches the fetal spine, it is most likely renal in origin. Other cystic structures may pose greater diagnostic difficulty. If the cyst is lower in the abdomen and the fetus is female, ovarian cyst is considered even though such cysts may be visualized quite "high" in the abdominal cavity (Fig. 9–47). Some ovarian cysts have achieved such great size (up to 11 cm in diameter) that they have extended from the pelvis to the liver, impressing upon the diaphragm and thorax.[153, 154] They may be simple, without internal echoes, or contain septations. They may be complicated by torsion or hemorrhage,[155] but

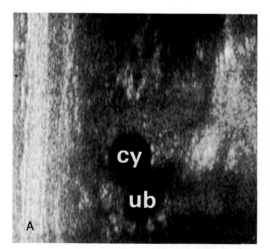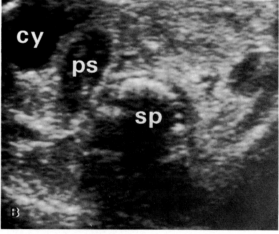

Figure 9–47. Fetal ovarian cyst. A, Coronal view demonstrates a cyst (cy) above the bladder (ub). B, Postpartum axial view of the abdomen of the same patient. sp, spine; ps, psoas muscle; cy, cyst.

fetal ovarian cysts are nearly always benign.[156] They may be unilateral or bilateral and have been associated with polyhydramnios in 10 percent of the cases. Ovarian cysts have been reported in association with fetal hypothyroidism.[157] Theca-lutein cysts are felt to result from elevated circulating hCG and have been associated with diabetes in pregnancy.[158] Small follicular cysts, although common in autopsy specimens (33 percent), are generally too small to be seen on fetal sonography.[159]

The differential diagnosis of fetal abdominal cyst should include mesenteric, gut duplication, choledochal, and urachal cyst, and cystic teratoma, as well as cysts of renal origin. Choledochal cysts, as described previously, generally appear in the right upper quadrant near the expected location of the common bile duct. Urachal cysts occur near the ventral apex of the bladder wall and tend to be associated with the ventral abdominal wall. Cysts of renal origin tend to be located more dorsally and in close proximity to the spine. Occasionally, a dilated ureter may be confused with colon or vice versa.

Mesenteric cysts, on the other hand, are thought to be lymphatic in origin and have been reported to occur most commonly in the mesentery of the small bowel.[160, 161] There is some confusion regarding the nomenclature of a lymphangioma and mesenteric cyst, and although the two may be distinguished histologically using current electron micrographic techniques, these distinctions have not always been drawn in the literature. Takiff and colleagues, in a study of surgical cases including children and adults, found lymphangiomas to be rare, more frequently multilocular, larger, more commonly symptomatic, and usually in children.[162] Alternatively, mesenteric cysts in this series appeared to be more common, smaller, more localized to the omentum, asymptomatic, unilocular, and most often in adults. Mesenteric cysts, when discovered in childhood, are reported to be uniformly benign.[163] Regardless, mesenteric cysts or lymphangiomas are extremely rare lesions and, despite their inclusion in the differential diagnosis of a fetal abdominal cyst, to the authors' knowledge have not been described on antenatal sonography.

Exquisite detail in the fetal abdomen may now be discerned during antenatal sonogra-

phy. Although anomalies of the thorax and abdomen are uncommon, attention to the available normal anatomic information in the fetal chest and abdomen alerts the sonographer to even minor alterations in morphology that may have a major impact on the health, development, and management of the fetus and newborn infant.

References

1. Moore KL: Development of body cavities, primitive mesenteries, and the diaphragm. In The Developing Human: Clinically Oriented Embryology, 4th Ed. Philadelphia, WB Saunders Co, 1988.
2. Jeanty P, Romero R, Hobbins JC: Fetal pericardial fluid: A normal finding in the second half of gestation. Am J Obstet Gynecol 149:529, 1984.
3. Yagel S, Hurwitz A: Fetal pericardial fluid. (Letter to the editor.) Am J Obstet Gynecol 152:721, 1985.
4. Jeanty P, Romero R, Hobbins JC: Vascular anatomy of the fetus. J Ultrasound Med 3:113, 1984.
5. Cooper C, Mohony BS, Bowie JD, et al: Ultrasound evaluation of the normal fetal upper airway and esophagus. J Ultrasound Med 4:343, 1985.
6. Fried AM, Loh FK, Umer MA, et al: Echogenicity of fetal lung: Relation to fetal age and maturity. AJR 145:591, 1985.
7. Gayea PD, Grant DC, Doubilet PM, et al: Prediction of fetal lung maturity: Inaccuracy of study using conventional ultrasound instruments. Radiology 155:473, 1985.
8. Birnholz JC, Farrell EE: Fetal lung development: Compressibility as a measure of maturity. Radiology 154:495, 1985.
9. Nimrod C, Davies D, Stanislaw W, et al: Ultrasound prediction of pulmonary hypoplasia. Obstet Gynecol 68:495, 1986.
10. Devore GR, Horenstein J, Platt LD: Fetal echocardiography: Assessment of cardiothoracic disproportion—A new technique for the diagnosis of thoracic hypoplasia. Am J Obstet Gynecol 155:1066, 1986.
11. Chitkara U, Rosenberg J, Chervenak FA, et al: Prenatal sonographic assessment of the fetal thorax: Normal values. Am J Obstet Gynecol 156:1069, 1987.
12. Bovicelli L, Rizzo N, Orsini LF, et al: Ultrasonic real-time diagnosis of fetal hydrothorax and lung hypoplasia. J Clin Ultrasound 9:253, 1981.
13. Schumacher RE, Farrell PM: Congenital diaphragmatic hernia: A major remaining challenge in neonatal respiratory care. Perinatol Neonatol 9:29, 1985.
14. Nakayama DK, Harrison MR, Chinn DH, et al: Prenatal diagnosis and natural history of the fetus with a congenital diaphragmatic hernia: Initial clinical experience. J Pediatr Surg 20:118, 1985.
15. Puri P, Gorman F: Lethal nonpulmonary anomalies associated with congenital surgery. J Pediatr Surg 19:29, 1984.
16. Farrant P: The antenatal diagnosis of oesophageal atresia by ultrasound. Br J Radiol 53:1202, 1980.
17. Harrison MR, Golbus MS, Filly RA: Congenital

diaphragmatic hernia. *In* The Unborn Patient. Orlando, FL, Grune & Stratton, 1984, pp 237–276.

18. Gilsanz V, Emons D, Hansmann M, et al: Hydrothorax, ascites, and right diaphragmatic hernia. Radiology 158:243, 1986.

19. Harrison MR, Adzick NS, Nakayama DK, et al: Fetal diaphragmatic hernia: Fatal but fixable. Semin Perinatol 9:103, 1985.

20. Harrison MR, Bjordal RI, Landmark F, et al: Congenital diaphragmatic hernia: The hidden mortality. J Pediatr Surg 13:227, 1979.

21. Vintzileos AM, Campbell WA, Nochimson DJ: Antenatal evaluation and management of ultrasonically detected fetal anomalies. Obstet Gynecol 69:640, 1987.

22. Adzick NS, Harrison MR, Glick PL, et al: Fetal cystic adenomatoid malformation: Prenatal diagnosis and natural history. J Pediatr Surg 20:483, 1985.

23. Johnson JA, Rumack CM, Johnson ML, et al: Cystic adenomatoid malformation: Antenatal demonstration. AJR 142:483, 1984.

24. Pezzuti RT, Isler RJ: Antenatal ultrasound detection of cystic adenomatoid malformation of lung: Report of a case and review of the recent literature. J Clin Ultrasound 11:342, 1983.

25. Graham D, Winn K, Dex W, et al: Prenatal diagnosis of cystic adenomatoid malformation of the lung. J Ultrasound Med 1:9, 1982.

26. Mayden KL, Tortora M, Chervenak F: The antenatal sonographic detection of lung masses. Am J Obstet Gynecol 143:349, 1984.

27. Miller RK, Sieber WK, Yunis EJ: Congenital adenomatoid malformation of the lung: A report of 17 cases and a review of the literature. Path Ann 1:387, 1980.

28. Stocker JT, Madewell JE, Drake RM: Congenital cystic adenomatoid malformation of the lung. Hum Pathol 8:155, 1977.

29. Van Dijk C, Wagenvoort CA: The various types of congenital adenomatoid malformations of the lung. J Pathol 110:131, 1973.

30. Wolf SA, Hertzler JH, Philippart AI: Cystic adenomatoid dysplasia of the lung. J Pediatr Surg 15:925, 1980.

31. Fraser RG, Paré JAP: Pulmonary abnormalities of developmental origin. *In* Diagnosis of Diseases of the Chest, 2nd Ed. Philadelphia, WB Saunders Co, 1977, pp 602–628.

32. Thomas CS, Leopold GR, Hilton S, et al: Fetal hydrops associated with extralobar sequestration. J Ultrasound Med 5:668, 1986.

33. Mariona F, McAlpin G, Zador I, et al: Sonographic detection of fetal extrathoracic pulmonary sequestration. J Ultrasound Med 5:283, 1986.

34. Romero R, Chervenak FA, Kotzen J, et al: Antenatal sonographic findings of extralobar pulmonary sequestration. J Ultrasound Med 1:131, 1982.

35. Buntain WL, Woolley MM, Mahour GH, et al: Pulmonary sequestration in children: A twenty-five year experience. Surgery 81:413, 1977.

36. Levine MM, Nudel DB, Gootman N, et al: Pulmonary sequestration causing congestive heart failure in infancy: A report of two cases and review of the literature. Ann Thorac Surg 34:581, 1981.

37. DeParedes CG, Pierce WS, Johnson DG, et al: Pulmonary sequestration in infants and children: A 20-year experience and review of the literature. J Pediatr Surg 5:136, 1970.

38. Paré JAP, Fraser RG: Synopsis of Diseases of the Chest. Philadelphia, WB Saunders Co, 1983, pp 239–242.

39. Dumontier C, Graviss ER, Silberstein MJ, et al: Bronchogenic cysts in children. Clin Radiol 36:431, 1985.

40. McAlister WH, Wright JR, Crane JP: Main-stem bronchial atresia: Intrauterine sonographic diagnosis. AJR 148:364, 1987.

41. Harrison MR, Golbus MS, Filly RA: Management of the fetus with nonimmune hydrops. *In* The Unborn Patient. Orlando, FL, Grune & Stratton, 1984, pp 193–216.

42. Hutchinson AA, Drew JH, Yu VYH, et al: Non-immunologic hydrops fetalis: A review of 61 cases. Obstet Gynecol 59:347, 1982.

43. Mahony BS, Filly RA, Callen PW, et al: Severe non-immune hydrops fetalis: Sonographic evaluation. Radiology 151:757, 1984.

44. Frigoletto FD, Greene MF, Benacerraf BR: Ultrasonographic fetal surveillance in the management of the isoimmunized pregnancy. N Engl J Med 315:430, 1986.

45. Benacerraf BR, Frigoletto FD: Mid-trimester fetal thoracentesis. J Clin Ultrasound 13:202, 1985.

46. Vain NE, Swarner OW, Cha CC: Neonatal chylothorax: A report and discussion of nine consecutive cases. J Pediatr Surg 15:261, 1980.

47. Chernick V, Reed MH: Pneumothorax and chylothorax in the neonatal period. J Pediatr 76:624, 1970.

48. Petres RE, Redwine FO, Cruikshank DP: Congenital bilateral chylothorax: Antepartum diagnosis and successful intrauterine surgical management. JAMA 248:1360, 1982.

49. Lange IR, Manning FA: Antenatal diagnosis of congenital pleural effusion. Am J Obstet Gynecol 140:839, 1981.

50. Brodman RF: Congenital chylothorax. NY State J Med 75:553, 1975.

51. Seeds JW, Bowes WA: Results of treatment of severe fetal hydrothorax with bilateral pleuroamniotic catheters. Obstet Gynecol 68:577, 1986.

52. Rahmani MR, Fong KW, Connor RP: The varied sonographic appearance of cystic hygromas in utero. J Ultrasound Med 5:165, 1986.

53. Caudle MR, Buschi AJ, Glenbridge AN, et al: Sonographic diagnosis of a cystic lymphangioma in utero. Effect on obstetrical management. J Reprod Med 26:49, 1981.

54. Chervenak FA, Isaacson G, Blakemore KJ, et al: Fetal cystic hygroma: Cause and natural history. N Engl J Med 309:822, 1983.

55. Sheth S, Nussbaum AR, Hutchins GM, et al: Cystic hygromas in children: Sonographic-pathologic correlation. Radiology 162:821, 1987.

56. Fryns JP, Vanderberghe K, Moerman PH, et al: Cystic hygroma and multiple pterygium syndrome. Ann Genet 27:252, 1984.

57. Benacerraf BR, Frigoletto FD: Prenatal sonographic diagnosis of isolated congenital cystic hygroma, unassociated with lymphedema or other morphologic abnormality. J Ultrasound Med 6:63, 1987.

58. Crelin ES: Functional Anatomy of the Newborn. New Haven, Yale University Press, 1973, pp 47–69.

59. Gross BH, Callen PW, Filly FA: Ultrasound appearance of the fetal greater omentum. J Ultrasound Med 1:67, 1982.

60. Moore KL: The placenta and fetal membranes. *In*

The Developing Human: Clinically Oriented Embryology, 4th Ed. Philadelphia, WB Saunders Co, 1988.

61. Lyons EA, Levi CS: Ultrasound in the first trimester of pregnancy. In Callen PW (ed): Ultrasonography in Obstetrics and Gynecology. Philadelphia, WB Saunders Co, 1983, pp 10–11.

62. Moore KL: The digestive system. In The Developing Human: Clinically Oriented Embryology, 4th Ed. Philadelphia, WB Saunders Co, 1988.

63. Moore KL: The urogenital system. In The Developing Human: Clinically Oriented Embryology, 4th Ed. Philadelphia, WB Saunders Co, 1988.

64. Currarino G: The genitourinary tract. In Silverman FN (ed): Caffey's Pediatric X-Ray Diagnosis, Vol II, 8th Ed. Chicago, Year Book Med Pubs, 1985, pp 1671–1672.

65. Ney C, Friedenberg RM: Radiographic Atlas of the Genitourinary System. Philadelphia, JB Lippincott Co, 1981, pp 1359–1360.

66. Moore KL: The digestive system. In The Developing Human: Clinically Oriented Embryology, 4th Ed. Philadelphia, WB Saunders Co, 1988.

67. Grand RJ, Watkins JB, Torti FM: Development of the human gastrointestinal tract. Gastroenterology 70:790, 1976.

68. Cyr DR, Mack LA, Schoenecker SA, et al: Bowel migration in the normal fetus: US detection. Radiology 161:119, 1986.

69. Schmidt W, Yarkoni S, Crelin ES, et al: Sonographic visualization of physiologic anterior abdominal wall hernia in the first trimester. Obstet Gynecol 69:911, 1987.

70. Harman CR: Specialized applications of obstetrical ultrasound: Management of the alloimmunized pregnancy. Semin Perinatol 9:184, 1985.

71. Witter FR, Graham D: The utility of ultrasonically measured umbilical vein diameters in isoimmunized pregnancies. Am J Obstet Gynecol 146:225, 1983.

72. Rudolph AM: Hepatic and ductus venosus blood flows during fetal life. Hepatology 3:254, 1983.

73. Moore KL: The digestive system. In The Developing Human: Clinically Oriented Embryology, 4th Ed. Philadelphia, WB Saunders Co, 1988.

74. Nguyen DL, Leonard JC: Ischemic hepatic necrosis: A cause of fetal liver calcification. AJR 147:596, 1986.

75. Blanc WA, Berdon WE, Baker DH, et al: Calcified portal vein thromboemboli in newborn and stillborn infants. Radiology 88:287, 1967.

76. Friedman AP, Hally JO, Boyer B, Looper R: Calcified portal vein thromboemboli in infants: Radiography and sonography. Radiology 140:381, 1981.

77. Krandel K, Williams CH: Ultrasound case report of hepatic teratoma in newborns. J Clin Ultrasound 12:98, 1984.

78. Namakoto SK, Dreilinger A, Dattel B, et al: The sonographic appearance of hepatic hemangiomas in utero. J Ultrasound Med 2:239, 1983.

79. Dehner LP: Hepatic tumors in the pediatric age group: A distinctive clinicopathologic spectrum. In Rosenberg HS, Bolande RP (eds): Prospectives in Pediatric Pathology, Vol IV. Chicago, Year Book Med Pubs, 1978, pp 217–268.

80. Edmonson HA: Differential diagnosis of tumors and tumor-like lesions of the liver in infancy and childhood. Am J Dis Child 91:168, 1956.

81. Chung WM: Antenatal detection of hepatic cyst. J Clin Ultrasound 14:217, 1986.

82. Longmire WP, Mandrola SA, Gordon HE: Congenital cystic disease of the liver and biliary system. Ann Surg 174:711, 1971.

83. Foucar E, Wilhamson RA, Yiu-Chin V, et al: Mesenchymal hamartoma of the liver identified by fetal sonography. AJR 140:970, 1983.

84. Davies CH, Stringer DA, Whyte H, et al: Congenital hepatic fibrosis with saccular dilatation of intrahepatic bile ducts and infantile polycystic kidney disease. Pediatr Radiol 16:302, 1986.

85. Ishak KG, Glunz PR: Hepatoblastoma and hepatocellular carcinoma in infancy and childhood. Report of 47 cases. Cancer 20:396, 1967.

86. Jouppila P, Heikkinen J, Kirkinen P: Contractibility of maternal and fetal gallbladder: An ultrasonic study. J Clin Ultrasound 13:461, 1985.

87. Elrad H, Mayden KL, Ahart S, et al: Prenatal ultrasound diagnosis of choledochal cyst. J Ultrasound Med 4:553, 1985.

88. Frank JL, Hill MC, Chirathivat S, et al: Antenatal observation of a choledochal cyst by sonography. AJR 137:166, 1981.

89. Beretsky I, Lankin DH: Diagnosis of fetal cholelithiasis using real time high resolution imaging employing digital detection. J Ultrasound Med 2:381, 1983.

90. Dewbury KC, Aluwihare M, Birch SJ, et al: Prenatal ultrasound demonstration of a choledochal cyst. Br J Radiol 53:906, 1980.

91. Yamaguchi M: Congenital choledochal cyst. Am J Surg 140:653, 1980.

92. Lilly JR: Choledochal cyst and "correctable" biliary atresia. J Pediatr Surg 20:299, 1985.

93. Kamath KR: Abnormalities of the biliary tree. Clin Gastroenterol 15:157, 1986.

94. Andrews HG, Zwiren GT, Caplan DB, et al: Biliary atresia: An evolving perspective. South Med J 79:581, 1986.

95. Moore TC, Hyman PE: Extrahepatic biliary atresia in one human leukocyte antigen identical twin. Pediatrics 76:604, 1985.

96. Green D, Carroll BA: Ultrasonography in the jaundiced infant: A new approach. J Ultrasound Med 5:323, 1986.

97. Schmidt W, Yarkoni S, Jeanty P, et al: Sonographic measurements of the fetal spleen: Clinical implications. J Ultrasound Med 4:667, 1985.

98. Potter EL: Pathology of the Fetus and Infant. Chicago, Year Book Med Pubs, 1961, p 14.

99. Gruenwald P, Minh HN: Evaluation of body and organ weights in perinatal pathology. Am J Clin Pathol 34:247, 1960.

100. Mittlestaedt CA: Ultrasound of the spleen. Semin Ultrasound 2:233, 1981.

101. Eliezer S, Feldman E, Ehud W, et al: Fetal splenomegaly, ultrasound diagnosis of cytomegalovirus infection: A case report. J Clin Ultrasound 12:520, 1984.

102. Lawson TL, Foley WD, Berland LL, et al: Ultrasonic evaluation of fetal kidneys. Radiology 138:153, 1981.

103. Netter NH: Endocrine System and Selected Metabolic Diseases. Summitt, NJ, CIBA, 1965, pp 77–81.

104. Robbins SL, Cotran RS: Pathologic Basis of Diseases, 2nd Ed. Philadelphia, WB Saunders Co, 1979, pp 1387–1388.

105. Rosenberg ER, Bowie JD, Andreotti RF, et al: Sonographic evaluation of fetal adrenal glands. AJR 139:1145, 1982.

106. Co CS, Filly RA: Normal fetal adrenal gland location. (Letter to the editor.) J Ultrasound Med 5:117, 1986.

107. Giulian BB, Chang CCN, Yoss BS: Prenatal ultrasonographic diagnosis of fetal adrenal neuroblastoma. J Clin Ultrasound 14:225, 1986.

108. Villee DB: The development of steroidogenesis. Am J Med 53:533, 1972.

109. Moore KL: The digestive system. In The Developing Human: Clinically Oriented Embryology, 4th Ed. Philadelphia, WB Saunders Co, 1988.

110. Grand RJ, Watkins JB, Torti FM: Development of the human gastrointestinal tract. Gastroenterology 70:790, 1976.

111. Pritchard JA: Fetal swallowing and amniotic fluid volume. Obstet Gynecol 28:606, 1966.

112. Kimura RE, Warshaw JB: Intrauterine development of gastrointestinal tract function. In Lebenthal E (ed): Textbook of Gastroenterology and Nutrition in Infancy, Vol I. New York, Raven Press, 1981, pp 39–46.

113. Abramovich DR: Fetal factors influencing the volume and composition of liquor amnii. J Obstet Gynaecol Br Commonw 77:865, 1970.

114. Zilianti M, Fernández A: Correlation of ultrasonic images of fetal intestine with gestational age and fetal maturity. Obstet Gynecol 62:569, 1983.

115. Bustamante S, Koldovsky O: Synopsis of development of the main morphological structures of the human gastrointestinal tract. In Lebenthal E (ed): Textbook of Gastroenterology and Nutrition in Infancy. New York, Raven Press, 1981, pp 49–55.

116. Fakhry J, Reiser M, Shapiro LR, et al: Increased echogenicity in the lower fetal abdomen: A common normal variant in the second trimester. J Ultrasound Med 5:489, 1986.

117. Manco LG, Nunan FA, Sohnen H, et al: Fetal small bowel simulating abdominal mass at sonography. J Clin Ultrasound 14:404, 1986.

118. Nyberg DA, Mack LA, Patten RM, et al: Fetal bowel, normal sonographic findings. J Ultrasound Med 6:3, 1987.

119. Fakhry J, Shapiro LR, Schechter A, et al: Fetal gastric pseudomasses. J Ultrasound Med 6:177, 1982.

120. Moore KL: The respiratory system. In The Developing Human: Clinically Oriented Embryology, 4th Ed. Philadelphia, WB Saunders Co, 1988.

121. Pretorius DH, Meier PR, Johnson ML: Diagnosis of esophageal atresia in utero. J Ultrasound Med 2:475, 1983.

122. Duenhoelter JH, Santos-Ramos R, Rosenfeld CR, et al: Prenatal diagnosis of gastrointestinal tract obstruction. Obstet Gynecol 47:618, 1976.

123. Jassani MN, Gauderer MWL, Fanaroff AA, et al: A perinatal approach to the diagnosis and management of gastrointestinal malformations. Obstet Gynecol 59:33, 1982.

124. Eyheremendy E, Fister M: Antenatal real-time diagnosis of esophageal atresia. J Clin Ultrasound 11:395, 1983.

125. Nelson LH, Clark CE, Fishburne JI, et al: Value of serial sonography in the in utero detection of duodenal atresia. Obstet Gynecol 59:657, 1982.

126. Moore KL: The digestive system. In The Developing Human: Clinically Oriented Embryology, 4th Ed. Philadelphia, WB Saunders Co, 1988.

127. Loveday BJ, Barr JA, Atkens J: The intra-uterine demonstration of duodenal atresia by ultrasound. Br J Radiol 48:1031, 1975.

128. Boychuk RB, Lyons EA, Goodhard TK: Duodenal atresia diagnosed by ultrasound. Radiology 127:500, 1978.

129. Zimmerman HB: Prenatal demonstration of gastric and duodenal obstruction by ultrasound. J Can Assoc Radiol 29:138, 1978.

130. Lees RF, Alford BA, Brenbridge NAG, et al: Sonographic appearance of duodenal atresia in utero. AJR 131:701, 1978.

131. Weinberg B, Diakoumalis EE: Three complex cases of foregut atresia: Prenatal sonographic diagnosis with radiographic correlation. J Clin Ultrasound 13:481, 1985.

132. Touloukian RJ: Intestinal atresia. Clin Perinatol 5:3, 1978.

133. Kirkpatrick JA, Wagner ML, Pilling GP: A complex of anomalies associated with tracheoesophageal fistula and esophageal atresia. AJR 95:208, 1965.

134. Girvan DP, Stephens CA: Congenital intrinsic duodenal obstruction: A twenty-year review of its surgical management and consequences. J Pediatr Surg 9:833, 1974.

135. Bovicelli L, Rizzo N, Orsini LF, et al: Prenatal diagnosis and management of fetal gastrointestinal abnormalities. Semin Perinatol 7:109, 1983.

136. Goldstein RB, Filly RA: Diagnosis of meconium ileus in utero. J Ultrasound Med 6:663, 1987.

137. Groli C, Zucca S, Cesaretti A: Congenital chloridorrhea: Antenatal ultrasonographic appearance. J Clin Ultrasound 14:293, 1986.

138. Kirkinen P, Jouppila P: Prenatal ultrasonic findings in congenital chloride diarrhoea. Prenat Diagn 4:457, 1984.

139. Hon EH: The foetal heart rate. In Carey HM (ed): Modern Trends in Human Reproductive Physiology. London, Butterworth, 1963, p 245.

140. Saling E, Schneider D: Biochemical supervision of the foetus during labour. J Obstet Gynaecol Br Commonw 74:799, 1967.

141. Fenton AN, Steer CM: Fetal distress. Am J Obstet Gynecol 83:354, 1962.

142. Matthews TG, Warshaw JB: Relevance of the gestational age distribution of meconium passage in utero. Pediatrics 64:30, 1979.

143. Harris RD, Nyberg DA, Mack LA, Weinberger E: Anorectal atresia: Prenatal sonographic diagnosis. AJR 149:395, 1987.

144. Vermesh M, Mayden KL, Confino E, et al: Prenatal sonographic diagnosis of Hirschsprung's disease. J Ultrasound Med 5:37, 1986.

145. Mahony BS, Callen PW, Filly RA: Fetal urethral obstruction: US evaluation. Radiology 157:221, 1985.

146. Hashimoto BE, Filly RA, Callen PW: Fetal pseudoascites: Further anatomic observations. J Ultrasound Med 5:151, 1986.

147. Dillard JP, Edwards DU, Leopold GR: Meconium peritonitis masquerading as fetal hydrops. J Ultrasound Med 6:49, 1987.

148. Farouhar E: Meconium peritonitis: Pathology, evolution and diagnosis. Am J Clin Pathol 78:208, 1982.

149. Heydenrych JJ, Marcus PB: Meconium granuloma of the tunica vaginalis. J Urol 115:596, 1976.

150. McGahan JP, Hanson F: Meconium peritonitis with accompanying pseudocyst: Prenatal sonographic diagnosis. Radiology 148:125, 1983.
151. Martin L: Meconium peritonitis. In Ravitch MM, Welch KJ, Benson CD, et al (eds): Pediatric Surgery, Vol II, 3rd Ed. Chicago, Year Book Med Pubs, 1979, pp 952–955.
152. Brugman S, Bjelland JC: Cancer of the mouth. Ariz Med 35:802, 1978.
153. Suita S, Ikeda K, Koyamagi T, et al: Neonatal ovarian cyst diagnosed antenatally: Report of two patients. J Clin Ultrasound 12:517, 1984.
154. Landrum B, Ogburn PL, Feinberg S, et al: Intrauterine aspiration of a large fetal ovarian cyst. Obstet Gynecol 68:11S, 1986.
155. Preziosi P, Fariello G, Moiorana A, et al: Antenatal sonographic diagnosis of complicated ovarian cysts. J Clin Ultrasound 14:196, 1986.
156. Tabsh KM: Antenatal sonographic appearance of a fetal ovarian cyst. J Ultrasound Med 1:329, 1982.
157. Jafri SZH, Bree RL, Silver TM, et al: Fetal ovarian cysts: Sonographic detection and association with hypothyroidism. Radiology 150:809, 1984.
158. Nguyen KT, Reid RL, Sauerbrei E: Antenatal sonographic detection of a fetal theca lutein cyst: A clue to maternal diabetes mellitus. J Ultrasound Med 5:665, 1986.
159. DeSa DJ: Follicular ovarian cysts in stillbirths and neonates. Arch Dis Child 50:45, 1975.
160. Haller JO, Schneider M, Kassner EG, et al: Sonographic evaluation of mesenteric and omental masses in children. AJR 130:269, 1978.
161. Girdany BR: The abdomen and gastrointestinal tract. In Silverman FN (ed): Caffey's Pediatric X-Ray Diagnosis, Vol II, 8th Ed. Chicago, Year Book Med Pubs, 1985, pp 1398–1399.
162. Takiff H, Calabria R, Yin L, et al: Mesenteric cysts and intraabdominal cystic lymphangiomas. Arch Surg 120:1266, 1985.
163. Kurtz RJ, Heimann TM, Beck AR, et al: Mesenteric and retroperitoneal cysts. Ann Surg 203:109, 1986.

10

ABDOMINAL WALL DEFECTS

David A. Nyberg, M.D.
Laurence A. Mack, M.D.

ABDOMINAL WALL DEFECTS

Abdominal wall defects represent a relatively common group of fetal anomalies, occurring in approximately one in 2500 births. Knowledge of these defects and of their clinical significance has grown tremendously over the last 30 years. Gastroschisis and omphalocele, the two most common types of abdominal wall defects, are clearly distinguished on the basis of their distinct etiologies, pathologic findings, and prognoses.[1-6] The distinction between omphalocele and gastroschisis has been further clarified on prenatal sonograms.[9, 10] In recent years, other complex abdominal wall defects have been recognized and identified by prenatal sonography including cloacal exstrophy,[11, 12] ectopia cordis,[13] amniotic band syndrome,[14] and limb–body wall complex.[15]

Prenatal sonographic diagnoses of omphalocele and gastroschisis were first reported in the late 1970s.[16, 17] In conjunction with widespread maternal alpha-fetoprotein (AFP) screening, the sonographic diagnosis of abdominal wall defects has become increasingly common.[18] In addition to detecting these anomalies, sonography can identify the specific type of abdominal wall defect, secondary bowel complications, and concurrent malformations.[19] This informa-

tion is important for guiding appropriate obstetric management of affected pregnancies. If the decision is made to continue the pregnancy, knowledge of an abdominal wall defect should influence the time, mode, and place of delivery.[1, 20] Prenatal awareness of the defect will also alert pediatricians and surgeons so that prompt treatment and corrective surgery can be accomplished after birth.

Gastroschisis

Gastroschisis is a relatively small (2 to 4 cm) defect involving all layers of the abdominal wall. It is nearly always located just to the right of the umbilicus, although left-sided defects have rarely been observed (Fig. 10–1).[6, 7] Although the incidence of gastroschisis appears to be increasing, it is uncertain whether this represents a true increase or is simply due to a greater recognition of its presence.[1, 21, 22] Gastroschisis is reportedly more common than omphalocele in live-born infants but is less common in fetal autopsy series.[23] It also occurs more commonly among children of younger women than does omphalocele.

The most widely accepted etiology of gastroschisis, as proposed by DeVries, suggests

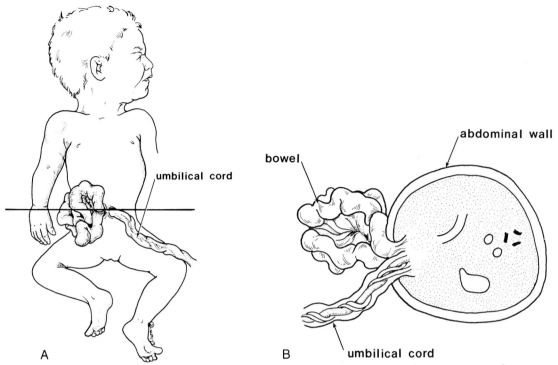

umbilical cord

bowel

abdominal wall

umbilical cord

A

B

Figure 10–1. Typical features of gastroschisis, shown on external examination *(A)* and on cross-sectional view *(B)*.

that the defect results from abnormal involution of the right umbilical vein, which normally occurs 28 to 33 days after conception (42 to 47 menstrual days).[6] Other authors suggest that the defect is caused by disruption of the omphalomesenteric artery.[24] A minority opinion suggests that gastroschisis represents an omphalocele that has ruptured before or during delivery.[25, 26] In any event, the defect of gastroschisis is sporadic, and no genetic association or recurrence risks have been described.

Anomalies other than bowel abnormalities rarely occur with gastroschisis. For example, cardiovascular malformations have been reported in 0 to 8 percent of fetuses with gastroschisis, compared with 20 to 40 percent of fetuses with an omphalocele.[5, 27] On the other hand, bowel abnormalities are much more common with gastroschisis. By definition, the small bowel is nonrotated and lacks secondary fixation to the dorsal abdominal wall. Intestinal atresia or stenosis occurs in 7 to 30 percent of cases and is thought to develop from intestinal and mesenteric ischemia caused by compression from the relatively small abdominal wall defect.[1, 2, 5, 28]

Survival of infants with gastroschisis has

steadily and dramatically improved during the last three decades.[1–5, 22, 29] Perinatal mortality was as high as 82 percent in 1960 but was less than 10 percent in 1984. This remarkable achievement can be attributed to improved perinatal management, including use of total parenteral nutrition and improved surgical technique. The greatest improvement has been shown in infants who weigh more than 2500 gm. The major causes of neonatal death today are prematurity, sepsis, and intestinal complications related to bowel ischemia.[1, 29]

The long-term outcome of survivors with gastroschisis is excellent. Infants tend to grow slowly during infancy but exhibit normal growth and development after 5 years of age.[30] Most patients remain asymptomatic, although some develop recurrent bowel obstruction or esophageal reflux. Infants with bowel atresia and infants who required small bowel resection during the neonatal period are more likely to develop these complications.

The essential sonographic features of gastroschisis are compared with those of omphalocele and the limb–body wall complex in Table 10–1. In gastroschisis, the full-thickness abdominal wall defect is located

Table 10–1. ESSENTIAL FEATURES OF GASTROSCHISIS, OMPHALOCELE, AND LIMB–BODY WALL COMPLEX (LBWC).

	Gastroschisis	Omphalocele	LBWC
Location	Right paraumbilical	Midline	Lateral
Umbilical cord site	Normal	Apex of defect	Involved in defect
Size of defect	Small (2–4 cm)	Large (2–10 cm)	Large
Membrane	No	Yes	Involved in defect
Liver involvement	Rare to never	Common	Common
Ascites	No	Common	Common
Bowel thickening	Common at term	Rarely (ruptured)	No
Bowel atresia	Common (15%)	Rare	Yes
Ischemia	Common (15%)	Rare	Rare
Cardiac anomalies	Rare (ASD, PDA)	Common (complex)	Common (complex)
Cranial anomalies	Rare	Occasionally (holoprosencephaly)	Common (encephalocele)
Limb anomalies	Rare	Occasionally	Common
Scoliosis	No	No	Common
Chromosomal abnormalities	No	Common (15%)	No

ASD, atrial septal defect; PDA, patent ductus arteriosus.

just to the right of a normal umbilical cord insertion site. Intra-abdominal organs protrude through the defect and are exposed to the surrounding amniotic fluid, Externalized structures appear disproportionately large relative to the small defect (Fig. 10–2). The most common extruded organs, in decreas-

ing order of frequency, include the small bowel, large bowel, stomach, genitourinary system, and, rarely, portions of the liver. The abdominal cavity is reduced in size, depending on the proportion of eviscerated structures. Polyhydramnios has been reported in less than one-half of the cases. As

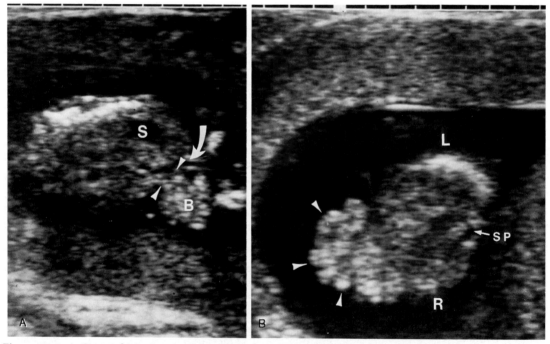

Figure 10–2. *A*, Gastroschisis. Longitudinal sonogram of the fetus at 16 weeks, performed because of an elevated maternal serum AFP level, shows bowel (B) herniated through a small abdominal wall defect *(arrowheads)* just to the right of the umbilical cord insertion site *(curved arrow)*. S, stomach. *B*, Transverse sonogram again shows bowel protruding through a right-sided abdominal wall defect and floating in the amniotic fluid. Note the absence of limiting membrane *(arrowheads)*. SP, spine; L, left; R, right.

concurrent anomalies are unusual, their presence should suggest a diagnosis other than gastroschisis, such as the amniotic band syndrome or the limb–body wall complex.[14, 15]

Although the reported accuracy of sonography for distinguishing gastroschisis from omphalocele varies, the authors believe that awareness of their respective findings permits an accurate diagnosis in nearly all cases. The distinction of gastroschisis from omphalocele may actually be easier by sonography than by clinical means, since the surrounding membrane of omphalocele may rupture during delivery[3] but rarely ruptures in utero. Rupture of omphaloceles during delivery may help explain why some cases of "gastroschisis" have been previously associated with chromosomal abnormalities (Trisomy 13 or 18) or externalized liver.[2, 25]

With increasing menstrual age, eviscerated bowel loops tend to appear thickened and matted on sonography (Fig. 10–3). Correspondingly, the bowel looks edematous and foreshortened at birth and is covered with a fibrinous peel on the serosal surface. This appearance is thought to represent a chemical peritonitis induced by fetal urine in the amniotic fluid,[31] and is the probable cause of the prolonged postoperative ileus experienced by many infants with gastroschisis. This fibrinous peel usually resolves within four weeks after surgical correction.[30]

Mild dilatation of both the small and large bowel is commonly seen sonographically (Fig. 10–3). However, marked bowel dilatation, which may be either external or internal to the abdominal cavity, may indicate bowel obstruction or ischemia (Fig. 10–4). Ischemia, which is thought to develop from compression of the bowel and mesentery through the relatively small abdominal wall defect, may lead to bowel atresia or stenosis, perforation, and gangrene (Fig. 10–5).[28] The importance of bowel ischemia to the clinical outcome of gastroschisis is emphasized by two large neonatal series of 170 cases in which half of the 23 infants who presented with ischemia or gangrene subsequently died.[1, 2]

Although the management of fetuses who are diagnosed with gastroschisis varies from institution to institution,[32] the authors have developed a successful approach based on their experience with 17 fetuses with gastroschisis who were evaluated during the last five years.[20] When the sonographic diagnosis of gastroschisis is certain, amniocentesis for chromosomal analysis is not indicated. Patients who elect to continue the pregnancy are followed with serial sonograms to evaluate fetal growth and to detect possible bowel complications. The infants are delivered at a referral center staffed with experienced surgeons to promptly correct these defects after delivery. Cesarean delivery is preferred because of the risk of contaminating eviscerated bowel through vaginal delivery;[1, 20] this is controversial, however.

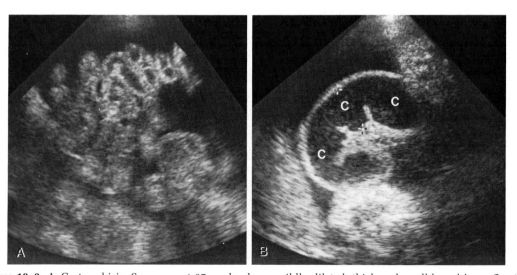

Figure 10–3. A, Gastroschisis. Sonogram at 37 weeks shows mildly dilated, thickened small bowel loops floating in the amniotic fluid. B, The same fetus shows a loop of mildly dilated colon (C) with haustral markings.

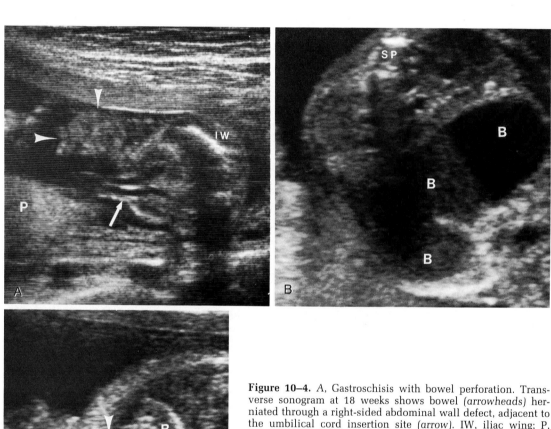

Figure 10–4. A, Gastroschisis with bowel perforation. Transverse sonogram at 18 weeks shows bowel (*arrowheads*) herniated through a right-sided abdominal wall defect, adjacent to the umbilical cord insertion site (*arrow*). IW, iliac wing; P, placenta. B, Repeat sonogram at 27 weeks shows a dilated bowel loop (B) with a fluid-debris layer, suggesting bowel obstruction. SP, spine. C, Follow-up sonogram four weeks later shows that the bowel loop (B) has decompressed. Multiple calcific foci (*arrowheads*) on the peritoneal surface of the bowel, and extending through the defect, suggest meconium peritonitis. At birth, meconium peritonitis, associated with multiple bowel perforations, was confirmed.

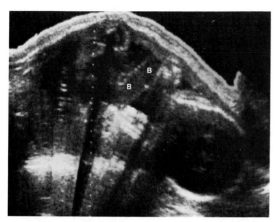

Figure 10–5. Gastroschisis with bowel infarction. Longitudinal sonogram at 34 weeks shows multiple dilated loops of small bowel (B) floating in the amniotic fluid. This proved to be infarcted bowel and contributed to intrauterine fetal demise, found one week later.

The abdominal wall defect should be repaired or covered as soon as possible after birth to minimize complications of bacterial contamination, sepsis, hypothermia, and metabolic acidosis. Primary closure of the abdominal wall defect is performed whenever possible, although staged reduction and closure of the defect by a Silastic prosthesis may be necessary for larger defects. At the authors' institution, primary repair of gastroschisis is usually accomplished within two hours of delivery. After surgery, infants are treated with parenteral nutrition until normal bowel function resumes. In most cases, the infants are discharged within four weeks after delivery.

Omphalocele

Omphalocele has a reported incidence of about one in 4000 births. An increased incidence has been observed with advancing maternal age.[20] Simply stated, omphalocele may be considered a persistence of the primitive body stalk that forms during early embryologic development but normally resolves by 12 weeks.[6] A midline defect of abdominal muscles, fascia, and skin at the umbilicus results in the herniation of intra-abdominal structures into the base of the umbilical cord. Unlike gastroschisis, the defect of omphalocele is limited by a "membrane" that is comprised of the intact peritoneum and amnion, separated by Wharton's jelly (Fig. 10–6).[6]

Omphalocele may be an isolated anomaly or may be associated with other major malformations. The overall reported frequency of associated anomalies ranges from 29 to 66 percent.[5, 20, 32] As with gastroschisis, malrotation or nonrotation of the bowel is present

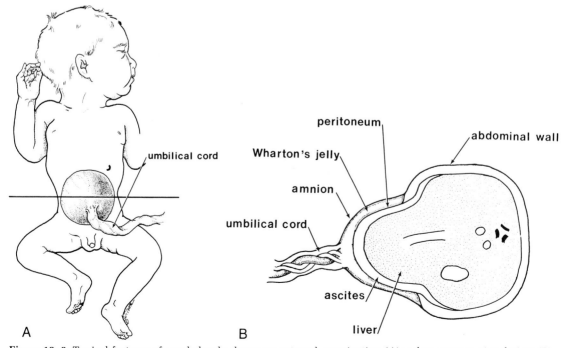

Figure 10–6. Typical features of omphalocele shown on external examination (A) and on cross-sectional view (B).

in almost all cases. Excluding bowel abnormalities, the most frequent associated anomalies involve the cardiovascular and genitourinary systems. Groups of severe anomalies may be categorized into recognized syndromes:

1. Pentalogy of Cantrell. This is characterized by a large upper abdominal omphalocele, an anterior diaphragmatic hernia, a sternal cleft, ectopia cordis, and a variety of cardiovascular malformations. Ventricular septal defect is the most common associated cardiac malformation, followed by tetralogy of Fallot.

2. Cloacal exstrophy. This consists of a low omphalocele, bladder or cloacal exstrophy, and frequently other caudal anomalies including anal atresia, spinal abnormalities or meningomyelocele, and lower limb anomalies.[11, 12] Most affected fetuses have a single umbilical artery.

3. Beckwith-Wiedemann syndrome. This autosomal dominant disorder may show an omphalocele (12 percent of cases) or an umbilical hernia, gigantism, macroglossia, and pancreatic hyperplasia (resulting in neonatal hypoglycemia).[33] Affected patients have an increased incidence of Wilms' tumors, renal anomalies, and hemihypertrophy.

4. Trisomy syndromes. Trisomies 13 to 15 and 16 to 18 and, less frequently, Trisomy 21 are associated with omphalocele.[33, 34] Approximately one-third of fetuses with Trisomy 13 and 10 to 50 percent of fetuses with Trisomy 18 will have an omphalocele.[33] Fetuses with an omphalocele and major concurrent anomalies, particularly cardiovascular and intracranial malformations, are likely to have a chromosomal abnormality.[19, 33]

The prognosis for fetuses with omphalocele depends primarily on the presence and severity of concurrent anomalies.[1, 21, 33] For this reason, the overall mortality rate for fetuses with omphaloceles during the last two decades (20 to 30 percent) has not improved as much as that for those with gastroschisis.[1, 3] If at least one other anomaly is present, perinatal mortality approaches 80 percent,[5, 35] whereas the presence of a chromosomal abnormality and a major cardiovascular malformation increases the mortality rate to nearly 100 percent.[19] When no other anomalies are present, however, the mortality rate drops to nearly 10 percent, which is similar to that for fetuses with gastroschisis.[5, 22, 33]

In addition to associated anomalies, the size of the defect and the number of eviscerated organs may also be of prognostic significance. Large defects have been associated

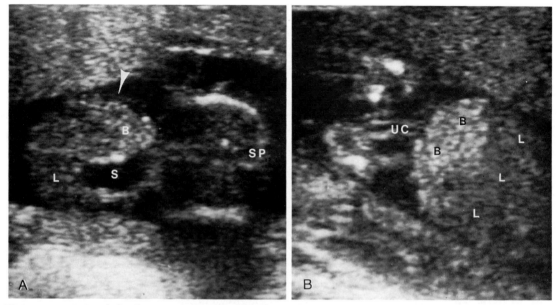

Figure 10–7. *A,* Omphalocele. Transverse sonogram at 16 weeks shows herniation of the liver (L), stomach (S), and small bowel (B) through a large midline abdominal defect. Note the presence of a surrounding membrane *(arrowhead).* Sp, spine. *B,* Slightly lower scan shows the umbilical cord (UC) inserting into the apex of the eviscerated structures. B, bowel; L, liver.

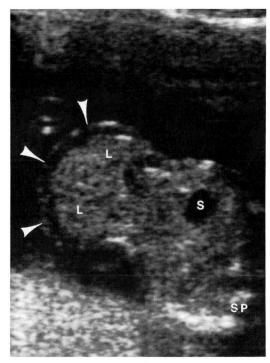

Figure 10–8. Omphalocele. Sonogram of another patient at 18 weeks better shows the membrane (arrowheads) surrounding the eviscerated liver (L) and a small amount of ascites. S, stomach; SP, spine.

with a higher mortality rate in some series[5] but not in others.[1, 33] More importantly than the absolute size of the defect, however, herniation of specific organs may adversely

affect outcome. For example, herniation of the spleen and heart have been associated with neonatal death in nearly all cases.[27] On the other hand, evisceration of the liver has been inconsistently associated with greater mortality.[27, 32]

Sonographically, an omphalocele appears as a midline abdominal wall defect, limited by a "membrane" (Figs. 10–7, 10–8). Occasionally, both components of the membrane (peritoneum and amnion) can be visualized, separated by tissue representing Wharton's jelly (Fig. 10–9). The surrounding membrane can sometimes be difficult to demonstrate, particularly in the presence of oligohydramnios or a large amount of ascites, in which case an omphalocele can be mistaken for gastroschisis (Fig. 10–10). Although rupture of the membrane has been reported in 10 to 20 percent of omphaloceles in clinical series,[3, 22, 33] this complication rarely occurs in utero.[26]

The presence of a limiting membrane in omphalocele ordinarily prevents bowel from being exposed to amniotic fluid. Hence, bowel does not become thickened or matted as in gastroschisis.[8, 31] The presence of a membrane also means that omphaloceles are more likely to be associated with normal maternal serum AFP levels than gastroschisis.

Ultrasonographers should be aware of the possibility of producing an appearance that

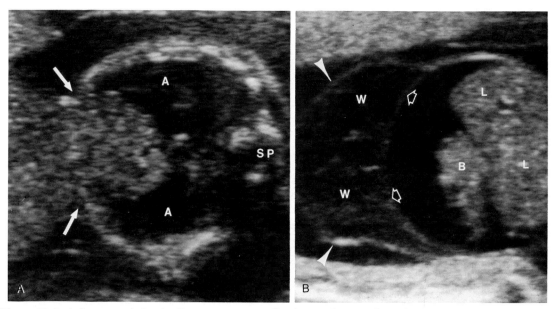

Figure 10–9. A, Large omphalocele. Sonogram at 22 weeks shows a large midline abdominal wall defect (arrows) with nearly complete evisceration of the abdominal organs. A, ascites; SP, spine. B, View of the eviscerated structures shows the liver (L), the bowel (B), and a large amount of ascites. Note that the covering membrane consists of both peritoneum (open arrows) and amnion (arrowheads), separated by Wharton's jelly (W).

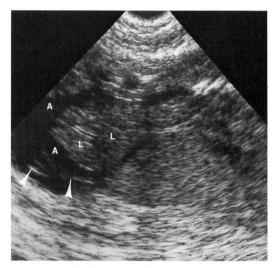

Figure 10–10. Omphalocele simulating gastroschisis. Sonogram at 26 weeks shows the liver (L) protruding from the fetal abdomen. Because of oligohydramnios and fetal ascites (A), this appearance could be mistakenly interpreted as gastroschisis. However, the presence of a surrounding membrane *(arrowheads)* helped confirm the diagnosis of omphalocele.

simulates an omphalocele by scanning in an oblique plane or by compressing the fetal abdomen (Fig. 10–11).[36, 37] Repeat scanning in a true transverse plane and using minimal compression should clarify any question of such a defect. Another potential pitfall in the diagnosis of an abdominal wall defect may occur during early pregnancy, between

six to 12 menstrual weeks, when bowel loops normally protrude into the base of the umbilical cord.[38] At this time, bowel grows faster than the abdominal cavity and so herniates into the base of the umbilical cord, where it undergoes a counterclockwise rotation. By 12 weeks, the bowel has re-entered the abdomen and has formed its normal adult configuration.[38]

The defect of omphalocele usually contains liver,[11] but smaller defects may contain bowel alone. Identification of eviscerated liver virtually always indicates that the abdominal wall defect represents an omphalocele and not gastroschisis. In one prenatal series, externalized liver was associated with an omphalocele in 13 of 14 cases.[8] In a larger clinical series, liver was herniated in 29 of 57 infants (51 percent) with omphalocele, compared with only three of 64 (5 percent) infants with gastroschisis who had only a portion of the liver "exposed" through the defect.[1]

A key distinguishing feature of omphalocele is the relationship of the umbilical cord insertion site to the abdominal wall defect. The umbilical cord inserts into the caudal-apical portion of the herniated sac. Demonstrating this relationship may be difficult on transverse scans alone, in which case sagittal or oblique scans may be helpful (Fig. 10–12). In one ultrasound series, the umbilical cord insertion site was shown in only 11 of

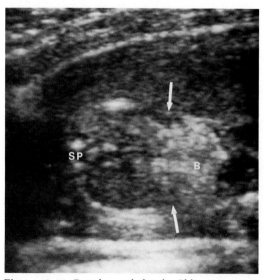

Figure 10–11. Pseudo-omphalocele. Oblique sonogram with compression, made at 16 weeks, produces an appearance that simulates an omphalocele *(arrows)*. SP, spine; B, bowel.

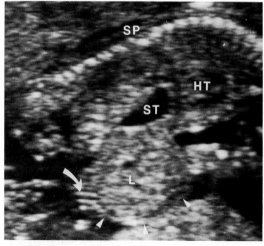

Figure 10–12. Omphalocele. Longitudinal sonogram at 17 weeks shows an omphalocele *(arrowheads)* containing liver (L). Note the umbilical cord insertion site at the caudal-apical portion of the eviscerated sac *(curved arrow)*. ST, stomach; HT, heart; SP, spine.

24 omphaloceles (46 percent).[8] Nevertheless, other features of an omphalocele (presence of a membrane, ascites, and herniation of the liver) usually permit a firm diagnosis without precise localization of the umbilical cord insertion site.

In addition to detection of omphaloceles, sonography can potentially identify major concurrent malformations. Cardiac anomalies, present in approximately 40 percent of fetuses with an omphalocele, are typically more complex and have a poorer prognosis than those occasionally seen in fetuses with gastroschisis (Fig. 10–13). Nevertheless, cardiac malformations may be difficult to identify during the second trimester. For these reasons, a careful fetal echocardiogram is recommended whenever an omphalocele is identified.[5] Cardiovascular malformations are more common in fetuses with Trisomy 18, whereas concurrent cranial malformations, particularly holoprosencephaly, suggest a diagnosis of Trisomy 13 (Fig. 10–14).[39]

The appropriate mode of delivery for fetuses who are found to have an omphalocele is controversial. Although an elective cesarean delivery has usually been the preferred mode of delivery, several authors have questioned the validity of this practice.[32, 35] Certainly when an omphalocele is associated with other major malformations, cesarean delivery may not be justifiable. However, when no other anomalies are present, prompt surgical repair has been reported to carry a low perinatal mortality rate. At the authors' institution, fetuses that are continued to term and are not associated with other anomalies are delivered by cesarean section to decrease the risk of infection and to avoid possible rupture of the sac during vaginal delivery. Following delivery, infants should undergo a thorough clinical examination and echocardiography. Infants who are thought to be suitable surgical candidates may then undergo surgical repair of the defect.

Amniotic Bands

The amniotic band syndrome (ABS) is a relatively common cause of defects involving the fetal abdominal wall and trunk, limbs, and craniofacial regions. Although the incidence of ABS has been reported to be as high as one in 1200 births, some of the previously reported cases may have represented more complex conditions, including the limb–body wall complex. The ABS is thought to be caused by rupture of the am-

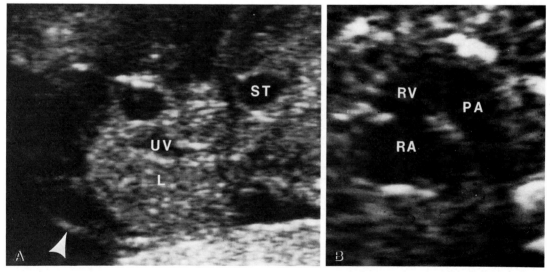

Figure 10–13. A, Omphalocele with complex cardiac malformation. Transverse sonogram of the abdomen at 20 weeks shows characteristic findings of omphalocele, including an eviscerated liver (L) and a surrounding membrane (arrowhead). UV, umbilical vein; ST, stomach (displaced anteriorly). B, Oblique sonogram of the heart shows an enlarged right atrium (RA) and right ventricle (RV) and marked dilatation of the pulmonary artery (PA). The left atrium and ventricle were markedly hypoplastic. A hypoplastic left heart was confirmed at autopsy. Chromosomal analysis was normal (46 XX).

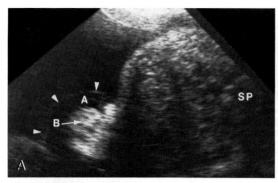

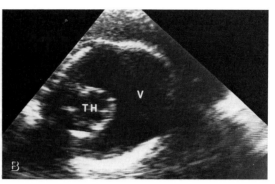

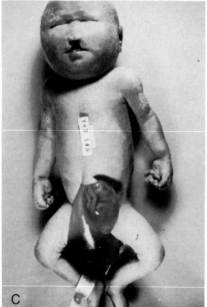

Figure 10–14. *A,* Trisomy 13. Transverse sonogram of the abdomen at 31 weeks shows an omphalocele containing bowel (B) but not liver. Note the presence of ascites (A) and a surrounding membrane *(arrowheads).* SP, spine. *B,* Transverse sonogram of the cranium shows characteristic findings of alobar holoprosencephaly, including the fused central thalami (TH), a single surrounding ventricle (V), and the absence of the falx and midline structures. *C,* Photograph of the fetal specimen, following neonatal death, confirms an omphalocele containing bowel and ascites. Also note the typical facial features of alobar holoprosencephaly, including hypotelorism and facial cleft. *(From* Nyberg DA, Mack LA, Bronstein A, et al: Holoprosencephaly: Prenatal sonographic diagnosis. AJNR 149:1051, 1987.)

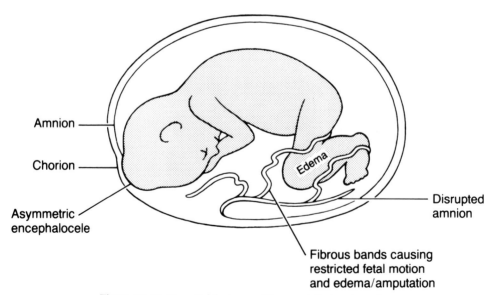

Figure 10–15. Essential features of the amniotic band syndrome.

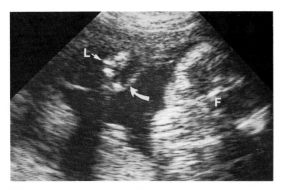

Figure 10–16. Amniotic band syndrome. Sonogram shows a fetal limb (L) trapped behind the amniotic membrane *(arrow)*. F, fetus. At birth, multiple anomalies were noted, including amniotic band, stricture of the left ankle, imperforate anus, and ambiguous genitalia. Chromosomal analysis revealed a normal male karyotype.

nion, leading to subsequent entanglement of fetal parts by the more "sticky" chorion (Fig. 10–15). Torpin, who first proposed this hypothesis, also suggested that the amnion normally protects the fetus from contact with the chorion.[40] Entrapment of fetal parts may cause amputation or slash defects in random sites, unrelated to embryologic development. Since development of amniotic bands is a sporadic event, there is no recurrence risk to subsequent pregnancies.

Although the sonographic findings of the ABS are variable, certain types of defects are characteristic of this disorder. Involvement of the abdominal wall can produce an appearance similar to gastroschisis. However, an atypical location of the defect or liver evisceration, which rarely occurs from simple gastroschisis, should suggest the diagnosis of ABS. The presence of both gastroschisis and other defects, such as an encephalocele, a facial cleft, or amputated fingers, also should strongly suggest the diagnosis of ABS.[14] Identification of a membrane contiguous with such a defect establishes the diagnosis of ABS (Fig. 10–16) or the limb–body wall complex.

Limb–Body Wall Complex

The limb–body wall complex (LBWC) is a complicated fetal malformation that is characterized by neural tube defects, lateral body wall defects, limb defects, and scoliosis. Owing to the severity of defects incompatible with extrauterine life, it is important to distinguish the LBWC from other types of abdominal wall defects.

The pathogenesis of the LBWC is uncertain. Some researchers have suggested that the primary defect involves body stalk dysmorphogenesis. Smith and others have suggested that the LBWC results from rupture of the amnion through vascular disruption or mechanical compression between the third and fifth weeks.[41] Still others consider the LBWC to simply represent a severe form

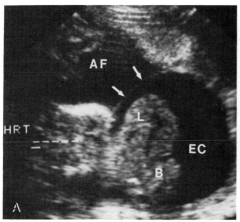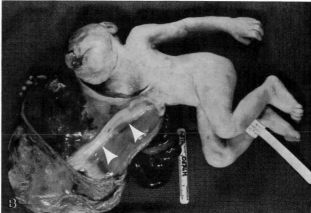

Figure 10–17. *A,* Limb–body wall complex. Transverse sonogram at the level of the thoracoabdominal junction demonstrates a large defect with extrusion of bowel (B) and liver (L) into the extraembryonic coelom (EC). Note the continuity of the amniotic membrane *(arrows)* with the body wall defect. AF, amniotic fluid; HRT, heart. *B,* Photograph of the fetal specimen shows the thoracoabdominal defect, facial cleft, and encephalocele. Note the umbilical cord *(arrowheads)* incorporated into the abnormal amniotic membrane. (*From Patten RM, Van Allen M, Mack LA, et al: Limb–body wall complex: In utero sonographic diagnosis of a complicated fetal malformation. AJR 146:1019. 1986. Copyright 1986, The American Roentgen Ray Society.)*

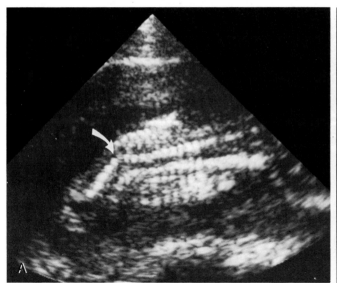
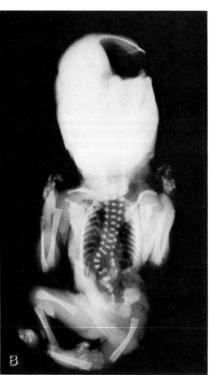

Figure 10–18. *A*, Limb–body wall complex. Coronal sonogram of the fetal spine shows abrupt and severe scoliosis *(arrow)*. *B*, Radiograph of the fetal specimen shows scoliosis, limb defects, and a slash defect of the cranium. (*From* Patten RM, Van Allen M, Mack LA, et al: Limb–body wall complex: In utero sonographic diagnosis of a complicated fetal malformation. AJR 146:1019, 1986. *Copyright* 1986, The American Roentgen Ray Society.)

of the ABS, although this does not entirely explain the presence of certain associated anomalies, such as the frequent occurrence of a single umbilical artery. Whatever its pathogenesis, it is clear that the LBWC is a sporadic event without sex or familial predilection or known recurrence risks. Karyotypes have also been normal in all reported cases.

The main features of the LBWC can be recognized on prenatal sonography. In a recent sonographic review of 13 fetuses with the LBWC, fetal trunk defects were seen in 12 cases (92 percent).[14] The defect may involve the thorax, abdomen, or both (Fig. 10–17). Abdominal and thoracic contents herniate through this defect into the extraembryonic coelom. Typically, the eviscerated organs form a complex bizarre-appearing mass entangled with membranes. Fetal membranes are contiguous with the body wall or neural tube defect. Cranial defects (anencephaly and encephalocele) are also common and were present in six cases in this series.[14] Spinal anomalies, including spinal dysraphic defects and scoliosis (which is often severe), are present in nearly all cases (Fig. 10–18). Distorted fetal position and the severity of the defects makes recog-

nition of normal fetal parts difficult. Specific limb anomalies may also be difficult to recognize, even though they are usually present on pathologic examination.

References

1. Mabogunje OOA, Mahour GH: Omphalocele and gastroschisis: Trends in survival across two decades. Am J Surg 148:679, 1984.
2. Luck SR, Sherman J, Raffensperger JG, Goldstein IR: Gastroschisis in 106 consecutive newborn infants. Surgery 98:677, 1985.
3. Martin LW, Torres AM: Omphalocele and gastroschisis. Symposium on pediatric surgery. Surg Clin North Am 65:1235, 1985.
4. King DR, Savrin R, Boles ET Jr: Gastroschisis update. J Pediatr Surg 15:553, 1980.
5. Mayer T, Black R, Matlak ME, Johnson DG: Gastroschisis and omphalocele. Ann Surg 192:783, 1980.
6. DeVries PA: The pathogenesis of gastroschisis and omphalocele. J Pediatr Surg 15:245, 1980.
7. Redford DH, McNay MB, Whittle MJ: Gastroschisis and exomphalos: Precise diagnosis by midpregnancy ultrasound. Br J Obstet Gynaecol 92:54, 1985.
8. Bair JH, Russ PD, Pretorius DH, et al: Fetal omphalocele and gastroschisis: A review of 24 cases. AJR 147:1047, 1986.
9. Osborne J: Gastroschisis and omphalocele. Prenatal ultrasonic detection and its significance. Australas Radiol 30:113, 1986.

10. Brown BSJ: The prenatal ultrasonographic features of omphalocele: A study of 10 patients. J Can Assoc Radiol 36:312, 1985.

11. Meizner I, Bar-Ziv J: In utero prenatal ultrasound diagnosis of a rare case of cloacal exstrophy. J Clin Ultrasound 13:500, 1985.

12. Mirk P, Calisti A, Fileni A: Prenatal sonographic diagnosis of bladder exstrophy. J Ultrasound Med 5:291, 1986.

13. Haynor DR, Shuman WP, Brewer DR, Mack LA: Imaging of fetal ectopia cordis: Role of sonography and computed tomography. J Ultrasound Med 3:25, 1984.

14. Mahony BS, Filly RA, Callen PW, Golbus MS: The amniotic band syndrome: Antenatal diagnosis and potential pitfalls. Am J Obstet Gynecol 152:63, 1985.

15. Patten RM, Van Allen M, Mack LA, et al: Limb–body wall complex: In utero sonographic diagnosis of a complicated fetal malformation. AJR 146:1019, 1986.

16. Giulian BB, Alvear DT: Prenatal ultrasonographic diagnosis of fetal gastroschisis. Radiology 129:473, 1978.

17. Cameron GM, McQuown DS, Modanlou HD, et al: Intrauterine diagnosis of an omphalocele by diagnostic ultrasonography. Am J Obstet Gynecol 131:821, 1978.

18. Dibbins AW, Curci MR, McCrann DJ Jr: Prenatal diagnosis of congenital anomalies requiring surgical correction. Am J Surg 149:528, 1985.

19. Crawford DC, Chapman MG, Allan LD: Echocardiography in the investigation of anterior abdominal wall defects in the fetus. Br J Obstet Gynaecol 92:1034, 1985.

20. Lenke RR, Hatch EI: Fetal gastroschisis: A preliminary report advocating the use of cesarean section. Obstet Gynecol 67:395, 1986.

21. Grosfeld JL, Dawes L, Weber TR: Congenital abdominal wall defects: Current management and survival. Surg Clin North Am 61:1037, 1981.

22. Schwaitzenberg SD, Pokorny WJ, McGill CW, Harberg FJ: Gastroschisis and omphalocele. Am J Surg 144:650, 1982.

23. Fink IJ, Filly RA: Omphalocele associated with umbilical cord allantoic cyst: Sonographic evaluation in utero. Radiology 149:473, 1983.

24. Hoyme HE, Higginbottom MC, Jones KL: The vascular pathogenesis of gastroschisis: Intrauterine interruption of the omphalomesenteric artery. J Pediatrics 98:228, 1981.

25. Shaw A: The myth of gastroschisis. J Pediatr Surg 10:235, 1975.

26. Glick PL, Harrison MR, Adzick S, et al: The missing link in the pathogenesis of gastroschisis. J Pediatr Surg 20:406, 1985.

27. Sermer M, Benzie RJ, Pitson L, et al: Prenatal diagnosis and management of congenital defects of the anterior abdominal wall. Am J Obstet Gynecol 156:308, 1987.

28. Tibboel D, Raine M, McNee M, et al: Developmental aspects of gastroschisis. J Pediatr Surg 21:865, 1986.

29. Stringel G, Filler RM: Prognostic factors in omphalocele and gastroschisis. J Pediatr Surg 14:515, 1979.

30. Swartz KR, Harrison MW, Campbell JR, Campbell TJ: Long-term follow-up of patients with gastroschisis. Am J Surg 151:546, 1986.

31. Kluck P, Tibboel D, Van Der Kamp AWM, Molenaar JC: The effect of fetal urine on the development of bowel in gastroschisis. J Ped Surg 18:47, 1983.

32. Kirk EP, Wah R: Obstetric management of the fetus with omphalocele or gastroschisis: A review and report of one hundred twelve cases. Am J Obstet Gynecol 146:512, 1983.

33. Knight PJ, Sommer A, Clatworthy HW: Omphalocele: A prognostic classification. J Ped Surg 16:599, 1981.

34. Hauge M, Bugge M, Nielsen J: Early prenatal diagnosis of omphalocele constitutes indication for amniocentesis. Lancet 2:507, 1983.

35. Hasan S, Hermansen MC: The prenatal diagnosis of ventral abdominal wall defects. Am J Obstet Gynecol 155:842, 1986.

36. Salzman L, Kuligowska E, Semine A: Pseudoomphalocele: Pitfall in fetal sonography. AJR 146:1283, 1986.

37. Lindfors KK, McGahan JP, Walter JP: Fetal omphalocele and gastroschisis: Pitfalls in sonographic diagnosis. AJR 147:797, 1986.

38. Cyr DR, Mack LA, Schoenecker SA, et al: Bowel migration in the normal fetus: US detection. Radiology 161:119, 1986.

39. Nyberg DA, Mack LA, Bronstein A, et al: Holoprosencephaly: Prenatal sonographic diagnosis. AJNR 149:1051, 1987.

40. Torpin R: Fetal Malformations: Caused by Amnion Rupture During Gestation. Springfield, IL, Charles C Thomas, 1968, pp 1–76.

41. Smith DW: Recognizable Patterns of Human Malformation, 3rd Ed. Philadelphia, WB Saunders Co, 1981, pp 488–496.

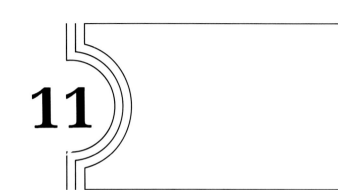

THE GENITOURINARY SYSTEM

Barry S. Mahony, M.D.

Before the advent of sonography, attempts to outline the fetal genitourinary (GU) system were so frequently unrewarding that diagnosis of abnormalities typically did not take place until after birth. Antenatal ultrasonography has now revolutionized the assessment of the GU system. It readily demonstrates the normal GU system and enables accurate identification and characterization of numerous fetal urinary tract abnormalities. Furthermore, ultrasound may provide functional information about the fetal kidneys. The information pertaining to fetal GU anomalies yielded by antenatal sonography, therefore, often dramatically alters obstetric and neonatal management.

Fetal GU lesions, most of which are cystic or obstructive, constitute the major cause of neonatal abdominal masses. Because ultrasound can reliably detect and accurately depict fluid-filled pathologic lesions as small as 1 to 2 mm in utero, careful evaluation of the fetal abdomen will identify many GU abnormalities. Significant diminution or absence of amniotic fluid heralds the presence of the many lethal GU abnormalities and alerts the sonographer to examine this system carefully. Since many fetal GU anomalies are discovered as incidental findings, however, only a complete fetal ultrasound examination will reveal most of these diagnostically important defects that would otherwise go undetected until later in life.

Following detection of a fetal GU anomaly, thorough evaluation of each of the components of the GU system often enables an accurate antenatal diagnosis. Knowledge of the normal sonographic appearance of the fetal GU system and of the expected sonographic features of the different anomalies assists in this task. The antenatal sonographic detection of fetal GU anomalies alerts the parents, obstetrician, urologist, and pediatrician to potential problems and assists them in prompt efficacious postnatal management.[1] In addition, antenatal sonography may help in the selection of which fetuses might benefit from in utero diversion of significant obstructive urinary tract lesions.[2-4] For all these reasons, every second or third trimester obstetric ultrasound should include assessment of amniotic fluid volume, documentation of the fetal urinary bladder, and evaluation of the fetal kidneys.[5]

THE NORMAL URINARY TRACT

At approximately six menstrual weeks, the ureteral bud begins as an out-pouching of the mesonephric (wolffian) duct from the urogenital sinus.[6] Several days later, the caudal part of the urogenital sinus, called the cloaca, narrows and elongates to form the urethra and the neck of the bladder. The remainder of the bladder derives from the allantois, which ends as the urachus, extending anteriorly to the umbilicus. The ureteral bud grows and branches in a dichotomous pattern for 15 generations and becomes the ureter, renal pelvis, calyces, and collecting tubules. Through interaction with the metanephric blastema, the ureteral bud also plays a crucial role in nephron induction; without a ureteral bud, the kidney will not develop.[7] Nephrons first appear at approximately ten menstrual weeks, after three to five branchings of the ureteral bud. Urine formation begins early in the second trimester of pregnancy when ultrasound first detects fluid in the urinary bladder. Before 16 menstrual weeks, the kidneys contribute little tó amniotic fluid dynamics, but their role becomes increasingly important such that in the second half of gestation, fetal urination produces most of the amniotic fluid.[8]

An assessment of the quantity of amniotic fluid correlated with menstrual age, therefore, constitutes the initial step in the evaluation of the fetal urinary tract (Fig. 11–1). Although before 16 menstrual weeks a normal amount of amniotic fluid may be present in the absence of renal function, a normal amount of amniotic fluid in the second half of gestation implies at least one functioning kidney, especially in the absence of features that would otherwise lead to polyhydramnios, i.e., central nervous system anomalies or upper gastrointestinal obstruction. Conversely, decreased amniotic fluid volume in the absence of other common causative factors (fetal demise, growth retardation, rupture of the membranes, or post-term gestation) must alert the sonographer to search diligently for urinary tract anomalies.

The factors that regulate the dynamics of amniotic fluid volume remain incompletely understood.[9] Nevertheless, the author employs the following fairly subjective guidelines in the sonographic assessment of diminished amniotic fluid volume. Near the end of the second trimester, the volume occupied by the fetus approximates that of the amniotic fluid; the fetus occupies relatively less volume before that time and relatively more as gestation progresses. Determination of mild diminution in amniotic fluid volume is especially subjective, but significant alterations from the normal amount are readily apparent. Significant diminution of amniotic fluid volume typically compresses and crowds the fetus, restricting its motion. Oligohydramnios in the second trimester carries a very poor prognosis because of the associated pulmonary hypoplasia.[10]

Although the variations in fetal positioning and the lack of contrast between kidney and surrounding tissues occasionally do not permit identification of both fetal kidneys, normal ones often become visible in their paraspinous location as early as 14 menstrual weeks. Depending upon fetal positioning, sonography clearly defines at least 90

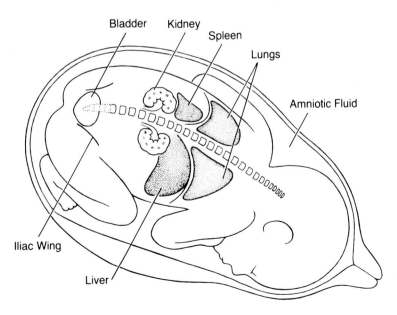

Figure 11–1. Normal renal function permits adequate amniotic fluid volume and normal lung development. The normal kidney spans approximately four to five vertebrae in length, even in utero, when its proportions approximate those of the adult.

percent of fetal kidneys by approximately 20 menstrual weeks.[11] Longitudinally, the kidneys exhibit an elliptical shape, and in transverse section, they have a circular appearance, adjacent to the lumbar spinal ossification centers. As gestation progresses, echogenic retroperitoneal fat surrounding the kidneys delineates their outlines clearly, and the echogenic central sinus becomes apparent.[12] The hypoechoic fetal renal pyramids orient in anterior and posterior rows, in a configuration corresponding to the calyces around the central sinus (Fig. 11–2). The relative hypoechoic intensity of the renal pyramids contrasts with the echotexture of the normal fetal renal cortex, which usually approximates or may even be slightly greater than that of the surrounding tissues. Identification of the characteristic configuration of the pyramids in anterior and posterior rows permits positive identification of the kidney and avoids any potential confusion between renal pyramids and parenchymal cysts.

Standard measurements for renal circumference, volume, thickness, width, and length have been reported as a function of menstrual age.[13-15] These measurements increase throughout gestation and correspond with those of renal size obtained on stillborn fetuses postnatally. Renal length and anteroposterior diameter represent the technically easiest measurements of renal size to obtain. A good rule of thumb is that the menstrual age in weeks approximates the normal fetal kidney length in millimeters or twice the anteroposterior diameter in millimeters. The ratio of kidney circumference to abdominal circumference remains constant at 0.27 to 0.33 throughout pregnancy but is technically more difficult to obtain and reproduce. Significant deviation from this pattern (in the absence of ascites or other rarer causes of abdominal circumference enlargement) enables antenatal detection of renal enlargement. Diminution in renal size may be more difficult to detect because the exact renal border may be hard to discern.

Nondilated fetal ureters are not routinely visualized. However, sonography readily identifies a dilated ureter. A useful guideline in identification of the fetal urinary tract and differentiation between it and other abdominal structures is the following: an abdominal structure or mass that touches the fetal spine most likely originates within the retroperitoneal urinary tract. This rule holds true in correct identification of ureters, kidneys, and abnormal perirenal masses (urinomas). One should beware of the normal hypoechoic psoas muscle that touches the spine and may occasionally mimic a distended ureter. Observation of its characteristic location and triangular configuration should avoid any confusion with a distended ureter.

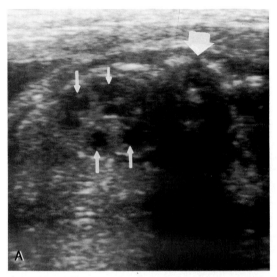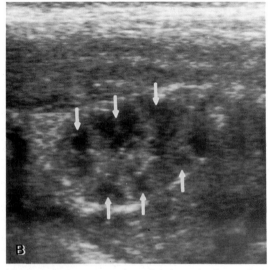

Figure 11–2. Transverse and sagittal sonograms of the fetal kidney at 37 menstrual weeks show the hypoechoic pyramids arranged in anterior and posterior rows *(arrows)*. This constitutes positive identification of the kidneys. *Wide arrow,* spine.

Shortly after the commencement of fetal urine production, ultrasound visualizes fluid within the fetal urinary bladder. The normal bladder has a very thin or virtually invisible wall and occupies an anterior midline position within the fetal pelvis. When distended, the urinary bladder becomes spherical or elliptical in configuration. Changes in volume over time differentiate the urinary bladder from other cystic pelvic structures. The fetus normally fills and empties the bladder every 30 to 45 minutes. During the course of a sonographic examination, therefore, the bladder may increase in size and empty. At term, the maximal normal bladder volume is approximately 40 ml.[16] Fetal urinary production, calculated by the change in bladder volume over time, increases from 9.6 ml/hr at 30 weeks to 27.3 ml/hr at term but may vary in a normal circadian rhythm.[17, 18] Visualization of filling and emptying of the fetal bladder confirms that the fetus produces urine but does not indicate the quality of urine produced.

The nondilated urethra is difficult to detect in females, and in males is imaged at a time when the penis is flaccid but appears as an echogenic line extending the length of an erect penis. After 20 menstrual weeks, the pulsating dorsal arteries of the penis can occasionally be seen. Sonography may also detect streaming of urine into the amniotic fluid during voiding.

URINARY TRACT ABNORMALITIES

Congenital malformations of the urinary tract occur with high frequency, probably because of the complicated embryologic development of this organ system. The sonographer plays a crucial role in the evaluation of the fetal urinary tract by detecting, localizing, and characterizing the severity of anomalies in an attempt to predict prognosis and to optimize perinatal management.

Fortunately, only a limited range of urinary tract anomalies manifest in utero. Although the underlying etiology of many urinary tract abnormalities remains uncertain, knowledge of the basic embryology of the urogenital sinus and of the dichotomous branching pattern of the ureteral bud provides a developmental model that renders understanding of seemingly diverse morpho-logic abnormalities relatively straightforward.[7]

The vast majority of primary urinary tract abnormalities manifest in utero, including (1) renal agenesis or severe hypoplasia; (2) urethral level obstruction; (3) ureterovesical junction (UVJ) obstruction, usually with a duplex collecting system; (4) primary megaureter; (5) ureteropelvic junction (UPJ) obstruction; (6) multicystic dysplastic kidney, either global or segmental; (7) autosomal recessive (infantile) polycystic kidney disease; and (8) rare renal tumors (mesoblastic nephroma). One can view urethral level obstruction as a cloacal abnormality, and each of the others as anomalous development of the ureteral bud system. Secondary manifestations of these primary abnormalities often dominate the sonographic features, including renal parenchymal cysts, urinary ascites, and paranephric urinomas from obstructive uropathy. Other rare in utero urinary tract manifestations might include megacalyces, autosomal dominant (adult type) polycystic kidney disease, medullary sponge kidney, simple renal cyst, or metabolic storage diseases such as tyrosinosis or glycogen storage disease.

A systematic approach to the abnormal urinary tract will most often permit accurate antenatal diagnosis and assessment of prognosis. This approach includes (1) assessment of the appropriateness of amniotic fluid volume, (2) localization and characterization of urinary tract abnormalities, and (3) search for associated abnormalities. Oligohydramnios during the second trimester, either from decreased urinary production or decreased egress of urine into the amniotic fluid, carries a very poor prognosis.[10] Conversely, normal amniotic fluid volume in the setting of a urinary tract abnormality typically signifies a good prognosis, although the urinary tract finding warrants follow-up.[19] Polyhydramnios in association with a urinary tract anomaly characteristically occurs with a mesoblastic nephroma or with associated abnormalities of the central nervous system or gastrointestinal tract.[20–22] Occasionally and paradoxically, polyhydramnios may occur with incomplete obstruction at the level of the UPJ, which presumably impairs the renal concentrating ability and leads to increased renal output.[23] Isolated mesoblastic nephroma or UPJ obstruction has a good prognosis; the prognosis for cases with concomitant abnormalities varies depending on the associated findings.

Assessment of unilaterality or bilaterality and of symmetry of urinary tract involvement also assists in prediction of diagnosis and, occasionally, of prognosis. Unilateral disease occurs at or proximal to the ureteral bud and has a good prognosis. Bilateral but asymmetric disease implies either involvement at the level of the cloaca (urethral level) or asymmetric ureteral bud abnormality with obstruction or reflux. Bilateral symmetric disease often heralds a genetic abnormality (autosomal recessive polycystic kidney disease) or other severe abnormalities involving both ureteral bud systems (bilateral multicystic dysplastic kidney or renal agenesis). In cases of urinary tract dilatation, determination of distribution and degree of dilatation helps to localize and assess the severity of the disease.[24, 25] Even in the absence of dilatation, observation of bladder wall abnormalities (thickening or calcification), renal size and echogenicity, or focal parenchymal cysts provides very helpful diagnostic and prognostic information, as delineated subsequently.[4, 26] Finally, detection of certain urinary tract abnormalities may herald the presence of other abnormalities or syndromes, such as clubfoot, encephalocele (Meckel's syndrome with cystic kidneys), or VACTERL (Vertebral, Anal, Cardiac, TracheoEsophageal fistula, Renal, and Limb) abnormalities.

Renal Agenesis

Absence of ureteral bud formation occurs in approximately one in 4000 births and causes bilateral renal agenesis and death from pulmonary hypoplasia.[27, 28] The lack of urine production results in severe oligohydramnios and absence of a demonstrable urinary bladder, the only constant sonographic features of this uniformly lethal entity (Figs. 11–3, 11–4). A small midline urachal diverticulum may mimic the bladder, but its lack of filling and emptying distinguishes it from the bladder. Identification of a normal bladder excludes this diagnosis. Nonvisualization of the bladder is more significant than apparent visualization of the kidneys because, in renal agenesis, the adrenal glands may assume an oval or reniform shape, or bowel in the renal fossae may simulate kidneys.[29] The most reliable feature that discriminates a kidney from bowel or an adrenal gland is identification of hypoechoic medullary pyramids. Bilateral severe renal hypoplasia exhibits a similar clinical course and similar sonographic features to that of renal agenesis, although the small kidneys may be identified.

When one does not visualize the fetal urinary bladder over a period of approximately two hours, 30 to 60 mg of furosemide may be given intravenously to the mother. This may induce fetal diuresis and the subsequent appearance of urine in the bladder

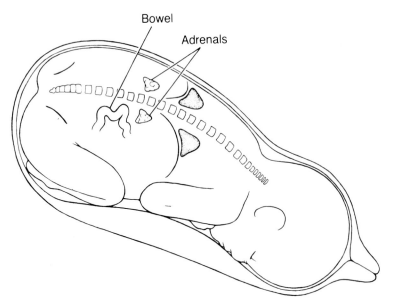

Figure 11–3. Bilateral renal agenesis or severe hypoplasia results in severe oligohydramnios, pulmonary hypoplasia, Potter's facies, and contractures. Bowel or adrenals in the renal fossa should not be mistaken for kidneys.

Figure 11–4. Scans of a fetus with bilateral renal agenesis demonstrate severe oligohydramnios in the second trimester as well as the absence of urinary bladder visualization, even following maternal administration of furosemide. The lack of visualization of the fetal kidneys represents an unreliable sign of renal agenesis. *Curved arrow,* fetal pelvis; *straight arrow,* fetal head; S, spine; Bl, maternal urinary bladder.

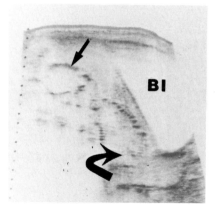
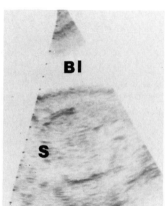

about 15 to 45 minutes after administration;[30] if this occurs, the fetus can produce urine, and bilateral renal agenesis is excluded. Conversely, absence of urine in the fetal bladder following furosemide challenge is *not* a reliable indicator of bilateral renal agenesis. For example, severe intrauterine growth retardation with normal postnatal renal function may produce identical sonographic findings.[31, 32] As a result, this test has recently fallen out of favor.

Unilateral renal agenesis occurs four times more commonly than does bilateral agenesis.[29] This can be a very difficult diagnosis to confirm antenatally because the adrenal or bowel in the renal fossa may simulate the kidney. Nevertheless, the bladder fills and empties normally, and unilateral renal agenesis has a good prognosis. Crossed renal ectopia occurs less frequently (one in 7000) but may mimic unilateral renal agenesis. In crossed-fused ectopia, the ectopic kidney is abnormally large and bilobed, unlike the contralateral kidney in unilateral agenesis.[33] Compensatory contralateral renal hyperplasia does not occur with unilateral renal agenesis in utero. Renal ectopia may cause obstructive uropathy or reflux and may accompany other cardiovascular or gastrointestinal anomalies.

Urinary Tract Dilatation

Dilatation of the fetal urinary tract frequently, but not necessarily, signifies obstruction.[24, 25, 34, 35] Conversely, a fetus can have obstructive uropathy in the absence of urinary tract dilatation.[26, 36] Nevertheless, after 19 weeks, measurements of the anteroposterior diameter of the fetal renal pelvis (PD) and of the kidney (KD) and assessment of the degree of calyectasis provide important clinical information that often permits early and effective postnatal surgical reconstruction. A fluid-filled PD measuring less than 5 mm occurs frequently and is probably physiologic.[37] High levels of circulating maternal hormones, resulting in relaxation of the smooth muscle of the urinary tract, both fetal and maternal, may be the predominant factor leading to this finding. A PD of 5 to 9 mm and a PD to KD ratio of less than 50 percent in the absence of rounded calyces also is probably physiologic and rarely progresses (Fig. 11–5).[24, 25] For example, Grignon and associates reported that only one in 29 fetuses had a mild UPJ obstruction and did not require postnatal therapy.[25] On the other hand, a PD of more than 10 to 15 mm with a PD/KD of more than 50 percent and with rounded calyces represents significant pelvocalyectasis that rarely regresses, often progresses, and frequently requires surgical management.[25] Even when the PD/KD is less than 50 percent, rounded calyces usually indicate hydronephrosis.[23]

When antenatal sonography demonstrates unequivocal pelvocalyectasis, a normal neonatal ultrasound in the first 48 hours after birth should not alter this assessment. Confirmation of in utero findings at five to seven days post partum avoids the confusion introduced by the dehydration typically present in the first 48 hours after birth.[38] Although urinary tract dilatation may occur with reflux, nonobstructive megacystis, or megacalyces, it almost always implies an intrinsic GU abnormality. Hydrocolpos or other pelvic masses, e.g., intrapelvic sacrococcygeal

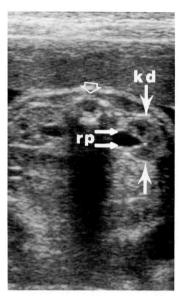

Figure 11–5. Transverse sonogram of the fetal kidneys in the third trimester shows bilateral fluid-filled renal pelves measuring 5 to 9 mm in anteroposterior diameter with a pelvic diameter/kidney diameter of less than 50 percent. In the absence of calyectasis, this degree of pelvic distention is probably physiologic and rarely progresses. *Open arrow*, spine; rp, renal pelvis; kd, kidney diameter. (Courtesy of Peter W Callen, MD, University of California, San Francisco, CA.)

teratoma, represent rare causes for urinary tract obstruction and dilatation.[39–41]

Urethral Level Obstruction.[26] Distal urinary tract obstruction, most commonly from posterior urethral valves, produces a variable and often insidious clinical presentation. Nevertheless, antenatal diagnosis followed by prompt postnatal therapy improves the outcome in many cases, and some fetuses may benefit from in utero diversion of the obstructed urinary tract.[1, 42–44]

Urethral level obstruction produces a broad spectrum of sonographic features antenatally, but the cardinal signs include (1) persistent dilatation of the urinary bladder and proximal urethra and (2) thickening of the bladder wall (Figs. 11–6, 11–7).[26] Documentation of the dilated proximal urethra, which resembles a keyhole extending from the bladder toward the fetal perineum, constitutes convincing (but not always demonstrable) evidence of urethral obstruction. A dilated urinary bladder fills the true pelvis (and frequently extends into the false pelvis and abdomen) and does not empty during the course of the examination. Since the normal urinary bladder wall is almost im-

perceptibly thin, a pathologically thickened bladder wall has a finite thickness of more than approximately 2 mm. In fetuses with urethral obstruction but a nondilated bladder, the bladder wall characteristically thickens to approximately 10 to 15 mm.

When considering the diagnosis of urethral level obstruction, the sonographer should examine the fetal perineum to determine the sex. Documentation of male external genitalia provides strong evidence that the urethral level obstruction results from posterior urethral valves. If male genitalia cannot be documented in fetuses with massive distention of the urinary bladder, one must consider caudal regression anomaly, urethral atresia, or megacystis intestinal hypoperistalsis syndrome. Each of these occurs in either gender, but the latter occurs more commonly in females. In such cases, and in fetuses with posterior urethral valves, the urethral level obstruction may dilate the

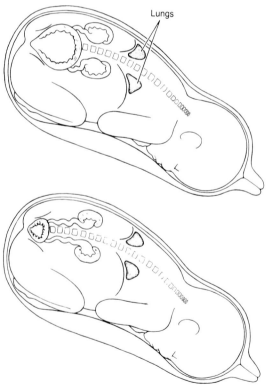

Figure 11–6. Although the sonographic features of urethral level obstruction vary, the cardinal signs include a thick-walled, dilated bladder and a dilated proximal urethra. The degree of pelvocalyectasis, ureterectasis, and megacystis varies and may be mild. Oligohydramnios, when present, leads to pulmonary hypoplasia and a poor prognosis.

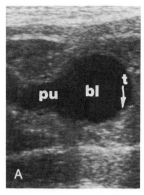 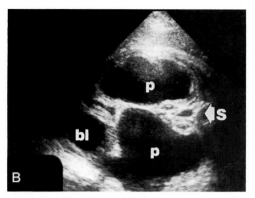 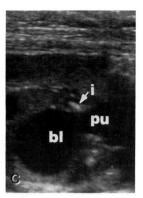

Figure 11–7. Representative sonograms of urethral level obstruction show: *A*, a dilated, trabeculated urinary bladder with a dilated proximal urethra; and *B*, a nondilated but thick-walled bladder with severe bilateral pelvocalyectasis. In an unusual case *(C)*, the bladder has prolapsed partially through the perineum. Each case exhibits oligohydramnios. bl, bladder; pu, proximal urethra; i, iliac wing; t, trabeculations; p, pelvocalyectasis; S, spine.

bladder to the point that it extends the fetal abdomen and elevates the hemidiaphragms and may contribute to the lax abdominal musculature characteristic of the prune-belly syndrome.[45]

Other features indicative of fetal urinary tract obstruction, such as oligohydramnios, ureterectasis, and calyectasis, assist in the diagnosis of obstructive uropathy. Their absence should not preclude the diagnosis, however, since they do not occur uniformly. Oligohydramnios occurs in approximately 50 percent of fetuses with urethral level obstruction, whereas only 40 percent of affected fetuses have associated pyelocalyectasis or ureterectasis. Several observations explain the apparent discrepancy between urinary tract obstruction and absence of oligohydramnios, ureterectasis, or calyectasis. Because egress of urine from the bladder may potentially occur, except in the presence of urethral atresia, lack of oligohydramnios does not preclude the diagnosis of urethral obstruction. Calyectasis and proximal ureterectasis may be absent because urethral obstruction most prominently affects the organs most proximal to the site of obstruction (i.e., the bladder and distal ureters), probably from reflux of urine under high pressure from the hypertrophied bladder into the ureters.[46] Furthermore, in approximately 10 to 20 percent of fetuses with urethral obstruction, the urinary bladder may spontaneously decompress through rupture of the urinary tract or development of a paranephric pseudocyst.[4, 47] Finally, diminution or cessation of urine production may result from renal dysplasia caused by increased intraluminal pressure within the urinary tract during nephrogenesis.[48]

Just as absence of urinary tract dilatation does not preclude an obstructive uropathy, its presence does not necessarily imply obstruction. In a rare case of massive vesicoureteral reflux without obstruction, for example, the bladder may appear persistently dilated because it empties but rapidly refills with refluxed urine.[35] Nevertheless, even in the absence of one or two of the cardinal signs of urethral level obstruction, the sonographer can frequently diagnose fetal urethral obstruction confidently, especially in the presence of a constellation of findings including oligohydramnios and evidence of spontaneous urinary tract decompression (perirenal urinoma, urinary ascites, or dystrophic peritoneal calcification). Often, these associated features dominate the sonographic findings, and occasionally one must resort to percutaneous antegrade pyelography to confirm the diagnosis (Table 11–1).[49]

Oligohydramnios represents a poor prognostic sign in urethral obstruction, probably

Table 11–1. OBSTRUCTIVE UROPATHY—MANIFESTATIONS THAT MAY DOMINATE THE PICTURE IN UTERO

Oligohydramnios
Cystic dysplasia
Urinary tract rupture
   Urinary ascites—small, moderate, large
   Paranephric urinoma
   Dystrophic calcification
Massively dilated bladder
Pelvocalyectasis/ureterectasis

because it leads to pulmonary hypoplasia.[50] Approximately 95 percent of fetuses with urethral level obstruction and oligohydramnios will not survive the neonatal period.[26] Conversely, one may predict a good prognosis for fetuses with obstructive uropathy but with a normal amount of amniotic fluid.[19] Other sonographic signs, such as lack of calyectasis or a large amount of ascites and dystrophic calcifications, also indicate a poor prognosis.[26] Lack of calyectasis in the absence of urinary tract decompression suggests the presence of renal dysplasia resulting in diminution of urine production. A large amount of urinary ascites from spontaneous urinary tract decompression is also a poor prognostic indicator, perhaps secondary to elevation of the fetal diaphragms, which may contribute to the pulmonary hyperplasia. Occasionally, the sonographer may detect dystrophic bladder wall calcification at the site of bladder perforation; this finding also correlates with a poor prognosis for survival beyond the neonatal period, probably because it indicates prior high pressure within the urinary tract that may lead to dysplasia.

In urethral level obstruction, oligohydramnios probably represents the overriding feature that indicates a poor prognosis, as it does in any circumstance, especially during the second trimester of pregnancy. The absence of calyectasis or the presence of a large amount of ascites or dystrophic calcification lends corroborative evidence for a poor prognosis.

Ureterovesical Junction Obstruction.[51, 52] Duplication of the renal collecting system occurs in up to 4 percent of the population and represents the most common major GU anomaly. In ureteral duplication, presumably from anomalous initial division of the ureteral bud, the upper pole moiety characteristically obstructs, whereas the lower pole moiety refluxes (Fig. 11–8).

Documentation of the dilated upper pole moiety with a normal lower pole intrarenal collecting system represents the key feature that permits accurate sonographic diagnosis of an obstructed duplex collecting system (Fig. 11–9). The dilated upper renal pole moiety may enlarge to the point that it displaces the nondilated lower pole of the kidney inferiorly and laterally. The associated thin-walled and fluid-filled ectopic ureterocele within the bladder may be very difficult to detect in utero, as is visualization of two distinct ureters and collecting systems. Often, however, the dilated ureter (either from reflux or from obstruction) manifests as a serpentine fluid-filled structure that may mimic bowel. Documentation that the structure touches the fetal spine, originates from the renal pelvis, and extends into a retrovesicular position without debris distinguishes a dilated ureter from fluid-filled bowel. Ectopic ureterocele occurs bilaterally in approximately 15 percent of cases. The amniotic fluid volume should be appropriate unless the obstruction is severe bilaterally.

Unlike ureterectasis associated with a duplex collecting system, which frequently requires postnatal surgery, primary megaureter represents a benign congenital anomaly that typically requires no therapy (Fig. 11–10).[53] Localized dysfunction of the distal ureter

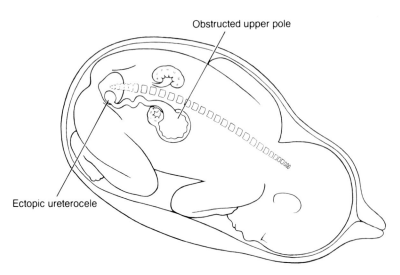

Obstructed upper pole

Ectopic ureterocele

Figure 11–8. An ectopic ureterocele typically produces an obstructed upper pole moiety.

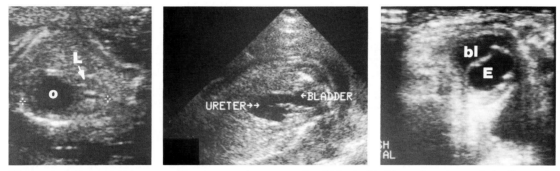

Figure 11–9. Representative scans show an ectopic ureterocele within the bladder and ureterectasis leading to the obstructed upper pole moiety. Note that the obstructed upper pole resembles a solitary cyst, but its thick rind is continuous with and displaces the parenchyma of the lower pole inferiorly. The ureterocele and ureterectasis frequently are not evident. bl, bladder; E, ectopic ureterocele; o, obstructed upper pole moiety; L, displaced lower pole moiety. (Courtesy of Jack H Hirsch, MD, Swedish Hospital Medical Center, Seattle, WA.)

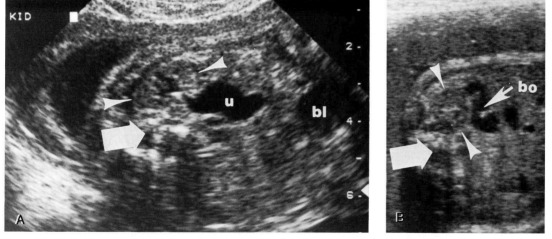

Figure 11–10. *A,* Primary megaureter at 26 menstrual weeks shows a normal-sized bladder with no dilatation of the distal ureter but with fusiform dilatation of the ureter proximally. There is no pelvocalyectasis, and the amniotic fluid volume is normal. *B,* A fluid-filled segment of bowel should not be confused with a dilated ureter. Unlike the ureter, bowel typically does not touch the fetal spine, cannot be traced to the renal pelvis, and frequently coexists with polyhydramnios. bl, bladder; u, ureter; bo, bowel; *arrowheads,* kidney; *wide arrow,* spine.

produces predominant distal ureteral dilatation not associated with obstruction, reflux, or bladder dysfunction. Proximal dilatation of the renal collecting structures occurs only rarely. Documentation that the dilated ureter arises symmetrically from the kidney should avoid confusion between this entity and the more common duplex collecting system.

Ureteropelvic Junction Obstruction. Tracing the ascent of the ureteral bud system proximally, obstruction frequently occurs at the level of the UPJ, the site of the first bifurcation of the ureteral bud (Figs. 11–11, 11–12). This represents the most common cause of neonatal hydronephrosis.[54] Since 85 to 90 percent of affected neonates may appear entirely normal on physical examination, antenatal detection of UPJ obstruction permits early therapy of a correctable lesion that may otherwise remain unrecognized for years.[55]

In unilateral UPJ obstruction, the renal pelvis, infundibula, and calyces are dilated, and the PD/KD is greater than 50 percent. In more severe cases of UPJ obstruction, one visualizes only a single fluid-filled structure representing the dilated renal pelvis with a thin rim of surrounding parenchyma. In dramatic cases, the renal pelvis may dilate to create a giant abdominal cyst without recognizable parenchyma. It may distend the abdomen and compress the thorax.[56] In UPJ obstruction, the nondilated ureters are not visible. In rare instances, the renal pelvis and infundibula may be stenotic, such that only the calyces dilate.[57] The nonobstructed contralateral kidney produces a normal amount of amniotic fluid, and the urinary bladder fills and empties normally, even if the degree of obstruction causes renal dysplasia of the ipsilateral kidney. In cases with UPJ obstruction, the degree of dilatation rarely progresses in utero and frequently exceeds that observed postnatally, presumably because of circulating maternal hormones that relax smooth muscle.[23] This discrepancy should not preclude the antenatal diagnosis.

Unilateral UPJ obstruction may be associated with contralateral multicystic dysplasia or renal agenesis, both of which may produce profound oligohydramnios if the UPJ obstruction is severe. Bilateral UPJ obstruc-

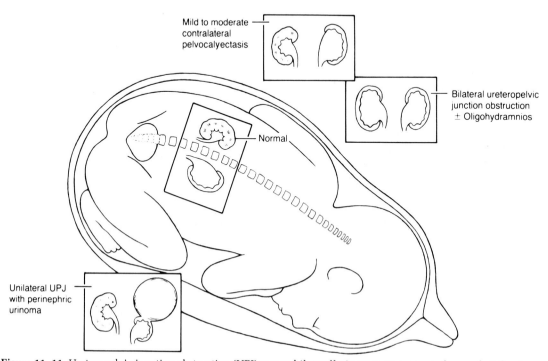

Figure 11–11. Ureteropelvic junction obstruction (UPJ) occurs bilaterally in 10 to 30 percent of cases, but the degree of obstruction usually is not symmetric. If severe, UPJ can cause extreme thinning of the renal parenchyma, or the kidney may rupture, resulting in a urinoma.

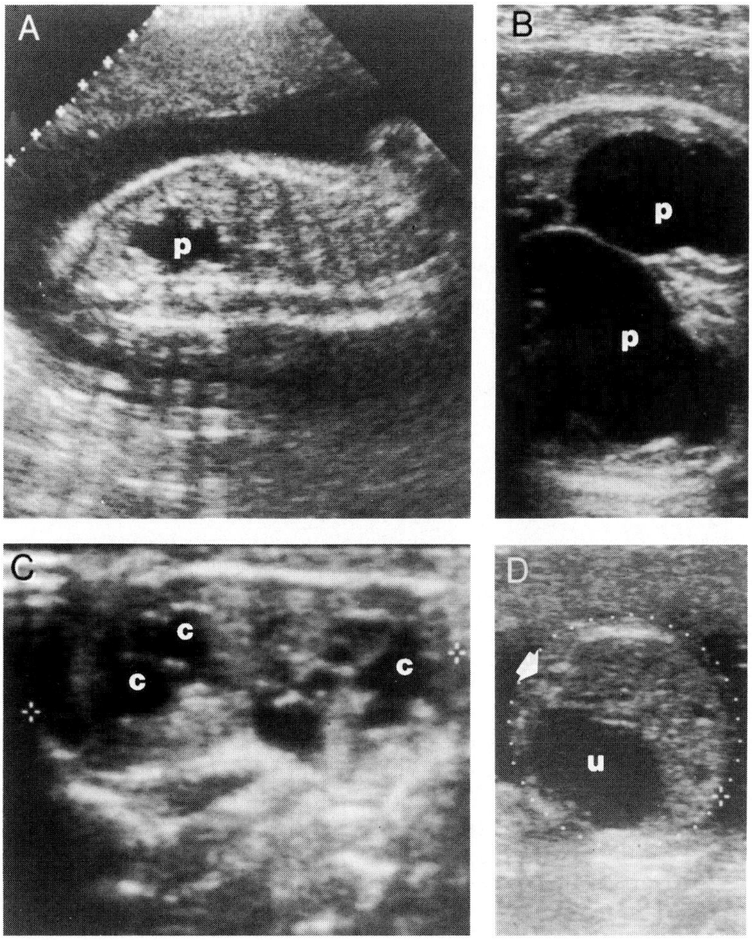

Figure 11–12. The degree of dilatation in ureteropelvic junction obstruction varies. Case *A* has moderate unilateral pelvocalyectasis, but in *B*, only a thin rim of tissue surrounds the markedly dilated renal pelves bilaterally. Occasionally, stenosis of the pelves and infundibula *(C)* produces dilatation predominantly of the calyces. Urinary tract obstruction may lead to rupture and formation of a perinephric urinoma *(D)*, a unilocular paraspinous fluid-filled mass. p, renal pelves; c, calyces; u, urinoma; *arrow*, spine.

tion occurs in approximately 10 to 30 percent of cases;[23] fortunately, involvement is usually asymmetric, and severe obstruction rarely occurs. Although cases with severe bilateral UPJ obstruction may result in oligohydramnios and an empty urinary bladder, milder forms are unlikely to be fatal.[23] UPJ obstruction may paradoxically result in polyhydramnios in up to 25 percent of cases.[23] Visualization of a paranephric urinoma from rupture of the collecting system correlates with severe obstruction and a low probability of residual renal function. A paranephric urinoma appears as a large unilocular cystic flank mass that touches the fetal spine.[47]

Renal Dysplasia

Renal dysplasia results from anomalous differentiation of metanephric tissue and implies irreversible renal damage.[58, 59] The functional capacity of an affected kidney depends upon the extent and severity of the dysplasia. Disorganized epithelial structures and abundant fibrous tissue characterize renal dysplasia histologically; cortical cysts frequently, but not necessarily, occur in renal dysplasia and represent the key feature to search for sonographically.

Approximately 90 percent of dysplastic kidneys result from urinary tract obstruction during nephrogenesis. The severity of obstruction as well as the patterns of dysplasia correspond with the site of obstruction.[59, 60] Bernstein classifies renal dysplasia into four major groups: (1) multicystic dysplasia, usually caused by ureteropelvic atresia; (2) focal and segmental cystic dysplasia, typically resulting from obstruction or atresia of one of the ureters leading from a duplex kidney; (3) cystic dysplasia associated with nonatretic urinary tract obstruction, most commonly from posterior urethral valves; and (4) heredofamilial cystic dysplasia.[58] Only the relatively uncommon heredofamilial cystic dysplasias result from nonobstructive causes.

Obstructive Renal Dysplasia

Multicystic Dysplastic Kidney. Multicystic dysplastic kidney (MCDK) disease probably occurs during embryogenesis, resulting from atresia of the ureteral bud system at the level of the upper third of the ureter, with concomitant atresia of the renal pelvis and infundibula. Rarely, segmental atresia of the proximal third of the ureter without atresia of the renal pelvis and infundibula produces the hydronephrotic type of MCDK.[60] Ureteral atresia of a duplex kidney causes segmental MCDK involving the collecting system supplied by the atretic ureter.[61] The ureteral atresia in MCDK prevents the metanephric blastema from inducing formation of nephrons, such that an MCDK characteristically has no normal renal parenchyma proximal to the atretic ureter. The collecting tubules distributed randomly throughout the anomalous kidney become cystically enlarged to variable degrees, without macroscopic intercommuni-

cations. Since the drastic reduction in nephron formation is seldom absolute, an MCDK may exhibit some (usually very minimal) residual urine formation. For practical purposes, however, an MCDK represents a functionless kidney.[62]

The sonographic appearance of an MCDK correlates well with the pathologic appearance (Figs. 11–13, 11–14).[63] The renal pelvis and the ureter are usually atretic and not visible. Occasionally, however, the renal pelvis may be dilated in cases with isolated ureteral atresia. Multicystic dysplasia typically visualizes as a paraspinous flank mass, characterized by numerous cysts of variable sizes without identifiable communication or anatomic arrangement. The large cysts frequently distort the contour of the mass, and no normal renal parenchyma exists. Any tissue resembling possible renal parenchyma localizes as small islands of echogenic material interspersed between these cysts.

An MCDK may change markedly in size and appearance as gestation progresses.[62] The MCDK and its cysts may undergo progressive enlargement or diminution or may initially enlarge then decrease in size later in pregnancy. Minimal residual capacity for glomerular filtration explains this variable appearance of the MCDK. As progressive

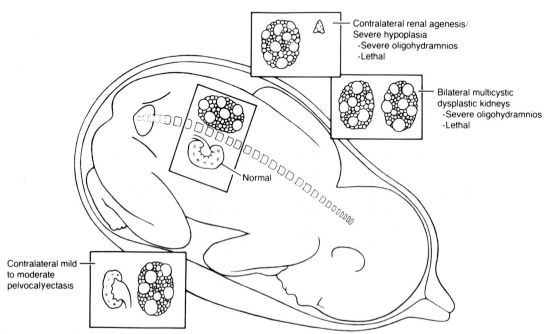

Contralateral renal agenesis/ Severe hypoplasia
-Severe oligohydramnios
-Lethal

Bilateral multicystic dysplastic kidneys
-Severe oligohydramnios
-Lethal

Normal

Contralateral mild to moderate pelvocalyectasis

Figure 11–13. The multicystic dysplastic kidney is essentially nonfunctional. Attention must be focused on the contralateral kidney since it is the only potentially functional kidney.

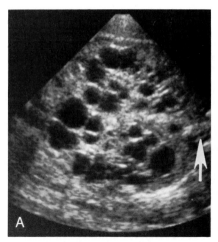
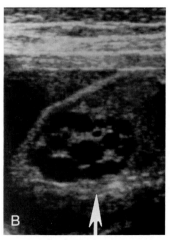
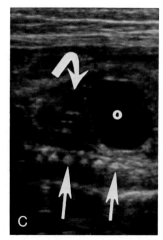

Figure 11–14. Bilateral multicystic dysplastic kidneys (MCDK) *(A)* cause profound oligohydramnios and multiple cysts of varying sizes without demonstrable communication or anatomic arrangement. This is a lethal entity. Unilateral MCDK *(B)* with a normal amount of amniotic fluid presumes a functioning contralateral kidney that must be followed closely. In this case, the renal contour is relatively preserved. Segmental MCDK *(C)* occurs with atresia of one of the ureters leading from a duplex kidney. o, obstructed upper pole moiety; *straight arrows,* spine; *curved arrow,* multicystic dysplastic lower pole of duplex kidney.

fibrosis of nephrons occurs, the MCDK ceases to grow then involutes.

Once the sonographer has confirmed the diagnosis of MCDK, assessment of the contralateral kidney assumes primary importance, since the MCDK produces little filtrate and no urine that reaches the amniotic fluid. Contralateral renal anomalies occur in approximately 40 percent of fetuses with an MCDK.[64] If overlying fetal parts obscure the contralateral renal region, an appropriate amount of amniotic fluid and normal emptying and filling of the fetal urinary bladder imply normal contralateral renal function. Profound oligohydramnios and absence of fetal urinary bladder filling, on the other hand, imply lethal fetal renal disease, which occurs in 30 percent of fetuses with MCDK, from either bilateral multicystic dysplasia (20 percent) or contralateral renal agenesis (10 percent). Typical multicystic flank masses should be readily visible in bilateral MCDK disease. When only a unilateral MCDK is visible, the sonographer can infer the diagnosis of contralateral renal agenesis or severe hypoplasia in the setting of profound oligohydramnios with absence of urinary bladder filling. Approximately 10 percent of patients with a unilateral MCDK have contralateral hydronephrosis, usually from obstruction at the UPJ. In such cases, the degree of obstruction determines the amount of amniotic fluid, since the obstructed kidney is the only potentially functional one. For this reason, one must obtain close follow-up of the contralateral kidney to watch for progression of dilatation or diminution of amniotic fluid that might necessitate interventive measures. Minimal contralateral renal pelvic distention occurs with approximately the same frequency as in fetuses without an MCDK and lacks clinical significance.[64]

Since MCDK and hydronephrosis constitute the two most common causes of a neonatal (and presumably fetal) abdominal mass and because their potential function and perinatal management differ dramatically, distinction between these two entities is critical.[65] In cases with mild pelvocalyectasis or a typical MCDK, this distinction is elementary. Differentiation between the atypical cases of the hydronephrotic form of MCDK and cases of hydronephrosis with predominant calyceal dilatation, but without multicystic dysplasia, may be much more difficult.[57, 66] The latter maintains the reniform contour, with renal parenchyma arranged at the periphery of the dilated calyces that are of uniform size, communicate with each other centrally, and align in anterior and posterior rows.

Cystic Renal Dysplasia. Experiments in fetal lambs demonstrate that urethral obstruction in the first half of gestation produces renal dysplasia.[48, 67] The dysplasia associated with urinary tract obstruction represents irreversible renal damage that probably results from elevated pressures within the developing nephron system.[59] In humans, cystic renal dysplasia occurs most frequently with urethral level obstruction but may also occur with obstruction at the level of the UPJ (Fig. 11–15). Although the severity of renal dysplasia varies, extensive renal dysplasia correlates with drastically reduced renal functional capacity. For this reason, sonographic detection of cystic renal dysplasia in a fetus with urinary tract obstruction provides useful prognostic information regarding renal function.

Among fetal kidneys with obstructive uropathy, sonographic demonstration of cortical cysts effectively indicates the presence of cystic renal dysplasia as early as 21 menstrual weeks (Fig. 11–16).[4] Since not all dysplastic kidneys have cysts or the cysts may be smaller than sonographic resolution capabilities, one cannot accurately predict the absence of dysplasia when cortical cysts

are not visible. Dysplastic kidneys tend to exhibit greatly increased echogenicity relative to surrounding fetal structures, presumably from the abundant fibrous tissue. Assessment of renal echogenicity is quite subjective, however, and not all echogenic kidneys are dysplastic. Furthermore, one cannot predict the absence of dysplasia with normal renal echogenicity. Assessment of renal echogenicity in obstructive uropathy, therefore, offers only limited predictive value for dysplasia.[4] Aspiration and catheter measurement of fetal urine provide corroborative quantitative information about fetal renal function.[3] One can predict a poor prognosis for a fetus with bilateral obstructive uropathy and decreased output of isotonic urine. Conversely, a fetus with an output of more than 2 ml/hr of normal hypotonic urine has a good prognosis. Normal hypotonic fetal urine implies intact glomerular and tubular function (Table 11–2).[3]

Just as the differentiation between an MCDK and hydronephrosis may be difficult,

RENAL PARENCHYMAL RESPONSES TO OBSTRUCTION

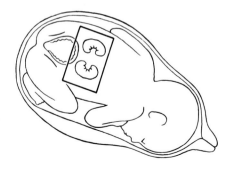
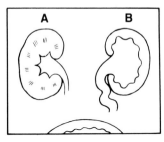

A. Normal
B. Thinned, normal echogenicity: no cysts

C. Increased echogenicity with cysts – dysplasia
D. Thinned, increased echogenicity with cysts – dysplasia

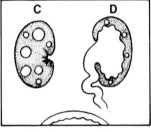
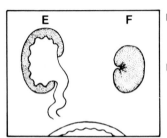

E. Thinned, increased echogenicity: no cysts – probable dysplasia
F. Small, increased echogenicity: no cysts – probable dysplasia

Figure 11–15. Urinary tract obstruction produces a varied response from the kidneys. *A*, The kidney may remain normal in urethral obstruction, without reflux. *B*, Pelvocalyectasis may attentuate the parenchymal thickness. *C*, The kidney may suffer cystic dysplasia (parenchymal cysts), become fibrotic (increased echogenicity), and cease to function (lack of pelvocalyectasis). *D*, Alternatively, it may undergo cystic dysplasia with parenchymal cysts and increased echogenicity but continue to have pelvocalyectasis and a thinned parenchyma. If no cysts are visible, but the parenchyma is of greatly increased echogenicity, either with *(E)* or without *(F)* pelvocalyectasis, dysplasia is probably, but not invariably, present.

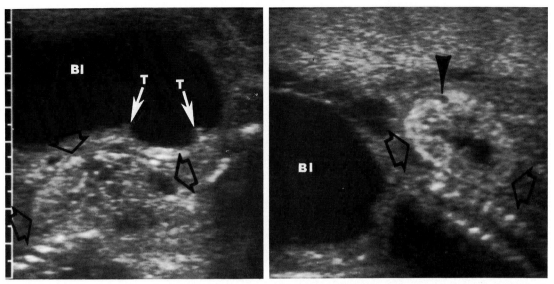

Figure 11–16. This case of urethral level obstruction produced bilateral renal cysts indicative of cystic dysplasia and irreversible damage. The number of parenchymal cysts in each kidney varies markedly. Greatly increased renal echogenicity provides corroborative but nondiagnostic information regarding dysplasia. T, trabeculations of bladder wall; Bl, bladder; *open arrows*, kidneys; *arrowhead*, parenchymal cyst (the contralateral kidney has numerous parenchymal cysts).

the distinction between MCDK and cystic renal dysplasia associated with urinary tract obstruction (but not ureteral atresia) may also be difficult, especially in the absence of hydronephrosis. As delineated previously, however, documentation of one of several of the cardinal signs of urethral level obstruction (the most common cause of cystic renal dysplasia) assists in this distinction. Furthermore, in MCDK, only small islands of tissue localize between predominant cysts,

whereas in cystic dysplasia from urinary tract obstruction, recognizable parenchyma surrounds the relatively small cysts. In addition, cystic dysplasia from distal urinary tract obstruction frequently involves both kidneys, but bilateral MCDK disease occurs in only 20 percent of cases. Obstruction at the level of the UPJ may result in cystic renal dysplasia that would typically be unilateral.[4, 23] The distinction between MCDK disease and cystic dysplasia from urinary tract obstruction, although helpful in terms of diagnosis, may be somewhat artificial in terms of prognosis, since in either case, the affected kidney typically maintains only minimal functional capacity.

Heredofamilial Cystic Dysplasia[58]

Several rare inherited syndromes may produce cystic dysplasia from nonobstructive causes and be associated with detectable sonographic features. Detection of the multiple renal cysts with the features associated with each syndrome, especially in the setting of familial risk for recurrence, permits confident antenatal diagnosis (Fig. 11–17). Meckel-Gruber syndrome, for example, is a lethal entity that recurs in an autosomal recessive manner (25 percent recurrence risk for subsequent pregnancies). Characteristic

Table 11–2. PROGNOSTIC INDICATORS IN FETAL BILATERAL OBSTRUCTIVE UROPATHY

Poor prognosis
  Decreased urine output < 2 ml/hr
  Isotonic urine
    Osmolarity > 210 mOsm
    Sodium > 100 mEq/ml
    Chloride > 90 mEq/ml
  Cystic dysplasia
Good prognosis
  Urine output > 2 ml/hr
  Hypotonic urine
    Osmolarity < 210 mOsm
    Sodium < 100 mEq/ml
    Chloride < 90 mEq/ml

From Glick PL, Harrison MR, Golbus MS, et al: Management of the fetus with congenital hydronephrosis II: Prognostic criteria and selection for treatment. J Pediatr Surg 20:376, 1985.

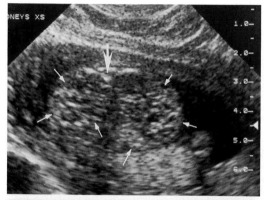

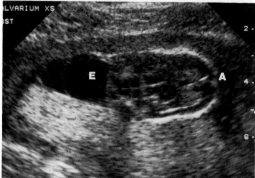

Figure 11–17. Multiple small renal cysts in conjunction with an encephalocele imply Meckel-Gruber syndrome. *Small arrows*, kidneys; *large arrow*, spine; E, encephalocele; A, anterior. (Courtesy of Robert A Schor, MD, Swedish Hospital Medical Center, Seattle, WA.)

features, the presence of at least two of which enables definitive diagnosis, include (1) bilateral nonobstructive MCDK disease (95 percent of cases), (2) occipital encephalocele (80 percent of cases), and (3) postaxial polydactyly (75 percent of cases).[68] In a fetus with a familial risk for Meckel-Gruber syndrome, the sonographer must focus on these regions to search for recurrence. Conversely, detection of an occipital encephalocele or of multiple bilateral cysts in the absence of a positive family history mandates careful search for other features indicative of the syndrome.

Jeune's syndrome (asphyxiating thoracic dystrophy), short-rib polydactyly syndrome, and Trisomy 13 may also manifest antenatally with nonobstructive cystic renal dysplasia (see Chap. 7 on the fetal musculoskeletal system). Visualization of multiple renal cysts in a fetus with a familial risk for Jeune's or short-rib polydactyly syndrome and with shortened extremities, a noticeably small thorax, and polydactyly provides con-

vincing evidence for recurrence. Multiple renal cysts may also occur in a fetus with holoprosencephaly and a fisted hand with clinodactyly, indicative of Trisomy 13.

Autosomal Recessive Polycystic Kidney Disease

Bilateral medullary ectasia, producing innumerable 1 to 2 mm cysts of nonobstructive renal collecting tubules, occurs in autosomal recessive (infantile) polycystic kidney disease.[7] Although this entity may be visible pathologically as early as 48 to 50 days of gestation, it expresses variably, depending upon the degree of renal involvement,[69–71] the severity of which correlates inversely with proliferation of bile ducts and hepatic fibrosis. Severely affected fetuses and neonates have a very high mortality rate, usually from pulmonary hypoplasia secondary to oligohydramnios from diminished renal function.

The diagnosis of autosomal recessive (infantile) polycystic kidney disease can be made as early as 16 menstrual weeks on the basis of oligohydramnios and characteristic renal abnormalities seen on the antenatal sonogram, especially when the sonogram is performed because of a familial risk for the disorder (Figs. 11–18, 11–19). This entity typically causes bilaterally enlarged fetal kidneys that maintain their reniform shape but exhibit increased echogenicity. Early in pregnancy, the renal cortex may appear echogenic, whereas the medullae appear echopenic. Later in pregnancy, the pattern reverses, and a peripheral rim of hypoechoic

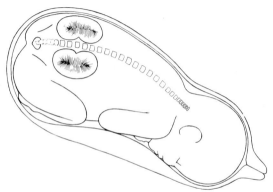

Figure 11–18. Autosomal recessive (infantile) polycystic kidney disease produces enlarged, echogenic kidneys, often with oligohydramnios.

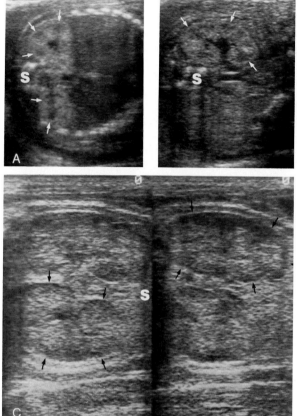

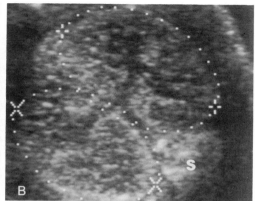

Figure 11–19. These scans demonstrate the variable appearance of autosomal recessive polycystic kidney disease in utero. *A*, Typically, the kidneys are enlarged and echogenic. *B*, Recent technology now occasionally permits visualization of the innumerable 1 to 2 mm cysts as early as 16 menstrual weeks. *C*, Later in pregnancy, a peripheral sonolucent rim may become evident. *Small arrows* or *outlines*, kidneys; S, spine.

renal cortex surrounds the echogenic medullae. Diminished renal function usually produces nondilated renal pelves, ureters, and bladder, with a decreased amount of amniotic fluid. Although the numerous tiny cysts are usually smaller than the limit of sonographic resolution, the multiple interfaces produced by these cysts result in the characteristic diffusely increased renal echogenicity. Newer technology now often permits visualization of innumerable 1 to 2 mm cysts scattered throughout symmetrically enlarged kidneys. The enlarged kidneys may lead to dystocia.[71]

When bilaterally enlarged and very echogenic kidneys occur in a fetus at risk for autosomal recessive (infantile) polycystic kidney disease, one can strongly suspect the diagnosis of recurrence. However, biologic variability of this disease may prevent accurate diagnosis in all cases, and a normal sonogram of a fetus at risk for autosomal recessive (infantile) polycystic kidney disease does not ensure absence of this genetic disease.[70, 71] Usually, but not always, the sonogram shows evidence for recurrence by approximately 24 menstrual weeks. In the absence of a genetic risk for this entity, sonographic visualization of enlarged fetal kidneys most likely indicates autosomal recessive polycystic kidney disease. Autosomal dominant (adult) polycystic kidney disease rarely manifests antenatally, but when it does, one to several macroscopic cysts representing dilated nephrons are evident. Examination of the parents in such cases should demonstrate innumerable renal cysts in at least one parent and differentiate autosomal dominant (adult) from autosomal recessive (infantile) polycystic kidney disease. In an extremely rare case, a macroscopic simple renal cyst may also manifest antenatally as an incidental finding.[72] Other very rare possibilities that the sonographer could conceivably confuse with autosomal recessive polycystic kidney disease include bilateral renal tumors, medullary sponge kidney, medullary cystic disease, or congenital metabolic diseases (i.e., glycogen storage disease or tyrosinosis). Oligohydramnios and absence of urine within the urinary bladder would favor autosomal recessive (infantile) polycystic kidney disease over all of these other rare entities.

Renal Tumors

Congenital renal tumors occur only rarely. Mesoblastic nephroma represents the most common congenital renal neoplasm (Fig. 11–20).[20–22] It is a solitary hamartoma with a usually benign course. Although rare reports of recurrence after nephrectomy exist, curative therapy usually consists of nephrectomy alone. Antenatal detection of a mesoblastic nephroma, therefore, should not necessitate preterm delivery. Nevertheless, mesoblastic nephroma frequently coexists with polyhydramnios, which may contribute to premature labor. The reason for a clear association between mesoblastic nephroma and polyhydramnios remains unclear.

Mesoblastic nephroma visualizes as a large, solitary, predominantly solid, retroperitoneal mass arising from and not separable from adjacent normal kidney. It does not have a well-defined capsule and may contain cystic areas. Its predominantly solid texture distinguishes mesoblastic nephroma from an unusual case of UPJ obstruction with polyhydramnios. Although its sonographic appearance resembles a Wilms' tumor, the age of presentation provides an important differentiating factor. Whereas mesoblastic nephroma is the most common congenital renal neoplasm, Wilms' tumor is exceptionally rare in the neonate. Identification of a predominantly solid fetal renal mass in the presence of polyhydramnios provides convincing evidence for a mesoblastic nephroma.

Fetal Gender

Determination of fetal gender is by no means a trivial matter. Attempts to document fetal gender in utero serve numerous purposes, especially during the second trimester of pregnancy.[73] Gender determination among fetuses at risk for severe X-linked disorders assumes paramount importance since unequivocal identification of a female fetus excludes the possibility of the disorder. Documentation of different genders in twin pregnancy permits accurate assessment of dizygosity, which precludes the possibility of twin-twin transfusion syndrome, cord entanglement, or conjoined twins.[74] It also confirms that both sacs have been sampled in amniocentesis. In cases with discrepant so-

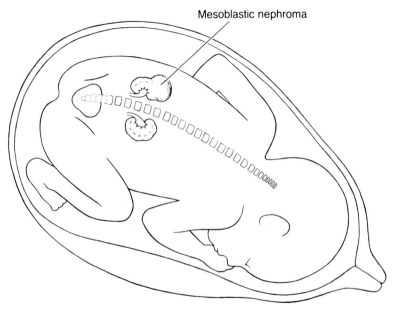

Mesoblastic nephroma

Figure 11–20. A mesoblastic nephroma is a solitary, predominantly solid, benign renal tumor associated with polyhydramnios.

nographic and amniocentesis data, ultrasound may detect an intersex state such as testicular feminization with male karyotype but female external genitalia.[75] Even without amniocentesis data, careful analysis of the fetal perineum may detect ambiguous genitalia.[76] Furthermore, whether verbalized or not, determination of fetal gender constitutes one of the prime expectations the parents have during their sonogram. The physician's duty of full disclosure and the parents' right to know may create a complicated ethical and moral problem.[73]

Accurate sonographic assessment of fetal gender requires adequate perineal visualization to permit unequivocal distinction between the labia and scrotum. Only documentation of testicles within the scrotum provides 100 percent reliability in gender assessment, but this is not possible in utero until approximately 28 to 34 menstrual weeks.[77] Unfortunately, inopportune fetal positioning precludes perineal visualization in approximately 30 percent of fetuses, especially before 24 menstrual weeks.[73, 77] Even after adequate perineal visualization, ultrasonography incorrectly assigns fetal gender in approximately 3 percent of cases.[73]* The sonographer should bear in mind this small but definite error rate and avoid using sonography as the sole method for gender determination.[73]

---

*One study reports adequate pelvic visualization in 97.1 percent of fetuses at 12 menstrual weeks and thereafter, with 99.9 percent correct gender assignment.[78]

Antenatal sonography usually visualizes the ovaries, uterus, and vagina only when these organs enlarge and produce a pelvic mass. Hydrometrocolpos, for example, produces a hypoechoic mass posterior to the bladder, extending to the abdomen in female fetuses with vaginal obstruction.[39–41] In approximately 55 percent of patients, the hydrometrocolpos compresses the urinary tract and causes hydronephrosis or hydroureter.[40] Ovarian cysts, on the other hand, typically do not compress the urinary tract but may obstruct small bowel.[79–81] Documentation that the ovarian cyst is separate from the normal urinary tract assists in the diagnosis but does not differentiate it from an enteric duplication, a mesenteric cyst, or a urachal cyst. However, duplication cysts tend to be more tubular, and urachal cysts extend to the umbilicus. In a female fetus, a multiseptated intra-abdominal cystic mass strongly suggests ovarian cysts, especially if bilateral (Fig. 11–21). Fetal ovarian cysts probably result from maternal hormonal stimulation and are characteristically benign but may be associated with hypothyroidism.[79] Furthermore, large but benign ovarian cysts may cause dystocia and require prompt perinatal surgical management, since they may lead to torsion, rupture, or intestinal obstruction.

A careful sonographic examination of the fetal abdomen and pelvis often permits detection of a variety of GU abnormalities that dramatically change obstetric and perinatal management. The sonographer may detect hydronephrosis that may otherwise go clinically undetected after birth. Antenatal so-

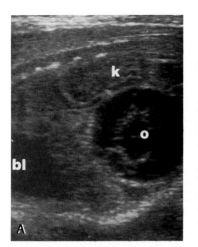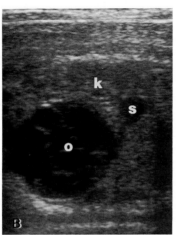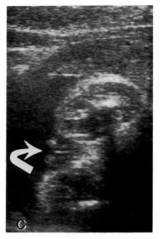

Figure 11–21. Visualization of a multiseptated lower abdominal mass, separate from the kidneys, bladder, and stomach in a female fetus, provides strong evidence of an enlarged ovarian cyst. o, ovary; k, kidney; s, stomach; bl, bladder; *curved arrow,* labia.

nographic delineation of the site of obstruction and assessment of potential reversibility of renal damage assist the urologist in patient selection and in timing surgical procedures. Detection of bilateral obstructive uropathy without evidence for severe irreversible renal damage suggests that the anomaly may be amenable to early postnatal or, possibly, prenatal therapy. In addition, the sonographer may identify fetuses with distention of the fetal abdomen from urinary ascites or from a massively distended urinary bladder. These fetuses may benefit from prenatal paracentesis or bladder drainage. Alternatively, one may consider elective cesarean section to optimize perinatal care. Conversely, early detection of lethal disorders, such as bilateral renal agenesis, bilateral MCDK disease, or severe autosomal recessive (infantile) polycystic kidney disease, may provide the parents with the option of elective termination.

References

1. Schwoebel MG, Sacher P, Bucher HU, et al: Prenatal diagnosis improves the prognosis in children with obstructive uropathy. J Pediatr Surg 19:187, 1984.
2. Harrison MR, Golbus MS, Filly FA, et al: Fetal surgery for congenital hydronephrosis. N Engl J Med 306:591, 1982.
3. Glick PL, Harrison MR, Golbus MS, et al: Management of the fetus with congenital hydronephrosis II: Prognostic criteria and selection for treatment. J Pediatr Surg 20:376, 1985.
4. Mahony BS, Filly RA, Callen PW: Fetal renal dysplasia: Sonographic evaluation. Radiology 152:143, 1984.
5. American Institute of Ultrasound in Medicine: Official Guidelines and Statements on Obstetrical Ultrasound, October 1985.
6. Moore KL: The urinary system. In The Developing Human: Clinically Oriented Embryology, 4th Ed. Philadelphia, WB Saunders Co, 1988.
7. Mellins HZ: Cystic dilatations of the upper urinary tract: A radiologist's developmental model. Radiology 153:291, 1984.
8. Abramovich DR: The volume of amniotic fluid and its regulating factors. In Fairweather DVI, Eskes TKA (eds): Amniotic Fluid Research and Clinical Application. 2nd Ed. Amsterdam, Excerpta Medica, 1978, pp 31–49.
9. Seeds AE: Current concepts of amniotic fluid dynamics. Am J Obstet Gynecol 138:575, 1980.
10. Barss VA, Benacerraf BR, Frigoletto FD: Second trimester oligohydramnios, a predictor of poor fetal outcome. Obstet Gynecol 64:608, 1984.
11. Lawson TL, Foley WD, Berland LL, et al: Ultrasonic evaluation of fetal kidneys: Analysis of normal size and frequency of visualization as related to stage of pregnancy. Radiology 138:153, 1981.
12. Bowie JD, Rosenberg ER, Andreotti MD, et al: The changing sonographic appearance of fetal kidneys during pregnancy. J Ultrasound Med 2:505, 1983.
13. Bertagnoli L, Lalatta F, Gallicchio MD, et al: Quantitative characterization of the growth of the fetal kidney. JCU 11:349, 1983.
14. Jeanty P, Dramaix-Wilmet M, Elkhazen N: Measurement of fetal kidney growth on ultrasound. Radiology 144:159, 1982.
15. Grannum P, Bracken M, Silverman R, et al: Assessment of fetal kidney size in normal gestation by comparison of ratio of kidney circumference. Am J Obstet Gynecol 136:249, 1980.
16. Campbell S, Wladimiroff JW, Dewhurst CJ: The antenatal measurement of fetal urine production. J Obstet Gynaecol Br Commonw 80:680, 1973.
17. Wladimiroff JW, Campbell S: Fetal urine-production rates in normal and complicated pregnancy. Lancet 1:151, 1974.
18. Chamberlain PF, Manning FA, Morrison I, et al: Circadian rhythm in bladder volumes in the term human fetus. Obstet Gynecol 64:657, 1984.
19. Hellstrom WJG, Kogan BA, Jeffrey RB, et al: The natural history of prenatal hydronephrosis with normal amounts of amniotic fluid. J Urol 132:947, 1984.
20. Ehman RL, Nicholson SF, Machin GA: Prenatal sonographic detection of congenital mesoblastic nephroma in a monozygotic twin pregnancy. J Ultrasound Med 2:555, 1983.
21. Guilian BB: Prenatal ultrasonographic diagnosis of fetal renal tumors. Radiology 152:69, 1984.
22. Geirsson RT, Ricketts NEM, Taylor DJ, et al: Prenatal appearance of a mesoblastic nephroma associated with polyhydramnios. JCU 12:488, 1985.
23. Kleiner B, Callen PW, Filly RA: Sonographic analysis of the fetus with ureteropelvic junction obstruction. AJR 148:359, 1987.
24. Arger PH, Coleman BG, Mintz MC, et al: Routine fetal genitourinary tract screening. Radiology 156:485, 1985.
25. Grignon A, Filion R, Filiatrault D, et al: Urinary tract dilatation in utero: Classification and clinical applications. Radiology 160:645, 1986.
26. Mahony BS, Callen PW, Filly RA: Fetal urethral obstruction: US evaluation. Radiology 157:221, 1985.
27. Dubbins PA, Kurtz AB, Wapner RJ, et al: Renal agenesis: Spectrum of in utero findings. JCU 9:189, 1981.
28. Romero R, Cullen M, Crannum P, et al: Antenatal diagnosis of renal anomalies with ultrasound. III. Bilateral renal agenesis. Am J Obstet Gynecol 151:38, 1985.
29. Austin CW, Brown JM, Friday RO: Unilateral renal agenesis presenting as a pseudomass in utero. J Ultrasound Med 3:177, 1984.
30. Wladimiroff JW: Effect of furosemide on fetal urine production. Br J Obstet Gynaecol 82:221, 1985.
31. Rosenberg ER, Bowie JD: Failure of furosemide to induce diuresis in a growth-retarded fetus. AJR 142:485, 1984.
32. Harmon CR: Maternal furosemide may not provoke urine production in the compromised fetus. Am J Obstet Gynecol 150:322, 1984.
33. Greenblatt AM, Beretsky I, Lankin DH, et al: In utero diagnosis of crossed renal ectopia using high-resolution real-time ultrasound. J Ultrasound Med 4:105, 1985.

34. Blane CE, Koff SA, Baverman RA, et al: Non-obstructive hydronephrosis: Sonographic recognition and therapeutic implications. Radiology 147:95, 1983.

35. Reuter KL, Lebowitz RL: Massive vesicoureteral reflux mimicking posterior urethral valves in a fetus. JCU 13:584, 1985.

36. Glazer GM, Filly RA, Callen PW: The varied sonographic appearance of the urinary tract in the fetus and newborn with urethral obstruction. Radiology 144:563, 1982.

37. Hoddick WK, Filly RA, Mahony BS, Callen PW: Minimal fetal renal pyelectasis. J Ultrasound Med 4:85, 1985.

38. Laing FC, Burke VD, Wing VW, et al: Postpartum evaluation of fetal hydronephrosis: Optimal timing for follow-up sonography. Radiology 152:423, 1984.

39. Hill SJ, Hirsch JH: Sonographic detection of fetal hydrometrocolpos. J Ultrasound Med 4:323, 1985.

40. Davis GH, Wapner RJ, Kurtz AB, et al: Antenatal diagnosis of hydrometrocolpos by ultrasound examination. J Ultrasound Med 3:371, 1984.

41. Russ PD, Zavitz WR, Pretorius DH, et al: Hydrometrocolpos, uterus didelphys, and septate vagina: An antenatal sonographic diagnosis. J Ultrasound Med 5:211, 1986.

42. Harrison MR, Golbus MS, Filly RA: Congenital hydronephrosis. In The Unborn Patient. Orlando, Grune & Stratton, 1984, pp 277–348.

43. Glick PL, Harrison MR, Adzick NS, et al: Correction of congenital hydronephrosis in utero. IV: In utero decompression prevents renal dysplasia. J Pediatr Surg 19:649, 1984.

44. Shalev E, Weiner E, Feldman E, et al: External bladder—Amniotic fluid shunt for fetal urinary tract obstruction. Obstet Gynecol 63:31S, 1984.

45. Meizner I, Bar-Ziv J, Katz M: Prenatal ultrasonic diagnosis of the extreme form of prune belly syndrome. JCU 13:581, 1985.

46. Rattner WH, Meyer R, Bernstein J: Congenital abnormalities of the urinary system. IV. Valvular obstruction of the posterior urethra. J Pediatr 63:84, 1963.

47. Callen PW, Bolding D, Filly RA, et al: Ultrasonographic evaluation of fetal paranephric pseudocysts. J Ultrasound Med 2:309, 1983.

48. Beck AD: The effect of intrauterine urinary obstruction upon the development of the fetal kidney. J Urol 105:784, 1971.

49. Gore RM, Callen PW, Filly RA, et al: Prenatal percutaneous antegrade pyelography in posterior urethral valves: Sonographic guidance. AJR 139:994, 1982.

50. Thomas IT, Smith DW: Oligohydramnios: Cause of the non-renal features of Potter's syndrome, including pulmonary hypoplasia. J Pediatr 84:811, 1974.

51. Jeffrey RB, Laing FC, Wing VW, et al: Sonography of the fetal duplex kidney. Radiology 153:123, 1984.

52. Montana MA, Cyr DR, Lenke RR, et al: Sonographic detection of fetal ureteral obstruction. AJR 145:595, 1985.

53. Dunn V, Glasier CM: Ultrasonographic antenatal demonstration of primary megaureters. J Ultrasound Med 4:101, 1985.

54. Lebowitz RL, Griscomb NT: Neonatal hydronephrosis—146 cases. Radiol Clin North Am 15:49, 1971.

55. Grignon A, Filiatrault D, Homsy Y, et al: Ureteropelvic junction stenosis: Antenatal ultrasonographic diagnosis, postnatal investigation, and follow-up. Radiology 160:649, 1986.

56. Jaffe R, Abramowicz J, Fejgin M, et al: Giant fetal abdominal cyst: Ultrasonic diagnosis and management. J Ultrasound Med 6:45, 1987.

57. Lucaya J, Enriquez G, Delgado R, et al: Infundibulopelvic stenosis in children. AJR 142:471, 1984.

58. Bernstein J: A classification of renal cysts. In Gardner KD (ed): Cystic Diseases of the Kidney. New York, John Wiley & Sons, 1976, pp 7–30.

59. Bernstein J: The morphogenesis of renal parenchymal maldevelopment (renal dysplasia). Pediatr Clin North Am 18:395, 1971.

60. Felson B, Cussen LJ: The hydronephrotic type of unilateral congenital multicystic disease of the kidney. Semin Roentgenol 10:113, 1975.

61. Diard F, LeDosseur P, Cadier L, et al: Multicystic dysplasia in the upper component of the complete duplex kidney. Pediatr Radiol 14:310, 1984.

62. Hashimoto BE, Filly RA, Callen PW: Multicystic dysplastic kidney in utero: Changing appearance on US. Radiology 159:107, 1986.

63. Stack KJ, Koff SA, Silver TM: Ultrasonic features of multicystic dysplastic kidney: Expanded criteria. Radiology 143:217, 1982.

64. Kleiner B, Filly RA, Mack L, et al: Multicystic dysplastic kidney: Observations of contralateral disease in the fetal population. Radiology 161:27, 1986.

65. Sanders RC, Hartman DS: The sonographic distinction between neonatal multicystic kidney and hydronephrosis. Radiology 151:621, 1984.

66. Garcia CJ, Taylor KJW, Weiss RM: Congenital megacalyces: Ultrasound appearance. J Ultrasound Med 6:163, 1987.

67. Glick PL, Harrison MR, Noall RA, et al: Correction of congenital hydronephrosis in utero. III. Early mid-trimester ureteral obstruction produces renal dysplasia. J Pediatr Surg 18:681, 1983.

68. Pardes JG, Engel IA, Blomquist, et al: Ultrasonography of intrauterine Meckel's syndrome. J Ultrasound Med 3:33, 1984.

69. Vinaixa F, Gotzens VJ, Tejedo-Mateu A: Tubular gigantism of the kidney in a 41 mm, Streeter's 23rd horizon, human fetus with a comparative study of renal structures in normal human fetuses at a similar stage of development. Eur Urol 10:331, 1984.

70. Mahony BS, Callen PW, Filly RA, et al: Progression of infantile polycystic kidney disease in early pregnancy. J Ultrasound Med 3:277, 1984.

71. Luthy DA, Hirsch JH: Infantile polycystic kidney disease: Observations from attempts at prenatal diagnosis. Am J Med Genet 20:505, 1985.

72. Steinhardt GF, Slovis TL, Perlmutter AD: Simple renal cysts in infants. Radiology 155:349, 1985.

73. Elejalde BR, de Elejalde MM, Heitman T: Visualization of the fetal genitalia by ultrasonography: A review of the literature and analysis of its accuracy and ethical implications. J Ultrasound Med 4:633, 1985.

74. Mahony BS, Filly RA, Callen PW: Amnionicity and chorionicity in twin pregnancies: Prediction using ultrasound. Radiology 155:205, 1985.

75. Stephens JD: Prenatal diagnosis of testicular feminization. Lancet 2:1038, 1984.

76. Cooper C, Mahony BS, Bowie JD, et al: Prenatal ultrasound diagnosis of ambiguous genitalia. J Ultrasound Med 4:433, 1985.

77. Birnholz JC: Determination of fetal sex. N Engl J Med 309:942, 1983.

78. Natsuyama E: Sonographic determination of fetal sex from twelve weeks of gestation. Am J Obstet Gynecol 149:748, 1984.

79. Jafrie SZH, Bree RL, Silver TM, et al: Fetal ovarian cysts: Sonographic detection and association with hypothyroidism. Radiology 150:809, 1984.

80. Sandler MA, Smith SJ, Pope SG, et al: Prenatal diagnosis of septated ovarian cysts. JCU 13:55, 1985.

81. Holzgreve W, Winde B, Willital GH, et al: Prenatal diagnosis and perinatal management of a fetal ovarian cyst. Prenat Diagn 5:155, 1985.

ULTRASOUND EVALUATION OF HYDROPS FETALIS

Daryl H. Chinn, M.D.

Hydrops fetalis is the condition character-ized by excessive fluid accumulation within fetal extravascular compartments and body cavities. This serious condition, which pre-sents with varying degrees of fetal anasarca, ascites, pericardial effusion, pleural effu-sion, placental edema, and polyhydramnios, was first described nearly 100 years ago by Ballantyne.[1] In 1939, Levine discovered that maternal sensitization to a fetal blood group antigen played a major role in the develop-ment of hydrops fetalis.[2] In 1940, Landstei-ner and Weiner discovered the sensitizing antigen, the Rh factor.[3] In 1943, Potter iden-tified a subgroup of hydrops fetalis in which maternal Rh sensitization was not present.[4] With these observations, hydrops fetalis was categorized into those cases caused by an immunologic response, *immune hydrops fe-talis*, and those cases not caused by an im-munologic response, *nonimmune hydrops fetalis*. These two entities will be discussed separately.

IMMUNE HYDROPS FETALIS

In order to best appreciate the role of ultrasound in the evaluation of pregnancies complicated by immune hydrops fetalis, one must understand the revolutionary changes that have occurred in the diagnosis, manage-ment, and prevention of this disease.

After the discovery of the Rh blood group, distinct antigens (D, C, and E) were identi-fied within this system. The Rh(D) antigen initially accounted for 98 percent of all cases of immune hydrops fetalis. Other blood group antigens, such as E and C of the Rh system, K of the Kell system, and Fy[a] of the Duffy system, have less frequently been the cause of severe immune hydrops fetalis.[5]

Pathophysiology

The pathogenesis of immune hydrops fe-talis depends upon the presence of maternal serum IgG antibody against one of the fetal red blood cell antigens. A maternal serum antibody to a red blood cell antigen will develop if the mother is exposed to red blood cell antigens different from her own. Typi-cally, this occurs during the release of fetal red blood cells into the maternal circulation at the time of delivery of a prior newborn. Other sensitizing events can be fetal–mater-nal hemorrhage, which can occur sponta-neously, associated with amniocentesis, or from an abortion (spontaneous or therapeu-tic). Transfusion of mismatched blood oc-

277

casionally occurs, resulting in maternal sensitization.

Maternal IgG will cross the placental–fetal barrier and enter the fetal circulation, bind to surface antigens on the fetal red blood cell, and promote fetal red blood cell hemolysis. If the concentration of maternal IgG is sufficiently high to result in significant fetal hemolysis, fetal anemia will result.

The following pathophysiologic interactions, although not absolutely proven, represent the current accepted theory for the development of immune hydrops: extramedullary erythropoiesis follows fetal anemia; erythropoietic and fibroblastic tissues replace the normal liver parenchyma and create hepatomegaly; and portal venous hypertension follows and results in fetal ascites. The elevated umbilical vein pressure decreases placental perfusion; placental edema and enlargement follows. Impaired placental diffusion of amino acids, combined with the decreased protein synthesis by an abnormal fetal liver, results in severe fetal hypoproteinemia, which leads to hydrops fetalis (Fig. 12–1).[6, 7]

Although intuitively one might predict that severe fetal anemia might cause fetal congestive heart failure and thereby result in fetal hydrops, this does not appear to be the case. Studies of blood volume in fetuses and neonates with immune hydrops fetalis demonstrate a normal blood volume.[8, 9] This sequence of pathologic events emphasizes the complex interaction of multiple mechanisms. Additionally, there is no constant relationship between fetal venous hematocrit and the presence or absence of immune hydrops fetalis.[7] Some fetuses become hydropic with hemoglobin greater than 7 gm per 100 ml, and some fetuses are not hydropic with hemoglobin less than 3 gm per 100 ml.[10] Additionally, isolated severe fetal hypoproteinemia, as present with analbuminemia and congenital nephrotic syndrome, does not always result in fetal hydrops.[7, 9]

For the sonographer, the above-noted mechanisms offer a framework with which one can organize sonographic observations and attempt to assign significance to these findings.

Prophylaxis Against Rh(D) Sensitization: Intrauterine Transfusion

Since 1960, medical advances have greatly reduced the impact of Rh(D) sensitization in the development of immune hydrops fetalis. Effective Rh(D) sensitization prophylaxis, effective screening for the isoimmunized pregnancy, and fetal therapy for immune hydrops fetalis now exist.

With the administration of Rh(D) immune globulin (RhoGAM) to Rh(D)-negative women at the time of their potential sensitization to the antigen, the incidence of Rh(D)-sensitized women has been significantly reduced. Bowman has reported a decreased incidence of sensitization from 10.6 to 2.7 per 1000.[11] With this decrease, the incidence of non-Rh(D) sensitization due to other atypical antibodies, such as Rh(E), Rh(C), K of the Kell system, and Fy[a] of the Duffy system, has risen from 2 to 10 percent of the cases of immune hydrops fetalis.[5]

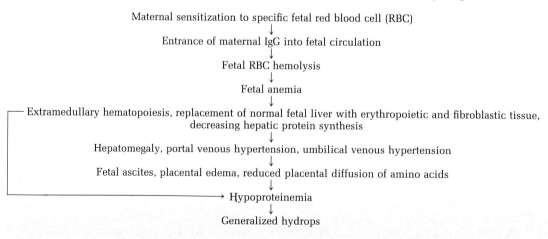

Maternal sensitization to specific fetal red blood cell (RBC)
↓
Entrance of maternal IgG into fetal circulation
↓
Fetal RBC hemolysis
↓
Fetal anemia
↓
Extramedullary hematopoiesis, replacement of normal fetal liver with erythropoietic and fibroblastic tissue, decreasing hepatic protein synthesis
↓
Hepatomegaly, portal venous hypertension, umbilical venous hypertension
↓
Fetal ascites, placental edema, reduced placental diffusion of amino acids
↓
Hypoproteinemia
↓
Generalized hydrops

Figure 12–1. Sequence of events leading to immune hydrops fetalis.

Prenatal screening for the presence of maternal atypical antibodies is routinely performed. If atypical antibodies are present, they are subsequently identified and quantified. The father's blood will be tested for the corresponding antigen. In the case of anti-Rh(D) antibody, a titer greater than 1:8 is considered above the "critical value" and renders the fetus at risk for immune hydrops fetalis.

In 1961, Liley established the relationship between amniotic fluid spectrophotometric determination of bilirubin and the severity of fetal hemolysis at 27 to 41 weeks' gestation. Before the development of ultrasound, the determination of amniotic fluid bilirubin was the primary means of fetal assessment in the isoimmunized pregnancy.[12]

In 1963, Liley ushered in the era of fetal intervention with the revolutionary concept of intrauterine transfusion of compatible blood into the peritoneal cavities of fetuses suffering from Rh(D)-immune hydrops fetalis.[13]

In the 1970s, with the development of ultrasound, this technology was applied to the clinical problem of immune hydrops fetalis to improve guidance and control of obstetric interventional techniques and to assess the severity of immune hydrops fetalis.[14–16]

Ultrasound Assessment

As experience with the Liley technique for evaluating the severity of immune hydrops fetalis grew, it became clear that Liley curves extrapolated into the second trimester were poor predictors of the severity of fetal hemolysis.[17, 18] Furthermore, in the third trimester, amniotic fluid determination

of bilirubin, while reflecting the severity of fetal hemolysis, fails to account for possible fetal compensatory mechanisms that may be accompanying the hemolytic process. Numerous authors have described cases of normal amniotic fluid bilirubin in which severe immune hydrops fetalis was present.[19, 20] For these reasons, ultrasound plays a major role in assessment of the physiologic status of the fetus at risk for immune hydrops fetalis in both the second and third trimester.

Upon review of the pathophysiology of immune hydrops fetalis delineated in Figure 12–1, one would predict that ultrasound would display a number of morphologic manifestations, including profound skin thickening, placental thickening, serous cavity effusions, hepatomegaly, and polyhydramnios.

Integumentary thickening is considered abnormal when measuring greater than 5 mm. Measurements of this type, however, are quite subjective, and observation of subtle amounts of skin edema is extremely difficult to quantify (Figs. 12–2, 12–3). Additionally, anasarca is considered to be one of the late features of hydrops fetalis.[18]

Similarly, placental thickness is often reported as abnormal when greater than 4 cm (Figs. 12–4, 12–5). However, this measurement varies with gestational age, and with volume of amniotic fluid.[21] Qualitatively, placental edema has been described as having a ground glass appearance, with disappearance of the chorionic plate, buckling of the fetal surface, and loss of the cotyledon definition.[22] However, identification of early placental edema is very difficult sonographically owing to the subjectivity of the observation.

Total intrauterine volume estimations are conceptually appealing since this measure-

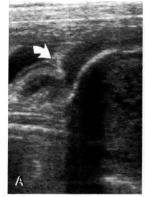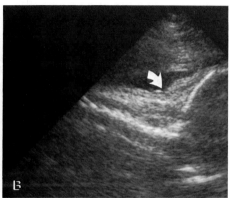

Figure 12–2. *A,* Longitudinal view of nuchal region, demonstrating markedly edematous integument *(arrow). B,* Normal integument *(arrow)* for comparison.

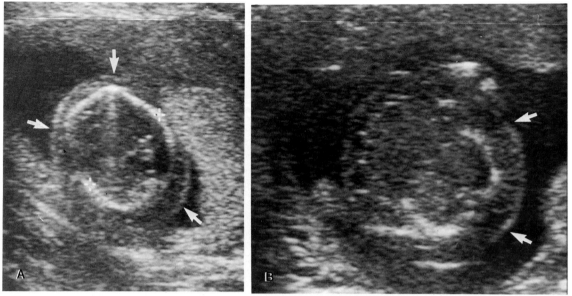

Figure 12–3. *A*, Transverse axial view of hydropic fetal head, depicting scalp edema *(arrows)*. *B*, Transverse axial image of hydropic fetal thorax, demonstrating chest wall edema *(arrows)*.

Figure 12–4. Longitudinal ultrasonogram demonstrating a massive placental thickening (P) and scalp edema (e) in a fetus with immune hydrops fetalis.

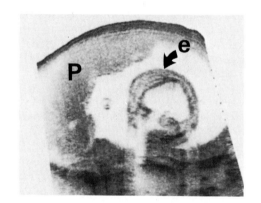

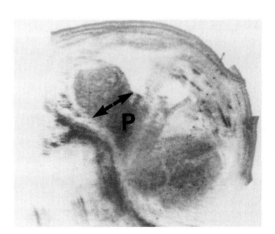

Figure 12–5. Longitudinal ultrasonogram demonstrating edematous placenta (P) with homogeneous texture, and buckling of the placental surface.

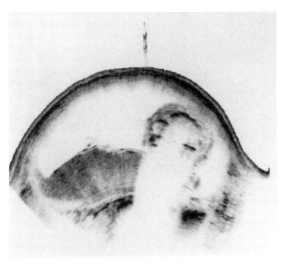

Figure 12–6. Longitudinal ultrasonogram demonstrating markedly thickened placenta, polyhydramnios, and facial integumentary edema in a fetus with immune hydrops fetalis secondary to maternal Kell sensitization.

ment would combine placental edema, fetal anasarca, and polyhydramnios (Fig. 12–6). This measurement has not proven useful as an indication of the overall status of the isoimmunized pregnancy.[17]

A review of the pathophysiology of immune hydrops fetalis (Fig. 12–1) suggests that fetal ascites might appear before anasarca and pleural effusions. This is consistent with clinical observations. In a case report, a small amount of ascites is reported to be the earliest ultrasound sign of impending decompensation in immune hydrops fetalis.[24] Small amounts of ascites are identi-

fied as fluid between bowel loops (Fig. 12–7). If the diagnosis of hydrops is considered, one should be aware of the potential pitfall of "pseudoascites." Frequently, a sonolucent band is seen adjacent to the anterior abdominal wall in a normal fetus. This finding is often due to the poorly echogenic integument of the anterior abdominal wall and should not be misinterpreted as representing peritoneal fluid (Fig. 12–8).[25]

DeVore and coworkers have proposed that pericardial effusion is the earliest sign of decompensation in immune hydrops fetalis. In a small series using M-mode real-time ultrasound, they identified pericardial effusion before the development of ascites, pleural effusion, or anasarca.[26] This observation has not been confirmed by others.

Pleural effusions are usually readily identified. They appear as fluid outlining the lungs in a supraphrenic location (Fig. 12–9).

Umbilical vein diameter had been proposed as a useful measurement for early fetal decompensation in immune hydrops fetalis;[27, 28] however, subsequent series have contradicted this observation.[17, 23, 29]

Consistent with the author's understanding of pathophysiology, fetal liver enlargement as a result of extramedullary hematopoiesis is an early event in the decompensation of the isoimmunized fetus. Although hepatomegaly is frequently identified in immune hydrops fetalis, attempts to quantify fetal liver size using abdominal circumference,[17, 23] abdominal circumference ratios,[18] and intraperitoneal volumes[17] have not been successful. Correlation of the sagittal length of the liver's right lobe with immune hydrops fetalis appears promising and may represent an early sonographic feature of impending decompensation.[23] Biophysical profiles, discussed in Chapter 15, are used in many laboratories for an assessment of the physiologic status of the fetus.

In summary, a consistent early sonographic sign of impending fetal decompensation in immune hydrops fetalis has not been found. Owing to the inexact correlation between spectrophotometric determination of amniotic fluid bilirubin and the physiologic status of the fetus, clinicians continue to rely on ultrasound and biophysical profiles, as well as amniotic fluid bilirubin, in their assessment of the isoimmunized fetus. In fetuses requiring intrauterine transfusions, serial ultrasound studies are very use-

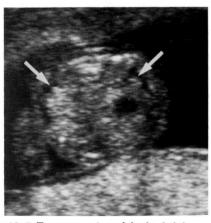

Figure 12–7. Transverse view of the fetal abdomen with a small amount of fetal ascites *(arrows)* interposed between echogenic bowel loops.

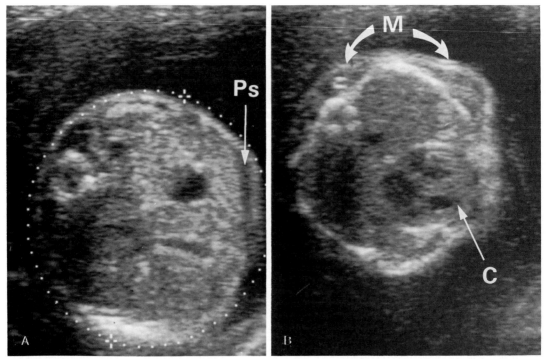

Figure 12–8. Pitfalls in sonographic diagnosis of hydrops fetalis. *A*, Pseudoascites (Ps). *B*, Pseudo–body wall edema. M, normal fetal musculature; C, cardiac structures.

ful in evaluating the immediate effectiveness of therapy.[22]

The Role of Ultrasound in Management of Immune Hydrops Fetalis

Ultrasound is a significant improvement over radiographic and fluoroscopic tech-niques previously used for locating the fetus during intrauterine transfusions (Fig. 12–10); it permits continuous monitoring of the dynamic situation without ionizing radia-tion. Use of ultrasound led to improved precision of intrauterine transfusion and re-duction in morbidity and mortality from the procedure.[22] Further refinements in the qual-ity of ultrasound, as well as refinements in its precision, have led to percutaneous um-

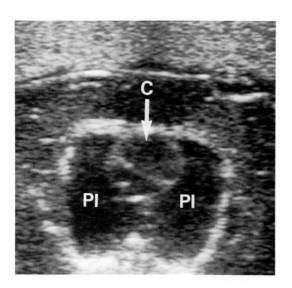

Figure 12–9. Transverse axial image through the fetal thorax, depicting massive pleural effusions (Pl) sur-rounding the cardiac structures (C).

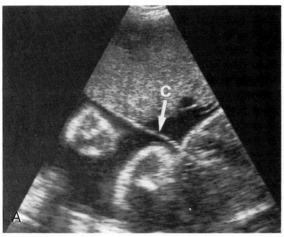 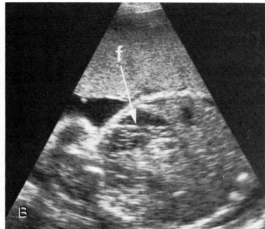

Figure 12–10. Intraperitoneal blood transfusion in a fetus with immune hydrops fetalis. *A,* Catheter (c) traversing the amniotic fluid and entering the fetal peritoneal cavity. *B,* Intraperitoneal bubbles and fluid (f) following intraperitoneal transfusion.

bilical vein sampling and direct intrauterine transfusion into the umbilical vessels (Figs. 12–11, 12–12).[15, 16] Ultrasound localization of the placenta also plays a crucial role in directing amniocentesis in the Rh(D)-negative mother. Decreasing the incidence of placental injury reduces the incidence of fetal–maternal hemorrhage and therefore the risk of maternal sensitization.

Prognosis

As stated above, Bowman and associates have accomplished a fourfold reduction in the incidence of Rh sensitization by the

administration of Rh(D) immune globulin to Rh(D)-negative women at the time of their delivery of Rh(D)-positive newborns, at the time of abortion, at the time of amniocentesis, and at the 28th week of pregnancy to prevent sensitization by clinically silent fetal–maternal hemorrhage.[11]

These investigators currently report fetal survival rates in Rh-sensitized pregnancies to be 100 percent for nonhydropic fetuses, 75 percent for hydropic fetuses, and 92 per-

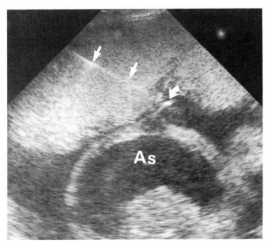

Figure 12–11. Intravascular transfusion in a fetus with immune hydrops fetalis. Note the needle *(straight arrows)* traversing the thickened placenta and entering the umbilical cord *(curved arrow).* As, ascites.

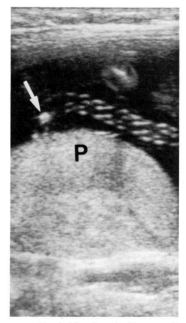

Figure 12–12. Fetal blood sampling needle *(arrow)* entering the umbilical vessel at the cord insertion site. P, placenta.

cent overall for all sensitized fetuses (Fig. 12–13). These excellent results are attributed to the extensive use of real-time ultrasound, which permits precise control of the intrauterine transfusion procedure, thereby reducing transfusion-related mortality from 51 to 0 percent. These investigators also credit ultrasound for a more exact assessment of fetal pathophysiology, permitting optimal timing for transfusion and immediate evaluation of the effectiveness of transfusion.[22]

The clinical problem of immune hydrops fetalis has significantly changed over the last 20 years owing to the development of effective prophylaxis, routine screening for atypical antibodies, availability of intrauterine therapy, and development of ultrasound. Despite Rh(D) prophylaxis, immune hydrops fetalis will continue because of instances of unsuccessful prophylaxis and continued cases of non–Rh(D)-immune hydrops fetalis. Ultrasound and amniotic fluid determinations of bilirubin provide complementary techniques for evaluating the pathophysiologic status of the fetus and directing management. Additional improvement in the prognosis of immune hydrops fetalis is anticipated.

NONIMMUNE HYDROPS FETALIS

In 1943, Potter described a clinical entity that affected non–Rh-sensitized pregnancies and was characterized by fetal anasarca, placental edema, and, often, fetal serous effusions. Potter recognized that this entity, since termed nonimmune hydrops fetalis, did not represent a specific disease but

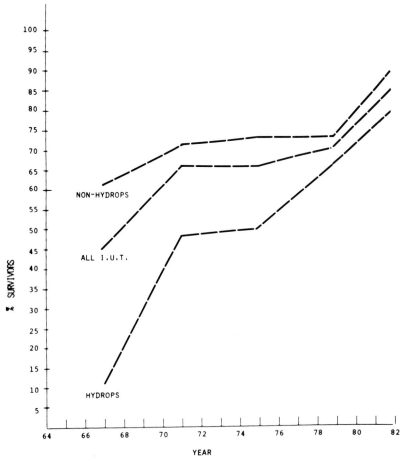

Figure 12–13. Line graphs of the percentage of surviving fetuses undergoing first intrauterine transfusion (IUT) for nonhydropic disease, all stages of disease, and hydrops. (*From* Harmon CR, Manning FA, Bowman JM, Lange IR: Severe Rh disease: Poor outcome is not inevitable. Am J Obstet Gynecol 145:823, 1983.)

rather a late manifestation of many severe diseases.[4]

When Potter first described nonimmune hydrops fetalis, this entity represented less than 20 percent of all the cases of hydrops fetalis; however, since the advent of effective prophylaxis against Rh(D) sensitization, the relative frequency of nonimmune hydrops fetalis has risen to 90 percent.[18]

Depending upon the clinical series and patient referral patterns, the incidence of nonimmune hydrops fetalis ranges from one in 14,000 to one in 7000.[30–32] The mortality rate for nonimmune hydrops fetalis ranges from 50 to 98 percent.[30, 33]

Unlike the situation with immune hydrops fetalis, there are no sensitive laboratory tests to screen pregnancies at risk for nonimmune hydrops fetalis. Ultrasound, if performed, will detect nearly all cases. Unfortunately, approximately 30 percent of pregnancies with nonimmune hydrops fetalis are clinically uneventful, and ultrasound is not obtained.[31]

Even when routine ultrasound is not performed, the identification of a pregnancy complication often leads to an ultrasound examination. In most series, polyhydramnios is the most frequent maternal complication, presenting as a size-date discrepancy. Polyhydramnios occurs in 50 to 75 percent of patients with nonimmune hydrops fetalis.[31, 33] Pregnancy-induced hypertension occurs in 15 to 46 percent of patients.[31, 32] Maternal anemia occurs in approximately 7 to 45 percent, depending on the definition of anemia and demographics of the particular study.[33, 34] Maternal hypoalbuminemia occurs in 7 to 67 percent.[31, 33] Other less frequent maternal complications included urinary tract infections, antepartum hemorrhage, and gestational diabetes mellitus.[31, 33] Clinical evidence for fetal arrhythmia was present in 15 percent of one series of patients with nonimmune hydrops.[35]

Etiology

The etiologies of nonimmune hydrops are extremely numerous; Table 12–1 represents a list of conditions associated with nonimmune hydrops fetalis.[36] Our knowledge of which conditions listed in Table 12–1 are truly causative of nonimmune hydrops fetalis is extremely limited. For instance, homozygous alpha-thalassemia causes nonimmune hydrops fetalis through its precipitation of severe fetal anemia, initiating the pathophysiologic cascade similar to immune hydrops fetalis (Fig. 12–1). Homozygous alpha-thalassemia is clearly etiologic in the development of nonimmune hydrops fetalis. However, pulmonary hypoplasia, which is listed in many tables as etiologic in the development of nonimmune hydrops fetalis, is rather, in most cases, a consequence of this condition. The pleural effusions that frequently accompany nonimmune hydrops fetalis do not permit proper development of the fetal lungs, and pulmonary hypoplasia results.[35]

Although homozygous alpha-thalassemia and fetal pulmonary hypoplasia are clear-cut examples of a cause and associated result of nonimmune hydrops fetalis, an attempt to separate Table 12–1 into causes and results of nonimmune hydrops would be difficult at this point. Likely, a third category of *associated* entities exists, which are neither etiologic nor a direct result of nonimmune hydrops fetalis.

The sonographic criteria for nonimmune hydrops differs between authors, and therefore case selection varies.[37, 38] Furthermore, authors differ in their willingness to consider an identified abnormality as causative of nonimmune hydrops, and subsequently the number of cases considered idiopathic in the etiology of nonimmune hydrops varies from 20 to 50 percent.[39, 40] It is inevitable that further associations with nonimmune hydrops fetalis will be observed.

Of the categories delineated in Table 12–1, among the Southeast Asian population, the major cause of nonimmune hydrops fetalis is homozygous alpha-thalassemia. Among North American and northern European populations, the leading cause of nonimmune hydrops fetalis is cardiac anomalies, both structural defects and arrhythmias, accounting for 20 to 76 percent of cases.[18, 41]

Pathophysiology

Owing to the diverse associations with nonimmune hydrops fetalis, knowledge of the pathophysiology in most cases is limited. As stated above, homozygous alpha-thalassemia and immune hydrops fetalis share a common cause and pathophysiology of fetal

Table 12–1. CONDITIONS ASSOCIATED WITH NIHF

Categories	Individual Conditions
Cardiovascular	Tachyarrhythmia Complex dysrhythmia Congenital heart block Anatomic defects (atrial septal defect, ventricular septal defect, hypoplastic left heart, pulmonary valve insufficiency, Ebstein's subaortic stenosis, aortic valve stenosis, subaortic stenosis, atrioventricular canal defect with mitral regurgitation, single ventricle, tetralogy of Fallot, premature closure of the foramen ovale or of the ductus arteriosus, subendocardial fibroelastosis, dextrocardia in combination with pulmonic stenosis) Calcified aortic valve Coronary artery embolus Cardiomyopathy Myocarditis (Coxsackie virus or CMV) Atrial hemangioma Intracardial rhabdomyoma Endocardial teratoma
Chromosomal	Down's syndrome (Trisomy 21) Other trisomies Turner's syndrome XX/XY mosaicism Triploidy
Malformation syndromes	Thanatophoric dwarfism Arthrogryposis multiplex congenita Asphyxiating thoracic dystrophy Hypophosphatasia Osteogenesis imperfecta Achondrogenesis Saldino-Noonan syndrome Neu-Laxova syndrome Francois syndrome, Type 3 Recessive cystic hygroma Pena-Shokier syndrome, Type 1
Twin pregnancy Hematologic	Twin-twin transfusion syndrome Alpha-thalassemia Arteriovenous shunts (e.g., large vascular tumors) Fetal Kasabach-Merritt syndrome In utero closed space hemorrhage Vena cava, portal vein, or femoral obstruction (e.g., thrombosis) G6PD deficiency
Urinary	Urethral stenosis or atresia Posterior urethral valves Bladder neck obstruction Spontaneous bladder perforation Congenital nephrosis (Finnish type) Neurogenic bladder with reflux Ureterocele Prune-belly syndrome

Table 12–1. CONDITIONS ASSOCIATED WITH NIHF *Continued*

Categories	Individual Conditions
Respiratory	Diaphragmatic hernia Cystic adenoma of the lung Pulmonary lymphangiectasia Hamartoma of the lung Mediastinal teratoma Pulmonary hypoplasia Hemangioma of the lung
Gastrointestinal	Jejunal atresia Midgut volvulus Malrotation of the intestines Duplication of the intestinal tract Meconium peritonitis
Liver	Hepatic calcifications Hepatic fibrosis Cholestasis Polycystic disease of the liver Biliary atresia Hepatic vascular malformations Familial cirrhosis
Maternal	Severe diabetes mellitus Severe anemia Hypoproteinemia
Placenta-umbilical cord	Chorioangioma Chorionic vein thrombosis Fetomaternal transfusion Placental and umbilical vein thrombosis Umbilical cord torsion True cord knots Angiomyxoma of the umbilical cord Aneurysm of the umbilical artery
Medications	Antepartum indomethacin (taken to stop premature labor, causing fetal ductus closure and secondary NIHF)
Infections	CMV Toxoplasmosis Syphilis Congenital hepatitis Herpes simplex, Type 1 Rubella Leptospirosis Chagas' disease
Miscellaneous	Congenital lymphedema Congenital hydro- or chylothorax Polysplenia syndrome Congenital neuroblastoma Tuberous sclerosis Torsion of an ovarian cyst Fetal trauma Sacrococcygeal teratoma

From Holzgreve W, Holzgreve B, Curry JR: Nonimmune hydrops fetalis: Diagnosis and management. Semin Perinatol 9:52, 1985.

hydrops, that of severe fetal anemia (Fig. 12–1).

Although heart failure has been shown not to be a dominant mechanism for the development of hydrops in immune hydrops fetalis,[8, 9] it undoubtedly plays a role in the development of nonimmune hydrops fetalis in fetuses with cardiac arrhythmias and gross cardiac malformations. However, the exact pathologic mechanism for the development of nonimmune hydrops fetalis in the vast majority of cases is purely speculative.

Although it is intuitively appealing to classify the pathologic mechanisms in nonimmune hydrops fetalis based on knowledge of the neonate's pathophysiology (elevated intravascular pressure, heart failure, decreased plasma oncotic pressure, increased capillary permeability, and obstruction to lymphatic flow),[32] these classifications are purely speculative. This approach does, however, provide an organization framework (Table 12–2).

Table 12–2. CLASSIFICATION OF HYDROPS FETALIS BASED ON SPECULATIVE PATHOPHYSIOLOGIC MECHANISMS

Increased intravascular hydrostatic pressure (due to hemodynamic disturbances)
  Primary myocardial failure
    Arrhythmia (e.g., paroxysmal atrial tachycardia, familial heart block)
    Severe anemia (e.g., G6PD deficiency, alpha-thalassemia)
    Twin transfusion syndrome
    Myocarditis (e.g., Coxsackie virus, TORCH)
    Cardiac malformation
  High-output failure
    Parabiotic syndrome
    Arteriovenous shunt
  Obstruction of venous return
    Congenital neoplasm/other space-occupying lesions (e.g., neuroblastoma, retroperitoneal fibrosis, vena caval thrombosis)
Decreased plasma oncotic pressure
  Decreased albumin formation (e.g., congenital cirrhosis, hepatitis)
  Increased albumin excretion (e.g., congenital nephrotic syndrome of Finnish type)
Increased capillary permeability
  Anoxia (e.g., congenital infection, placental edema)
Obstruction of lymph flow (e.g., Turner's syndrome)

From Im SS, Rizos N, Joutsi P, et al: Nonimmunologic hydrops fetalis. Am J Obstet Gynecol 148:566, 1984.

Clinical Evaluation

Ultrasound is the primary means for identifying the hydropic fetus. Once identified, immune hydrops fetalis can be excluded by the indirect Coombs test, which, in the case of nonimmune hydrops fetalis, would demonstrate the absence of atypical antibodies in the maternal serum. Further testing to determine the cause or conditions associated with nonimmune hydrops fetalis is listed in Table 12–3. Tests are organized in levels of diagnostic invasiveness. In addition to its use in diagnosing the hydropic state, ultrasound is listed in Table 12–3 as a major diagnostic means for identifying the conditions associated with nonimmune hydrops fetalis.

Sonographic Evaluation

The sonographic identification of the fetus with nonimmune hydrops is conceptually identical to the identification of immune hydrops fetalis discussed previously. The sonographer searches for the classic findings of skin thickening greater than 5 mm, placental enlargement greater than 4 cm, ascites, pericardial effusion, pleural effusion, and polyhydramnios. In some studies, ascites alone is considered diagnostic of nonimmune hydrops fetalis.[38] Other studies are purposely skewed to severe nonimmune hydrops fetalis, requiring serous effusions in two body cavities or a serous effusion in one body cavity in addition to anasarca for the diagnosis.[37] This lack of precision leads to variation in the cases included in series of nonimmune hydrops fetalis. Furthermore, variation in the assigned significance of skin thickening (i.e., whether secondary to maternal diabetes or redundant integument in short-limbed dwarfism) will affect whether that fetus and the associated findings are included in series of nonimmune hydrops fetalis.

Although it is true that ascites can be seen in the hydropic state, when it occurs alone, it is often from a local rather than a generalized condition. Ascites has often been noted to occur with urinary and intestinal tract obstruction (Figs. 12–14, 12–15).[42] Fetuses displaying only ascites, unassociated with generalized hydrops, generally have a better prognosis and should be considered separately.

It is the author's belief that the diagnosis of nonimmune hydrops fetalis should be

Table 12–3. DIAGNOSTIC STEPS IN THE PRENATAL EVALUATION OF NIHF

Levels of Diagnostic Invasiveness	Diagnostic Test	Possible Etiology of NIHF
Noninvasive	Complete blood count and indices	Hematologic disorders (alpha-thalassemia)
	Hemoglobin electrophoresis	Alpha-thalassemia
	Blood chemistry (e.g., maternal G6PD, pyruvate kinease carrier status)	Possibility of fetal red cell enzyme deficiency
	Betke-Kleihauer stain	Fetomaternal transfusion
	Syphilis (VDRL) and TORCH titers	Fetal infection
	Ultrasound	Assessment of NIHF and its progression, exclusion of multiple pregnancy and congenital malformations
	Fetal echocardiography (two-dimensional pulsed Doppler and M-mode)	Congenital heart defects Rhythm disturbances of the fetal heart
	Oral glucose tolerance test	Maternal diabetes mellitus
Amniocentesis	Fetal karyotype	Chromosomal abnormalities
	Amniotic fluid culture	CMV
	Alpha-fetoprotein	Congenital nephrosis, sacrococcygeal teratomas
	Specific metabolic tests	Gaucher, Tay-Sachs, GM_1 gangliosidosis, etc.
	Restriction endonuclease tests	Alpha-thalassemia
Fetal blood aspiration	Rapid karyotype and metabolic tests	Chromosomal or metabolic abnormalities
	Hemoglobin chain analysis	Thalassemias
	Fetal plasma analysis for specific IgM	Intrauterine infection
	Fetal plasma albumin	Hypoalbuminemia

From Holzgreve W, Holzgreve B, Curry JR: Nonimmune hydrops fetalis: Diagnosis and management. Semin Perinatol 9:52, 1985.

made only when there are either serous effusions in two body cavities or a serous effusion in one body cavity in addition to anasarca (Figs. 12–16 to 12–18). With these criteria, when a diagnosis of nonimmune hydrops is made, the poor prognosis reported to the parents is likely to be realistic. In contradistinction, when the isolated finding of ascites or minor integumentary thickening is discovered, the ultimate prognosis may not be as severe.

Isolated pericardial effusion has been proposed by DeVore as the earliest sonographic finding of developing hydrops in fetuses with structural cardiac anomalies.[43] DeVore stresses the use of real-time M-mode in the identification of fetal pericardial effusions (Fig. 12–19). These observations have not been independently confirmed (see Chap. 8).

Pleural effusion can be diagnosed when fluid is demonstrated in a supradiaphragmatic location within the thorax. This ap-

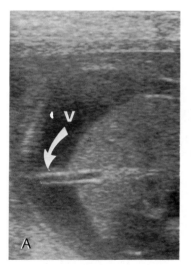 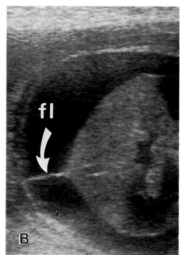 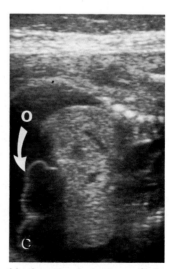

Figure 12–14. Potentially confusing structures in the presence of a large amount of fetal ascites. A, Ascites outlining the umbilical vein (v). B, Ascites outlining the falciform ligament (fl). C, Fluid in the greater and lesser peritoneal cavities, separated by the omentum (o).

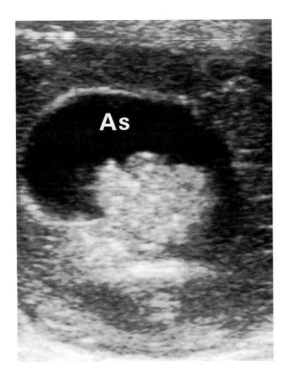

Figure 12–15. Large amount of ascites (As) outlines echogenic bowel.

pearance, however, can be mimicked by ascites that is present in a diaphragmatic hernia. Several studies have concluded that pulmonary hypoplasia is a major cause of death in fetuses with nonimmune hydrops fetalis.[33, 35, 44] Pulmonary hypoplasia secondary to in utero pulmonary compression by thoracic masses has been demonstrated in laboratory animals.[45] It has been proposed that the pleural effusions that frequently accompany nonimmune hydrops fetalis in many cases are responsible for pulmonary hypoplasia. Therefore, the sporadic in utero removal of fetal pleural effusions has been attempted to ameliorate the development of pulmonary hypoplasia. These interventions have met with mixed results.[44, 46]

Placental thickening greater than 4 cm is considered abnormal; however, in the presence of polyhydramnios, abnormal placental thickness may be present with measurements less than 4 cm. Placental thickening appears to correlate with disorders having abnormal umbilical blood flow, such as he-

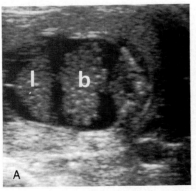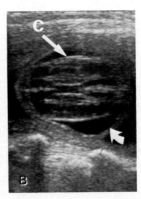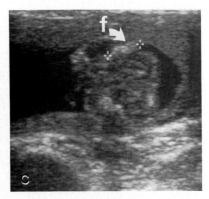

Figure 12–16. Severe nonimmune hydrops fetalis in hypophosphatasia dwarfism. *A*, Coronal view of the fetal abdomen, displaying ascites surrounding the liver (l) and bowel (b). *B*, Transverse axial images of the fetal head, depicting massive scalp edema *(arrow)*. Note the poorly mineralized calvaria (c) due to hypophosphatasia. *C*, Short, poorly mineralized femur (f).

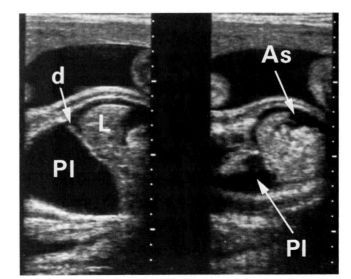

Figure 12–17. Sagittal images of the chest and abdomen, depicting a large pleural effusion (Pl) and ascites (As). Diaphragm, d; liver, L.

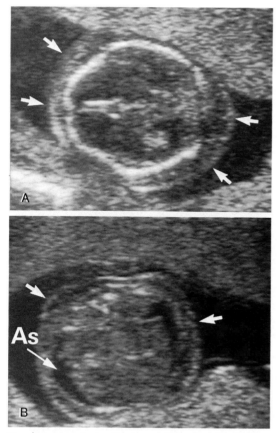

Figure 12–18. A, Axial images of the fetal head, demonstrating scalp edema *(arrows).* B, Axial images of the upper abdomen, demonstrating integumentary edema *(arrows)* and a rim of ascites (As).

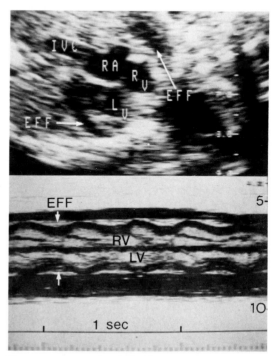

Figure 12–19. Pericardial effusion. Two-dimensional and M-mode ultrasound evaluation of a fetus with a pericardial effusion (EFF). IVC, inferior vena cava; RA, right atrium; RV, right ventricle; LV, left ventricle.

Table 12–4. STRUCTURAL ANOMALIES ASSOCIATED WITH HYDROPS FETALIS THAT MAY HAVE SONOGRAPHIC MANIFESTATIONS

	Sonographic Manifestation	Abnormality
Fetus		
Head	Intracranial mass, associated with congestive heart failure and microcephaly	Arteriovenous malformation, vein of Galen aneurysm, cytomegalic inclusion virus, toxoplasmosis
Neck	Cystic neck masses	Lymphatic dysplasias
Thorax	Poorly contracting heart	Congestive heart failure
	Pericardial effusion, tachycardia	Cardiac anomaly
	Asystole	Demise
	Mediastinal mass	Tumor
	Chest mass	Cystic adenomatoid malformation, pulmonary sequestration
	Small thorax	Dwarfism
	Cystic masses crossing diaphragm	Diaphragmatic hernias
Extremities	Short arms, legs	Dwarfism*
	Contractures	Arthrogryposis
	Fractures	Osteogenesis imperfecta
Placenta	Mass	Chorioangioma
Amniotic cavity	Number of fetuses, relative size, amniotic membrane	Twin-twin transfusion
	Umbilical cord anomalies	Single umbilical artery, umbilical cord torsion

*Redundant skin folds from shortened limbs should not be mistaken for edema.
Modified from Fleischer AC, Killam AP, Boehm FH, et al: Hydrops fetalis: Sonographic evaluation and clinical implications. Radiology 141:163, 1981.

matologic, vascular, or cardiac anomalies.[37] The association of placental thickening and in utero infection is also well established.

Polyhydramnios is identified in up to 75 percent of fetuses with nonimmune hydrops fetalis.[33] Polyhydramnios may play a role in the development of the high incidence of prematurity among fetuses with nonimmune hydrops (95 percent delivered at less than 37 weeks' gestation).[32] Oligohydramnios associated with nonimmune hydrops has a very poor prognosis.[38]

In addition to identifying the hydropic status of the fetus, ultrasound will identify associated fetal structural anomalies in 25 to 40 percent of cases.[32, 35] Since nearly every organ of the fetus may display an abnormality that has been associated with nonimmune hydrops fetalis, careful systematic sonographic evaluation is required. Organized by anatomic region, Table 12–4 represents a brief list of abnormalities that might be detected sonographically. Special attention must be given to the cardiovascular system

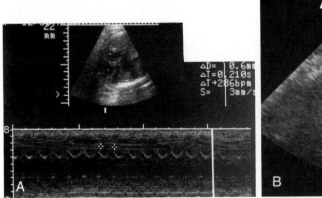
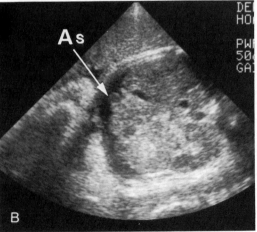

Figure 12–20. Nonimmune hydrops fetalis in a fetus with supraventricular tachycardia. *A*, Four-chamber heart view/M-mode demonstrating tachyrhythmia with a heart rate equal to 286 beats/min. *B*, Transverse view of the fetal abdomen, demonstrating ascites (As).

owing to the high frequency of structural abnormalities and arrhythmias (Figs. 12–20, 12–21). Many arrhythmias are intermittent, requiring prolonged inpatient monitoring for detection.[47] Identification of fetal cardiac arrhythmias is particularly rewarding as these are among the most treatable causes of nonimmune fetal hydrops.

The use of ultrasound in directing fetal blood sampling will likely play a greater role in the analysis of nonimmune hydrops fetalis. As in immune hydrops fetalis, improved success rates and decreased morbidity and mortality rates are expected with percutaneous umbilical vein sampling than with fetoscopic blood sampling.[48]

Prognosis

Prognosis of nonimmune hydrops fetalis is very poor. The mortality rate ranges from 50 to 98 percent.[30, 33] The sonographic identification of a fetal structural abnormality indicates a perinatal risk of mortality approaching 100 percent.[32, 35, 49] Generalized lymphangiectasia is nearly always lethal (Figs. 12–22, 12–23).

Two series evaluated the utility of sonographic findings to predict fetal outcome. Based on collective experience with immune hydrops fetalis, one would have anticipated a worse prognosis in nonimmune hydrops fetalis in those fetuses displaying anasarca and large serous effusions; however, in two analyses of sonographic features, prognosis

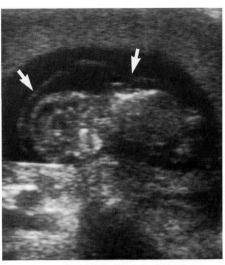

Figure 12–22. Nonimmune hydrops fetalis secondary to generalized lymphangiectasia. Longitudinal scan in a fetus of 11 to 12 menstrual weeks. Note the severe integumentary edema (arrows).

could not be predicted.[37, 38] The above analyses, however, were based on a single observation, and serial sonographic evaluations of the fetus with nonimmune hydrops fetalis remain useful to identify improvement or worsening of the fetal pathophysiologic state.

Despite the dismal clinical outcome for fetuses with nonimmune hydrops fetalis, it is useful to keep in mind several instances of spontaneous resolution of fetal ascites and sonographically severe nonimmune hydrops fetalis.[50–53]

Although nonimmune hydrops fetalis remains poorly understood, a few generalizations concerning the utility of ultrasound can be made.

1. Ultrasound is the pivotal examination in identifying nonimmune hydrops fetalis.

2. A sonographically demonstrated structural fetal anomaly in the setting of nonimmune hydrops fetalis implies a very poor prognosis. Generalized congenital lymphangiectasia is virtually always lethal.

3. The cardiovascular system is the most frequent organ system affected in identifiable causes of nonimmune hydrops fetalis among North American and northern European populations. Arrhythmias are among the fetal anomalies that are most amenable to therapy. Careful sonographic scrutiny of the heart is warranted.

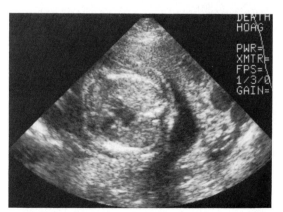

Figure 12–21. Nonimmune hydrops fetalis in a fetus with a hypoplastic left heart. Axial view of the fetal thorax, demonstrating integumentary edema. Note the absence of the left ventricular cavity on the "four-chamber view."

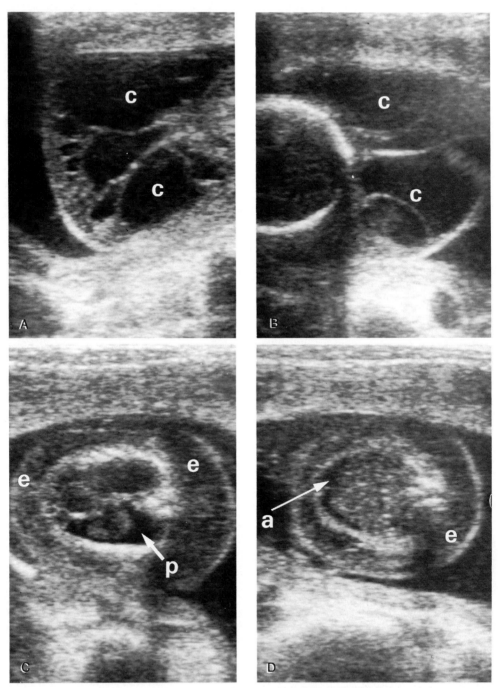

Figure 12–23. Diffuse lymphangiectasia. Large cystic hygromas (c) in *(A)* nuchal and *(B)* occipital regions. C, Transverse axial view of the fetal thorax, demonstrating integumentary edema (e) and pleural effusions (p). D, Transverse axial view of the fetal abdomen, demonstrating integumentary edema (e) and a thin rim of ascites (a).

References

1. Ballantyne JW: The Diseases of the Fetus. Edinburgh, Oliver & Boyd, 1892. *Cited in* Potter EL: Universal edema of the fetus unassociated with erythroblastosis. Am J Obstet Gynecol 46:130, 1943.
2. Levine P, Burnham L, Katzin EM, Vogel P: The role of isoimmunization in the pathogenesis of erythroblastosis fetalis. Am J Obstet Gynecol 42:925, 1941.
3. Landsteiner K, Weiner AS: Agglutinable factor in human blood recognized by immune sera for rhesus blood. Proc Soc Exper Biol Med 43:223, 1940.
4. Potter EL: Universal edema of the fetus unassociated with erythroblastosis. Am J Obstet Gynecol 46:130, 1943.
5. Frigoletto FD, Umansky I: Erythroblastosis fetalis: Identification, management, and prevention. Clin Perinatol 6:321, 1979.
6. James LS: Shock in the newborn in relation to hydrops. Annali Di Obstetricia, Ginecologia, Medicina Perinatale 92:599, 1971
7. Barnes SE: Hydrops fetalis. Molecular Aspects of Medicine 1:244, 1977.
8. Nicolaides KH, Clewell WH, Rodeck CA: Measurement of human fetoplacental blood volume in erythroblastosis fetalis. Am J Obstet Gynecol 157:50, 1987.
9. Phibbs RH, Johnson P, Tooley WH: Cardiorespiratory status of erythroblastotic newborn infants: II. Blood volume, hematocrit, and serum albumin concentration in relation to hydrops fetalis. Pediatrics 53:13, 1974.
10. Bowman JM: The management of Rh-isoimmunization. Obstet Gynecol 52:1, 1978.
11. Bowman JM: Suppression of Rh-isoimmunization. Obstet Gynecol 52:385, 1978.
12. Liley AW: Liquor amnii analysis in the management of the pregnancy complicated by rhesus sensitization. Am J Obstet Gynecol 82:1359, 1961.
13. Liley AW: Intrauterine transfusion of foetus in hemolytic disease. Br Med J 2:1107, 1963.
14. Cooperberg PL, Carpenter CW: Ultrasound as an aid in intrauterine transfusion. Am J Obstet Gynecol 128:239, 1977.
15. Berkowitz RL, Chikara U, Goldberg JD, et al: Intravascular transfusion in utero: The percutaneous approach. Am J Obstet Gynecol 154:622, 1986.
16. deCrespigny L, Robinson HP, Quinn M, et al: Ultrasound-guided fetal blood transfusion for severe rhesus isoimmunization. Obstet Gynecol 66:529, 1985.
17. Nicolaides KH, Rodeck CH, Bibashan RS, Kemp JR: Have Liley charts outlived their usefulness? Am J Obstet Gynecol 155:90, 1986.
18. Warsof SL, Nicolaides KH, Rodeck C: Immune and non-immune hydrops. Clin Obstet Gynecol 29:533, 1986.
19. Scott JR, Kochenour NK, Larkin RM, Scott MJ: Changes in the management of severely Rh-immunized patients. Am J Obstet Gynecol 149:336, 1984.
20. Hobbins J, Winsberg F, Berkowitz R: Ultrasonography in Obstetrics and Gynecology, 2nd Ed. Baltimore, Williams and Wilkins, 1983, p 84.
21. Hoddick WK, Mahony BS, Callen PW, Filly RA: Placental thickness. J Ultrasound Med 4:479, 1985.
22. Harman CR, Manning FA, Bowman JM, Lange IR: Severe Rh disease: Poor outcome is not inevitable. Am J Obstet Gynecol 145:823, 1983.
23. Vintzileos A, Campbell WA, Storlazzi E, et al: Fetal liver ultrasound measurements in isoimmunized pregnancies. Obstet Gynecol 68:162, 1986.
24. Benacerraf BR, Frigoletto FD: Sonographic sign for the detection of early fetal ascites in the management of severe isoimmune disease without intrauterine transfusion. Am J Obstet Gynecol 152:1039, 1985.
25. Hashimoto BE, Filly RA, Callen PW: Fetal pseudoascites: Further anatomic observations. J Ultrasound Med 5:151, 1986.
26. DeVore G, Donnerstein R, Kleinman C, et al: Fetal echocardiography, II. The diagnosis and significance of a pericardial effusion in the fetus using real-time directed M-mode ultrasound. Am J Obstet Gynecol 144:693, 1982.
27. DeVore G, Mayden K, Tortora M, et al: Dilatation of the fetal umbilical vein in rhesus hemolytic anemia: A predictor of severe disease. Am J Obstet Gynecol 141:464, 1981.
28. Mayden K: The umbilical vein diameter in Rh isoimmunization. Med Ultrasound 4:119, 1980.
29. Witter FR, Graham D: The utility of ultrasonically measured umbilical vein diameters in isoimmunized pregnancies. Am J Obstet Gynecol 146:225, 1983.
30. Etches PC, Lemons JA: Nonimmune hydrops fetalis: Report of 22 cases including three siblings. Pediatrics 64:326, 1979.
31. Graves GR, Baskett TF: Nonimmune hydrops fetalis. Antenatal diagnosis and management. Am J Obstet Gynecol 148:563, 1984.
32. Im SS, Rizos N, Joutsi P, et al: Nonimmunologic hydrops fetalis. Am J Obstet Gynecol 148:566, 1984.
33. Hutchison A, Drew JA, Yu V, et al: Nonimmunologic hydrops fetalis: A review of 61 cases. Obstet Gynecol 59:247, 1982.
34. Brown B: The ultrasonographic features of non-immune hydrops fetalis: A study of 30 successive patients. J Can Assoc Radiol 37:164, 1986.
35. Castillo RA, DeVoe LD, Hadi HA, et al: Nonimmune hydrops fetalis: Clinical experience and factors related to poor outcome. Am J Obstet Gynecol 155:812, 1986.
36. Holzgreve W, Holzgreve B, Curry JR: Nonimmune hydrops fetalis: Diagnosis and management. Semin Perinatol 9:52, 1985.
37. Mahony BS, Filly RA, Callen PW, et al: Severe nonimmune hydrops fetalis: Sonographic evaluation. Radiology 151:757, 1984.
38. Fleischer AC, Killam AP, Boehm FH, et al: Hydrops fetalis: Sonographic evaluation and clinical implications. Radiology 141:163, 1981.
39. Buttino L: Idiopathic non-immune hydrops: A common entity. Letter to the editor. Am J Obstet Gynecol 152:606, 1985.
40. Golbus M: Idiopathic non-immune hydrops: A common entity. Reply to letter to the editor. Am J Obstet Gynecol 152:607, 1985.
41. Kleinman C, Donnerstein, DeVore G, et al: Fetal echocardiography for evaluation of in utero congestive heart failure. NEJM 306:568, 1982.
42. Hadlock FP, Deter RL, Garcia-Pratt J, et al: Fetal ascites not associated with Rh incompatibility: Recognition and management with sonography. AJR 134:1225, 1980.
43. DeVore G: The prenatal diagnosis of congenital

heart disease: A practical approach for the actual sonographer. JCU 13:229, 1985.

44. Watson J, Campbell S: Antenatal evaluation and management in nonimmune hydrops fetalis. Obstet Gynecol 67:589, 1986.

45. Harrison MR, Bressack MA, Chung AM, deLoriner AA: Correction of congenital diaphragmatic hernia in utero, II. Simulated correction permits lung growth with survival at birth. Surgery 88:260, 1980.

46. Weiner C, Varner M, Pringle K, et al: Antenatal diagnosis and palliative treatment of nonimmune hydrops fetalis secondary to pulmonary extralobar sequestration. Obstet Gynecol 68:275, 1986.

47. Allan LD, Crawford DC, Sheridan R, Chapman MC: Aetiology of nonimmune hydrops: The value of echocardiography. Br J Obstet Gynaecol 93:223, 1986.

48. Hseih FJ, Chang FM, Ko TM, Chen HU: Percutaneous ultrasound-guided fetal blood sampling in management of non-immune hydrops fetalis. Am J Obstet Gynecol 157:44, 1987.

49. Vintzileos A, Campbell WA, Nochimson DJ, Weinbaum PJ: Antenatal evaluation and management of ultrasonically detected fetal anomalies. Obstet Gynecol 69:640, 1987.

50. Robertson L, Ott A, Mack L, Brown Z: Sonographically documented disappearance of non-immune hydrops fetalis associated with maternal hypertension. West J Med 143:382, 1985.

51. Kirkinen P, Jouppila P, Leisti J: Transient fetal ascites and hydrops with a favorable outcome. Reprod Med 32:379, 1987.

52. Shapiro I, Scharf M: Spontaneous intrauterine remission of hydrops fetalis in one identical twin: Sonographic diagnosis. JCU 13:427, 1985.

53. Mueller-Heuback E, Mazer J: Sonographically documented disappearance of fetal ascites. Obstet Gynecol 61:253, 1983.

13

ULTRASOUND EVALUATION OF THE PLACENTA

David A. Nyberg, M.D.
Peter W. Callen, M.D.

During the past decade, knowledge of the anatomy, physiology, and pathology of the human placenta has increased dramatically. This is in no small part due to the ability of diagnostic ultrasound to peer into the uterus to observe the developing fetus and membranes.

What follows is a discussion of the normal and abnormal development of the placenta. While the perspective will be that of the sonographer, the embryology and clinical information ultimately relevant to the diagnostician will be covered as well. The reader is encouraged to review the normal development of the fetus and placenta in the first trimester covered in Chapter 3.

THE NORMAL PLACENTA

Development

The placental unit is derived from two components: the maternal *decidua* and the fetal *chorion*. The decidua represents endometrium, which, under hormonal influence, is altered to allow for implantation of the developing blastocyst as well as for the subsequent placental formation. The decidua itself is often described on the basis of its location in respect to the implanted embryo. That portion of the decidua lying between the fetal unit and the myometrium is referred to as the *decidua basalis*. At the time of parturition, the placenta is shed, cleaving in the spongy zone of the decidua basalis. The *decidua capsularis* is that portion of the decidua that covers the implanted embryonal unit. As pregnancy progresses, the embryo and its surrounding fluid enlarge, expanding the decidua capsularis into the uterine cavity. At approximately 20 to 22 weeks, the decidua capsularis will fuse with the remaining decidual lining, the *decidua parietalis (decidua vera)*, and ultimately degenerate. It is these decidual layers that are responsible for the sonographic appearance of the gestational sac in the first trimester (Fig. 13–1) (see Chap. 3).

The Fetal Component (The Chorion)

At approximately 5 days after fertilization, the *trophoblastic* cells differentiate from those that will form the embryo. The trophoblast itself is differentiated into two cell types: the *syncytiotrophoblast,* an outer layer of multinuclear cells that are respon-

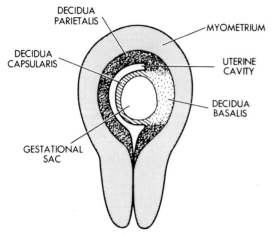

Figure 13–1. Diagram of the decidual layers of a first trimester gestational sac. (*From* Nyberg DA, Laing FC, Filly RA, et al: Ultrasonographic differentiation of the gestational sac of early intrauterine pregnancy from the pseudo-gestational sac of ectopic pregnancy. Radiology 146:755, 1983.)

sible for proteolytic invasion into the decidua as well as the secretion of human chorionic gonadotropin (hCG), and the *cytotrophoblast*, a mononuclear inner layer of cells.

The fusion of the trophoblast and the extraembryonic mesenchyme results in the *chorion* (derived from the Greek word meaning membrane).[1] The term chorion from the second trimester until term is often used synonymously with the *placenta*. Thus, as will be discussed later, in a *dichorionic* pregnancy, there are two placentas.

The major functioning unit of the placenta is the chorionic villus. Its development begins as a result of the somewhat random invasion of the syncytiotrophoblast into the decidua at approximately two weeks after fertilization (Fig. 13–2).[2] The spaces that are left adjacent to the trophoblast will become the intervillous spaces. Shortly thereafter,

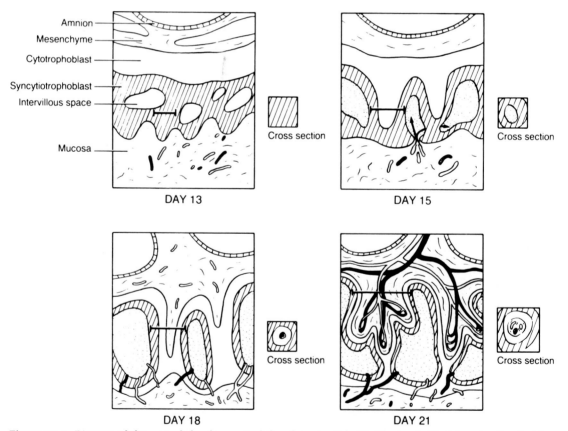

Figure 13–2. Diagram of the normal development of the placenta. *Day 13,* The trophoblast invades the decidua; the spaces not occupied by trophoblast represent the intervillous spaces. *Day 15,* Maternal blood enters the intervillous spaces, establishing the maternal blood supply to the villous unit. *Day 18,* A mesenchymal core of vascular islets enters the trophoblast core. *Day 21,* A vascular tuft is established within the chorionic villus, with connection to the fetus via the umbilical cord. (*Modified from* Tuchmann-Duplessis H, David G, Haegel P: Illustrated Human Embryology, Vol I: Embryogenesis. New York, Springer Verlag, 1982.)

blood from the maternal spiral arteries enters the intervillous space, establishing the maternal blood supply of the placenta (Fig. 13–2). At two and one-half weeks after fertilization, a mesenchymal core enters the villous structure in which vascular islets appear (Fig. 13–2). At three weeks after fertilization, the fetal vascular supply, from the umbilical cord down to the end-organ villus, is complete; this includes the fetal component of the placental circulation (Fig. 13–2). It should be mentioned that the amnion, which expands to fill the uterine cavity, invests the umbilical cord down to its insertion into the fetal abdomen.

Two steps occur concurrently with the above developmental stages and complete the final form of the placenta. First, atrophy of the villi associated with the decidua capsularis results in the *chorion laeve*. The remaining chorionic villi will establish the placental site, the *chorion frondosum*. Failure of atrophy may result in a succenturiate lobe or in placenta membranacea (Fig. 13–3). Succenturiate lobes occur in approximately one in 5000 pregnancies.[3, 4] Retention of one of the lobes may result in hemorrhage and infection. The second step in the completion of the placenta is partitioning of the villi by infolding of the decidua basalis upward but not into contact with the chorionic plate (Fig. 13–4). These septa divide the fetal component of the placenta into 10 to 30 areas called *cotyledons*.

The final term placenta is approximately 15 to 20 cm in diameter, discoid in shape, with an approximate weight of 600 gm. The thickness is said to be approximately 3 cm. It should be remembered, however, that placental thickness is a function of gestational age (Fig. 13–5).[5] As a general rule, the thickness of the placenta should be commensurate with the menstrual age in weeks; a placenta from a 23 week gestation should measure 23 mm. The normal placenta should never exceed 4 cm.[5]

Ultrasound Appearance

As was mentioned above, the future site of the placenta, the chorion frondosum, can be recognized early in the first trimester of pregnancy (Fig. 13–6). Thereafter, throughout pregnancy, the placenta can be recognized by its more echogenic soft tissue layer adjacent to the less echogenic myometrium

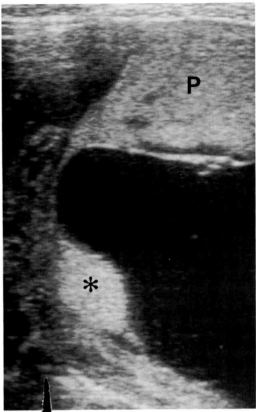

Figure 13–3. Succenturiate lobe of the placenta. The major portion of the placenta lies anteriorly (P). A small island of placental tissue (*asterisk*) is seen to lie in the fundus posteriorly.

and draining veins (Fig. 13–7).[6] This complex of echoes is often helpful in defining the placental site, particularly when only a portion of the placenta is seen. One should be aware of reverberation artifact and transient myometrial contractions, both of which may simulate the placenta (Fig. 13–8).

As noted earlier, the normal placenta rarely is greater than 3 cm in thickness in its normal state. In hydropic states, infection, and diabetes mellitus, the placenta may increase in thickness (Fig. 13–9). In cases of polyhydramnios, the placenta may be thinner than normal by virtue of the increased intrauterine volume.

The Placenta and Membranes in Multiple Gestation Pregnancies

Thus far the discussion has centered upon the development of the placenta in singleton

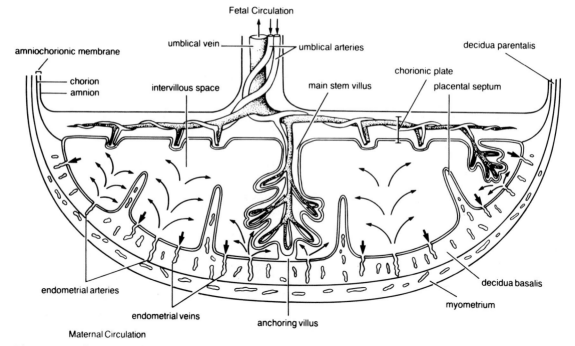

Figure 13–4. Illustration of a term placenta. The infolding of the decidual septa establishes the cotyledons in the term placenta. (*From Moore KL: The Developing Human: Clinically Oriented Embryology, 4th Ed. Philadelphia, WB Saunders Co, 1988.*)

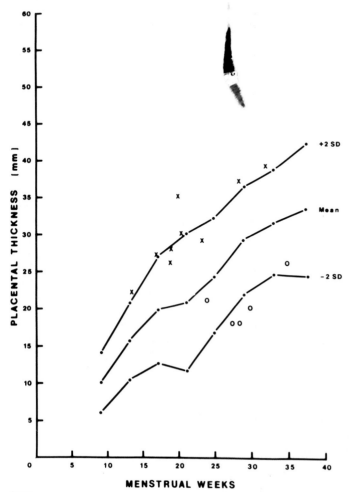

Figure 13–5. Relationship of placental thickness to menstrual age. The mean thickness of the placenta in millimeters is approximately equal to the menstrual age in weeks. (*From Hoddick WK, Mahony BS, Callen PW, Filly RA: Placental thickness. J Ultrasound Med 4:479, 1985.*)

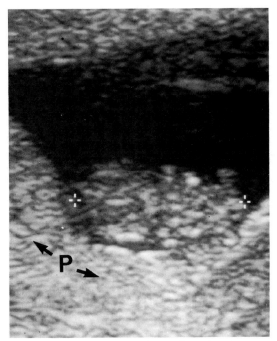

Figure 13–6. Ultrasonogram from a first trimester pregnancy. At this early stage of pregnancy, the placental site (P) is well seen.

pregnancies. In multiple gestations, the evaluation of the amnionicity (number of amniotic sacs) and the chorionicity (number of placentas) is important.

In twin gestations, the resulting pregnancy will be either *dizygotic* (two fertilized eggs [fraternal twins]) or *monozygotic* (a single fertilized egg that divides [identical twins]). Dizygotic twins are diamniotic and dicho-

rionic. The amnionicity and chorionicity of monozygotic twins depend upon the time of cleavage of the zygote.

Several embryologic facts help one better understand the resultant chorionicity and amnionicity of monozygotic twins (Fig. 13–10):

1. Once a tissue differentiates, it is no longer capable of division.

2. The trophoblast differentiates at approximately four to six days after fertilization.

3. The amnion differentiates at approximately eight days after fertilization.

Thus, if the zygote in a monozygotic pregnancy divides before the time of trophoblast differentiation, a *dichorionic-diamniotic* form of placentation will result. This is uncommon, occurring in approximately one-third of monozygotic twins. If the zygote divides after trophoblast differentiation but before differentiation of the amnion (between four and eight days), a *monochorionic-diamniotic* twin will result. This is the most common form of twinning, occurring in approximately two-thirds of monozygotic twins. If division occurs after the eighth day, a *monochorionic-monoamniotic* twin results (< 1 percent).

The determination of the chorionicity and amnionicity in multiple gestation pregnancies is more than academic. Monochorionic pregnancies carry the risk of placental vascular anastomoses. These, if severe, may result in conditions such as the "twin-twin transfusion syndrome" and be seen in cases

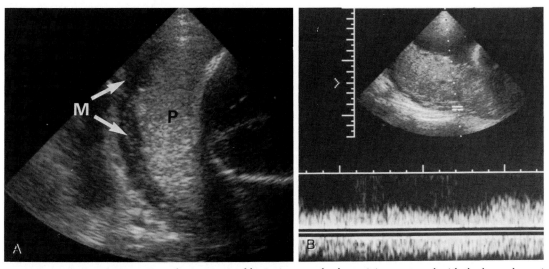

Figure 13–7. *A*, The placenta (P) is often recognized by its increased echogenicity compared with the less echogenic myometrium (M). *B*, Doppler venous flow study. The poor echogenicity of the region adjacent to the placenta is in large part due to veins at the junction of the decidua basalis and myometrium.

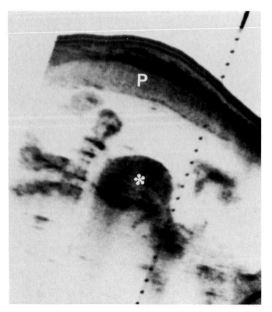

Figure 13–8. Transient contractions of the myometrium may appear echogenic and simulate the appearance of the placenta (P). The lack of the associated complex of the more echogenic placenta and less echogenic myometrium suggests that this tissue is myometrium (asterisk).

of parabiotic twinning (acephaly-acardia). In addition, monoamniotic twins are at risk of entanglement of the umbilical cords and vascular compromise of both fetuses.[7]

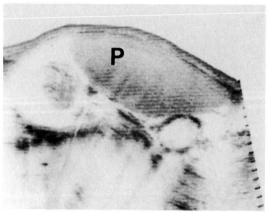

Figure 13–9. Thickened placenta (P) in a patient with hydrops fetalis. When the placenta is edematous, it often has a "ground glass" appearance with decreased echogenicity.

During the past several years, there has been a great interest in determining the amnionicity and chorionicity through ultrasound. This is particularly true in some cases of dichorionic pregnancies where the placentas are adjacent to one another and appear as a single placental site. Such features as the number of placental sites, fetal gender, and presence and thickness of a membrane have all been useful in making this determination (Tables 13–1, 13–2, Fig. 13–11).[8, 9]

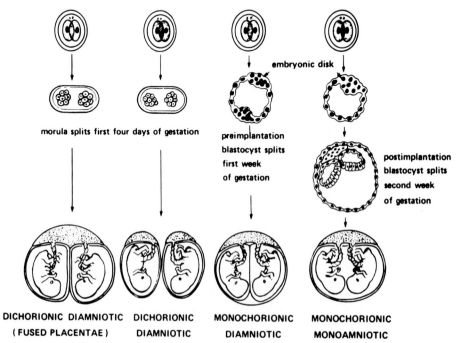

Figure 13–10. Diagram of the development and placentation of monozygotic twins. (*From* Fox H: Pathology of the Placenta. London, WB Saunders Co, 1978.)

Table 13–1. HELPFUL FEATURES IN ANTENATAL SONOGRAPHIC PREDICTION OF CHORIONICITY, AMNIONICITY, AND ZYGOSITY IN TWIN PREGNANCIES

| Sonographic Findings | | | Chorionicity | | | Amnionicity | | | Zygosity | | | Recommendation |
Placental Sites	Membrane Seen	Other Findings	Di	Mono	Either	Di	Mono	Either	Di	Mono	Either	
2	Yes		X			X					X	Check gender (male + female = dizygosity)
2	No			X			X				X	Membrane must be present but not observed; check gender
2	Yes or no	Hydropic twin, normal twin	X			X					X	Not twin transfusion syndrome; consider other causes for nonimmune hydrops fetalis
1	Yes				X	X					X	Check gender

From Mahony BS, Filly RA, Callen PW: Amnionicity and chorionicity in twin pregnancies: Prediction using ultrasound. Radiology 155:208, 1985.

Table 13–2. HELPFUL SONOGRAPHIC FEATURES IN THE PREDICTION OF CHORIONICITY, AMNIONICITY, AND ZYGOSITY IN TWIN PREGNANCIES WHEN ONLY ONE PLACENTAL SITE IS EVIDENT AND NO MEMBRANE IS SEEN SEPARATING THE FETUSES

| Sonographic Observations | Chorionicity | | | Amnionicity | | | Zygosity | | | Impression |
	Di	Mono	Either	Di	Mono	Either	Di	Mono	Either	
Male + female genitalia	X			X			X			Membrane present but not observed
"Stuck" twin			X			X			X	Confirms oligohydramnios in one sac
Hydropic twin; growth-retarded twin		X				X		X		Presumptive diagnosis TTS; check for unobserved membrane or "stuck" twin
Parabiotic twin		X				X		X		Check for unobserved membrane or "stuck" twin
Intertwined umbilical cords		X			X			X		
Conjoined twins		X			X			X		
>3 vessels in umbilical cord		X			X			X		

TTS, twin transfusion syndrome.

From Mahony BS, Filly RA, Callen PW: Amnionicity and chorionicity in twin pregnancies: Prediction using ultrasound. Radiology 155:208, 1985.

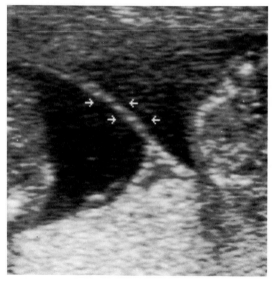

Figure 13–11. Ultrasound determination of chorionicity by assessment of membrane thickness. In this dichorionic twin gestation, a thick membrane *(arrows)* is seen separating the two amniotic sacs. This membrane is derived from two layers of amnion and two layers of chorion.

THE ABNORMAL PLACENTA

Placenta Previa

Placenta previa, defined as a portion of the placenta that covers all or part of the internal cervical os, is found in approximately one in 200 pregnancies at the time of delivery.[3, 10–13] A *complete* (total) previa covers the entire internal cervical os and occurs in one-fifth of cases, whereas a *partial* (marginal) previa partially covers the internal os but is not attached on all sides (Fig. 13–12). A *low-lying* placenta is diagnosed clinically when the placental edge can be palpated by the examiner's finger but does not cover the cervical os. Because of its speed, safety, and accuracy in localizing the placenta and because it also provides important information about the fetus, sonography is now universally accepted as the imaging method of choice for evaluating placenta previa.[14, 15] However, although placental localization is taken for granted today, it should be remembered that before ultrasonography, more invasive imaging methods, including angiography and nuclear scintigraphy, were required for this purpose.

The incidence of placenta previa increases with maternal age, multiparity, and prior uterine operations, including cesarean section.[3, 11, 12] In these situations, suboptimal placental attachment or decidualization is thought to induce the placenta to cover a disproportionately large surface area of the uterus, thereby increasing the likelihood that it will also cover the cervical os. In a similar manner, multiple pregnancies probably increase the risk of placenta previa because of the increased surface area of the placenta.

Painless vaginal bleeding is the clinical hallmark of placenta previa and eventually occurs in nearly all clinically significant cases.[3] Conversely, 3 to 5 percent of all pregnancies are complicated by third trimester bleeding, and of these, 7 to 11 percent are due to placenta previa.[3] Bleeding usually occurs during the third trimester because of uterine thinning and cervical effacement that leads to placental detachment and tears of the basilar and marginal veins. In 30 percent of cases, however, vaginal bleeding initially presents before the third trimester.[3] Although typically intermittent at first, vaginal bleeding can be sudden and life threat-

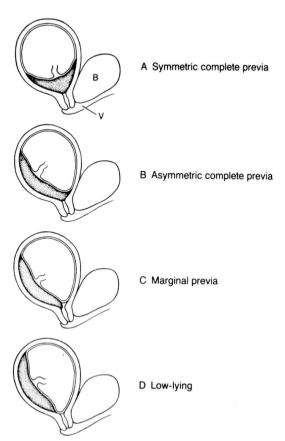

A Symmetric complete previa

B Asymmetric complete previa

C Marginal previa

D Low-lying

Figure 13–12. Classification of placental location.

ening. For this reason, prenatal diagnosis of a complete previa precludes vaginal delivery and pelvic examinations. In some institutions, a diagnosis of placenta previa after the time of fetal viability (24 weeks) also necessitates hospitalization until delivery.

In addition to maternal hemorrhage, major complications of placenta previa include premature delivery, intrauterine growth retardation (IUGR), and perinatal death.[3, 13] These complications, which are greater for complete previas than for marginal ones, are secondary to premature detachment of the placenta from the lower uterine segment. Perinatal mortality was as high as 40 percent before 1950, but was less than 5 percent in the 1970s owing in part to improved perinatal detection of placenta previa, as well as to improved neonatal management.[3]

Sonographic evaluation of placenta previa requires accurate localization of the internal cervical os relative to the placenta.[10] On sagittal scans, the cervical canal is recognized as an echogenic line representing the mucosal interface and mucous plug, surrounded by a hypoechoic zone of variable thickness representing submucosal glands (Fig. 13–13A). Because the uterus frequently deviates from a true sagittal orientation, slightly off-axis scans may be necessary to obtain this view. The echogenic mucosal interface of the vagina is also a useful land-mark leading to the cervix. The internal cervical os itself can be identified at the point of a slight "V" configuration or "funneling" of the amniotic fluid leading to the cervical canal.

Most sonographers begin scanning through a moderately distended urinary bladder since it provides an acoustic window for visualizing the cervix and because it places the cervical canal in a longitudinal orientation that is nearly perpendicular to the ultrasound beam. However, because an overly distended bladder can produce a false-positive impression of a placenta previa by compressing the lower uterine walls together,[16] some authorities recommend scanning through an empty urinary bladder (Fig. 13–13A).[17] Scanning through an empty bladder results in fewer false-positive diagnoses of placenta previa but produces a nearly vertical orientation of the cervix that may be difficult for the uninitiated observer to recognize.[17]

Sonographically, a complete placenta previa is diagnosed when the placenta covers the entire cervical os (Fig. 13–14), although a partial previa is suggested when the lower placental margin appears to extend to, but not across, the internal cervical os (Fig. 13–15). It has been suggested that a low-lying placenta should be diagnosed on sonography when the lower placental mar-

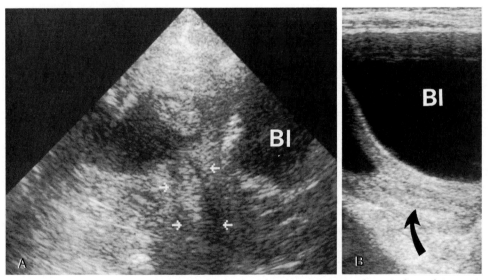

Figure 13–13. *A,* Normal cervical canal. Longitudinal scans demonstrate a normal cervical canal *(arrows),* which is in a nearly vertical orientation because of an empty urinary bladder (Bl). *B,* With a full urinary bladder (Bl), the cervical canal *(arrow)* is in a more horizontal orientation. Also note that the cervical canal and lower uterine segment are artificially lengthened from compression by a distended urinary bladder.

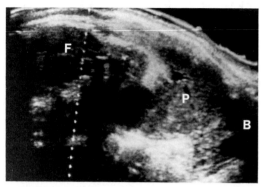

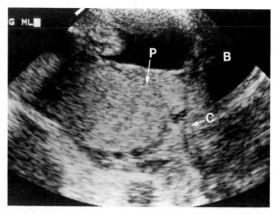

Figure 13–14. Placenta previa. Longitudinal scan shows the placenta (P) implanted over the lower uterine segment, completely covering the region of the cervical os. Note that the fetus (F) is in a breech presentation. B, urinary bladder.

Figure 13–16. Asymmetric complete placenta previa. Longitudinal scan demonstrates a placenta (P) that is predominantly posterior in location but which completely covers the cervical os (C). B, urinary bladder.

gin comes within 2 cm of the internal cervical os.[18] Identification of a complete placenta previa is easiest when the placenta is directly implanted over the os, forming a central or "symmetric" previa. In most cases, however, a complete previa results from an "asymmetric" placental location in which the placenta is located predominantly on the anterior, posterior, or lateral uterine wall (Fig. 13–16).[19] In either situation, a complete previa is commonly associated with a transverse or breech fetal lie since the bulk of the placenta prevents the fetal head from entering the pelvis. In some cases of complete or partial previas, hemorrhage can be identified

beneath the placenta and overlying the cervical os (Fig. 13–17).

Distinguishing an extremely asymmetric complete previa from a partial previa or a very low-lying placenta can be difficult. Traction or a Trendelenburg position may be useful for elevating fetal parts out of the pelvis.[20] Careful parasagittal as well as oblique scanning with varying degrees of bladder filling is usually necessary. In some cases, however, delineation of anatomic relationships may not be possible using conventional ultrasonography alone. Recently, transvaginal and transperineal sonography have been used for distinguishing a placenta

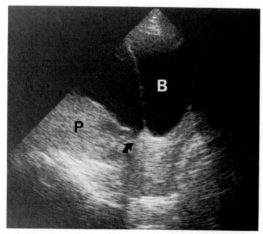

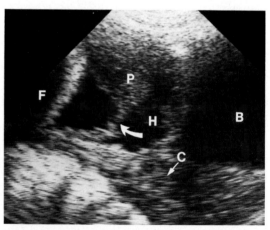

Figure 13–17. Partial placenta previa with underlying hematoma. Longitudinal scans demonstrate a hematoma (H) overlying the cervical os (C) and elevating the margin of the placenta (curved arrow). The placenta (P), which is in a predominantly anterior location, appears to form a partial previa. B, urinary bladder; F, fetus.

Figure 13–15. Partial palcenta previa. Longitudinal scan shows a posterior placenta (P) partially covering the cervical os (arrow) but not attached on the opposite myometrial surface. B, urinary bladder.

previa from a low-lying placenta,[21] although the potential benefits and risks of these procedures are currently unknown. Magnetic resonance imaging has also been reported to be useful for imaging posterior placentas that may be obscured by fetal parts on sonography.[22] Finally, if there is any question regarding the presence of a placenta previa, the obstetrician can physically examine the cervix after appropriate precautions have been taken ("double set-up").[23]

The reported accuracy of ultrasonography for diagnosing placenta previa varies widely. Although false-negative diagnoses are rare, false-positive diagnoses are relatively common, depending on (1) the gestational age at the time of the sonogram, (2) the sonographic technique employed, (3) the type of previa (complete versus partial), and (4) the patient's symptoms.[24–28] For example, some authors have reported no false-positive diagnoses for women who present with vaginal bleeding during the third trimester.[27] In contrast, ultrasound studies during the second trimester have reported a placenta previa in 2.5 to 7.5 percent of all pregnancies, compared with an actual frequency of only 0.5 percent at the time of delivery.[28, 29] Earlier ultrasound studies reported an even higher rate of false-positive diagnoses (up to one-half of all second trimester pregnancies), although many of these were due to technical factors.[24, 25]

The frequency of false-positive diagnoses of placenta previa during the second trimester can usually be attributed to two factors: (1) technical artifacts, primarily resulting from an overdistended urinary bladder (Fig. 13–18) or focal uterine contractions (Fig. 13–19), and (2) "placental migration."[28, 29] An overdistended bladder can be suspected when the apparent length of the cervix is much longer than normal (> 3.5 to 4.0 cm), and a focal uterine contraction can be suspected when the myometrial wall is abnormally thick (> 1.5 cm).[29] Rescanning after the patient has partially voided in the former situation or following a 30 to 60 minute delay in the latter will usually resolve normal anatomic relationships. However, even with the awareness of these technical artifacts, a study by Townsend and associates showed that 93 percent of women with a suspected marginal placenta previa seen before 20 weeks were ultimately found not to have a previa at the time of delivery, and two-thirds of false-positive diagnoses could be attributed to technical artifacts.[29] Importantly, no false-positive diagnoses were made of complete previas.

Placental "migration" is a term that attempts to explain the apparent ascension of the placenta during pregnancy.[30] These changes do not result from actual movement of the placenta itself but rather from differential growth of the lower uterine segment (Fig. 13–20). At 20 weeks, the placenta covers approximately one-fourth of the myometrial surface. Hence, low-lying placentas or suspected partial previas noted during the second trimester may appear completely normal in location during the third trimes-

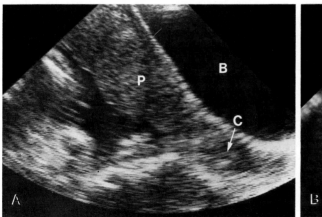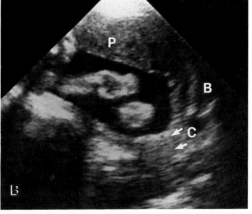

Figure 13–18. *A,* False-positive previa due to a distended bladder. Longitudinal scan with a distended urinary bladder (B) suggests that the anterior placenta (P) is partially covering the cervical os (C). *B,* Repeat sonogram with an empty bladder shows that the placenta (P) clearly does not form a previa. Note the nearly vertical orientation of the cervix (C).

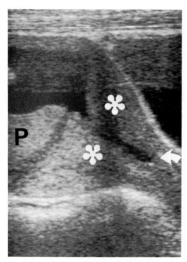

Figure 13–19. False-positive previa due to uterine contractions. A contraction of the lower uterine segment *(asterisks)* simulates a low-lying or marginal previa. In fact, the true cervical os *(arrow)* lies more distal. P, placenta.

ter. However, differential growth of the lower uterine segment cannot change the relationship of complete previas, which remain attached to all sides of the internal cervical os early in gestation.

The risks of overdiagnosing placenta previa should be weighed against the rare,

but potentially disastrous, error of missing a true previa. False-positive diagnoses can lead to unnecessary additional sonograms, greater expense, emotional stress, hospitalization, and even needless cesarean section. Since nearly every placental previa eventually produces vaginal bleeding, one could argue whether a diagnosis of a low-lying placenta or a partial placenta previa should be made at all in asymptomatic women scanned before 20 weeks. On the other hand, previas should probably continue to be over-interpreted in women with vaginal bleeding or when a complete placenta previa is suspected at any time in gestation.

Abruption and Hemorrhage

As the placenta is an extremely vascular organ, it is not surprising that hemorrhage is one of its most frequently encountered complications. Fox and others have described pathologically various sites of hemorrhage found in and around the placenta.[31] Retroplacental and marginal hemorrhages are associated with placental abruption, whereas other sites of hemorrhage include "subchorial," subamniotic, and intraplacental ("intervillous thrombosis") locations (Fig. 13–21).

In recent years, obstetric sonography has greatly contributed to knowledge of the placenta and placental hemorrhage. Sites of hemorrhage that were initially described pathologically can also be identified on sonography, although their terminology and observed frequency may vary. Unlike the pathologic examination that must await delivery of the placenta, ultrasonography has the ability to examine the placenta in vivo and throughout gestation. This information may

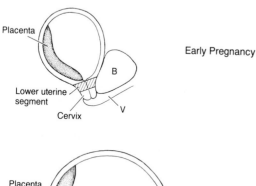

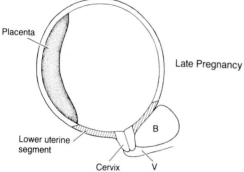

Figure 13–20. Differential growth of the lower uterine segment during pregnancy, explaining placental "migration."

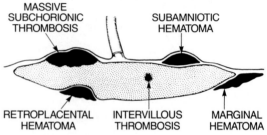

Figure 13–21. Sites of hemorrhage in and around the placenta, which have been described pathologically. *(From* Fox H: Pathology of the Placenta. London, WB Saunders Co, 1978, pp 107–157.)

help bridge the well-recognized gap between pathologic and clinical diagnoses of placental hemorrhage. By determining the size and location of placental hemorrhages, ultrasonography can also provide important prognostic information. In the following section, the authors will review the usual sonographic and clinical features of placental hemorrhage and attempt to correlate sonographic observations with previously described pathologic findings.

Placental abruption is defined as premature separation of a normally located placenta.[3, 32] It is clinically recognized in 1 percent of pregnancies, although evidence suggests that less severe cases occur much more frequently.[32, 33] Risk factors of placental abruption include hypertension, vascular disease, smoking, drugs (including cocaine), fibroids, trauma, and fetal malformations; however, in most cases, no specific cause can be identified. One of the strongest risk factors of placental abruption is a previous history of abruption, perinatal death, or preterm delivery. Women with placental abruption have five times the usual frequency of prior perinatal death and three times the frequency of prior preterm delivery.[3, 34–36]

Placental abruptions can be separated into *retroplacental* or *marginal* by their primary area of detachment (Fig. 13–22). Retroplacental abruptions result in hemorrhage predominantly beneath the placenta, whereas marginal abruptions involve only the placental margin.[32–39] Because blood from marginal abruptions tends to dissect beneath the placental membranes, most women experience vaginal bleeding. Up to 15 to 20 percent of third trimester vaginal bleeding is attributed to placental abruption, although many of the "idiopathic" causes of vaginal bleeding may also be due to small marginal abruptions.[32, 36]

Distinguishing retroplacental from marginal placental abruptions is important and is done on the basis of their distinctive etiologies, clinical symptoms, sonographic findings, and prognosis. Retroplacental hemorrhages usually result from rupture of spiral arteries, producing "high pressure" bleeds, whereas marginal hemorrhages appear to result from tears of marginal veins, producing "low pressure" bleeds.[32, 39] Retroplacental abruption has been most strongly associated with hypertension and vascular disease, whereas marginal abruption has been

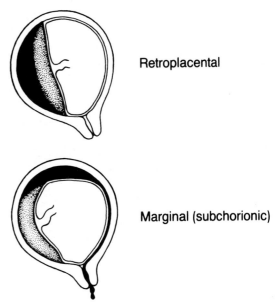

Retroplacental

Marginal (subchorionic)

Figure 13–22. Locations of retroplacental and marginal abruptions.

strongly associated with decidual necrosis due to cigarette smoking.[34] Large retroplacental hemorrhages are more likely to produce "classic" clinical symptoms of placental abruption, including a tense and painful uterus, precipitous delivery, coagulopathy, and fetal demise.[35–37] In contrast, the clinical symptoms of marginal placental abruption are often mild, requiring a high index of clinical suspicion.[39, 41]

Pathologic findings of placental abruption are variable and may not correspond to the clinical symptoms.[33, 36, 38] As all deliveries are traumatic events to some degree, distinguishing those placentas that detached prematurely from those that delivered normally can be difficult. Retroplacental hematomas are found in up to 4.5 percent of placentas at the time of delivery, although most are small and are not associated with significant clinical symptoms.[31] Conversely, acute abruptions do not show an adherent hematoma when the blood has not had time to clot. Older hemorrhages may have completely resolved by the time of delivery, leaving only associated findings of fibrin deposition, decidual necrosis, placental infarction, or thrombosis of marginal veins.[31, 38–40] Marginal placental separation is particularly difficult to diagnose pathologically but probably occurs more commonly than retroplacental abruptions.[37, 38]

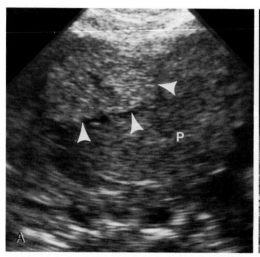
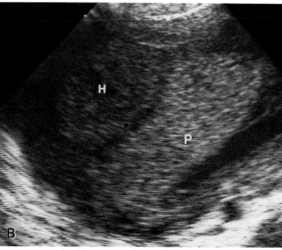

Figure 13–23. *A,* Retroplacental hematoma. Initial sonogram at 25 weeks demonstrates a large hyperechoic hematoma *(arrowheads)* beneath the placenta (P). *B,* Repeat sonogram one week later shows that the hematoma (H) has become hypoechoic relative to the placenta (P). The fetus suffered intrauterine fetal demise approximately one week following this sonogram. (*From* Hurd WW, Miodovnik M, Hertzberg V, Lavin JP: Selective management of abruption placenta: A prospective study. Obstet Gynecol 61:467, 1983.)

The major clinical threat of placental abruption, apart from potential maternal morbidity and rare maternal mortality, is the high rate of fetal death.[40–42] Overall, placental abruption has a perinatal mortality rate of 20 to 60 percent, depending on its severity, and accounts for up to 15 to 25 percent of all perinatal deaths.[42] In comparison, placenta previa is responsible for less than 4 percent of perinatal deaths.[34] Fetal death results from acute hypoxia produced by placental detachment and secondary infarction and so depends on the amount of placenta involved.[31, 41, 43] Owing to the "functional" reserve of the placenta, fetal demise does not usually occur from detachments involving less than 30 percent of the placenta.[31] Subacute abruptions associated with placental infarction may also result in chronic fetal hypoxia and intrauterine growth retardation.[33–37]

Both marginal and retroplacental hemorrhages frequently result in preterm labor and delivery, probably because the irritating effect of intrauterine blood stimulates uterine contractions.[37–39, 42, 44] This idea is supported by a recent sonographic study that found that nearly all intrauterine hematomas large enough to visualize after 20 weeks were associated with uterine contractions or preterm labor.[45] Sustained uterine contractions induced by intrauterine hemorrhage can further worsen hypoxia produced by the pla-

cental detachment, explaining the improved fetal outcome for cesarean section compared with vaginal delivery in many patients.[42, 44]

Sonographic findings of placental abruption are variable, depending on the location and size of the hematoma and the time interval since the acute hemorrhage.[46–50] An acute hemorrhage is hyperechoic to isoechoic relative to the placenta and becomes nearly sonolucent with two weeks if bleeding does not recur (Fig. 13–23).[50] As the sonographic findings are variable, correlation with the clinical history and repeat sonograms may be necessary for establishing the correct diagnosis. Both clinical and sonographic studies have stressed that a placental abruption should be strongly considered in any woman with vaginal bleeding, especially one who also experiences uterine contractions or irritability.[41, 50]

Ideally, a retroplacental abruption would be seen as a well-defined hematoma located between the placenta and uterus (Figs. 13–23, 13–24). Often, however, acute retroplacental hematomas may be difficult to recognize because they dissect into the placenta or myometrium and are similar in echogenicity to the placenta. Such large acute retroplacental hematomas have a particularly high fetal mortality rate. In these cases, sonography may demonstrate only a thickened heterogeneous-appearing placenta,[47, 50, 51] as well as nonspecific findings of rounded pla-

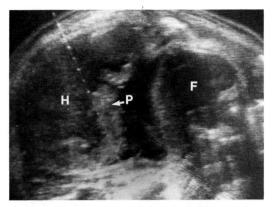

Figure 13–24. Retroplacental abruption. Sonogram from a 26 year old patient, who experienced vaginal bleeding followed by preterm labor, shows a large hematoma (H) beneath the placenta (P). The patient was resistant to tocolytic therapy, and one week later vaginally delivered a compromised baby with Apgar scores of 1 and 5 at one and five minutes, respectively. A 30 percent placental abruption was noted at delivery. F, fetus.

cental margins and intraplacental sonolucencies (Fig. 13–25). Jaffe and associates found that the placenta may measure up to 9 cm in thickness from acute retroplacental abruption, compared with a normal maximal thickness of 4 cm.[47] This appearance is not specific for retroplacental hemorrhage, however, and may have other causes, including diabetes, fetal hydrops, and triploidy (Fig. 13–26). A thickened placenta may also be seen from "chronic" abruptions probably due to secondary villous hyperplasia.

It is important not to confuse the normal subplacental venous complex for a retroplacental hemorrhage. Pathologically, the subplacental venous complex consists of large veins, located within the decidua basalis and adjacent myometrium, that carry blood from the placenta. It is characteristically seen as a sonolucent multiseptated area between the placenta and myometrium and is better appreciated beneath posterior than anterior placentas (Fig. 13–27).[52] Unlike retroplacental hematomas, the subplacental venous complex is relatively uniform in thickness, lacks a mass effect, and, importantly, demonstrates venous flow on real-time sonography (Fig. 13–7B).

Subchorionic (marginal) hemorrhage is by far the most common type of placental abruption seen on sonography, especially before 20 weeks.[33, 50] Although it is thought that nearly all subchorionic hematomas probably arise from the placental margin, in about only one-half the cases can the actual placental detachment be demonstrated (Figs. 13–28 to 13–30).[40, 50] Blood usually extends for a variable distance beneath the placental membranes (chorion and amnion), presumably because they are more easily detached from the myometrium than the placenta itself. The resulting hematoma may accumulate at a site separate from the placenta and can mimic other mass lesions, including a myoma, succenturiate lobe, chorioangioma, or placenta previa (Figs. 13–31, 13–32).[50, 53]

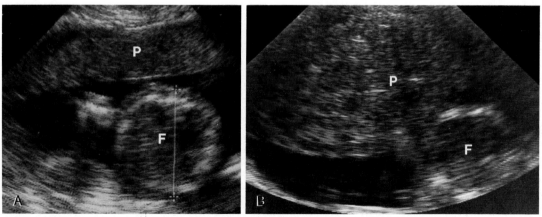

Figure 13–25. A, Retroplacental abruption. Initial sonogram at 23 weeks, performed to confirm the fetal age in a woman with a history of cocaine abuse and cigarette smoking, demonstrates a normal-appearing anterior placenta (P). F, fetus. B, Repeat sonogram one week later, after the patient presented with acute, intense abdominal tenderness, demonstrates a markedly thickened and heterogeneous placenta (P) representing a large retroplacental abruption. Fetal demise occurred shortly after this sonogram, and a large retroplacental hematoma was found at delivery. F, fetus.

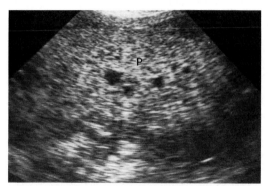

Figure 13–26. Triploidy. Sonogram at 18 weeks demonstrates a markedly thickened and heterogeneous placenta (P) with multiple small cystic areas. Compare with Figure 13–25B.

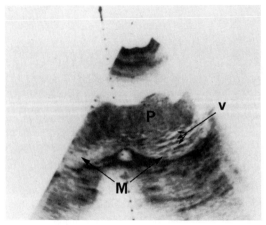

Figure 13–27. Subplacental venous complex. Prominent veins (v) at the decidua basalis and myometrium (M) should not be mistaken for retroplacental hemorrhage. P, placenta. (*From* Callen PW, Filly RA: The placental-subplacental complex: A specific indicator of placental position on ultrasound. JCU 8:21, 1980. *Copyright* © 1980, John Wiley & Sons. *Reproduced by permission of* John Wiley & Sons, Inc.) See Figure 13–7B.

As subchorionic hemorrhage resolves, it becomes nearly sonolucent in appearance so that, eventually, only the detached placental membrane may be identified. Intra-amniotic hemorrhage also frequently occurs from subchorionic hemorrhage, probably because blood dissects through the amnion.

Some authors have found that the size of subchorionic hematomas has prognostic significance,[54] whereas others have found that even large hematomas may have a normal outcome when only the placental margin is detached (Fig. 13–33).[43] Overall, approximately 80 percent of subchorionic hematomas seen before 20 menstrual weeks result in a normal term delivery.[43, 55] After 20 weeks, preterm labor and delivery frequently result from both retroplacental and subchorionic hematomas that are large enough to be visualized sonographically (Figs. 13–28, 13–34).[43]

When subchorionic hemorrhage occurs, the elevated membrane (consisting of the fused chorion and amnion) can be followed to the placental margin where the chorion becomes firmly adherent to the fetal placental surface as the chorionic plate. This de-

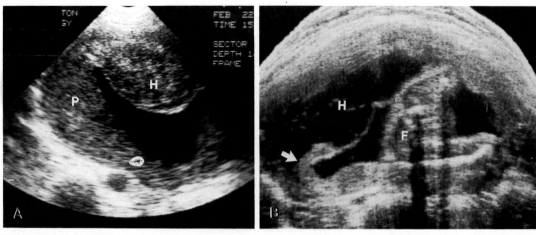

Figure 13–28. A, Subchorionic hematoma. Initial sonogram, performed at 24 weeks for vaginal bleeding, demonstrates a large subchorionic hematoma (H) extending to the margin of the placenta (P). Preterm labor developed shortly after this sonogram. B, Repeat sonogram two weeks later demonstrates that the hematoma (H) has become nearly sonolucent in appearance and elevates the margin of the placenta (*arrow*). One day later, the patient prematurely delivered a 780 gm baby boy with Apgars of 2 and 4 at one and five minutes, respectively. A large hematoma (300 ml) was noted at the time of delivery. F, fetus.

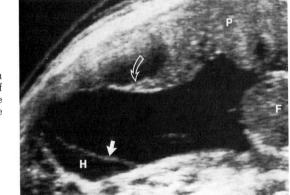

Figure 13–29. Marginal placental abruption. Sonogram at 28 weeks shows a hematoma elevating the margin of the placenta *(open arrow)* and extending beneath the chorionic membranes on the opposite uterine surface *(straight arrow)*. H, hematoma; P, placenta; F, fetus.

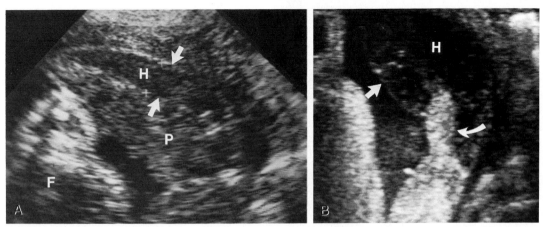

Figure 13–30. *A,* Marginal placental abruption. Sonogram at 18 weeks, performed for vaginal bleeding, demonstrates a hematoma (H, *arrows*) beneath the margin of the placenta (P). F, fetus. *B,* Repeat sonogram two weeks later demonstrates that the hematoma (H) is now nearly sonolucent in appearance and elevates the placental margin *(curved arrow)* and placental membranes *(straight arrow)*.

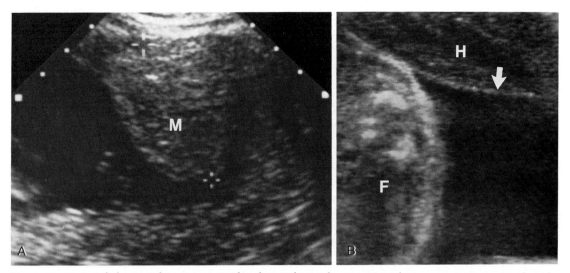

Figure 13–31. *A,* Subchorionic hematoma mistaken for a "placental tumor." Initial sonogram at 16 menstrual weeks demonstates a subchorionic mass (M) that was mistaken for a chorioangioma at another institution. *B,* Repeat sonogram seven weeks later demonstrates that the subchorionic hematoma (H) has almost completely resolved and is more sonolucent in appearance. *Arrow,* detached amnion and chorion; F, fetus.

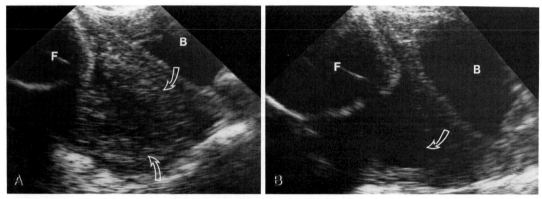

Figure 13–32. *A*, Subchorionic hematoma simulating placenta previa. Sonogram at 27 weeks in a patient with vaginal bleeding and preterm labor demonstrates a large mass *(curved arrows)* in the lower uterine segment that could be confused for a placenta previa. B, urinary bladder; F, fetus. *B*, However, this sonogram one day earlier in the same patient shows a dilated, empty cervical os *(arrows)*, confirming that the mass represented hemorrhage.

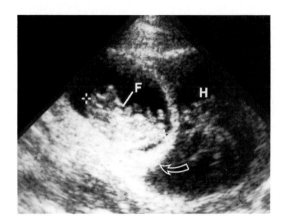

Figure 13–33. Early subchorionic hematoma. Sonogram at ten weeks, performed for vaginal bleeding, demonstrates a large subchorionic hematoma (H) elevating the placental margin *(open arrow)*. F, fetus. The subsequent pregnancy was unremarkable, and the patient delivered at term.

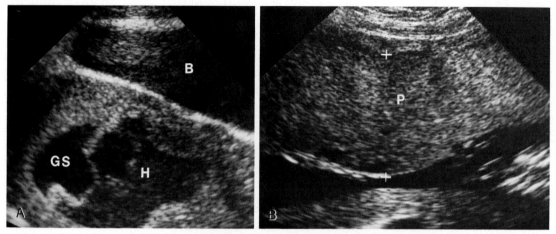

Figure 13–34. *A*, Early subchorionic hematoma. Initial sonogram, performed at ten menstrual weeks for vaginal bleeding, demonstrates a relatively large hematoma (H) distorting the adjacent gestational sac (GS). B, urinary bladder. *B*, The patient continued to experience vaginal bleeding, and a repeat sonogram at 25 weeks shows a thickened placenta (P). The patient prematurely delivered at 31 weeks.

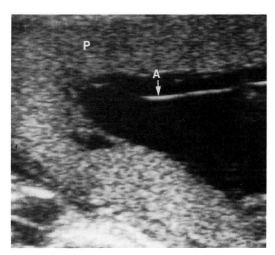

Figure 13–35. Chorioamniotic separation. Sonogram at 18 weeks demonstrates separation of the thin amnion (A) from the chorion and placenta (P) following amniocentesis.

tached membrane should be easily distinguished from the very thin amnion that, when visualized, can be followed to the base of the umbilical cord. Also, the amnion normally fuses with the chorion by 16 weeks, although chorioamniotic separation may be identified later, resulting from polyhydramnios, congenital anomalies, or prior amniocentesis (Fig. 13–35).

Other Sites of Hemorrhage

Another location of hemorrhage that may be occasionally detected on sonography is "preplacental" hemorrhage, located between the placenta and the amniotic fluid (Fig. 13–36).[50] Pathologically, hemorrhages seen here may be either *subamniotic* or subchorionic *("subchorial")* in location (Fig. 13–21), although it may be impossible to distinguish these on the basis of sonography. Although the etiology of subamniotic hemorrhages is unknown, some authors believe they result from rupture of vessels on the placental surface owing to temporary occlusion of the umbilical vein.[56] Since subamniotic hemorrhage does not communicate with the subchorionic space, vaginal bleeding may be absent.

Large hematomas seen in a "preplacental" location may be clinically significant and probably correspond to the "massive subchorial" hematomas (Breus' mole) that have been well described in the pathologic literature.[31, 57] Although the origin and significance of massive subchorial hematomas have been debated, clinical symptoms of vaginal bleeding, spontaneous abortion, preterm delivery, and hypertension are similar to those observed from placental abruptions. Although placental detachment apparently does not occur from hemorrhages at this site, fetal demise may result from large hematomas caused by compression of the umbilical cord, which must traverse between the placenta and fetus.[43]

Intervillous thrombosis is another frequent pathologic finding, seen in 36 percent of the placentas.[31] Intervillous thrombi apparently result from intraplacental hemorrhage caused by breaks in villous capillaries. Pathologically, these lesions are composed of coagulated blood originating from both the maternal and fetal systems.[31] As the lesions age, blood is replaced by fibrin, re-

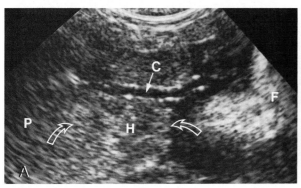

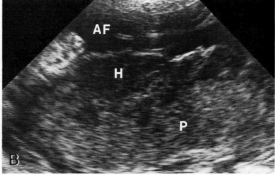

Figure 13–36. *A,* Sonogram at 30 weeks demonstrates an isoechoic "preplacental" hemorrhage (H, *arrows*) located between the placenta (P) and the fetus (F). Note that the hemorrhage also surrounds the umbilical cord (C). *B,* Repeat sonogram one week later demonstrates that an evolving hemorrhage (H) is now hypoechoic relative to the placenta (P). AF, amniotic fluid.

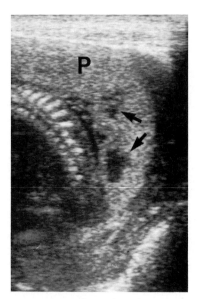

Figure 13–37. Intervillous thrombi. Sonogram performed at 18 menstrual weeks, because of an elevated maternal serum alpha-fetoprotein level, demonstrates several prominent sonolucencies *(arrows)* within the placenta (P), representing intervillous thrombi. No fetal anomalies were observed on sonography or following delivery.

sulting in a white laminated lesion. Adjacent villi are compressed and may show coagulation necrosis. Although intervillous thrombi are not a significant threat to the fetus, they are associated with Rh sensitization and elevated maternal alpha-fetoprotein (AFP) levels from fetal-maternal hemorrhage.[58-60]

Sonographically, intervillous thrombi are seen as intraplacental sonolucencies (Fig. 13–37).[62] They are observed with increasing frequency as the placenta matures. Similar sonolucencies may demonstrate flowing blood, in which case they have been termed "maternal lakes."[62] Although the pathologic correlate of "maternal lakes" is unclear, some may represent sites of prior hemorrhage that have resolved and now communicate with the intervillous space (Fig. 13–38).

Other Abnormalities

INFARCT. Small *placental infarcts* are observed pathologically in up to 25 percent of normal placentas at term.[31] Large infarcts or infarcts that occur early in pregnancy usually indicate underlying uteroplacental dysfunction from hypertension, renal disease, or vascular disease (Fig. 13–39). A submu-

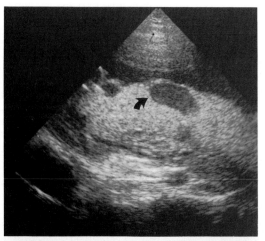

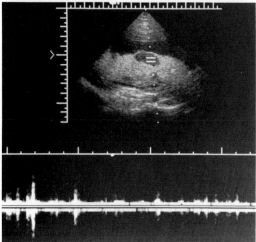

Figure 13–38. Subchorionic "lakes." Sonogram at 25 weeks, performed for fetal age determination, shows a subchorionic fluid collection *(arrow)*. Doppler evaluation reveals flow within the collection.

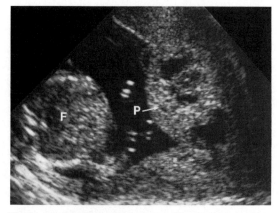

Figure 13–39. Placental infarcts. Sonogram from a 20 year old patient with long-standing systemic lupus erythematosus demonstrates confluent sonolucencies throughout the placenta (P) at 19 weeks, representing multiple infarcts. F, fetus. Intrauterine fetal demise occurred three weeks after the sonogram.

cous myoma may also be the cause of infarction in some cases. Placental infarction has been diagnosed prenatally as an intraplacental sonolucency, although it is usually not possible to distinguish this finding from intervillous thrombi.

PLACENTA ACCRETA/INCRETA/PERCRETA. Placenta accreta is an abnormally adherent placenta in which the chorionic villi grow into the myometrium.[3] Villi that extend through the myometrium are called *placenta increta*, and villi that penetrate the uterine serosa are termed *placenta percreta* (Fig. 13–40). This complication apparently results from underdeveloped decidualization. The most common predisposing factor is a uterine scar from previous cesarean section. The major potential clinical problem is retained placental tissue that may cause persistent bleeding after delivery. In severe cases, unsuccessful manual extraction of the placenta may even require hysterectomy.

Placenta accreta or increta is rarely recognized by sonography.[63] Occasionally, the diagnosis can be suspected when myometrium is not identified beneath the placenta, an observation that is best demonstrated for anterior placentas. Placenta percreta can be suggested when the placenta is seen extending through the myometrium into the urinary bladder.

CHORIOANGIOMA. Chorioangioma is a benign vascular malformation that acts as an arteriovenous shunt, bypassing normal placental tissue. Pathologically, small chorioan-

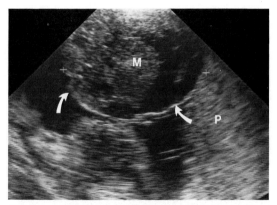

Figure 13–41. Chorioangioma. Sonogram shows a large complex mass (M, *arrows*), contiguous with the placenta (P), which proved to be a chorioangioma that resulted in fetal demise.

giomas can be identified in 1 percent of placentas, but these are not large enough to be clinically significant.[31] Tumors that are large enough to produce clinical symptoms and be visualized on sonography are much less common, occurring in one in 3500 to 20,000 births. Complications of chorioangioma include polyhydramnios, hemorrhage, preterm labor, fetal hydrops, IUGR, and fetal demise. Chorioangiomas can also be the source of elevated maternal serum AFP levels.

Sonographically, chorioangiomas are usually seen as circumscribed solid or complex masses protruding from the fetal surface of the placenta (Fig. 13–41).[64] Rarely, pedunculated lesions simulating a succenturiate lobe can also occur. Many reported masses are located near the umbilical cord insertion site (Fig. 13–42). Large lesions are often associated with fetal hydrops and polyhydramnios (Fig. 13–43).

UMBILICAL CORD ANOMALIES. The umbilical cord is the fetal lifeline that connects to the placenta. Because it is bathed by amniotic fluid, the umbilical cord can be readily visualized on sonography as two umbilical arteries, a larger umbilical vein, and a variable amount of myxomatous material called Wharton's jelly (Fig. 13–44). Fetal blood normally flows through the umbilical arteries, which branch into small capillaries within the chorionic villi, and returns via the umbilical vein. The placental insertion site of the umbilical cord can be demonstrated in nearly all fetuses and is important as a site for fetal blood sampling (Fig.

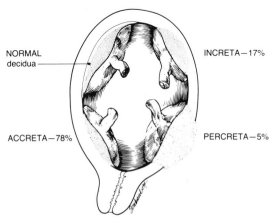

NORMAL
decidua

INCRETA—17%

ACCRETA—78%

PERCRETA—5%

Figure 13–40. Differences between normal decidualization, placenta accreta, placenta increta, and placenta percreta. (*From* Benedetti TJ: Obstetric hemorrhage. *In* Gabbe SG, Niebyl JR, Simpson JL (eds): Obstetrics: Normal and Problem Pregnancies. New York, Churchill Livingstone, 1986.)

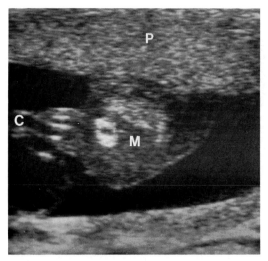

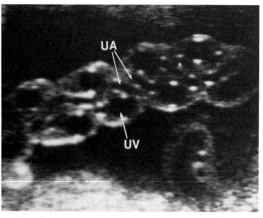

Figure 13–44. Normal umbilical cord. Longitudinal sonogram of the umbilical cord shows the uterine vein (UV) spiraling around the two smaller umbilical arteries (UA).

Figure 13–42. Chorioangioma of the umbilical cord. Sonogram at 16 weeks, performed for a markedly elevated maternal serum alpha-fetoprotein level (30 multiples of the median), demonstrates a mass (M) on the fetal surface of the placenta (P), intimately associated with the umbilical cord (C). This proved to be a chorioangioma.

13–45). At the fetal umbilicus, the two umbilical arteries converge from a location just lateral to the urinary bladder, whereas the vein courses in a cephalad direction into the fetal liver.

A variety of abnormalities may affect the umbilical cord. The most commonly encountered abnormality is a single umbilical artery (SUA), found in 0.2 to 1.0 percent of pregnancies.[65, 66] The reported frequency is higher among autopsy series but is lower among studies of live newborns. The clinical significance of a single umbilical artery is an association with other fetal malformations, reported in 14 to 62 percent of cases.[65, 67] This represents a 10 to 40 times greater risk of fetal malformations compared with the baseline risk.

Sonographically, a single umbilical artery is diagnosed when the umbilical cord contains two vessels instead of the usual three (Fig. 13–46). Typically, the single umbilical artery is larger than normal and is nearly as large as the umbilical vein. Since anomalous fetuses with a single umbilical artery tend to have multiple malformations involving

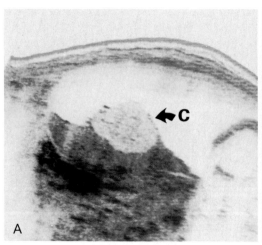

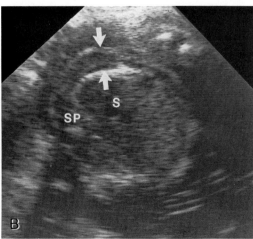

Figure 13–43. *A,* Chorioangioma. Sonogram at 30 weeks shows a large mass (C) protruding from the fetal surface of the placenta that proved to be a chorioangioma. *B,* Fetal hydrops was also noted, shown as marked soft tissue thickening *(arrows).* S, fetal stomach, SP, spine.

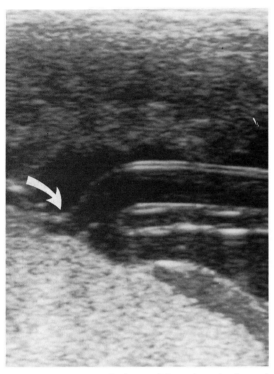

Figure 13–45. Normal placental insertion site *(arrow)* of the umbilical cord.

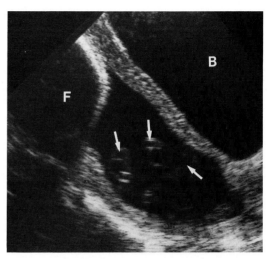

Figure 13–47. Prolapsed umbilical cord. Longitudinal sonogram at 30 weeks, performed for preterm labor, demonstrates the umbilical cord *(arrows)* prolapsed into a dilated cervix. F, fetal head, B, urinary bladder.

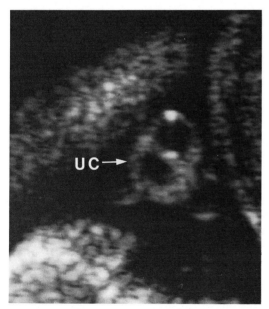

Figure 13–46. Single umbilical artery. Transverse sonogram demonstrates two vessels in the umbilical cord (UC) instead of the normal three. This fetus had multiple anomalies, including a large thoracolumbar meningomyelocele, facial cleft, single atrium, ventricular septal defect, and absent right kidney.

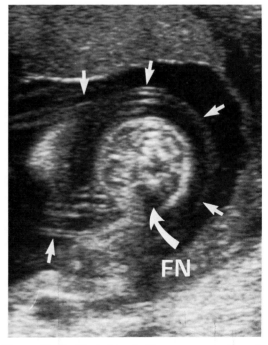

Figure 13–48. Nuchal cord. Transverse scan through the fetal neck (FN). The umbilical cord *(arrows)* can be seen to wrap around the fetal neck.

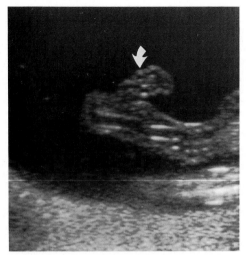

Figure 13–49. False cord knot. While a true knot of the umbilical cord is a potentially life-threatening situation, a false knot is not! Here, an extra loop of umbilical vessels *(arrow)* gives the appearance of a knot.

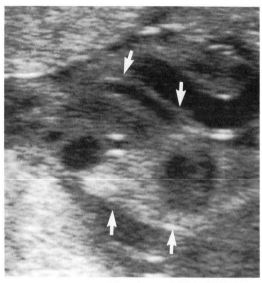

Figure 13–51. Normal large cord. An abundance of Wharton's jelly, rather than vascular dilatation, results in a large umbilical cord *(arrows)*.

multiple organ systems, detection of a single umbilical artery and at least one other malformation may help predict the presence of additional anomalies, many of which may not be visible. The presence of a single umbilical artery in association with other malformations also significantly increases the likelihood of an underlying chromosomal disorder.

In addition to an abnormal number of vessels, other umbilical cord abnormalities

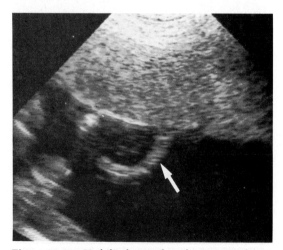

Figure 13–50. Umbilical vein thrombosis *(arrow)* in a dead fetus. (*Reprinted with permission from Abrams SL, Callen PW, Filly RA: Umbilical vein thrombosis: Sonographic detection in utero. J Ultrasound Med 4:283, 1985. Copyright 1985 by the American Institute of Ultrasound in Medicine.*)

that can be recognized on sonography include an abnormal location of the umbilical cord, umbilical vein thrombosis, umbilical cord edema, cysts, and tumors. Identification of a prolapsing umbilical cord or a nuchal cord places the fetus at risk for a vascular accident (Fig. 13–47, 13–48). Likewise, an umbilical cord knot also is a life-threatening event (Fig. 13–49). Umbilical vein thrombosis is invariably associated with fetal demise (Fig. 13–50). Although there appears to be little clinical significance to most umbilical cord cysts (representing allantoic cysts),[68] Fink and Filly noted an association between them and omphaloceles.[69]

Umbilical cord size varies widely.[70] This appears to be due to variation in the size of the umbilical vessels and in the amount of Wharton's jelly present (Fig. 13–51). Umbilical cord enlargement may occur from fetal hydrops. Other causes of umbilical cord enlargement include maternal diabetes, a hematoma, or umbilical cord tumors. Chorioangiomas on the placental surface often involve the umbilical cord (Fig. 13–43).

References

1. Moore KL: The Developing Human: Clinically Oriented Embryology, 4th Ed. Philadelphia, WB Saunders Co, 1988.
2. Tuchmann-Duplessis H, David G, Haegel P: Illustrated Human Embryology, Vol I: Embryogenesis. New York, Springer Verlag, 1982.

3. Goplerud CP: Bleeding in late pregnancy. In Danforth DN (ed): Obstetrics and Gynecology, 3rd Ed. Hagerstown, Maryland, Harper & Row, 1977, pp 378–384.

4. Jeanty P, Kirkpatrick C, Verhoogen C, Struyven J: The succenturiate placenta. J Ultrasound Med 2:9, 1983.

5. Hoddick WK, Mahony BS, Callen PW, Filly RA: Placental thickness. J Ultrasound Med 4:479, 1985.

6. Callen PW, Filly RA: The placental–subplacental complex: A specific indicator of placental position on ultrasound. JCU 8:21, 1980.

7. Nyberg DA, Filly RA, Golbus MS, Stephens JD: Entangled umbilical cords: A sign of monoamniotic twins. J Ultrasound Med 3:29, 1984.

8. Mahony BS, Filly RA, Callen PW: Amnionicity and chorionicity in twin pregnancies: Prediction using ultrasound. Radiology 155:205, 1985.

9. Hertzberg BS, Kurtz AE, Choi HY, et al: Significance of membrane thickness in the sonographic evaluation of twin gestations. AJR 148:151, 1987.

10. Laing FC: Ultrasound evaluation of obstetric problems relating to the lower uterine segment and cervix. In Sanders RC, James AE Jr (eds): The Principles and Practice of Ultrasonography in Obstetrics and Gynecology, 3rd Ed. Norwalk, Connecticut, Appleton-Century-Crofts, 1985, pp 355–367.

11. Hibbard LT: Placenta praevia. Am J Obstet Gynecol 104:172, 1969.

12. Crenshaw CJ, Jones DED, Parker RT: Placenta praevia: A survey of twenty years experience with improved perinatal survival by expected therapy and cesarean delivery. Obstet Gynecol Surv 28:461, 1975.

13. Naeye RL: Placenta previa: Predisposing factors and effects on the fetus and surviving infants. Obstet Gynecol 52:521, 1978.

14. Scheer K: Ultrasonic diagnosis of placenta previa. Obstet Gynecol 42:707, 1973.

15. Bowie JD, Rochester D, Cadkin AV, et al: Accuracy of placental localization by ultrasound. Radiology 128:177, 1978.

16. Zemlyn S: The effect of the urinary bladder in obstetrical sonography. Radiology 128:169, 1978.

17. Bowie JD, Andreotti RF, Rosenberg EF: Sonographic appearance of the uterine cervix in pregnancy: The vertical cervix. AJR 140:737, 1983.

18. Zemlyn S: The placenta. In Sarti D (ed): Diagnostic Ultrasound, 2nd Ed. Chicago, Illinois, Year Book Med Pubs, 1987, pp 839–856.

19. Newton R, Barss V, Certrulo CL: The epidemiology and clinical history of asymptomatic midtrimester placenta previa. Am J Obstet Gynecol 148:743, 1984.

20. Jeffrey RB, Laing FC: Sonography of the low-lying placenta: Value of Trendelenburg and traction scans. AJR 137:547, 1981.

21. Smeltzer JS, Parm R, Boone D: Benefit of perineal ultrasound for placental location. Presented to the Seventh Annual Meeting of the Society of Perinatal Obstetricians. Lake Buena Vista, Florida, February 5–7, 1987.

22. Powell MC, Buckley J, Price H, et al: Magnetic resonance imaging and placenta previa. Am J Obstet Gynecol 154:565, 1986.

23. Chervenak FA, Lee Y, Hendler MA, et al: Role of attempted vaginal delivery in the management of placenta previa. Obstet Gynecol 64:798, 1984.

24. Wexler P, Gottesfeld KR: Second trimester placenta previa: An apparently normal placentation. Obstet Gynecol 50:706, 1977.

25. Wexler P, Gottesfeld KR: Early diagnosis of placenta previa. Obstet Gynecol 54:231, 1979.

26. Mittelstaedt CA, Partain CL, Boyce IL Jr, Dainiel EB: Placenta praevia: Significant in the second trimester. Radiology 131:465, 1979.

27. Gillieson MS, Winer-Muran HT, Muran D: Low-lying placenta. Radiology 144:577, 1982.

28. Artis AA III, Bowie JD, Rosenberg ER, Rauch RF: The fallacy of placental migration: Effect of sonographic techniques. AJR 144:79, 1985.

29. Townsend RT, Laing FC, Nyberg DA, et al: Technical factors responsible for "placental migration": Sonographic assessment. Radiology 160:105, 1986.

30. King DL: Placenta migration demonstrated by ultrasonography. Radiology 109:167, 1973.

31. Fox H: Pathology of the Placenta. London, WB Saunders Co, 1978, pp 107–157.

32. Green-Thompson RW: Antepartum haemorrhage. Clin Obstet Gynaecol 9:479, 1982.

33. Douglas RG, Buchman MI, MacDonald FA: Premature separation of the normally implanted placenta. Br J Obstet Gynaecol 62:710, 1955.

34. Naeye RL: Abruptio placentae and placenta previa: Frequency, perinatal mortality, and cigarette smoking. Obstet Gynecol 55:701, 1980.

35. Hibbard BM, Jeffcoate TNA: Abruptio placentae. Obstet Gynecol 27:155, 1966.

36. Sexton LI, Hertig AT, Reid DE, et al: Premature separation of the normally implanted placenta. Am J Obstet Gynecol 59:13, 1950.

37. Gruenwald P, Levin H, Yousem H: Abruption and premature separation of the placenta. Am J Obstet Gynecol 102:604, 1968.

38. Harris BA: Marginal placental bleeding. Am J Obstet Gynecol 61:53, 1985.

39. Harris BA, Gore H, Flowers CE: Peripheral placental separation: A possible relationship to premature labor. Obstet Gynecol 66:774, 1985.

40. Naeye RL, Harkness WL, Utts J: Abruptio placentae and perinatal death: A prospective study. Am J Obstet Gynecol 128:740, 1977.

41. Hurd WW, Miodovnik M, Hertzberg V, Lavin JP: Selective management of abruption placenta: A prospective study. Obstet Gynecol 61:467, 1983.

42. Knab DR: Abruptio placentae. An assessment of the time and method of delivery. Obstet Gynecol 52:625, 1978.

43. Sher G: A rational basis for the management of abruptio placentae. J Reprod Med 31:123, 1978.

44. Odendaal HJ: The frequency of uterine contractions in abruptio placentae. S Afr Med J 50:2129, 1976.

45. Nyberg DA, Mack LA, Benedetti TJ, et al: Placental abruption and placental hemorrhage: Correlation of sonographic findings with fetal outcome. Radiology 164:357, 1987.

46. Spirt BA, Kagan EH, Rozanski RM: Abruptio placenta: Sonographic and pathologic correlation. AJR 133:877, 1979.

47. Jaffe MH, Schoen WC, Silver TM, et al: Sonography of abruptio placentae. AJR 137:1049, 1981.

48. McGahan JP, Phillips HE, Reid MH, Oi RH: Sonographic spectrum of retroplacental hemorrhage. Radiology 142:481, 1982.

49. Spirt BA, Gordon LP, Kagan EH: The placenta: Sonographic-pathologic correlations. Semin Roentgen 17:219, 1982.

50. Nyberg DA, Cyr DR, Mack LA, et al: Sonographic spectrum of placental abruption. AJR 148:161, 1987.
51. Mintz MC, Kurtz AB, Arenson R, et al: Abruptio placentae: Apparent thickening of the placenta caused by hyperechoic retroplacental clot. J Ultrasound Med 5:411, 1986.
52. Marx M, Caesola G, Scheible W, Deutsch A: The subplacental complex: Further sonographic observations. J Ultrasound Med 4:459, 1985.
53. Williams CH, VanBergen WS, Prentice RL: Extra-amniotic blood clot simulating placenta previa on ultrasound scan. JCU 5:45, 1976.
54. Sauerbrei EE, Pham DH: Placental abruption and subchorionic hemorrhage in the first half of pregnancy: Ultrasound appearance and clinical outcome. Radiology 160:109, 1986.
55. Goldstein SR, Subramanyan BR, Raghavendra BN, et al: Subchorionic bleeding in threatened abortion: Sonographic findings and significance. AJR 141:975, 1983.
56. Desa DJ: Rupture of fetal vessels on placental surface. Arch Dis Child 46:495, 1971.
57. Shanklin DR, Scott JS: Massive subchorial thrombohaematoma (Breus' mole). Br J Obstet Gynaecol 82:476, 1975.
58. Hoogland HJ, de Hann J, Vooys GP: Ultrasonographic diagnosis of intervillous thrombosis related to Rh isoimmunization. Gynecol Obstet Invest 10:237, 1979.
59. Javert CT, Reiss C: The origin and significance of macroscopic intervillous coagulation hematomas (red infarcts) of the human placenta. Surg Gynecol Obstet 94:257, 1985.
60. Perkes EA, Baim RS, Goodman KR, Macri JN: Second-trimester placental changes associated with elevated maternal serum alpha-fetoprotein. Am J Obstet Gynecol 144:935, 1982.
61. Spirt BA, Gordon LP, Kagan EH: Intervillous thrombosis: Sonographic pathologic correlation. Radiology 147:197, 1983.
62. Cooperberg PL, Wright VJ, Carpenter CW: Ultrasonographic demonstration of a placental maternal lake. JCU 7:62, 1979.
63. Pasto ME, Kurtz AB, Rijkin MD, et al: Ultrasonographic findings of placenta increta. J Ultrasound Med 2:155, 1983.
64. Rodan BA, Bean WJ: Chorioangioma of the placenta causing intrauterine fetal demise. J Ultrasound Med 2:95, 1983.
65. Benirschke K, Bourne GL: The incidence and prognostic implication of congenital absence of one umbilical artery. Am J Obstet Gynecol 79:251, 1960.
66. Bryne J, Blane WA: Malformations and chromosome anomalies in spontaneously aborted fetuses with single umbilical artery. Am J Obstet Gynecol 151:340, 1985.
67. Tortora M, Chervenak F, Mayden D, Hobbin JC: Antenatal sonographic diagnosis of single umbilical artery. Obstet Gynecol 63:693, 1984.
68. Sachs L, Fourcroy JL, Wenzel DJ, Nash JD: Prenatal detection of umbilical cord allantoic cyst. Radiology 145:445, 1982.
69. Fink IJ, Filly RA: Omphalocele associated with umbilical cord allantoic cyst: Sonographic evaluation in utero. Radiology 149:473, 1983.
70. Casola G, Scheible W, Leopold GR: Large umbilical cord: A normal finding in some fetuses. Radiology 156:181, 1985.

SONOGRAPHIC PREDICTION OF FETAL LUNG MATURITY

Frank P. Hadlock, M.D.

Normal fetal lung development is a sequential process that involves several phases. The important alveolar phase generally begins at the 24th menstrual week and extends into postnatal life. During this time, the alveolar cells secrete phospholipids (surfactant) that play a key role in the functional integrity of the fetal lung at delivery. If these phospholipids are not present in sufficient quantities at birth, the fetal alveoli will collapse, and the fetus will receive inadequate oxygenation. This form of respiratory embarrassment is called respiratory distress syndrome (RDS) or, more specifically, hyaline membrane disease (HMD). This condition usually affects fetuses that are born prematurely.

There are two major clinical situations in which it is useful to have an accurate assessment of fetal lung maturity in utero, since both may result in RDS secondary to premature delivery. One is the preterm patient who is at high risk of imminent delivery secondary to premature labor or in whom early delivery is mandated by maternal or fetal indications (e.g., a 34 week pregnancy with severe preeclampsia and growth retardation). The second category is the otherwise uncomplicated pregnancy with unknown dates in which a cesarean delivery is necessary. Assessment of fetal lung maturity in the former category is less critical, since maternal or fetal factors may dictate immediate delivery regardless of the fetal lung's status. In the latter case, however, knowledge of fetal lung maturity is necessary to avoid iatrogenic RDS due to unnecessary premature delivery.[22]

In such cases, fetal lung maturity can be accurately assessed by biochemical analysis of amniotic fluid samples obtained through amniocentesis.[15] Amniocentesis performed with ultrasound guidance is usually a benign procedure,[48] but it carries the potential for serious complications, such as premature separation of the placenta, premature rupture of membranes, premature labor, fetal or maternal bleeding, and even fetal death. Because of these possible complications, efforts have been made to use prenatal diagnostic ultrasound as a means of evaluating fetal lung maturity. The purpose of this chapter is to determine what role, if any, ultrasound can play in predicting fetal lung maturity in utero.

BIOCHEMICAL MARKERS

In 1971, Gluck and Kulovich demonstrated that the relationship between the surface-active phospholipids in amniotic fluid could be used to evaluate the maturity of the human fetal lung.[15] They demonstrated that in random pregnancies, both normal and abnormal, when the lecithin/sphingomyelin (LS) ratio was 2 or greater, there was an absence of RDS at birth, irrespective of age and weight.[16] They also noted that certain maternal conditions, such as diabetes mellitus (Classes A to C) and Rh incompatibility, may cause a delay in fetal lung maturation, whereas other maternal conditions, such as chronic hypertension or severe diabetes mellitus (Classes D, F, R), may actually accelerate the development of fetal lung maturity in utero.[16, 30]

Refinements in the evaluation of amniotic fluid phospholipids for determination of fetal lung maturity have resulted in a complete fetal *lung profile*,[30] which consists of the LS ratio, as well as percentages of disaturated (acetone-precipitated) lecithin, phosphati-

dylinositol (PI), and phosphotidylglycerol (PG). The relative changes in the concentration of these phospholipids in amniotic fluid over time can be seen in Figure 14–1. One should note that in normal pregnancies, the fetal lung is generally not mature before 34 weeks but is mature after 37 weeks. From 34 to 37 weeks, there is a transitional phase in which varying degrees of fetal lung maturity can be expected. Subsequent clinical experience has indicated that the lung profile predicts fetal lung maturity more accurately than it does immaturity; that is, there is a virtual absence of RDS in fetuses with a mature lung profile, whereas some fetuses with an immature lung profile will not develop RDS at delivery. Because of the ability of the mature lung profile to predict fetal lung maturity, it serves as a "gold standard" against which sonographic predictors of fetal lung maturity can be judged.

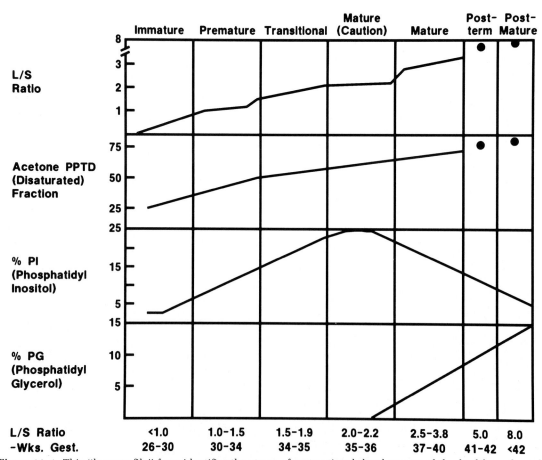

Figure 14–1. This "lung profile" form identifies the stages of maturational development of the fetal lung through amniotic fluid analysis. (*From* Kulovich MV, Hallman MB, Gluck L: The lung profile. I. Normal pregnancy. Am J Obstet Gynecol 135:57, 1979. Copyright: Regents of the University of California.)

SONOGRAPHIC PREDICTORS

Theoretical Considerations

If one were to design a study for evaluation of an ultrasound marker of fetal lung maturity, it would be important to test the marker in a large series of patients in the third trimester of pregnancy. Ideally, all patients would be scanned at weekly intervals from the 28th week, and cesarean delivery would be done on the day the marker is first identified, regardless of menstrual age. However, in view of the increased perinatal morbidity and mortality associated with premature (< 37 weeks) delivery, such a study would be both unethical and clinically unjustifiable.[22]

Because of these constraints, the design of any sonographic study for predicting fetal lung maturity will be limited in two major respects. First, although it is relatively easy to obtain a large sample of *term* patients who have undergone amniocentesis before cesarean delivery, it is virtually impossible to obtain a correspondingly large sample of *preterm* uncomplicated pregnancies, since there is no clinical indication for amniocentesis in this group. Thus, not only is the preterm population invariably smaller than the term population, but virtually all amniocenteses in the preterm period will be in patients with maternal or fetal complications that are known to accelerate fetal lung maturity (e.g., premature labor, ruptured membranes, maternal hypertension or toxemia, fetal growth retardation, nongestational diabetes mellitus, and steroid therapy). The results from the biochemical testing in this population will thus be skewed in favor of fetal lung maturity in comparison with a corresponding preterm control group.[22]

Second, since a sonographic study with development of RDS as an endpoint would not be ethical, one must evaluate sonographic markers of fetal lung maturity in terms of their ability to predict a mature biochemical lung profile. Based on reports to date,[22] the combination of an LS ratio equal to or greater than 2 and a PG concentration of at least 0.02 percent should predict fetal lung maturity in all nondiabetic patients, regardless of menstrual age. When the LS ratio is less than 2 and PG is absent, or present in a concentration less than 0.02 percent in the amniotic fluid, a high percentage of cases of fetal RDS can be expected

after immediate cesarean delivery in an uncomplicated nondiabetic pregnancy. The exact percentage of such fetuses in which RDS would develop if delivered immediately is not known, but it would relate in large part to the actual menstrual age at the time of delivery. Based on the available data,[8, 10, 16, 31, 47] the risk of RDS in such patients between 35 and 37 weeks would be 20 to 40 percent, whereas deliveries between 32 and 35 weeks would carry a risk of 40 to 85 percent. These risks are clearly unacceptable when the timing of cesarean delivery is elective.

Biparietal Diameter (BPD)

Early reports by Goldstein and associates[19] and Spellacy and colleagues[42] suggested that use of a BPD equal to or greater than 9.0 cm resulted in an unacceptably high false-positive rate (27 to 30 percent) in predicting fetal lung maturity as judged by an LS ratio greater than 2. Strassner and coworkers[43] subsequently confirmed this finding and demonstrated that in the presence of an immature LS ratio, a BPD equal to or greater than 9.0 cm provided no significant information on the presence or absence of PG in the amniotic fluid. Harman,[24] in a study of 235 third trimester patients, demonstrated that a BPD of at least 9.0 cm correlated with a mature LS ratio in only 79 percent of cases, whereas a BPD less than 9.0 cm was associated with a mature LS ratio in 80 percent of cases. The results of the study by Hadlock and coworkers[22] are quite similar (Table 14–1).

Hayashi and colleagues,[25] Golde and associates,[17] and Petrucha and coworkers[37] focused on the presence or absence of HMD at delivery as a standard against which to judge the prediction of fetal lung maturity. They suggested that a BPD greater than 9.2 cm is adequate evidence of fetal lung maturity in the absence of maternal diabetes mellitus. In Hayashi's sample population,[25] the menstrual age at the time of the sonogram was thought to be at least 38 menstrual weeks, an age known to be associated with fetal lung maturity, irrespective of the BPD.[16, 22] Golde[17] and Petrucha[37] concluded that a BPD of at least 9.2 cm had 100 percent predictive power for fetal lung maturity, but these studies were limited by failure to indicate the menstrual ages of the fetuses studied and by

Table 14–1. RELATION BETWEEN BPD AND FETAL LUNG MATURITY

Author	N	Age*	BPD	Index of Lung Maturity	False Positive (%)
Goldstein et al[19]	61	NG	≥9.0 cm	LS ≥ 2	29.5
Spellacy et al[42]	84	NG	≥9.0 cm	LS ≥ 2	27.3
	84	NG	≥9.3 cm	LS ≥ 2	14.3
Strassner et al[43]	83	NG	≥9.0 cm	LS ≥ 2	10.7
	55	NG	≥9.0 cm	PG+	31.0
Harman et al[24]	108	NG	≥9.0 cm	LS ≥ 2	21.3
Hayashi et al[25]	91	>38 wks	≥9.3 cm	RDS	0.0
Golde et al[17]	92	NG	≥9.2 cm	RDS	0.0
	57	NG	≥9.2 cm	LS ≥ 2; PG+	7.0
Petrucha et al[37]	124	NG	≥9.2 cm	RDS	0.0
Newton et al[35]	100	NG	≥9.2 cm	LS ≥ 2	17.0
			≥9.2 cm	OD650 > 0.15	19.0
			≥9.2 cm	LS ≥ 2; OD ≥ 0.15	9.0
Golde et al[18]	200	≈38 wks	≥9.2 cm	RDS	0.5
Hadlock et al[22]	105	≥37 wks	≥9.3 cm	LS ≥ 2; PG+	9.5
	7	<37 wks	≥9.3 cm	LS ≥ 2; PG+	85.6

RDS, respiratory distress syndrome; PG+, phosphatidylglycerol of at least 0.02%; LS, lecithin/sphingomyelin ratio; NG, not given; OD, optical density.

False positive (%) is the number of fetuses, predicted to have mature lungs by BPD, who actually had immature lungs on the basis of the index of lung maturity used.

*Age is the menstrual age at the time of study.

inclusion of patients with maternal and fetal problems known to be associated with accelerated fetal lung maturity. The importance of the age distribution of the fetal population tested is indicated in Figure 14–2. For example, if one evaluates only fetuses in the white zone (> 37 weeks), one would expect a virtual absence of RDS at delivery based on the well-known relation between fetal lung maturity and menstrual age.[16] However, if the sample of fetuses with a BPD equal to or greater than 9.3 cm included only the group in the gray zone (< 37 weeks), a high incidence of RDS would be expected, increasing as menstrual age decreases.[8, 10, 16, 22, 31, 47]

In another work by Golde and coworkers,[18] an effort was made to evaluate a BPD equal to or greater than 9.2 cm as a predictor of fetal lung maturity. The fetuses of their nondiabetic patient population were thought to be at least 38 weeks of gestational age based on the last menstrual period; RDS developed in only one fetus with a BPD equal to or greater than 9.2 cm when delivery was within one week of the ultrasound examination. Predictably, in this infant, the dates were incorrect; the actual fetal age based on neonatal examination was 34 weeks. It is meaningless to further test a BPD equal to or greater than 9.2 cm (or any sonographic marker) as a predictor of fetal lung maturity in fetuses known to be at least 38 menstrual weeks of age, since it is age and not the BPD

measurement that determines fetal lung maturity in such cases.[22] In the author's opinion, there is no BPD measurement above which one can be certain that the fetus has mature lungs.

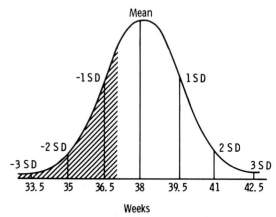

Figure 14–2. A normal bell-shaped curve that would be anticipated for the frequency distribution of menstrual ages for a biparietal diameter (BPD) of 9.3 cm in an unselected fetal population. Approximately 24 percent of these fetuses would be less than 37 menstrual weeks *(shaded area)*, and 14 percent of this group would be less than 35 weeks. Given the well-known relation between fetal lung maturity and advancing menstrual age, substantial differences would be expected if a BPD of 9.3 cm or greater was used to predict lung maturity in a study population limited to either the *white area* (greater than 37 weeks) or the *shaded area* (less than 37 weeks). (*From Hadlock FP, Irwin JF, Roecker E, et al: Ultrasound prediction of fetal lung maturity. Radiology 155:469, 1985.*)

Evaluation of Placental Maturity

In the original study by Grannum and colleagues (Fig. 14–3),[20] a Grade III placenta was associated with fetal lung maturity (as assessed by the LS ratio) in 100 percent of cases. A subsequent study[38] confirmed this finding, but the data on the menstrual ages of the fetuses and on maternal fetal complications that might accelerate lung maturity were inadequate; thus, one could not deduce how accurate a Grade III placenta would be in predicting lung maturity in an uncomplicated population undergoing cesarean delivery at varying menstrual ages. Several case reports that followed indicated that a Grade III placenta could be associated with biochemical fetal lung immaturity as well as RDS, and, not surprisingly, these concerned fetuses delivered preterm by cesarean section.[13, 29] In several studies, representing 349 cases with Grade III placentas, it has been shown that a Grade III placenta has less than 100 percent predictive power for fetal lung maturity (Table 14–2).[22] Moreover, the effect

of menstrual age demonstrated for the BPD has also been seen in these studies. For example, in the work of Kazzi and colleagues,[27] a Grade III placenta had 100 percent predictive power for fetal lung maturity when seen after 38 weeks, whereas the predictive power for the presence of PG before 38 weeks was only 15.8 percent. Such an age effect has also been demonstrated in the studies by Tabsh[44] and Hills and associates[26] and was confirmed in the study by Hadlock and coworkers[22] (Table 14–2). Subsequent to the author's study, a florid case of RDS was seen in the presence of a Grade III placenta in a fetus who was delivered at 32 weeks of a nondiabetic mother. As with the BPD, knowing that a Grade III placenta is associated with fetal lung maturity after 38 weeks is of limited clinical usefulness, since fetuses delivered after 38 weeks without Grade III placentas also have fetal lung maturity.[22]

In 1985, Destro and colleagues[9] reported data from what is, in the author's opinion, the definitive evaluation of the relation between placental grade and fetal lung maturity in the preterm fetus. They evaluated 32

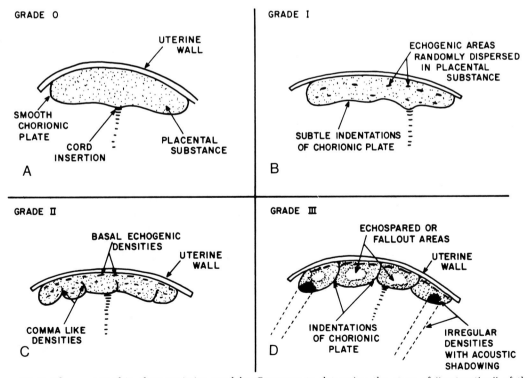

Figure 14–3. The sonographic characteristics used by Grannum to determine the stage of "maturation" of the placenta. A Grade III represents the most mature placenta. (*From* Grannum PA, Berkowitz RL, Hobbins JC: The ultrasonic changes in the maturing placenta and their relation to fetal pulmonic maturity. Am J Obstet Gynecol 133:915, 1979.)

Table 14–2. RELATION BETWEEN PLACENTA GRADE III AND
FETAL LUNG MATURITY

Author	N	Age*	Index of Fetal Lung Maturity	False Positive (%)
Grannum et al[20]	23	>35 wks	LS ≥ 2.0	0.0
Petrucha et al[38]	15	>37 wks	LS ≥ 2.0	0.0
	15	>37 wks	RDS	0.0
	13	>37 wks	PG+	8.0
Quinlan et al[39]	12	NG	LS ≥ 2.0	41.7
Harman et al[24]	130	30–44 wks	LS ≥ 2.0	7.0
	100	30–44 wks	PG+	25.0
Clair et al[7]	13	Near term	LS ≥ 2.0	7.7
Ragozzino et al[40]	12	>37 wks	LS ≥ 3.0	8.0
	12	>37 wks	RDS	0.0
Kazzi et al[27]	61	>38 wks	LS ≥ 2.0	0.0
	61	>38 wks	PG+	0.0
	19	<38 wks	LS ≥ 2.0	21.0
	19	<38 wks	PG+	84.2
	19	<38 wks	RDS	15.8
Tabsh[44]	68	>37 wks	LS ≥ 2.0	5.9
	7	<37 wks	LS ≥ 2.0	28.6
Hills et al[26]	17	>37 wks	LS ≥ 2.0	0.0
	10	<37 wks	LS ≥ 2.0	50.0
Hadlock et al[22]	51	>37 wks	LS ≥ 2.0; PG+	5.9
	2	<37 wks	LS ≥ 2.0; PG+	100.0

RDS, respiratory distress syndrome; PG+, phosphatidylglycerol of at least 0.02%; LS, lecithin/sphingomyelin ratio.

False positive (%) is the number of cases, predicted to be mature by placental grading, who actually had immature lungs on the basis of the index of lung maturity used.

*Age is the menstrual age at the time of study.

normal pregnant women between 29 and 33 menstrual weeks for determination of placental grade by ultrasound, with simultaneous biochemical evaluation of fetal lung maturity by LS ratio and Clements' foam stability test. A Grade I placenta was observed in ten cases, and in this group, there was only one mature LS ratio, which was in a patient at 33 menstrual weeks. A Grade II placenta was observed in the remaining 22 cases, and again only one mature LS ratio was seen, occurring in a patient at 33 menstrual weeks. No patients with a Grade III placenta were identified in this group. These authors concluded that placental grading is of no value in evaluating pulmonary maturity of the fetus before 34 weeks.

Fetal Epiphyseal Ossification Centers

Chinn and colleagues[6] and Mahony and associates[32, 33] demonstrated that sonographically visible lower extremity epiphyseal ossification centers in the distal femur and proximal tibia can be useful in the evaluation of fetal age and lung maturity by ultrasound (Figs. 14–4, 14–5). They demonstrated that sonographically visible distal femoral epiphyses (DFE) indicated a menstrual age of at least 33 weeks with 95 percent accuracy and that the presence of the proximal tibial epiphyses (PTE) indicated a menstrual age of at least 35 weeks with 95 percent accuracy (Fig. 14–5). Shortly thereafter, several investigators evaluated the presence of such ossification centers as indicators of fetal lung maturity. Gentili and coworkers[14] evaluated 51 normal pregnancies between 31 and 38 weeks and found a mature LS ratio in every case in which the distal femoral epiphyseal ossification center was equal to or greater than 6 mm in diameter. In the same year, Tabsh[45] evaluated 133 nondiabetic patients and demonstrated a mature LS ratio in 100 percent of cases in which the proximal tibial epiphysis was greater than 5 mm in diameter; he also noted that when a distal femoral epiphysis measured more than 5 mm in diameter, a mature LS ratio was present in 95 percent of the cases. In 1986, Mahony and coworkers[33] demonstrated that 100 percent of the fetuses

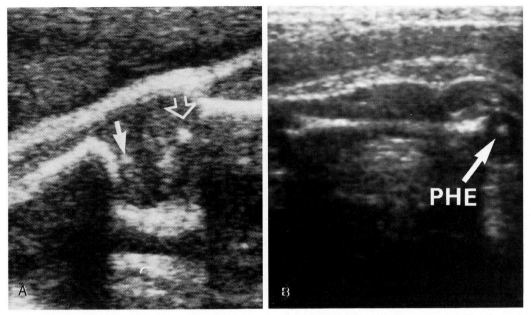

Figure 14–4. *A,* Typical sonographic appearance of the distal femoral epiphysis (DFE, *open arrow*) and proximal tibial epiphysis (PTE, *closed arrow*) in a 36 week fetus. *B,* Sonographic appearance of the proximal humeral epiphysis (PHE). (Courtesy of Barry S Mahony, MD.)

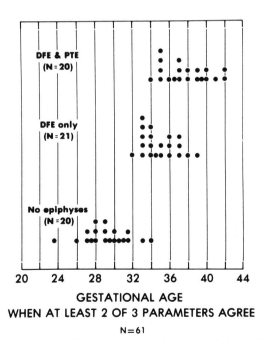

Figure 14–5. The appearance of the distal femoral epiphysis (DFE) and proximal tibial epiphysis (PTE) in a small series of patients in whom gestational age was confirmed by at least two parameters. (*From* Chinn DH, Bolding DB, Callen PW, et al: Ultrasonographic identification of fetal lower extremity epiphyseal ossification centers. Radiology 147:815, 1983.)

studied had a mature fetal lung profile when the combined diameters of the distal femoral epiphyses and proximal tibial epiphyses were greater than 11 mm. They also noted that when there was less than a 1 mm difference in the size of the distal femoral and proximal tibial epiphyses, similar results were obtained. In addition, Mahony demonstrated that 100 percent of fetuses studied had a mature lung profile when there were sonographically visible proximal humeral epiphyses (PHE).

What can be concluded from these studies about the use of epiphyseal ossification centers in predicting fetal lung maturity? Certainly, when one looks at the relation between the appearance time of these ossification centers and menstrual age, it is not surprising that they correlate relatively well with the presence of mature fetal lungs. In the author's opinion, the size of the distal femoral epiphysis should never be used alone as a predictor of fetal lung maturity. In addition, the presence of a proximal tibial epiphysis greater than 5 mm in diameter should be viewed with some suspicion, since, as indicated in the work of Tabsh,[45] epiphyses of this size can be seen as early as 35 menstrual weeks, a time in pregnancy when most, but not all, fetuses can be expected to have mature lungs.[16] The work of Mahony and coworkers[33] regarding the proximal humeral epiphyses is more provocative, because this marker generally occurs at approximately 38 weeks or thereafter, a point in pregnancy when virtually all fetuses can be expected to have mature lungs.[16] As Mahony cautions, however, great care must be used in the demonstration of the proximal humeral epiphyses, since other reflective structures (e.g., synovium or capsule) in this area may be mistaken for the proximal humeral epiphyses. Further, it should be noted that although the presence of the proximal humeral epiphyses may be an indication of fetal lung maturity, failure to demonstrate them does not necessarily imply immature fetal lungs; Mahony[33] noted that the predictive value of the proximal humeral epiphyses' absence with immature amniocentesis was only 24 percent.

Sonographically Detected Free-Floating Particles in Amniotic Fluid

In 1978, Bree[2] reported sonographic identification of reflective material in the amniotic fluid that he felt was fetal vernix, and he theorized that this material may be a marker of fetal maturity. In 1983, however, Parulekar[36] demonstrated that free-floating particles (FFP) may be seen in amniotic fluid as early as mid-trimester and concluded that they have no pathologic significance. Khaleghian,[28] on the other hand, in the same year, reported echogenic material in the amniotic fluid in the second trimester, which he considered a sign of fetal distress. Although there was some controversy about the significance of this material, there was no question that it could be identified using modern ultrasound equipment.

In 1985, Gross and coworkers[21] noted that the turbidity of amniotic fluid was related to the LS ratio in a positive way; that is, the proportion of mature LS ratio values in their study increased with increasing turbidity of the amniotic fluid. This prompted a second study in which the relationship between fetal lung maturity and the presence of FFP in amniotic fluid were evaluated. (This study used a strict definition of FFP, defined as multiple linear densities between 1 and 5

mm in length, suspended, but gradually settling, in the amniotic fluid. It was noted that fetal movement causes a swirling of these particles, giving the appearance of a blizzard.) In a study of 135 patients between 34 and 42 weeks, FFPs were present in 39 patients and absent in 96. When FFPs were present, the LS ratio was uniformly mature; however, when they were absent, the LS ratio was mature in 74 percent of patients.[21] A secondary finding in this study was that of increased FFP in association with large for gestational age (LGA) infants.

Gross and coworkers[21] concluded that the presence of FFP on real-time ultrasound in mothers greater than 38 weeks gestation can serve to confirm fetal maturity. Surely such a limited conclusion warrants caution in the use of FFP as a predictor of fetal lung maturity. In the author's experience, there have been fetuses with FFP in amniotic fluid who had immature lung profiles at amniocentesis, and the author therefore cautions against the use of this finding in evaluation of fetal lung maturity. This is particularly true since LGA infants, who are perhaps at greatest risk for iatrogenic prematurity, more commonly have FFP than normal or small infants of the same age.

Tissue Characterization of Fetal Lung

Because of the potential complications of amniocentesis and in part because of the failure of other sonographic methods in predicting fetal lung maturity, several authors[1, 3, 4, 5, 11, 34, 46] have attempted this estimation by direct sonographic evaluation of the fetal lung. This approach, which has considerable theoretical appeal, was first evaluated by Thieme and associates,[46] and later by Benson and colleagues,[1] Morris,[34] and Cayea and coworkers.[5] Thieme had noted that the developing alveolus can be thought of as a hollow sphere of tissue filled with fluid, the walls of which become thinner with maturity. Thus, the ratio of the volume of the central cavity containing fluid to the total volume of the sphere increases with maturity. Thieme[46] hypothesized that ultrasound should be able to detect an increase in fluid content by demonstrating enhanced through transmission of sound in the fetal lungs. Cayea further theorized that the reflectivity (echogenicity) of the fetal lung should increase with maturity because of the increased number of acoustic interfaces provided by the increased number of alveoli.[5]

Clinical research aimed at determining the utility of direct fetal lung evaluation has taken several forms. Benson and associates,[1] recognizing that much of the information present in the radio frequency signal is discarded during the formation of clinical sonographic images, theorized that analysis of the entire RF signal may yield sufficient data to distinguish between mature and immature fetal tissue. In their study, definite differences between mature and immature tissue were demonstrated for both fetal lung and the placenta, but correlations with objective predictors of the functional maturity of the fetal lung, such as the biochemical lung profile, were not provided; thus, the clinical utility of these data is not known at this time.[1]

In 1984, Morris[34] used a more subjective approach for sonographic evaluation of fetal lung maturity. Morris described a liver/lung ratio based on the observed reflectivity pattern in these two organs, considering the fetal lung to be mature when its reflectivity was greater than that of the fetal liver (Fig. 14–6). In a small group of patients, there was excellent correlation between a mature liver/lung ratio and a mature biochemical lung profile. Morris concluded that the liver/lung ratio alone (or in combination with vernix in the amniotic fluid and a mature placenta) correlates very well with a mature LS ratio but cautioned that confirmation of these results in a large prospective study is needed—at the present time, no such study has been forthcoming.[34]

In 1985, Cayea and associates[5] evaluated subjective sonographic signs of fetal lung maturity using conventional ultrasound in-

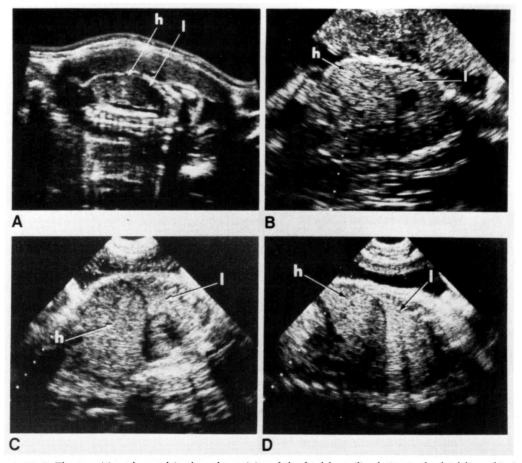

Figure 14–6. The transition observed in the echogenicity of the fetal lung (l) relative to the fetal liver (h). Some authors believe that fetal lung maturity can be assured when the fetal lung is more echogenic than the fetal liver, as noted in *D*. (*From* Fried AM, Loh FK, Umer MA, et al: Echogenicity of fetal lung: Relation to fetal age maturity. AJR 145:591, 1985. *Copyright by* The American Roentgen Ray Society, 1985.)

strumentation. They evaluated the fetal lung/liver ratio, in terms of both echogenicity and texture, as well as through transmission of sound by the fetal lung. In a group of 81 patients, these authors demonstrated no correlation between these sonographic indices of fetal lung maturity in comparison with objective standards, such as the LS ratio, or specific measurements of phosphatidylcholine. In 1985, Fried and coworkers[11] evaluated fetal lung echogenicity (see Fig. 14–6) in predicting fetal lung maturity as determined by the LS ratio and PG concentration obtained by amniocentesis. No clinically applicable relation was established in their study. In the same year, Birnholz and Farrell[3] evaluated lung compressibility noted on real-time sonograms and concluded that increased compressibility correlates rather well with lung maturity.

It is clear from the foregoing that the results of predicting fetal lung maturity by direct sonographic evaluation have been mixed. Carson and coworkers[4] have also been active in the investigation of the fetal lung through ultrasound, and they urge caution in drawing negative conclusions too early from preliminary studies. They note that technical problems can drastically affect experimental outcomes in such studies and have urged that future research in this area be done using consistent techniques, with regard to both experimental design and instrumentation. Until further research has been completed, however, one must conclude that this approach for predicting fetal lung maturity should not form the basis of clinical decision-making in obstetrics.

A Multiple Parameter Scoring System

In 1986, at the annual meeting of the American Institute of Ultrasound in Medicine, Salman and Quetel[41] described preliminary results from an ongoing study in which multiple observations and measurements were used to assess fetal lung maturity. In their scoring system, which is described in detail in Table 14–3, a score of five or greater out of a possible total of ten indicated fetal lung maturity in their initial study group of 104 patients. This approach has considerable theoretical appeal because it takes into account many sonographic parameters that,

Table 14–3. A COMPOSITE SCORING SYSTEM FOR FETAL LUNG MATURITY

Ultrasound Measurements and Observations	Lung Maturity Score
Composite age (by BPD, HC, AC, FL) (Hadlock et al[23])	
<35 wks	0
35–37 wks	1
>37 wks	2
Placenta grade (Grannum et al[20])	
0–I	0
II	1
III	2
Fetal bowel pattern (Zilianti and Fernandez[49])	
Stages 1–2	0
Stage 3	1
Stage 4	2
Lung/liver ratio (Morris[34])	
<1	0
1	1
>1	2
Distal femoral epiphysis (Chinn et al[6])	
Absent	0
Slitlike	1
Globular	2

BPD, biparietal diameter; HC, head circumference; AC, abdominal circumference; FL, femoral length.

From Salman F, Quetel T: Sonographic scoring of fetal pulmonary maturity. (Suppl.) J Ultrasound Med 5:145, 1985.

when used alone, have been demonstrated to have some relation to fetal lung maturity. In order to gain wide acceptance, however, this system must have its positive and negative predictive values evaluated in a large prospective study of series of patients throughout the third trimester age range.

At present, primarily because of the small number of fetuses studied and the possible effect of their ages on the results, no sonographic finding in the third trimester of pregnancy can be considered unequivocal evidence of fetal lung maturity. The presence of the proximal humeral epiphyses may prove to be the exception, but further evaluation of this finding will be necessary. The use of a combination of findings, as described by Salman and Quetel,[41] is a rational approach that also may prove sufficiently accurate to obviate the need for amniocentesis; it too will require further evaluation by other investigators before it can be used routinely in clinical practice.

Ultrasound at present is best used in one of the following ways: (1) in nondiabetic patients who present early in pregnancy, sonographic documentation of the fetal age allows elective delivery after 38 menstrual weeks with virtually no risk of RDS, and (2) in patients who present late in pregnancy with no validation of menstrual dates, ultrasound can be used to guide amniocentesis for determination of lung maturity by the fetal lung profile. In the future, however, some composite scoring system, such as that reported by Salman and Quetel,[41] will allow the prediction of functional maturity of the fetal lungs by prenatal sonography.

References

1. Benson DM, Waldroup LD, Kurtz AB, et al: Ultrasonic tissue characterization of fetal lung, liver, and placenta for the purpose of assessing fetal maturity. J Ultrasound Med 2:489, 1983.

2. Bree RL: Sonographic identification of fetal vernix in amniotic fluid. JCU 6:269, 1978.

3. Birnholz JC, Farrell EE: Fetal lung development: Compressibility as a measure of maturity. Radiology 157:495, 1985.

4. Carson PL, Meyer CR, Bowerman RA: Prediction of fetal lung maturity with ultrasound. Radiology 155:533, 1985.

5. Cayea PD, Grant DC, Doublet PM, et al: Prediction of fetal lung maturity: Inaccuracy of study using conventional ultrasound instruments. Radiology 155:473, 1985.

6. Chinn DH, Bolding DB, Callen PW, et al: Ultrasonographic identification of fetal lower extremity epiphyseal ossification centers. Radiology 147:815, 1983.

7. Clair MR, Rosenberg ET, Tempkin D, et al: Placental grading in the complicated or high risk pregnancy. J Ultrasound Med 2:297, 1983.

8. Collaborative Group on Antenatal Steroid Therapy: Effect of antenatal dexamethasone administration on the prevention of respiratory distress syndrome. Am J Obstet Gynecol 141:276, 1981.

9. Destro F, Calcagnile F, Ceccarello P: Placental grade and pulmonary maturity in premature fetuses. JCU 13:637, 1985.

10. Donald IR, Freeman RK, Goebelsmann U, et al: Clinical experience with the amniotic fluid lecithin-sphingomyelin ratio. I. Antenatal prediction of pulmonary maturity. Am J Obstet Gynecol 115:547, 1973.

11. Fried AM, Loh FK, Umer MA, et al: Echogenicity of fetal lung: Relation to fetal age maturity. AJR 145:591, 1985.

12. Frigoletto FD, Davies PM II, Ryan KJ: Avoiding iatrogenic prematurity with elective repeat cesarean section without the routine use of amniocentesis. Am J Obstet Gynecol 137:521, 1980.

13. Gast MJ, Ott W: Failure of ultrasonic placental grading to predict severe respiratory distress in a neonate. Am J Obstet Gynecol 145:464, 1983.

14. Gentili P, Trasimeni A, Giorlandino C: Fetal ossification centers as predictors of gestational age in normal and abnormal pregnancies. J Ultrasound Med 3:193, 1984.

15. Gluck L, Kulovich MV, Borer RD, et al: Diagnosis of the respiratory distress syndrome by amniocentesis. Am J Obstet Gynecol 109:440, 1971.

16. Gluck L, Kulovich MV: Lecithin-spingomyelin ratios in amniotic fluid in normal and abnormal pregnancy. Am J Obstet Gynecol 115:539, 1973.

17. Golde SH, Petrucha R, Meade KW, et al: Fetal lung maturity: The adjunctive use of ultrasound. Am J Obstet Gynecol 142:445, 1982.

18. Golde SH, Tahilramaney MP, Platt LD: Use of ultrasound to predict fetal lung maturity in 247 consecutive elective cesarean deliveries. J Reprod Med 29:9, 1984.

19. Goldstein P, Gershenson D, Hobbins JC: Fetal biparietal diameter as a predictor of a mature lecithin/sphingomyelin ratio. Obstet Gynecol 48:667, 1976.

20. Grannum PAT, Berkowitz RL, Hobbins JC: The ultrasonic changes in the maturing placenta and their relation to fetal pulmonic maturity. Am J Obstet Gynecol 133:915, 1979.

21. Gross TL, Wolfson RN, Kuhnert PM, et al: Sonographically detected free floating particles in amniotic fluid predict a mature lecithin-sphingomyelin ratio. J Clin Ultrasound 13:405, 1985.

22. Hadlock FP, Irwin JF, Roecker E, et al: Ultrasound prediction of fetal lung maturity. Radiology 155:469, 1985.

23. Hadlock FP, Deter RL, Harrist RB, et al: Estimating fetal age: Computer-assisted analysis of multiple fetal growth parameters. Radiology 152:497, 1984.

24. Harman CR, Manning FA, Sterns E, et al: The correlation of ultrasonic placental grading and fetal pulmonary maturation in five hundred sixty-three pregnancies. Am J Obstet Gynecol 143:941, 1982.

25. Hayashi RH, Berry JL, Castillo S: Use of ultrasound biparietal diameter in timing of repeat cesarean section. Obstet Gynecol 57:325, 1981.

26. Hills D, Tuck S, Irwin GAL: The unreliability of placental gradings as an indicator of lung maturity in the pre-term fetus. In Society of Perinatal Obstetricians Annual Meeting, San Antonio, Texas, 1984.

27. Kazzi GM, Gross TL, Rosen MG, et al: The relationship of placental grade, fetal lung maturity, and neonatal outcome in normal and complicated pregnancies. Am J Obstet Gynecol 148:54, 1984.

28. Khaleghian R: Echogenic amniotic fluid in the second trimester: A new sign of fetal distress. JCU 11:498, 1983.

29. Kollitz J, Dattel BJ, Key TC, et al: Acute respiratory distress syndrome in an infant with Grade III placental changes. J Ultrasound Med 1:205, 1982.

30. Kulovich MV, Hallman MB, Gluck L: The lung profile. I. Normal pregnancy. Am J Obstet Gynecol 135:57, 1979.

31. MacKenna J, Hodson CA, Brame RG: Clinical utility of fetal lung maturity profile. Obstet Gynecol 57:493, 1981.

32. Mahony BS, Callen PW, Filly RA: The distal femoral epiphyseal ossification center in the assessment of third trimester age: Sonographic identification and measurement. Radiology 155:201, 1985.

33. Mahony BS, Bowie JD, Killiam AP, et al: Epiphyseal ossification centers in the assessment of fetal maturity: Sonographic correlation with the amniocentesis lung profile. Radiology 159:521, 1986.

34. Morris SE: Ultrasound: A predictor of fetal lung maturity. Med Ultrasound 8:1, 1984.

35. Newton ER, Cetrulo CL, Kosa DJ: Biparietal diam-

eter as a predictor of fetal lung maturity. J Reprod Med 28:480, 1983.

36. Paruekar SG: Ultrasonographic demonstration of floating particles in amniotic fluid. J Ultrasound Med 2:107, 1983.

37. Petrucha RA, Golde SH, Platt LD: The use of ultrasound in the prediction of fetal pulmonary maturity. Obstet Gynecol 144:931, 1982.

38. Petrucha RA, Golde ST, Platt LD: Real-time ultrasound of the placenta in assessment of fetal pulmonic maturity. Am J Obstet Gynecol 142:463, 1982.

39. Quinlan RW, Cruz AC, Buhi WC, et al: Changes in placental ultrasonic appearance. I. Incidence of grade III changes in the placenta in correlation to fetal pulmonary maturity. Am J Obstet Gynecol 144:468, 1982.

40. Ragozzino MW, Hill LM, Breckle R, et al: The relationship of placental grade by ultrasound to markers of fetal lung maturity. Radiology 148:805, 1983.

41. Salman F, Quetel T: Sonographic scoring of fetal pulmonic maturity. (Suppl.) J Ultrasound Med 5:145, 1985.

42. Spellacy WN, Gelman SR, Wood SD, et al: Comparison of fetal maturity evaluation with ultrasonic biparietal diameter and amniotic fluid lecithin-sphingomyelin ratio. Obstet Gynecol 51:109, 1978.

43. Strassner HT, Platt LD, Whittle M: Amniotic fluid phosphatidylglycerol and real-time ultrasonic cephalometry. Am J Obstet Gynecol 135:804, 1979.

44. Tabsh KM: Correlation of real-time ultrasonic placental grading with amniotic fluid lecithin/sphingomyelin ratio. Am J Obstet Gynecol 145:504, 1983.

45. Tabsh KM: Correlation of ultrasonic epiphyseal centers and the lecithin-sphingomyelin ratio. Obstet Gynecol 64:92, 1984.

46. Thieme GA, Banjavic RA, Johnson ML, et al: Sonographic identification of lung maturation in the fetal lamb. Invest Radiol 18:18, 1983.

47. Whittle MJ, Wilson AI, Whitefield CR, et al: Amniotic fluid phosphatidylglycerol and the lecithin/sphingomyelin ratio in the assessment of fetal lung maturity. Br J Obstet Gynaecol 89:727, 1982.

48. Williamson RA, Varner MW, Grant SS: Reduction in amniocentesis risk using a realtime needle guide procedure. Obstet Gynecol 65:751, 1985.

49. Zilianti M, Fernandez S: Correlation of ultrasonic images of fetal intestine with gestational age and fetal maturity. Obstet Gynecol 62:569, 1983.

ASSESSMENT OF FETAL WELL-BEING: THE BIOPHYSICAL PROFILE

Harbinder S. Brar, M.D.
Lawrence D. Platt, M.D.
Greggory R. DeVore, M.D.

Obstetric ultrasound scanning has been used to assess fetal growth parameters that change over relatively long periods of time and also to diagnose congenital malformations. Assessing fetal well-being on the basis of biophysical parameters, such as fetal breathing movements, movements, and tone, has been yet another application of real-time ultrasound. Before this, the development and perfection of specific and accurate diagnostic tests for the identification of the fetus at risk for in utero damage or death was a major challenge for the clinical researcher. With the advent of real-time ultrasound and the development of external fetal heart rate monitoring, fetal medicine has shifted away from reliance on nonspecific maternal clinical and biochemical markers of potential fetal disease, such as fundal height measurement and maternal weight, to more specific and direct examination of the fetus with ultrasound. It is likely that pulsed and continuous wave Doppler ultrasound of the fetus to assess flow velocities will also prove useful in the future.

ASSESSMENT OF FETAL CONDITION AND RISK

The improvement in management of high-risk pregnancies and in neonatal care over the last two decades, as well as the prevention of and early recognition of perinatal asphyxia to improve neonatal survival, have added impetus to the development of accurate and reliable diagnostic tests for better assessment of fetal well-being.

Historically, initial attempts to assess fetal well-being relied heavily on measurement of various biochemical markers in maternal serum or urine, such as placental alkaline phosphatase, human placental lactogen, and estriol. "Placental function tests," such as those that measure the metabolic clearance rate of dehydroepiandrosterone sulfate (MCR_{DHEAS}) and DHEAS loading, assess the "fetoplacental unit" and are therefore an indirect measure of fetal well-being. These tests fell into disrepute not only because of difficulty in measurement and interpretation

335

but more importantly because they have a low sensitivity and specificity.

With the introduction of the nonstress test (NST), the contraction stress test (CST) to monitor fetuses at risk, and the concomitant improvement in neonatal care, perinatal mortality has fallen dramatically to less than 12 per 1000 live births. The ratio of stillbirth to neonatal death has changed from 1:2 in 1970 to 2:1 in 1980.[1] Thus, prevention of stillbirth has become a major challenge in modern obstetrics. These tests (NST and CST) predict normal outcome reasonably well; however, they are much less accurate in the prediction of poor outcome as judged by Apgar scores, fetal distress, and similar indicators. Both these tests have a low false-negative rate (1 percent or less) and a high false-positive rate (50 to 75 percent).[2, 3] The use of the CST presents both practical and theoretic difficulties, inasmuch as it is lengthy and cumbersome and it also has failed to identify a dying fetus in certain instances.[4]

The antepartum stillbirth rate in an unscreened population runs about eight per 1000 and accounts for at least 65 percent of all perinatal morbidity. The causes of stillbirth include chronic intrauterine asphyxia, congenital anomalies, and acute complications, e.g., placental abruption and infection. Clearly, accurate methods for the detection of developing fetal asphyxia, if available, will reduce both fetal and neonatal loss.

Therefore:

1. The ideal antepartum test should be highly sensitive and specific, since low sensitivity can result in asphyxial fetal death (a false-negative result) and low specificity can result in inappropriate intervention for the normal fetus (a false-positive result), leading in turn to possible iatrogenic fetal, neonatal, or maternal morbidity and mortality.

2. The test should also be capable of identifying a fetus with major anomalies incompatible with extrauterine life, avoiding unnecessary surgical intervention, especially since a high incidence of abnormal fetal heart rate patterns is seen in infants with major anomalies. Conversely, a high incidence of anomalies (up to 30 percent) is seen in selected populations whose antepartum fetal heart rates test abnormal.[5]

It should be emphasized, nonetheless, that patients who are at high risk for fetal malformations or who have a maternal complication should have an ultrasound performed in the second trimester, and serial ultrasound examinations should be initiated where appropriate.

The advantage of high-resolution ultrasound imaging is the ability to "see" the fetus and monitor its activities and responses to a variety of stimuli, allowing for the application of the time-honored principle of physical examination, albeit indirectly, to the fetus. With this, the fetus is now regarded as a "true patient."[6] This concept enables the physician to intervene, when appropriate, in those patients with fetuses at risk (e.g., delivery of a preterm patient with oligohydramnios).[7]

Fetal Biophysical Activities

The number of biophysical activities that can be studied by real-time B-scan ultrasound are numerous. To date they include:

1. General biophysical activities such as gross body movements, breathing movements, and fetal tone.[8]

2. Specific activities such as sucking, swallowing, micturition, and reflex motions.[9]

3. Sleep states, recognized by monitoring motion of the fetal eye.[10]

4. Fetal heart rate.[2]

5. Flow in umbilical vessels.[11]

6. The intrauterine environment in which these activities occur, including amniotic fluid volume;[12] placental architecture, grade, and pathology;[13] and cord position.

7. Peristaltic patterns, purposeful movements, and evoked fetal reflexes, such as the startle response, evoked using an artificial larynx.[14]

The extent of biophysical activities that may be incorporated is not limited by technical ability but by the practicality of time constraints.

Factors Affecting Biophysical Activities

The sensitivity of specific central nervous system (CNS) areas to hypoxemia is unknown, but it has been speculated[29] that variation may exist. The biophysical activities that appear first in fetal development are said to be the last to disappear under the influence of progressive asphyxia, which, when severe enough, causes all biophysical activities to cease. For example, the hypothesized fetal tone center (cortex-subcortical area), which is the earliest to function (7.5 to 8.5 weeks), is the last function to disappear during progressively worsening asphyxia. The absence of fetal tone (FT 0) is indeed associated with the highest perinatal death rate (42.8 percent). On the other hand, the fetal heart rate reactivity center matures only at about 28 weeks and therefore should be more sensitive to asphyxia and should be the first biophysical activity affected (Table 15–1).

The effect on the biophysical profile will depend on the extent, duration, chronicity, and frequency of the insult. With sustained fetal asphyxia, the redistribution of blood to the fetus may lead to reduced or total cessation of perfusion to the lungs and kidneys, with decreased urine production and lung liquid flow, resulting in oligohydramnios.[15, 16]

The effects of fetal asphyxia on biophysical variables are of two kinds:

1. Acute effects: After an acute insult, the fetus shows diminished fetal breathing movements, tone, movement, and heart rate reactivity (NST).

2. Chronic effects: After acute repetitive or chronic asphyxia, the fetus usually shows oligohydramnios as the only finding.

Drugs that depress CNS activity, such as sedatives (barbiturates, diazepam), analgesics (morphine, meperidine), and anesthetics (halothane), usually reduce or abolish fetal biophysical activities,[8] whereas CNS stimulants and hyperglycemia often result in increased fetal biophysical activities. A knowledge of drug use is therefore essential for proper interpretation of results.

Table 15–1. FETAL CENTRAL NERVOUS SYSTEM CENTERS

FT	Cortex (subcortical area?)		↑
FM	Cortex—nuclei		
FBM	Ventral surface of 4th ventricle	Embryogenesis	Hypoxia
NST	Posterior hypothalamus, medulla	↓	

FT, fetal tone; FM, fetal movements; FBM, fetal breathing movements; NST, nonstress test.

From Vintzileos AM, Campbell WA, Ingardia CJ, Nochimson DJ: The fetal biophysical profile and its predictive value. Ob Gyn 62:271, 1983. *Reprinted with permission from* The American College of Obstetricians and Gynecologists.

Fetal biophysical activities are initiated by complex integrated fetal brain electrical activity[17] that varies, depending on the sleep-wake cycle of the fetus. The presence of normal biophysical activity indicates that the portion of the CNS that controls the activity is intact and functioning and therefore nonhypoxemic. The absence of a given activity, however, is much more difficult to interpret, as it may reflect either pathologic depression or normal periodicity of sleep-wake cycles. The periodicity has been shown to be short term (20 to 80 minutes) or long term, similar to circadian (diurnal) rhythms seen in extrauterine life.

Single Biophysical Variable Tests

I. NONSTRESS TEST. The combination of fetal heart rate acceleration and fetal body movements has been associated with a high probability of a favorable perinatal outcome.[2] Movement precedes the onset of most acceleration, indicating some kind of reflex feedback mediated through the neurophysiologic pathways initiating the acceleration.[18] The false-negative rate (uncorrected for lethal anomalies) is around 6.80 per 1000, and with abnormal test results, the perinatal death rate is 12 percent.[19] The major advantage of the NST is the ease of the testing. The major disadvantages of any single test (including the NST) are as follows:

1. The frequency of abnormal test results is relatively high (9 to 10 percent).[2]

2. The true positive predictive accuracy of an abnormal test result is low (12 to 13 percent),[19] although it may be improved by extending the duration of the test[20] (to allow for sleep cycles) or by combining it with other tests like fetal breathing movements (FBM)[21] or the CST.[22]

3. The false-negative rate is relatively high (four to six per 1000).[19]

The high false-positive rate due to fetal sleep cycles may be reduced by using the acoustic stimulation test to arouse the fetus.[23] In a prospective randomized clinical study comparing the NST with the fetal biophysical profile (FBP), the frequency of abnormal test results was significantly higher with the nonstress test, and the positive predictive accuracy was lower,[24] although the negative predictive accuracy did not vary.

II. FETAL MOVEMENT

SUBJECTIVE. Clinical studies suggesting an association between subjective (maternal) reports of decreased fetal movement and adverse outcome have been confirmed.[25]

OBJECTIVE. These movements can be monitored by real-time ultrasound, and they occur in episodes of 30 minutes (with ten to 16 discrete movements) in each 90 minute period and appear to be related to sleepwake cycles.[26] In a prospective blind study of 216 high-risk pregnancies,[27] a low five minute Apgar score, fetal distress in labor, and perinatal mortality all significantly increased in incidence in inactive fetuses as compared with active ones.

III. FETAL BREATHING MOVEMENTS.

The occurrence of rhythmic episodes of breathing movements in utero as part of human fetal development has been documented.[21] Such movements are episodic, with bursts of fetal breathing interspersed among periods of apnea. Boddy and Dawes[28] showed that fetuses that spent less than 50 percent of their time breathing had poor outcomes; however, these researchers did not use real-time ultrasound. In another prospective study,[29] the presence of fetal breathing movements before delivery was a strong predictor of a normal nonstressed fetus (90 percent), whereas only 50 percent of fetuses with absent breathing were asphyxiated or depressed at birth. These results are similar to those for the NST in the sense that when abnormal, they are poor predictors of outcome. However, predictive accuracy improved markedly when the two tests were combined.[27]

IV. FETAL TONE.

Hypotonia, characterized by limb deflexion, unclasped hands, and loss of fist formation, is a usual finding in asphyxiated newborns. Normal fetal tone is defined as active flexion-deflexion of the limbs. Manning and associates suggest this can be assessed equally well by opening and closing of the fetal hand.[27] Fetal tone is considered abnormal if there is no return to a position of complete flexion after movement or if the fetus is in a deflexed position (partial or complete) without movement. In the previously mentioned prospective blind study,[27] absent fetal tone was associated with a high incidence of fetal distress in labor, a low five minute Apgar score, and perinatal morbidity as compared with their incidence in fetuses having normal tone on the last

test before delivery. A better objective method of detecting tone is to evoke a fetal startle response with acoustic stimulation.

V. PLACENTAL GRADE. Although in itself placental grade is not a biophysical variable, it does assess the environment of the fetus. Vintzileos and coworkers suggested that it be included in the composite biophysical profile scoring.[30] In their study, patients with Grade III placentas had an increased incidence of intrapartum abnormal fetal heart rate patterns and abruptio placentae.

VI. AMNIOTIC FLUID VOLUME (AFV). Decreased AFV, defined as a pocket of fluid less than 1[31] or 2 cm[12] as seen by real-time ultrasound, has been shown to be associated with intrauterine growth retardation and increased perinatal morbidity and mortality.[31] Other conditions associated with oligohydramnios include dysmaturity syndromes, such as postmaturity, and major congenital fetal anomalies, mostly involving the genitourinary tract (e.g., renal agenesis).[31]

The four-quadrant assessment of fluid volume with ultrasound has been used to diagnose oligohydramnios. The sum of the total depth of amniotic fluid in four quadrants has been called the Amniotic Fluid Index (AFI). A score of 5 or less is associated with a higher incidence of meconium, fetal distress in labor, and a low five minute Apgar score.[32]

Composite Fetal Biophysical Variable Monitoring

Using a single variable, a normal test result is a much more powerful predictor of a normal fetal condition than an abnormal test result is of fetal compromise. Individual variables continue to have both false-negative test results (at a rate of four to six per 1000 for the NST)[19] and an unacceptably high number of false-positive results (30 to 70 percent), presumably as a result of sleepwake cycles.

Since an abnormal test result can be due to asphyxia or the sleep-wake cycle, it is necessary to develop a test that can differentiate these two scenarios. This diagnostic dilemma may be resolved by observing multiple biophysical profiles while extending the period of observation beyond a sleepwake cycle. This hypothesis was intriguing enough to have led to the development of a combined biophysical profile of the fetus.

There are two different kinds of scoring systems in the literature:

1. The first is the one described by Manning and colleagues[27] in which each variable is scored either normal (2) or abnormal (0), as described in Table 15–2.

2. The second is the one described by Vintzileos and associates[30] in which each variable receives a score of 0, 1, or 2, as shown in Table 15–3.

ANTEPARTUM CLINICAL STUDIES. Table 15–4 represents a review of all studies published; the details are as follows:

In an initial study of 216 patients[27] in which only the NST was used for management purposes, there was a higher correlation between an abnormal score and low five minute Apgar scores, fetal distress in labor, and high antepartum and perinatal death rates; the lower the score, the greater the correlation.

Combining individual parameters of the profile always resulted in improved positive predictive accuracy for both normal and abnormal test results. The maximal positive predictive accuracy for a normal test result was achieved when all variables were normal, and the maximal predictive accuracy for an abnormal test result was achieved when all variables were abnormal. The perinatal death rate, when all variables were normal (a combined score of 10), was 0 as compared with 400 per 1000 when all variables were abnormal (a score of 0).

In a follow-up study of 1184 consecutive referred high-risk pregnancies,[26] 5182 fetal biophysical profile score results were used in clinical management according to the protocol in Table 15–5. Although the protocol was used in the study, it is probably better to individualize management schemes, e.g., intervention in a patient with oligohydramnios would depend on the condition's cause and the duration of gestation. Performing a CST in these patients might be a reasonable option to obtain more information about the status of the fetus. Only one fetus suffered unpredictable and unpreventable death (a true false-negative rate of 0.8 per 1000). Six perinatal deaths occurred, resulting in a corrected perinatal mortality rate of 5.06 per 1000, lower than the rate expected in even a low-risk population. In addition, 13 fetuses with major congenital anomalies (eight of them lethal) were detected.

Baskett and associates[33] reported a similar prospective study on 2400 high-risk pregnancies. The perinatal death rates ranged

Table 15–2. BIOPHYSICAL PROFILE SCORING: TECHNIQUES AND INTERPRETATION

Biophysical *Variable*	Normal *(Score = 2)*	Abnormal *(Score = 0)*
Fetal breathing movements (FBM)	The presence of at least 30 sec of sustained FBM in 30 min of observation.	Less than 30 sec of FBM in 30 min.
Fetal movements	Three or more gross body movements in 30 min of observation. Simultaneous limb and trunk movements are counted as a single movement.	Two or less gross body movements in 30 min of observation.
Fetal tone	At least one episode of motion of a limb from a position of flexion to extension and a rapid return to flexion.	Fetus in a position of semi- or full-limb extension with no return to flexion with movement. Absence of fetal movement is counted as absent tone.
Fetal reactivity	The presence of two or more fetal heart rate accelerations of at least 15 bpm and lasting at least 15 sec and associated with fetal movement in 40 min.	No acceleration or less than two accelerations of the fetal heart rate in 40 min of observation.
Qualitative amniotic fluid volume	A pocket of amniotic fluid that measures at least 1 cm in two perpendicular planes.	Largest pocket of amniotic fluid measures <1 cm in two perpendicular planes.
Maximal score	10	—
Minimal score	—	0

From Manning FA, Morrison I, Lange IR: Fetal biophysical profile scoring: A prospective study of 1,184 high risk patients. Am J Obstet Gynecol 140:289, 1981.

Table 15–3. CRITERIA FOR SCORING BIOPHYSICAL VARIABLES

Nonstress test
  Score 2 (NST 2): 5 or more FHR accelerations of at least 15 bpm in amplitude and at least 15 sec duration associated with fetal movements in a 20 min period.
  Score 1 (NST 1): 2 to 4 accelerations of at least 15 bpm in amplitude and at least 15 sec duration associated with fetal movements in a 20 min period.
  Score 0 (NST 0): 1 or fewer accelerations in a 20 min period.
Fetal movements
  Score 2 (FM 2): At least 3 gross (trunk and limbs) episodes of fetal movements within 30 min. Simultaneous limb and trunk movements were counted as a single movement.
  Score 1 (FM 1): 1 or 2 fetal movements within 30 min.
  Score 0 (FM 0): Absence of fetal movements within 30 min.
Fetal breathing movements
  Score 2 (FBM 2): At least 1 episode of fetal breathing of at least 60 sec duration within a 30 min observation period.
  Score 1 (FBM 1): At least 1 episode of fetal breathing lasting 30 to 60 sec within 30 min.
  Score 0 (FMB 0): Absence of fetal breathing or breathing lasting less than 30 sec within 30 min.
Fetal tone
  Score 2 (FT 2): At least 1 episode of extension of extremities with return to position of flexion and also 1 episode of extension of spine with return to position of flexion.
  Score 1 (FT 1): At least 1 episode of extension of extremities with return to position of flexion or 1 episode of extension of spine with return to position of flexion.
  Score 0 (FT 0): Extremities in extension. Fetal movements not followed by return to flexion. Open hand.
Amniotic fluid volume
  Score 2 (AF 2): Fluid evident throughout the uterine cavity. A pocket that measures 2 cm or more in vertical diameter.
  Score 1 (AF 1): A pocket that measures less than 2 cm but more than 1 cm in vertical diameter.
  Score 0 (AF 0): Crowding of fetal small parts. Largest pocket less than 1 cm in vertical diameter.
Placental grading
  Score 2 (PL 2): Placental grading 0, I, or II.
  Score 1 (PL 1): Placenta posterior difficult to evaluate.
  Score 0 (PL 0): Placental grading III.

NST, nonstress test; FHR, fetal heart rate; bpm, beats per minute; FM, fetal movements; FBM, fetal breathing movements; FT, fetal tone; AF, amniotic fluid; PL, placental grading.
Maximal score 12; minimal score 0.
From Vintzileos AM, Campbell WA, Ingardia CJ, Nochimson DJ: The fetal biophysical profile and its predictive value. Ob Gyn 62:271, 1983. *Reprinted with permission from* The American College of Obstetricians and Gynecologists.

Table 15–4. CUMULATIVE RESULTS OF FETAL BIOPHYSICAL PROFILE FOR ANTEPARTUM FETAL ASSESSMENT

Study Population	No. of Patients	High Risk (%)	No. Tests Total	Normal	Equivocal	Abnormal	Crude PNM No.	Rate	Corrected PNM* No.	Rate	False-Negative Rate† No.	Rate
Manitoba general population 1979–1982	65,979	20%	—		—	—	943	14.1	586	8.81	—	—
Manitoba prospective study	12,620	100%	26,257	97.52%	1.72%	0.76%	93	7.37	24	1.90	8	0.643
Baskett et al	2400	100%	5618	97.1%	1.70%	1.2%	23	9.20	11	4.40	1	0.500
Platt et al‡	286	100%	1112	94%	3.5%	2.4%	4	14.00	2	7.00	2	7.400
Schifrin et al‡	158	"Most"	240	—	—	—	7	44.00	2	12.60	1	6.300
Vintzileos et al	150	100%	342	94.9%	2%	3.1%	5	33.30	4§	26.60	0	0
Total	15,614	>90%	33,569	>95%	2%	1%	132	8.40	43	2.70	12	0.770

*The perinatal mortality (PNM) rate is corrected to exclude death due to lethal anomaly or Rh disease.
†Stillbirth within one week of a normal test result.
‡Modified use of biophysical profile scoring.
§All neonatal deaths.
From Manning FA: Assessment of fetal condition and risk: Analysis of single and combined biophysical variable monitoring. Semin Perinatol 9:168, 1985.

Table 15–5. BIOPHYSICAL PROFILE SCORING: MANAGEMENT PROTOCOL

Score	Interpretation	Management
10	Normal infant, low risk for chronic asphyxia	Repeat testing at weekly intervals. Repeat twice weekly in diabetics and patients $\geq$ 42 wks gestation.
8	Normal infant, low risk for chronic asphyxia	Repeat testing at weekly intervals. Repeat testing twice weekly in diabetics and patients $\geq$ 42 wks. Oligohydramnios an indication for delivery.
6	Suspect chronic asphyxia	Repeat testing in 4–6 hr. Deliver if oligohydramnios present.
4	Suspect chronic asphyxia	If $\geq$ 36 wks and favorable then deliver. If < 36 wks and L/S < 2.0, repeat test in 24 hr. If repeat score $\leq$ 4, deliver.
0–2	Strong suspicion of chronic asphyxia	Extend testing time to 120 min. If persistent score $\leq$ 4, deliver, regardless of gestational age.

L/S, amniotic fluid lecithin/sphingomyelin ratio.

From Manning FA: Assessment of fetal condition and risk: Analysis of single and combined biophysical variable monitoring. Semin Perinatol 9:168, 1985.

from 0.3 per 1000 when the score was 10 (false-negative rate) to 292 per 1000 when the score was 0. The corrected perinatal morbidity rate was 2.8 per 1000.

The largest reported antenatal experience has been described by Manning and coworkers[16] in 12,620 referred high-risk pregnancies. A total of 26,257 tests were performed. Ninety-three perinatal deaths occurred (a gross perinatal mortality rate of 7.37 per 1000) of which only 24 occurred among structurally normal nonisoimmunized fetuses, and these were presumed to be asphyxial in origin (a corrected perinatal mortality rate of 1.9 per 1000). Eight structurally normal fetuses died within one week of a normal test result (a corrected false-negative rate of 0.634 per 1000), 97.52 percent of tests were normal, and only 0.75 percent were scored 4 or less. The same authors managed 307 consecutive post-term patients with twice weekly biophysical profile scores. Twice weekly scores accurately differentiated normal fetuses from those at risk for intrauterine hypoxia. When the profile score is normal, waiting for spontaneous labor results in healthy neonates and a much lower cesarean rate (15 versus 42 percent for "prophylactic" induction).[7]

Vintzileos and colleagues[30] reported their experience with 342 examinations of 150 high-risk pregnancies. There was a high correlation of an abnormal score with abnormal intrapartum fetal heart rate patterns, meconium during labor, fetal distress, and peri-

natal mortality, but predictive values increased when variables were combined. The results confirm the highly predictive value of a normal test result for a good neonatal outcome. In contrast, each abnormal variable was associated with a high false-positive rate. The absence of fetal movements was the best predictor of abnormal heart rate patterns in labor (80 percent); the nonreactive nonstress test was the best predictor of meconium (33.3 percent); decreased amniotic fluid volume was the best predictor of fetal distress (37.5 percent); and poor fetal tone was the best predictor of perinatal death.

Platt and coworkers,[34] in their study of 286 fetuses, reported a corrected perinatal mortality rate of 7.0 per 1000 compared with 22.6 per 1000 for all patients in their institution. Although they confirmed the predictive values of the abnormal score, they challenged whether the predictive value of the normal score exceeds that of the NST. In this regard, it is interesting that the combined studies of FBP scoring from other institutions have consistently yielded a false-negative rate of less than one per 1000, whereas cumulative studies of the NST alone yield a false-negative rate of four to six per 1000.[50] In another study, Platt and associates[35] randomized patients into two groups, one managed by the NST and one managed by the FBP; 279 patients were randomized into the FBP group and 361 into the NST group. There was no significant difference in the negative predictive value, the sensitivity, or the specificity of the two tests in attempting to identify overall abnormal outcome as measured by the presence of perinatal mortality, fetal distress in labor, low five minute Apgar score, or small for gestational age babies. The corrected perinatal mortality rate in the biophysical profile was five per 1000 compared with seven per 1000 in the nonstress test group. A statistically significant difference was found only between the FBP and the NST for a positive predictive value in determining whether a patient will have any abnormal outcome.

AN EARLY PREDICTOR OF FETAL INFECTION. Vintzileos and colleagues[36] serially assessed the modified FBP in 73 patients with ruptured membranes who were not in labor. A score of 8 or more was associated with an infection rate of 2.7 percent, whereas a score of 7 or less was associated with a rate of 93.7 percent.

They suggested that rupture of membranes by itself should not alter the biophysical activity of the healthy fetus. A low score ($\leq$ 7) was a good predictor of impending fetal infection, and the biophysical activities were altered in this group, in a manner similar to uteroplacental insufficiency. The first manifestations of impending fetal infection were a nonreactive NST and absent fetal breathing. Loss of fetal motion and poor fetal tone were late signs. The presence of fetal breathing had the highest specificity in predicting the absence of infection, with no cases of fetal infection when breathing was present 24 hours before delivery. The hypothesized mechanism by which fetal infection diminishes biophysical activities seems to be that increasing fetal oxygen demands cause local tissue hypoxia, thereby altering the CNS centers that control reflex biophysical activities.

In a follow-up study[37] by the same authors, a comparison between the daily FBP and amniocentesis in predicting infection was prospectively studied in 58 patients with preterm rupture of the membranes. The FBP had a sensitivity, specificity, and positive and negative predictive value of 80, 97.6, 92.3, and 93.2 percent, respectively, in predicting infection outcome as compared with 60, 81.3, 52.9, and 85.3 percent, respectively, for Gram stain obtained at the time of amniocentesis.

SCOPE. Fetal assessment based on the FBP method offers several potential advantages in clinical practice. The test can be performed by specially trained personnel in about 20 minutes, and its use appears to result in a substantial decrease in false-positive results and has false-negative results comparable with the oxytocin challenge test (OCT). It also provides other useful information about the fetal number and position, risk of intrauterine growth retardation (IUGR) and placental location and grading; the impact of this information cannot be measured but is likely to be beneficial. It may identify major congenital anomalies not detected earlier in pregnancy, possibly altering obstetric management. It must be emphasized, however, that early ultrasound in the high-risk fetus is preferable and in many cases indicated. It can be widely applied to most high-risk pregnancies, and the assurance of fetal well-being in pregnancies at risk has allowed for conservative therapy, preventing early intervention and the associated risk of failed induction, iatrogenic prematurity, and cesarean delivery. The test potentially helps monitor patients with prematurely ruptured membranes for impending infection, preventing neonatal and maternal sepsis.

The long-term developmental sequelae for fetuses with low scores is still unknown, and the authors are unaware of long-term studies. The different CNS centers responsible for the individual biophysical activities have varying degrees of sensitivity. The duration and frequency of hypoxemia and their effect on the fetus is as yet unknown.

Evaluation of the Fetus with Doppler Ultrasound

With the advent of Doppler ultrasound, it is now possible to assess the fetoplacental and uteroplacental circulation in a noninvasive fashion. Because of the large standard deviations in volume flow using Doppler ultrasound, investigators have recently turned their attention to analysis of aortic and peripheral arterial waveforms in an attempt to evaluate fetuses at risk for increased peripheral resistance, subsequent fetal hypoxia, and growth retardation. The principle underlying this application is twofold. First, the relationship between the systolic and diastolic peaks of waveform, as well as the

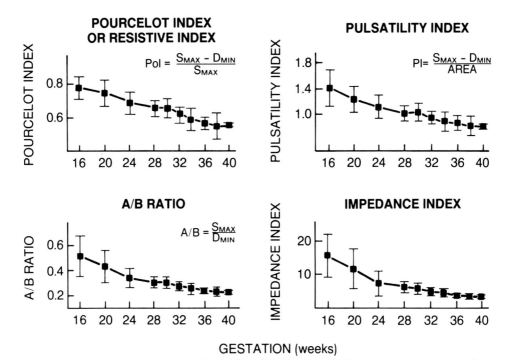

Figure 15–1. Doppler waveform analysis of the fetal umbilical artery. With advancing gestation and increasing compliance of the placenta, there is a progressive decrease in the S/D ratio, Pourcelot index (PoI), and pulsatility index (PI) of the umbilical artery that is the result of increased placental flow due to decreased resistance. (*Modified from* Erskine RLA, Ritchie JWK: Umbilical artery blood flow characteristics in normal and growth-retarded fetuses. Br J Obstet Gynaecol 92:605, 1985.)

$$\text{Systolic to Diastolic Ratio (S/D or A/B Ratio)* } = \frac{\text{Maximal Systolic Measurement}}{\text{Minimal Diastolic Measurement}}$$

$$\text{Pourcelot or Resistance Index (PoI) } = \frac{\text{Maximal Systolic Measurement } - \text{ Minimal Diastolic Measurement}}{\text{Maximal Systolic Measurement}}$$

$$\text{Pulsatility Index (PI) } = \frac{\text{Maximal Systolic Measurement } - \text{ Minimal Diastolic Measurement}}{\text{Area Under the Waveform Curve†}}$$

area under the curve, can be analyzed independent of the actual height of the Doppler frequency shift or the velocity waveform, both of which are dependent upon the angle of insonation. Second, angle-independent indices have been shown to reflect peripheral resistance.[38, 39]

Qualitative Assessment of Peripheral Resistance

In the peripheral vessels, as resistance increases, the diastolic flow progressively

*The above measurements are obtained from the waveform whether it is displayed in units of the Doppler frequency shift (Hz) or in velocity (cm/sec).

†The area under the waveform is obtained by integration and is equivalent to the temporal mean frequency shift or the temporal mean velocity.

decreases and, in more severe cases, is absent or shows reversal.

CLINICAL STUDIES. Laurin and coworkers studied 159 fetuses of which 74 had intrauterine growth retardation (IUGR). By classifying the waveforms qualitatively, they noted that, of the 27 cesarean sections done for fetal distress in the IUGR group, 25 (93 percent) had an abnormal waveform.[40]

Quantitative Assessment of Peripheral Resistance

The angle-independent methods for quantitation of peripheral resistance have been used by different investigators (Fig. 15–1).[38, 39] Although each of the above indices (S/D, PoI, and PI) increase as the diastolic flow is absent or reversed, only the PoI and PI maintain a numerical value, whereas the S/D becomes infinity.

Factors Affecting the Doppler Waveform

Once the qualitative and quantitative approaches of Doppler waveform analysis of the arterial system are understood, it is important to evaluate conditions, other than increased peripheral resistance, that could alter the waveform and lead to erroneous interpretation:

I. RESPIRATIONS. Fetal respirations affect the maximal systolic and diastolic values as well as the length of the cardiac cycle. Therefore, all waveform recordings for analysis require the fetus to be in a quiet nonrespiratory state.

II. HEART RATE

TACHYCARDIA. As a result of the rapid rate (greater than 180 beats/min), the waveform has an exaggerated diastolic component because there is not adequate "run-off" time.

BRADYCARDIA. This can result from heart block or premature atrial contractions with variable block. When either of the above occurs, the diastolic time is prolonged, and the maximal diastolic measurement is artifactually decreased.

III. BLOOD HEMATOCRIT. In Rh-sensitized pregnancies, there appears to be an increase in the fetal blood velocity with decreasing hematocrit.[41]

IV. BLOOD VISCOSITY. There appears to be an increase in the umbilical S/D ratio with an increase in whole blood viscosity at high shear, but not at low shear.[42, 43] Similarly, there is a significant negative correlation between umbilical venous blood flow and blood viscosity.[42]

Clinical Applications

INTRAUTERINE GROWTH RETARDATION

UMBILICAL ARTERY WAVEFORM. With advancing gestation and increasing compliance of the placenta, there is a progressive decrease in the S/D ratio, PoI, and PI of the umbilical artery that is the result of increased placental flow due to decreased resistance.[44–46] Giles and colleagues correlated placental microvascular anatomy with antenatal assessment of the S/D (A/B) ratio to validate the fact that the latter is an index of blood flow resistance.[47] They found that

the nodal small arterial vessel count in the tertiary stem villi of the placenta was significantly less (one to two arteries/field) in patients with high A/B ratios compared with patients with normal ratios (a count of seven to eight arteries/field). This suggested that the umbilical artery waveform identifies a specific microvascular lesion in the placenta characterized by obliteration of small muscular arteries in the tertiary stem villi. In a subsequent study by the same group of investigators, 32 of 43 (74 percent) patients delivering growth-retarded fetuses were found to have an increase in placental flow resistance as measured by the S/D ratio, with reduced, absent, or even reversed flow at end-diastole (Fig. 15–2).[48] Similar results identifying abnormal waveform in IUGR fetuses were also reported by Erskine and Ritchie and by Schulman and associates.[44, 49, 50] McCowan and coworkers performed umbilical artery Doppler studies on 15 singleton preterm growth-retarded pregnancies on the day of delivery and found abnormal PIs and S/D ratios in 14 of 15 patients (93 percent).[51] Additionally, a positive correlation was found between the degree of abnormality of the PI and S/D ratio and poor neonatal outcome.

Some studies[52] have pointed out that the PI in the umbilical artery may be raised several weeks or months before IUGR is clinically suspected. Although ultrasound measurements of the fetal upper abdomen have greatly improved the early detection of IUGR, whether PI changes in these vessels occur at a very early stage of placental insufficiency, and well before IUGR is clinically manifest, is as yet an untested hypothesis.

An elevated PI of the umbilical artery and a reduced PI ("brain-sparing effect") in the internal carotid artery are seen in patients with IUGR who do not have structural or chromosomal defects.[53] On the contrary, some recent evidence suggests that the "brain-sparing effect" might not occur in IUGR fetuses who have associated structural or chromosomal defects[54] but is a unique finding confined to asymmetric IUGR secondary to uteroplacental insufficiency and preferential shunting of blood to the brain.

Absent end-diastolic velocity in the umbilical artery represents the most extreme waveform abnormality and is associated with a high incidence of early delivery,

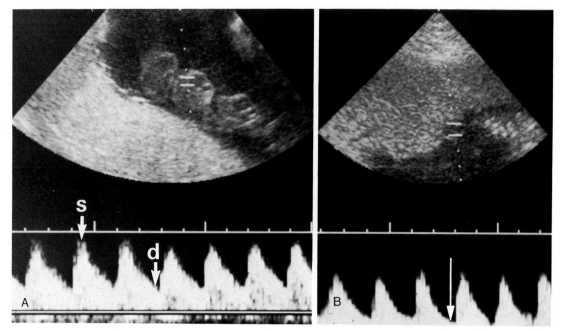

Figure 15–2. *A,* Qualitative Doppler evaluation of the umbilical artery from a normal fetus, demonstrating a normal systolic (s) to diastolic (d) relationship. *B,* Abnormal Doppler evaluation from a growth-retarded fetus, demonstrating little to no diastolic flow *(arrow).*

IUGR, oligohydramnios,[55] pregnancy-induced hypertension, cesarean section for fetal distress, neonatal intensive care unit admission, and low Apgar scores.[56] All these fetuses usually have evidence of acute or chronic hypoxia.[56]

UTERINE ARTERY. Schulman and associates[57] have shown the development of uterine (arcuate) artery compliance in pregnancy. With advancing gestation, there appears to be a fall in S/D ratios of the arcuate artery, with disappearance of diastolic notching in the second trimester. A uterine artery S/D ratio of more than 2.6 or the presence of a diastolic notch suggests increasing resistance in the uteroplacental circulation. Subsequently, the same group of investigators performed uterine and umbilical artery velocimetry on 71 women with hypertensive disorders of pregnancy that included chronic hypertension, preeclampsia, and superimposed preeclampsia.[58] Their results suggested that pregnancies with a uterine artery S/D ratio greater than 2.6 or with diastolic notching of the waveform were associated with a significantly higher complication rate as judged by stillbirth, premature birth, IUGR, and superimposed preeclampsia with positive and negative predictive values of 93 and 91 percent, re-

spectively. Cohen-Overbeek and coworkers,[59] in a similar study, found increased pulsatility and decreased diastolic velocity of the arcuate artery in proteinuric hypertensive pregnancies, and these changes preceded similar changes in fetal circulation by several weeks. This suggests arcuate artery changes precede umbilical artery changes and IUGR in the fetus.

Campbell and associates obtained the Pourcelot index[60] of the arcuate artery at 16 to 18 weeks using pulsed Doppler ultrasound to predict the development of pregnancy-induced hypertension, IUGR, and fetal asphyxia later in gestation. Thirty-one of the 126 high-risk pregnancies screened developed one or more of the above-mentioned complications, and the sensitivity, specificity, and positive and negative predictive values of this method were 68, 69, 42, and 87 percent, respectively. These results appear to be superior to existing techniques to predict IUGR in high-risk pregnancies. Trudinger and associates[61, 62] have shown similar results in their patient population with this method.

AORTA. Aortic velocity waveform in normal pregnancy was first described by Tonge and associates.[63] The same group of investigators then repeated the measurement of the pulsatility index in the thoracic aorta from a large series of IUGR infants and demonstrated it to be abnormal in 43 percent (42/74) of cases. Of the group with fetal distress and IUGR, the pulsatility index was abnormal in 67 percent (18/30).[40] One reason for the PI of the aorta being less specific for predicting IUGR is that it not only represents peripheral resistance of the umbilical artery but also of the vascular beds of the lower extremities and viscera. In another study, 29 of 82 consecutive IUGR fetuses with absent end-diastolic flow in the aorta had significantly greater severity of growth failure and a higher incidence of perinatal death, necrotizing enterocolitis, and hemorrhage compared with those with maintained end-diastolic flow.[64] In a recent study,[65] mean blood flow velocity in the fetal aorta was lower and the pulsatility index and rising slope were higher in pregnancies with IUGR compared with normal ones. Abnormal flow also correlated with adverse pregnancy outcome as judged by fetal distress, Apgar score, and umbilical cord pH. Characteristic changes in the fetal aortic blood velocity waveform with a decrease in diastolic blood velocity have also been found by multiple investigators, with a common conclusion that many such pregnancies show increased resistance in the placental vascular bed.[66–68] Even though the pulsatility index and velocity waveform of the descending aorta near term appears to have a large standard deviation secondary to the effect of the fetal behavioral state,[69] it holds promise as an adjunct to diagnosis and surveillance of pregnancies at risk for IUGR. In addition, there appears to be significant correlation between biochemical indicators of fetal compromise in IUGR fetuses and fetal aortic blood flow velocity. Soothill and colleagues[70] measured umbilical venous blood pO_2, pCO_2, pH, erythroblast count, and plasma lactate level in 29 fetuses with growth retardation. They found significant negative correlations between the severity of fetal hypoxia, hypercapnia, acidosis, and hyperlactacidemia and the mean velocity of blood in the fetal aorta measured by Doppler ultrasound. Jouppila and Kirkinen[71] also studied fetal blood velocity waveform of the descending thoracic aorta using duplex scanners in normal and hypertensive pregnancies. Hypertensive pregnancies complicated by IUGR had significantly higher resistance index, decreased mean velocity, and

end-diastolic velocity compared with controls and hypertensive pregnancies not complicated by IUGR, suggesting hemodynamic alterations in flow during developing hypoxia. Similar results were found by Tonge and coworkers[72] while comparing fetal aortic blood flow velocities in normal and growth-retarded fetuses.

CAROTID ARTERY. Wladimiroff and associates reported their experience from studying the cerebral blood flow in the fetus.[73] In 162 normal fetuses and 42 with IUGR, the pulsatility indices from the internal carotid artery and umbilical artery were obtained; in IUGR fetuses, the pulsatility index was increased in the umbilical artery and decreased in the internal carotid. This suggested a "brain-sparing effect." The sensitivities of the pulsatility index (greater than 2 SD from the mean) in the internal carotid artery ratio were 48, 60, and 70.[54] From their study, it would appear that the combination of the internal carotid and umbilical artery pulsatility indices was a better predictor of IUGR than either one alone.

Therefore, it appears that serial Doppler velocimetry of the aorta and the umbilical, uterine,[74] and carotid arteries reveals a relatively clear separation between normal and abnormal waveforms, a helpful adjunct in identifying pregnancies with IUGR and adverse pregnancy outcomes.

TWIN GESTATION

UMBILICAL ARTERY WAVEFORM. Farmakides and coworkers applied this principle to twin gestation to identify discordance.[75] In 43 pairs of twins studied, when the difference in the S/D ratio between fetuses averaged 0.4 or more, one could predict a weight difference of 349 gm or greater with a sensitivity and specificity of 73 and 82 percent, respectively. Two cases of twin-twin transfusion syndrome were also recognized by the simultaneous presence of high and low resistance values. In the study by Giles and associates, an S/D ratio difference of 1.57 or greater predicted a weight difference of 16.9 percent or greater.[76] In 33 of 65 twin pregnancies monitored using this method, one or both of the live-born fetuses were small for gestational age, and in 78 percent of these, at least one fetus had an elevated S/D ratio. Discordance in birth weight and the S/D ratio was associated with IUGR.

PLACENTA PREVIA

UMBILICAL ARTERY WAVEFORM. The authors have used the S/D ratio in the surveillance of pregnancies complicated with placenta previa.[77] Compared with controls, placenta previa patients with an elevated S/D ratio (> 3.0) were associated with a statistically higher incidence of adverse pregnancy outcome, with a sensitivity and specificity of 97.3 and 58.3 percent, respectively. The latter group included small for gestational age fetuses, meconium, and fetal distress in labor.

PREMATURE LABOR

UMBILICAL ARTERY WAVEFORM. There is growing evidence that the infant born prematurely is more likely to be small for gestational age than its counterpart of similar gestational age in utero. In a study that included 60 preterm labor patients, six of ten (60 percent) with elevated pretherapy umbilical S/D ratios failed tocolysis and delivered within 48 hours, compared with only eight (16 percent) of patients with normal ratios.[78] Therefore, elevated pretherapy S/D ratios may identify preterm labor patients with increased risk of failed therapy and preterm delivery.

OLIGOHYDRAMNIOS ASSOCIATED WITH POST-TERM PREGNANCIES

UMBILICAL ARTERY WAVEFORM. In the surveillance of pregnancies complicated with oligohydramnios, there also appears to be significant correlation of an elevated S/D ratio with an adverse pregnancy outcome as judged by meconium, fetal distress, and five minute Apgar (< 7 in the group where oligohydramnios is secondary to growth failure). However, no correlation was found in patients with oligohydramnios secondary to post-term or preterm rupture of the membranes.[79–81] Therefore, the value of Doppler velocimetry in post-term pregnancy appears to be of limited value.

DIABETES

UMBILICAL ARTERY WAVEFORM. Umbilical Doppler velocimetry has also been applied to diabetic pregnancies in which a significant positive correlation between the S/D ratio and serum glucose levels has been found. An elevated ratio was associated with an increased incidence of stillbirths, as well as neonatal morbidity.[82] Its clinical application, however, needs to be confirmed in larger studies.

ASSESSMENT OF FETAL WELL-BEING

UMBILICAL ARTERY WAVEFORM. Antepartum fetal surveillance using heart rate monitoring, although useful, can be misleading when normal or abnormal. The umbilical cord S/D ratio has been suggested as a means of assessing fetal well-being.[83] In a comparative study of the nonstress test (NST) and S/D ratios, the latter were found to be more selective in recognizing fetal compromise than the NST, with a sensitivity of 60 percent compared with 17 percent for the NST.[84] However, there was no difference in the specificity and the positive and negative predictive values of the two tests. In a subsequent randomized trial, patients undergoing surveillance with Doppler velocimetry were allowed to carry pregnancies longer and had lower incidences of fetal distress, cesarean section rates, and neonatal intensive care stays than control patients not undergoing surveillance. This suggests that availability of Doppler studies leads to better decision making during prenatal care.[85]

Comparison of Quantitative and Qualitative Methods

In their study, Giles and colleagues[86] estimated the fetal umbilical vein and aortic volume blood flow and compared it with umbilical artery flow velocity waveform analysis in 42 pregnancies. Umbilical artery S/D ratios were more sensitive, with a higher positive predictive value in the detection of IUGR fetus compared with that of volume flow, although the specificity was similar. Additionally, there was no difference when continuous wave was compared with pulsed Doppler ultrasound as a method of recording flow velocity waveforms.

In summary, it would appear, based on a cumulative experience of more than 15,000 patients from several centers, that the FBP scoring holds promise as an improved method of fetal risk detection. Antepartum detection, classification, determination of severity, and, ultimately, treatment of the fetus at risk for death and damage in utero form the very basis of modern perinatal medicine. It remains to be determined whether addition of further variables or refinement of existing variables will improve accuracy still further. The assessment of multiple biophysical variables and responses to intrinsic and extrinsic stimuli is most helpful in differentiating a normal sleeping fetus from an asphyxiated one.

References

1. Morrison I: Perinatal morbidity: Basic considerations. Semin Perinatol 9:155, 1985.
2. Phelan JP: The nonstress test: A review of 3,000 tests. Am J Obstet Gynecol 139:7, 1981.
3. Ray M, Freeman R, Pine S, et al: Clinical experiences with the oxytocin challenge test. Am J Obstet Gynecol 114:1, 1972.
4. Evertson LR, Gauthier RJ, Collea JV: Fetal demise following negative contraction stress tests. Obstet Gynecol 51:671, 1978.
5. Powell-Phillips WD, Towell ME: Abnormal fetal heart rate associated with congenital anomalies. Br J Obstet Gynaecol 87:270, 1980.
6. Manning FA: Assessment of fetal condition and risk: Analysis of single and combined biophysical variable monitoring. Semin Perinatol 9:168, 1985.
7. Johnson JM, Harman CR, Lange IR, Manning FA: Biophysical profile scoring in the management of the post term pregnancy. An analysis of 307 patients. Am J Obstet Gynecol 154:269, 1986.
8. Platt LD, Manning FA: Fetal breathing movements. An Update. Clin Perinatol 7:425, 1980.
9. Chamberlain PF, Manning FA, Morrison I, et al: Circadian rhythm in bladder volume in the term human fetus. Obstet Gynecol 674:657, 1984.
10. Martin CB Jr: On behavioral states in human fetus. J Reprod Med 26:425, 1981.
11. Campbell S, Griffin DR, Pearce JM, et al: New doppler technique for assessing utero placental blood flow. Lancet 1:675, 1983.
12. Chamberlain PFC, Manning FA, Morrison I, et al: Ultrasound evaluation of amniotic fluid volumes. I. The relationship of marginal and decreased amniotic fluid volumes to perinatal outcome. Am J Obstet Gynecol 150:245, 1984.
13. Grannum PAT, Berkowitz RL, Hobbins JC: The ultrasonic changes in the maturing placenta and their relationship to fetal pulmonic maturity. Am J Obstet Gynecol 133:915, 1979.
14. Divon MY, Plaatt LD, Cantrell CJ, et al: Evoked fetal startle response: A possible intrauterine neurological examination. Am J Obstet Gynecol 153:454, 1985.
15. Cohn HE, Sachs ET, Heyman MA, et al: Cardiovascular responses to hypoxemia and acidemia in fetal lambs. Am J Obstet Gynecol 120:817, 1974.
16. Manning FA, Morrison I, Lange IR, et al: Fetal assessment based on fetal biophysical profile scoring: Experience in 12,620 referred high risk pregnancies. I. Perinatal morbidity by frequency and etiology. Am J Obstet Gynecol 151:343, 1985.
17. Dawes GS, Fox HE, Leduc BM, et al: Respiratory movements and rapid eye movement sleep in the foetal lamb. J Physiol (London) 220:119, 1972.
18. Timor-Tritsch TE, Dierker LJ, Sador I, et al: Fetal movement associated with fetal heart rate acceleration and deceleration. Am J Obstet Gynecol 131:276, 1978.
19. Lavery JP: Non-stress fetal heart rate testing. Clin Obstet Gynecol 25:689, 1982.
20. Brown R, Patrick JE: The non-stress test: How long is enough? Am J Obstet Gynecol 141:645, 1981.
21. Manning FA, Platt LD, Sipos L, et al: Fetal breathing movements and the non-stress test in high risk pregnancies. Am J Obstet Gynecol 135:511, 1979.
22. Braly P, Freeman RK: The significance of fetal heart rate reactivity with a positive oxytocin challenge test. Obstet Gynecol 50:689, 1977.
23. Smith CV, Phelan JP, Paul RH: Fetal acoustic stimulation testing. III. The predictive value of a reactive test. (Abstract.) In Proceedings of the 6th Annual Meeting for the Society of Perinatal Obstetricians, San Antonio, Texas, 1986, p 54.
24. Manning FA, Lange IR, Morrison I, et al: Fetal biophysical profile score and the NST: A comparative trial. Obstet Gynecol 64:326, 1984.
25. Sadovsky E, Polishuk WZ: Fetal movements in utero. Obstet Gynecol 50:49, 1977.
26. Manning FA, Morrison I, Lange IR: Fetal biophysical profile scoring: A prospective study of 1,184 high risk patients. Am J Obstet Gynecol 140:289, 1981.
27. Manning FA, Platt LD, Sipos L: Antepartum fetal evaluation. Development of a fetal biophysical profile score. Am J Obstet Gynecol 136:787, 1980.
28. Boddy K, Dawes GS: Fetal breathing. Br Med Bull 31:1, 1975.
29. Platt LD, Manning FA, LeMay M: Fetal breathing movements: The relationship to fetal condition. Am J Obstet Gynecol 132:542, 1978.
30. Vintzileos AM, Campbell WA, Ingardia CJ, Nochimson DJ: The fetal biophysical profile and its predictive value. Obstet Gynecol 62:271, 1983.
31. Manning FA, Hill LM, Platt LD: Qualitative amniotic fluid volume determination by ultrasound: Antepartum detection of intrauterine growth retardation. Am J Obstet Gynecol 139:254, 1981.
32. Phelan JP, Smith CV, Broussard P, Small M: Amniotic fluid volume assessment using the four quadrant technique in the pregnancy between 36 and 42 weeks gestation. J Reprod Med 32:540, 1987.
33. Baskett TG, Gray JH, Prewett SJ, et al: Antepartum fetal assessment using a fetal biophysical profile score. Am J Obstet Gynecol 148:630, 1984.
34. Platt LD, Eglington GS, Sipos L, et al: Further experience with the fetal biophysical profile score. Obstet Gynecol 61:480, 1983.
35. Platt LD, Walla CA, Paul RH, et al: A prospective trial of fetal biophysical profile versus the nonstress test in the management of high-risk pregnancies. Am J Obstet Gynecol 153:624, 1985.
36. Vintzileos AM, Campbell WA, Nochimson DJ, et al: The fetal biophysical profile in patients with premature rupture of membranes—An early predictor of fetal infection. Am J Obstet Gynecol 152:510, 1985.
37. Vintzileos AM, Campbell WA, Nochimson DJ, et al: Fetal biophysical profile vs. amniocentesis in predicting infection in preterm premature rupture of the membrane. Obstet Gynecol 68:488, 1986.
38. Zwiebel WJ (ed): Introduction to Vascular Ultrasonography, 2nd Ed. New York, Grune & Stratton, 1986.
39. Hatle L, Angelsen B (eds): Doppler Ultrasound in Cardiology: Physical Principles and Clinical Applications, 2nd Ed. Philadelphia, Lea & Febiger, 1985.
40. Laurin J, Lingman G, Marsal K, Persson P: Fetal blood flow in pregnancies complicated by intrauterine growth retardation. Obstet Gynecol 69:895, 1987.
41. Rightmire DA, Nicolaides KH, Rodeck CH, et al: Fetal blood velocities in Rh isoimmunization. Re-

lationship to gestational age and to fetal hematocrit. Obstet Gynecol 68:233, 1986.

42. Giles WB, Trudinger BJ: Umbilical cord whole blood viscosity and the umbilical artery flow velocity time waveforms: A correlation. Br J Obstet Gynaecol 93:466, 1986.

43. Jouppila P, Kirkinen P, Purikka R: Correlation between umbilical vein blood flow and umbilical blood viscosity in normal and complicated pregnancies. Arch Gynecol 237:191, 1986.

44. Schulman H, Fleischer A, Stern W, et al: Umbilical velocity wave ratios in human pregnancy. Am J Obstet Gynecol 146:985, 1984.

45. Fitzgerald DE, Stuart B, Drumm JE, Duignan NM: The assessment of the feto-placental circulation with continuous wave Doppler ultrasound. Ultrasound Med Biol 10:371, 1984.

46. McCallum WD, Williams CS, Napel S, et al: Fetal blood velocity waveforms. Am J Obstet Gynecol 132:425, 1978.

47. Giles WB, Trudinger BJ, Baird PJ: Fetal umbilical artery flow velocity waveforms and placental resistance: Pathological correlation. Br J Obstet Gynaecol 92:31, 1985.

48. Trudinger BJ, Giles WB, Cook CM, et al: Fetal umbilical artery flow velocity waveforms and placental resistance: Clinical significance. Br J Obstet Gynaecol 92:23, 1985.

49. Erskine RLA, Ritchie JWK: Umbilical artery blood flow characteristics in normal and growth-retarded fetuses. Br J Obstet Gynaecol 92:605, 1985.

50. Fleischer A, Schulman H, Farmakides G, et al: Umbilical artery velocity waveforms and intrauterine growth retardation. Am J Obstet Gynecol 151:502, 1985.

51. McCowan LM, Erskine LA, Ritchie K: Umbilical artery Doppler blood flow studies in the preterm, small for gestational age fetus. Am J Obstet Gynecol 156:L655, 1987.

52. Reuwer PJHM, Bruinse HW, Stoutenbeek PH, et al: Doppler assessment of the fetoplacental circulation in normal and growth retarded fetuses. Eur J Obstet Gynaecol Reprod Biol 18:199, 1984.

53. Trudinger BJ, Cook CM: Umbilical and uterine artery flow velocity waveforms in pregnancy associated with major fetal abnormality. Br J Obstet Gynaecol 92:666, 1985.

54. Wladimiroff JW, Wijngaard JAGW, Degani S, et al: Cerebral and umbilical arterial blood flow velocity waveforms in normal and growth-retarded pregnancies. Obstet Gynecol 69:705, 1987.

55. Rochelson BL, Schulman H, Fleischer A, et al: The clinical significance of Doppler umbilical artery velocimetry in the small for gestational age fetus. Am J Obstet Gynecol 156:1223, 1987.

56. Rochelson BL, Schulman H, Farmakides G, et al: The significance of absent end diastolic velocity in umbilical artery velocity waveforms. Am J Obstet Gynecol 156:1213, 1987.

57. Schulman H, Fleischer A, Farmakides G, et al: Development of uterine artery compliance in pregnancy as detected by Doppler ultrasound. Am J Obstet Gynecol 155:1031, 1986.

58. Fleischer A, Schulman H, Farmakides G, et al: Uterine artery Doppler velocimetry in pregnant women with hypertension. Am J Obstet Gynecol 154:806, 1986.

59. Cohen-Overbeek T, Pearce JM, Campbell S: The antenatal assessment of uteroplacental and fetoplacental blood flow using Doppler ultrasound. Ultrasound Biol 11:329, 1985.

60. Campbell S, Pearce MF, Hackett G, et al: Qualitative assessment of uteroplacental blood flow: Early screening test for high-risk pregnancies. Obstet Gynecol 68:649, 1986.

61. Trudinger BJ, Giles WB, Cook C: Uteroplacental blood flow velocity time waveforms in normal and complicated pregnancy. Br J Obstet Gynaecol 92:39, 1985.

62. Trudinger BJ, Giles WB, Cook CM: Flow velocity waveforms in the maternal uteroplacental and fetal umbilical placental circulations. Am J Obstet Gynecol 152:155, 1985.

63. Tonge HM, Struyk PC, Custers P, et al: Vascular dynamics in the descending aorta of the human fetus in normal late pregnancy. Early Hum Dev 9:21, 1983.

64. Hackett GA, Campbell S, Gamsu H, et al: Doppler studies in the growth retarded fetus and prediction of neonatal enterocolitis, haemorrhage and neonatal morbidity. Br Med J 294:13, 1987.

65. Laurin J, Lingman G, Marsel K, et al: Fetal blood flow in pregnancies complicated by intrauterine growth retardation. Obstet Gynecol 69:895, 1987.

66. Lingman G, Laurin J, Marsal K: Circulatory changes in fetuses with imminent asphyxia. Biol Neonate 45:66, 1986.

67. Griffin D, Bilardo K, Masini L, et al: Doppler waveforms in the descending thoracic aorta of the human fetus in hypoxia. Br J Obstet Gynaecol 91:997, 1984.

68. Jouppila P, Kirkinen P: Increased vascular resistance in the descending aorta of the human fetus in hypoxia. Br J Obstet Gynaecol 91:853, 1984.

69. Van Eyck J, Wladimiroff JW, Noordam MJ, et al: The blood flow velocity waveform in the fetal descending aorta, its relationship to fetal behavioral states in normal pregnancy at 37–38 weeks. Early Hum Dev 12:137, 1985.

70. Soothill PW, Nicolaides KH, Bilardo CM, et al: Relation of fetal hypoxia in growth retardation to mean blood velocity in the fetal aorta. Lancet 2:1118, 1986.

71. Jouppila P, Kirkinen P: Blood velocity waveforms of the fetal aorta in normal and hypertensive pregnancies. Obstet Gynecol 67:856, 1986.

72. Tonge AM, Wladimiroff JW, Noodam MJ, et al: Blood flow velocity waveforms in descending fetal aorta: Comparison between normal and growth retarded pregnancies. Obstet Gynecol 67:851, 1986.

73. Wladimiroff JW, Tonge HM, Stewart PA: Doppler ultrasound assessment of cerebral blood flow in the human fetus. Br J Obstet Gynaecol 93:471, 1986.

74. Schulman H: The clinical implication of Doppler ultrasound analysis of the uterine and umbilical arteries. Am J Obstet Gynecol 156:889, 1987.

75. Farmakides G, Schulman H, Saldana LR, et al: Surveillance of twin pregnancy with umbilical arterial velocimetry. Am J Obstet Gynecol 153:789, 1985.

76. Giles WB, Trudinger BJ, Cook CM: Fetal umbilical artery flow velocity-time waveforms in twin pregnancies. Br J Obstet Gynaecol 92:490, 1985.

77. Brar HS, Platt LD, DeVore GR, et al: Surveillance

of pregnancies complicated by placenta previa using fetal umbilical velocimetry. Abstract presented at the 7th Annual Meeting of the Society of Perinatal Obstetricians, Lake Buena Vista, Florida, February 5–7, 1987.

78. Brar HS, Platt LD, DeVore GR, et al: Effect of tocolytics on uterine and umbilical vascular resistance using continuous wave Doppler ultrasound in patients with preterm labor. Abstract presented at the 34th Annual Meeting of the Society of Gynecologic Investigation, Atlanta, Georgia, March 18–21, 1987.

79. Brar HS, Platt LD, DeVore GR, et al: Placental vascular resistance using umbilical artery velocimetry in patients with oligohydramnios—An adjunct to antepartum fetal surveillance. Abstract presented at the 34th Annual Meeting of the Society of Gynecologic Investigation, Atlanta, Georgia, March 18–21, 1987.

80. Horenstein JH, Brar HS, Platt LD, et al: Cardiovascular evaluation of the post term fetus. Abstract presented at the 34th Annual Meeting of the Society for Gynecologic Investigation, Atlanta, Georgia, March 18–21, 1987.

81. Rightmire DA, Campbell S: Fetal and maternal Doppler blood flow parameters in postterm pregnancies. Obstet Gynecol 69:891, 1987.

82. Bracero L, Schulman H, Fleischer A, et al: Umbilical artery velocimetry in diabetes and pregnancy. Obstet Gynecol 68:654, 1986.

83. Friedman DM, Rutkowski M, Snyder JR, et al: Doppler blood velocity waveforms in the umbilical artery as an indicator of fetal well being. JCU 13:161, 1985.

84. Trudinger BJ, Cook CM, Jones L, et al: A comparison of fetal heart rate monitoring and umbilical artery waveforms in the recognition of fetal compromise. Br J Obstet Gynaecol 93:171, 1986.

85. Trudinger BJ, Cook CM, Giles WB, et al: Umbilical artery flow velocity waveforms in high risk pregnancy. Randomized, controlled trial. Lancet 1:188, 1987.

86. Giles WB, Lingman G, Marsal K, Trudinger BJ: Fetal volume blood flow and umbilical artery flow velocity waveforms analysis: A comparison. Br J Obstet Gynaecol 93:461, 1986.

16

THE ROLE OF COMPUTED TOMOGRAPHY AND MAGNETIC RESONANCE IMAGING IN OBSTETRICS

Shirley M. McCarthy, M.D., Ph.D.

The field of medicine has witnessed major technologic advances during the past decade in the area of diagnosis. Certainly, a major contribution has been the development of the computed tomographic (CT) and magnetic resonance imaging (MRI) scanner. Although this diagnostic equipment has mostly been used with nonobstetric patients, a number of obstetric applications have recently become apparent.

This chapter will focus on the diagnostic dilemmas in obstetrics for which this technology is presently useful, as well as future areas of investigation. In the case of CT, the major applications are in performing pelvimetry and, on occasion, helping to resolve the anatomy in cases of fetal malformations. The uses of MRI are in the assessment of the cervix, uterus, placenta, and adnexa when questions arise after diagnostic ultrasonography, as well as in the investigation of intrauterine growth retardation (IUGR) and in certain fetal anomalies.

PELVIMETRY

Although the value of pelvimetry in obstetric care continues to be debated, some obstetricians find it useful to judge safe passage of the fetus through the birth canal. The advances in ultrasound over the years have resulted in a dramatic decrease in the use of pelvimetry; however, a few current indications still exist: breech presentation, suspected face or brow presentation, suspected inadequate or deformed pelvis, unusually large fetus, and abnormal progress of labor.[1] Breech presentation is the most common reason why pelvimetry is requested.[6, 43] Although the clinician can in most cases judge pelvic adequacy, pelvimetry is the most accurate method of determining the dimensions of the bony pelvis.

Pelvic Anatomy

Anatomically, the pelvis is divided into the true and false pelvis. The linea terminalis (iliopectineal line) demarcates the false pelvis above from the true pelvis below. It is the true pelvis that is of prime obstetric concern (Fig. 16–1). Its superior boundaries, the pelvic inlet, are the sacral promontory and alae, the upper margins of the pubis, and the linea terminalis. Its inferior boundary, the pelvic outlet, is formed by the sacral

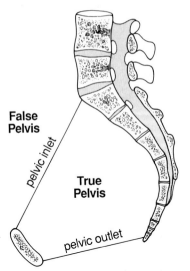

Figure 16–1. Midline sagittal section of the bony pelvis. The true pelvis is bordered superiorly by the pelvic inlet and inferiorly by the outlet. The false pelvis lies above the plane of the inlet.

tip, the ischial tuberosities, the pubic arch, and the sacrosciatic ligaments. The lateral boundaries, formed by the ischial bones, contain the anatomically important ischial spines. A line drawn between them represents the shortest diameter of the pelvis.

The distances (referred to as diameters) between certain anatomic locations within the true pelvis are used to assess pelvic adequacy. Important diameters obtained with radiographic pelvimetry include the anteroposterior (AP) pelvic inlet, the transverse pelvic inlet, and the bispinous diameter or transverse diameter of the midpelvis.[2, 25, 29]

There are actually three common AP measurements of the inlet. The *anatomic conjugate* is the distance between the sacral promontory and the superior surface of the pubic symphysis, whereas the *obstetric conjugate* is measured to the posterosuperior margin of the pubic symphysis (normal ≥ 10 cm). The latter dimension is the most important AP diameter of the inlet. The *diagonal conjugate*, which extends from the sacral promontory to the subpubic angle (normal ≥ 11.5 cm), is usually obtained manually to estimate the obstetric conjugate.

The transverse pelvic inlet is the maximum distance between the linea terminalis on each side (normal ≥ 11.5 cm). The bispinous diameter represents the distance spanning the ischial spines (normal ≥ 10.5

cm). This measurement lies in the plane of least pelvic dimensions, and it is here that most cases of arrest of delivery occur.

Measurements of the pelvic outlet are less critical and can also be approximated clinically. The AP diameter of the outlet is measured from the lower margin of the pubic symphysis to the tip of the sacrum. The transverse diameter of the outlet consists of the distance between the ischial tuberosities. The posterior sagittal diameter is measured from the tip of the sacrum to a right-angled intersection constructed with a line connecting the ischial tuberosities.

Conventional Radiographic Pelvimetry

Numerous methods of pelvimetry exist, but the four most common are the Thoms' perforated grid overlay, the Colcher-Sussman perforated rule modification of Weitzner, the orthometric method of Schwartz, and the triangulation method of Ball.[1] In general, anteroposterior and lateral radiographs of the pelvis are taken (Fig. 16–2). Numerical scales are radiographed with the patient in order to measure diameters directly on the film and thus correct for magnification.

Computed Tomographic Pelvimetry

The advent of CT has enabled development of a pelvimetric technique that offers many advantages over the conventional method.[9] It is simpler to perform and is more accurate. A standard set of radiographic factors are used, and images are stored electronically so that brightness and contrast can be manipulated after the study is finished. Since the measurements are obtained via computer, there is no need to correct for magnification nor to obtain manual time-consuming measurements directly from the radiograph. Most importantly, the radiation dose is less than that with conventional pelvimetry. The International Committee on Radiological Protection has recommended that the radiation dose to the fetus not exceed 1 rad.[30] X-ray pelvimetry is the most common single source of ionizing radiation exposure to the fetus. The Adrian committee

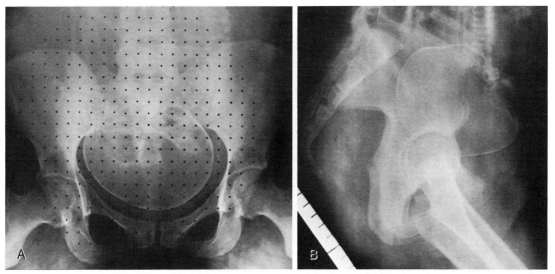

Figure 16–2. Conventional pelvimetry. *A,* Anteroposterior (AP) radiograph of the pelvis (Thomas' perforated grid overlay method), used to determine transverse pelvic dimensions. *B,* Lateral radiograph of the pelvis has a scale in the lower corner to obtain AP diameters.

in 1963 reported a mean fetal gonadal dose of 885 mrad.[24] Subsequent innovations such as rare earth screens, graphite cassettes, and high film speed have probably reduced the exposure. Nonetheless, the absorbed dose for the fetus and maternal gonads is only 20 mrad for each of the digital CT exposures, and the dose for the single axial CT section is 380 mrad.[9] The axial section, which is finely collimated, is taken caudal to the fetal and maternal gonads.

Computed tomographic pelvimetry can be performed in a matter of minutes. The patient's pelvis is centered in the gantry, whereupon AP and lateral digital radiographs (scout views) are obtained (Fig. 16–3). A single low-dose (approximately 40 mA) axial section is then obtained through the ischial spines. If they cannot be visualized, the fovea of the femoral heads are used instead, since they lie at the same level as the spines. At the console, using an electronic cursor, the radiographer can obtain any of the standard measurements directly from the images. Position of the fetus as well as degree of flexion or extension of the head is also ascertained.

In viewing the fetal skeleton during CT pelvimetry, care must be taken to avoid a potential pitfall.[4] Digital scanning beams can produce artifacts unlike those seen with conventional radiography. Motion typically causes blurring in the latter; however, with digital systems, each portion of the image is sequentially exposed so that anatomic borders can appear angled or wavy. Thus, an unusual appearance of the extremities is not necessarily abnormal.

Magnetic Resonance Imaging

Although the possible hazards of low-level diagnostic radiation remain unknown and quite controversial, measurement of the bony pelvis with a technique that entails no radiation is obviously most desirable. Some studies have indicated that ionizing radiation has carcinogenic potential and therefore should be avoided if possible.[2, 14, 23, 40] Magnetic resonance imaging is a new modality that entails no ionizing radiation. Images are created from the interaction of static magnetic fields, radio waves, and hydrogen nuclei. The energies involved are billions of times less than those necessary to generate an image with x-rays. There has been no evidence of any mutagenicity or adverse biologic effects associated with this new modality.[5, 7, 22, 31–33, 42, 44, 45] However, as this is a new technique, it is recommended that patients who undergo obstetric MRI are told that although there are no known hazards associated with this modality, there may be risks to the fetus in the future that are unforeseeable at this time.

Unlike CT — which measures one tissue property, electron density, to create a map

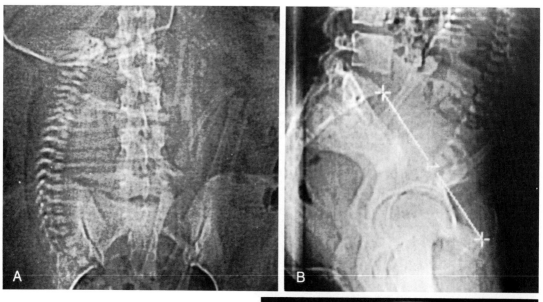

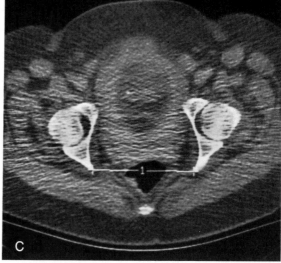

Figure 16–3. Computed tomography (CT) pelvimetry. *A*, AP scout view demonstrating the transverse pelvic inlet (1), measured with electronic cursors. *B*, Lateral scout view demonstrating the computer AP pelvic inlet (1). *C*, Axial section through the ischial spines shows the bispinous diameter (1).

of the body — MRI relies on four intrinsic tissue parameters: hydrogen density, its exponential time constants (T_1 and T_2), and bulk proton motion (flow). The range in tissue signal intensity permits contrast resolution that is far superior to any other technique. Combined with the ability to obtain multiplanar views, not only can the standard pelvimetric measurements be obtained, but also ample soft tissue information is available.[38] Cortical bone is a signal void or black (in contrast to marrow-containing bone) and thus serves as an easy landmark for electronic cursor measurements (Fig. 16–4). The relationship of the fetus to the placenta and internal os is also clearly demonstrated. Indeed, soft tissue dystocia,

which may be a cause of obstructed labor, may be better assessed in the future with MRI.

MATERNAL ANATOMY. The maternal deep pelvis is particularly well suited for MRI since the usual constraints with ultrasound, such as degree of bladder filling, bowel gas, and bone, are not impediments to its visualization.[19] A multiplanar global view of the pelvis can routinely be assessed. Furthermore, the superb contrast resolution of MRI enables visualization of discrete tissue layers within organs such as the uterus (Fig. 16–5).[16, 21] The internal os is clearly identified, enabling discrimination of cervix from corpus. The isthmus can be recognized as an area of lower signal intensity than myomet-

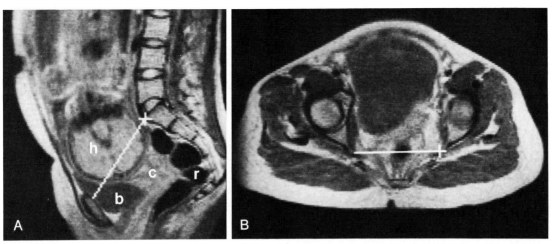

Figure 16–4. Magnetic resonance (MR) pelvimetry. *A,* Midline sagittal section through the maternal abdomen and pelvis, demonstrating the obstetric conjugate measurement. Note that the cortical bone is a signal void, whereas marrow-containing bone is bright. The fetal head (h) is juxtaposed to the cervix (c). The bladder (b) and rectum (r) are clearly seen. *B,* Axial section through the lower pelvis provides the bispinous diameter.

rium, owing to its higher fibrous content. The external os is separable from the vaginal fornices, canal, and walls. Within the cervix, mucus within the canal and epithelial glands has a different signal intensity than the surrounding fibrous tissue and presenting part (Fig. 16–6).

Since individual tissue layers can be recognized, the complex changes that the cervix undergoes during pregnancy can be seen. Early in pregnancy, the cervix is relatively elongated. The characteristic zonal architecture can be seen throughout pregnancy until labor (Fig. 16–6). Cervical ripening can be appreciated as shortening, dilatation, and loss of distinction of the fibrous stroma (Fig. 16–7). These visualized changes are probably due to stromal edema when inhibition of water occurs secondary to the increasing accumulation of extracellular noncollagenous protein.

Imaging of the cervix using MRI may in the future prove to be one of its most prom-

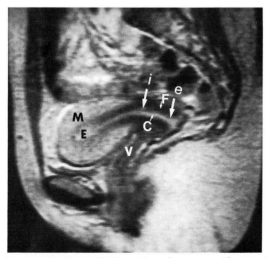

Figure 16–5. Sagittal MR section of a nongravid patient exhibits tissue layers within the uterus and vagina: endometrium (E), myometrium (M), endocervical canal (C), fibrous stroma (F), and vaginal canal and wall (V). The internal (i) and external (e) os are demarcated *(arrows).*

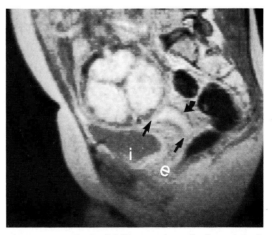

Figure 16–6. Sagittal MR scan through the pelvis, in late pregnancy. The fibrous stroma *(curved arrow),* endocervical canal, and internal (i) and external (e) os are well seen. The fetus is in cephalic presentation.

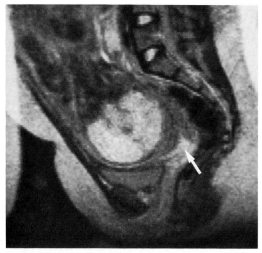

Figure 16–7. Sagittal MR section through the pelvis, demonstrating an effaced cervix *(arrow).* Note that the fibrous stroma is not discretely seen, and the cervix is shortened and dilated. *(From McCarthy SM, Stark DD, Filly RA, et al: Obstetrical magnetic resonance imaging: Maternal anatomy. Radiology 154:421, 1985.)*

ising obstetric uses. The present difficulties that ultrasound has in assessing the cervix — visualizing the true length unaffected by bladder filling, the internal cervical os unaffected by the fetal head, and the relationship of the internal cervical os to the placenta — are a few of the areas for which MRI appears to have superior imaging capability. In the future, MRI may be pivotal in assessing the cervix for the determination of incompetency and preterm labor.

The location of the placenta is well defined with MRI (Fig. 16–8). Its contrast resolution permits discrete separation of fetus, amniotic fluid, placenta, myometrium, and internal os.[10, 28, 36, 37] In a study of 25 women with placenta previa, MRI more accurately localized the placenta than ultrasound, particularly in cases of posterior placenta previa.[26] Both techniques determined position equally well; however, MRI was superior in determining the extent of previa. In two cases, the degree of previa was underestimated by ultrasound; in five of seven patients, the degree of previa was overestimated by ultrasound. In a subgroup of four women with marginal or partial placenta previa, sequential MR exams were obtained approximately eight weeks apart. Interestingly, the distance between the placental edge and internal os remained unchanged, not supporting the theory of "placental migration" due to differential myometrial growth.[26]

Placental pathology may be appreciated with MRI; however, insufficient data is available to ascertain whether or not MRI offers any advantage over ultrasound. Chorioangioma, retroplacental hematoma, and hydatidiform mole have been described.[27, 47, 48] In the last-named condition, one can appreciate, as with ultrasound, the typical cluster of grapes appearance and ovarian theca-lutein cysts (Fig. 16–9). Trophoblastic tissue can be distinguished from the normal myo-

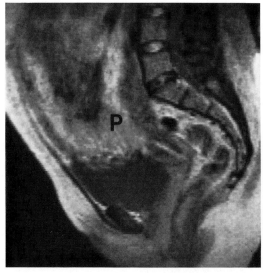

Figure 16–8. Sagittal MR scan through a patient with placenta previa. The placenta (P) occupies the anterior and posterior walls of the uterus and totally overlies the internal os *(arrow).*

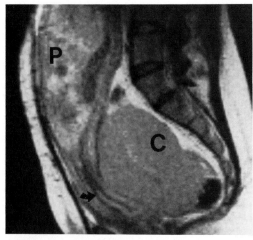

Figure 16–9. Sagittal MR scan of a 14 week gestation demonstrates a molar placenta (P) and displacement of the cervix *(arrow)* by a large theca lutein cyst (C).

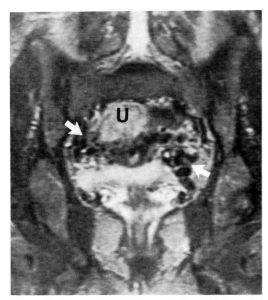

Figure 16–10. Coronal MR section through the pelvis of a patient with gestational trophoblastic neoplasia demonstrates obliteration of the normal uterine architecture (U) and numerous vessels within the adnexa and corpus *(arrows).*

metrium. Gestational trophoblastic neoplasia has been reported to have a characteristic appearance on MR scans.[12] The zonal architecture of the corpus is obliterated and numerous intra- and extrauterine vessels are seen (Fig. 16–10). The capability of directly visualizing the degree and extent of the vasculature is useful in deciding whether surgical management may be hazardous. Since vessels are readily identified without intravenous contrast, MRI allows appreciation of pathologic vasculature as well as the normal pelvic congestion that occurs in late pregnancy. The flattened cava, enlarged ovarian veins, and other pelvic collaterals are obvious.[19]

MATERNAL DISEASE. Although ultrasound is the standard screening technique for pelvic masses in the gravid patient, occasionally, certain limitations may result in an equivocal study. Obesity, overlying bowel gas or bone, poor bladder filling, and obscuration by the gravid uterus are the most common problems encountered. In such instances, MRI can be a useful adjunct because of the more global depiction of pelvic anatomy and the capability of tissue characterization. In the patient with myomatous disease, degenerated leiomyomas can be distinguished from nondegenerated ones, suggesting a cause for pelvic pain occurring

during pregnancy.[47] The number and location of leiomyomas, particularly their relationship to the fetus and birth canal, are also better documented with MRI. Hemorrhagic fluid collections can also be distinguished from simple fluid collections. In pregnant patients with medical or surgical disease who might ordinarily be exposed to ionizing radiation for diagnostic evaluation, MRI offers a relatively safe alternative (Fig. 16–11).[46]

FETAL ANATOMY. The limited MRI studies of the fetus that have been conducted demonstrate fetal anatomy to varying degrees. Fetal measurements such as biparietal diameter and crown-rump length are not as easily obtained as with ultrasound, since there is currently no real-time capability with MRI.[36, 37] Fetal soft tissue contrast is greater with MRI; however, fetal motion often prevents visualization of fine detail. As one might expect, fetal anatomy is better defined at later gestational ages. In one study containing a limited number of cases in the first trimester, only the head could be discerned.[49] In the second trimester, the head, heart, and liver could be identified. In 14 women in the last trimester, individual fetal organ systems could be identified in the majority of cases. In nine women examined

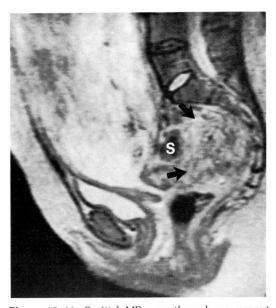

Figure 16–11. Sagittal MR scan through a pregnant patient with a suspected pelvic abscess demonstrates an inflammatory mass in the presacral space *(arrows)* that could not be visualized with sonography. The sigmoid colon (S) is displaced anteriorly.

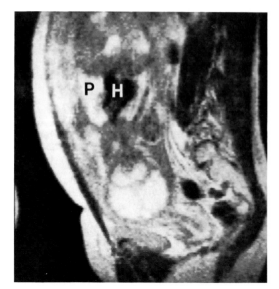

Figure 16–12. Sagittal MR section of a 36 week gestation demonstrates the fetus in a cephalic presentation and a coronal view of the heart (H) and lungs (P).

at 36 menstrual weeks, the fetal heart, lungs, liver, and brain were routinely depicted.[17] The heart was always identifiable owing to the characteristic signal void created by rapidly flowing blood (Fig. 16–12).[20] In some

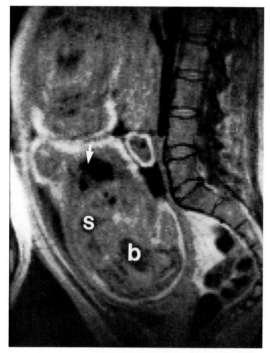

Figure 16–13. Sagittal MR scan of a 36 week gestation provides a coronal view of the fetus. The stomach (s) and bladder (b) contain fluid and are therefore obvious. Note that the left pulmonary artery can be identified (*arrow*).

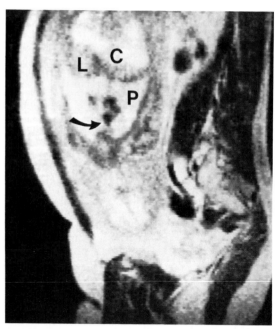

Figure 16–14. Sagittal MR scan of a 36 week fetus, demonstrating a coronal view of the liver (L), transverse colon (C), and lung (P). Mediastinal vascular structures are also seen (*arrow*).

cases, the individual cardiac chambers, pulmonary vessels, aorta, inferior vena cava, and portal and hepatic veins were demonstrated. The lungs were always well demarcated, presumably owing to the high signal intensity of fluid within alveoli. Similarly, other fluid-filled structures such as the stomach and the bladder were clearly seen (Fig. 16–13). The liver was easily recognized (Fig. 16–14), but rarely was the entire spine depicted (Fig. 16–15). Marrow-containing bone could be separated from cortical bone and

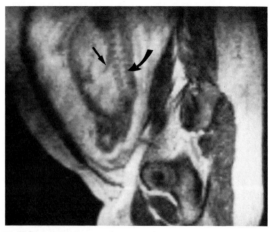

Figure 16–15. Sagittal MR scan of a 36 week fetus shows the fetal spine (*curved arrow*) and diaphragm (*straight arrow*).

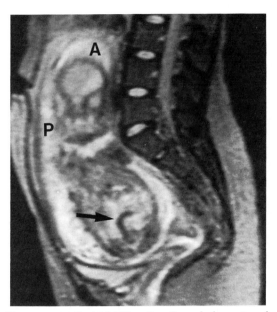

Figure 16–16. Sagittal MR section through the maternal abdomen and pelvis demonstrates the umbilical cord (*arrow*), amniotic fluid (A), and placenta (P).

surrounding muscles; however, extremity detail was particularly vulnerable to motion. The relative lack of myelination in utero could be appreciated; however, the occurrence and pattern of myelination has also been reported with MRI.[11, 13] Umbilical cord, placenta, and amniotic fluid were routinely visualized (Fig. 16–16).

Although fetal anatomy is demonstrable with MRI, the technique suffers from several disadvantages relative to ultrasound. The relatively long imaging times of MRI result in image degradation secondary to fetal motion. The real-time capability of ultrasound, combined with an unlimited number of transducer orientations, permits almost instantaneous investigation of fetal anatomy along any axis. With MRI, depiction of certain fetal structures, e.g., the spinal cord, is basically fortuitous, depending on fetal lie. Likewise, ultrasound has greater flexibility and is less costly. Thus, it is unlikely that MRI will replace ultrasound as the standard obstetric screening modality in the near future.

Magnetic resonance imaging may be a useful adjunct to sonography when the latter is equivocal in the identification of fetal dysmorphology.[18, 46] Sonographic evaluation is sometimes limited by a poorly positioned fetal head or oligohydramnios. The latter, with its associated decrease in fetal motion,

is actually an advantage for MRI. Central nervous system anomalies in particular may be a quite suitable application of MRI owing to the high natural contrast between brain tissue and cerebrospinal fluid (Fig. 16–17).[41]

It should be mentioned at this point that CT, while suffering from many of the same limitations as MRI, has been useful in the evaluation of some cases of fetal malformations. In the cases where sonography is indeterminate for renal agenesis, administration of intravenous iodinated contrast medium to the mother, followed by CT scans through the fetal abdomen, can prove useful in identifying the presence of functional kidneys via their contrast enhancement (Fig. 16–18).[35] Calvarial bony defects related to an encephalocoele are definable with CT.

Magnetic resonance imaging may prove particularly valuable in fetal diseases where sonographic accuracy is suboptimal, particularly in IUGR.[39] The diagnosis is usually suggested by ultrasound; however, sonographic misdiagnosis is common, with relatively high false-positive rates (30 to 65 percent).[8, 34] Serial measurements of fetal size as presently assessed with ultrasound may not be the most useful criteria in the diagnosis of IUGR, as size alone cannot distinguish the genetically small and normally nourished fetus from the malnourished one with IUGR. Since MRI is very sensitive and specific for fat, distribution and quantification of fetal fat may be used as a way of detecting IUGR (Fig. 16–19). Indeed, depletion of body fat occurs earlier than decreased body size in IUGR. In one study of fetuses aged 32 to 37 menstrual weeks, estimates of fetal fat stores correlated with neonatal outcome better than sonographic measurements of fetal growth parameters or actual birth weight.[39] Macrosomic fetuses of diabetic mothers could also be identified (Fig. 16–20). Further studies are necessary to define the exact role of MRI in IUGR.

In summary, the obstetric applications of MRI are relatively limited. Sonography readily satisfies the great majority of imaging indications in pregnancy. The ongoing rapid technical developments in MRI, however, will likely open new applications in the future. Much faster scanning times are enabling real-time imaging. MR spectroscopy, a metabolic rather than anatomic probe, offers promise in the study of fetal and maternal tissues at the subcellular level.

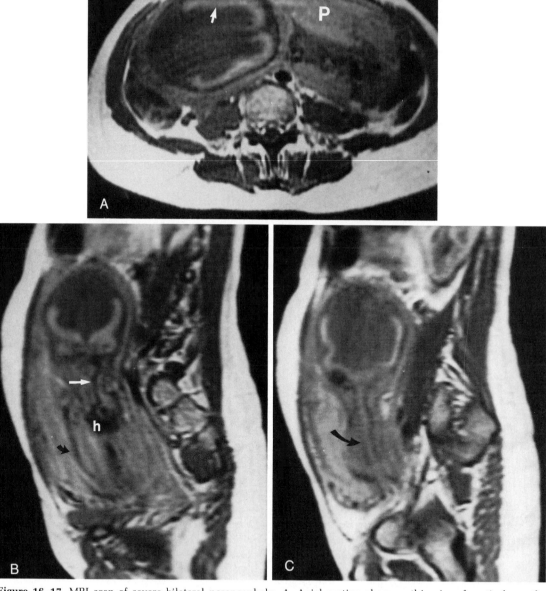

Figure 16–17. MRI scan of severe bilateral porencephaly. *A*, Axial section shows a thin rim of cortical mantle *(arrow)*. The placenta (P) is anterior. *B*, Coronal view of the fetal head again demonstrates abundant cerebrospinal fluid and little brain parenchyma. The carotid artery *(white arrow)*, heart (h), and umbilical cord *(black arrow)* are particularly well seen. *C*, A more posterior section demonstrates the entire spinal cord *(arrow)*. (Courtesy of Charles Carrasco, MD.)

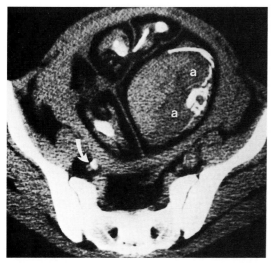

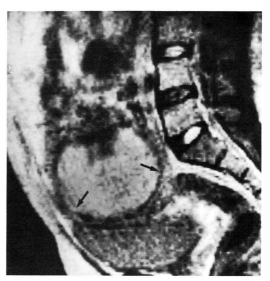

Figure 16–18. CT scan of the fetal abdomen shows soft tissue in the renal fossa (a) that proved to be adrenals at autopsy. The mother received intravenous contrast, and the maternal ureter *(arrow)* contains contrast; however, there are no enhancing structures in the fetal renal fossa to indicate that kidneys are present.

Figure 16–19. Sagittal MR scan through a fetus with intrauterine growth retardation (IUGR) demonstrates no fat around the fetal skull *(arrows)* or elsewhere.

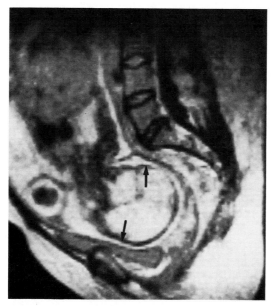

Figure 16–20. Sagittal MR scan through a macrosomic fetus exhibits abundant fat in the scalp *(arrows)* and remainder of the body. *(From Stark DD, McCarthy SM, Filly RA, et al: Evaluation of intrauterine growth retardation by magnetic resonance imaging. Radiology 155:425, 1985.)*

References

1. Bean WJ, Rodan BA: Pelvimetry revisited. Semin Roentgenol 3:164, 1982.
2. Benson RC: Handbook of Obstetrics and Gynecology, 8th Ed. Los Altos, Lange Med Publns, 1983, p. 379.
3. Bithell JR, Stewart AM: Prenatal irradiation and childhood malignancy: A review of British data from the Oxford Survey. Br J Cancer 31:271, 1975.
4. Brody AS, Saks BJ, Field DR, et al: Artifacts seen during CT pelvimetry: Implications for digital systems with scanning beams. Radiology 160:269, 1986.
5. Budinger RF: Nuclear magnetic resonance (NMR) in vivo studies: Known thresholds for health effects. J Comput Assist Tomogr 5:800, 1981.
6. Collea JV, Rabin SC, Weghorst GR, Quilligan EJ: The randomized management of term frank breech presentation: Vaginal delivery vs. cesarean section. Am J Obstet Gynecol 131:186, 1978.
7. Cooke P, Morris PG: The effects of NMR exposure on living organisms II. A genetic study of human lymphocytes. Br J Radiol 54:622, 1981.
8. Creasy RK, Resnick R: Intrauterine growth retardation. In Maternal-Fetal Medicine: Principles and Practice. Philadelphia, WB Saunders Co, 1984, pp. 491–510.
9. Federle MR, Cohen HA, Rosenwein MR, et al: Pelvimetry by digital radiography: A low-dose examination. Radiology 143:733, 1982.
10. Foster MA, Knight CH, Rimmington JE, Mallard JR: Fetal imaging by nuclear magnetic resonance: A study in goats. Radiology 149:193, 1983.
11. Holland B, Haas D, Norman D, et al: MRI of normal brain maturation. AJNR 7:201, 1986.
12. Hricak H, Demas BE, Braga CA, et al: Gestational trophoblastic neoplasm of the uterus: MR assessment. Radiology 161:11, 1986.
13. Johnson MA, Rennock JM, Bydder GM, et al: Clinical NMR imaging of the brain in children: Normal and neurologic disease. AJR 141:1005, 1983.
14. MacMahon B: Prenatal x-ray exposure and childhood cancer. JNCI 28:1173, 1982.
15. Mattison DR, Angtuaco T, Long C: Magnetic resonance imaging in obstetrics and gynecology. Contemp Ob/Gyn 29:48, 1987.
16. McCarthy S: Magnetic resonance imaging in obstetrics and gynecology. Magn Reson Imaging 4:59, 1986.
17. McCarthy SM, Filly RA, Stark DD, et al: Obstetrical magnetic resonance imaging: Fetal anatomy. Radiology 154:427, 1985.
18. McCarthy SM, Filly RA, Stark DD, et al: Magnetic resonance imaging of fetal anomalies in utero: Early experience. AJR 145:677, 1985.
19. McCarthy SM, Stark DD, Filly RA, et al: Obstetrical magnetic resonance imaging: Maternal anatomy. Radiology 154:421, 1985.
20. McCarthy S, Stark DD, Higgins CB: Demonstration of the fetal cardiovascular system by MR imaging. J Comput Assist Tomogr 8:1168, 1984.
21. McCarthy S, Tauber C, Gore J: Female pelvic anatomy: MR assessment of variations during the menstrual cycle and with use of oral contraceptives. Radiology 160:119, 1986.
22. McRobbie D, Foster MA: Pulsed magnetic field exposure during pregnancy and implications for NMR foetal imaging: A study with mice. Magn Reson Imaging 3:231, 1985.
23. Newcombe HB, McGregor JR: Childhood cancer following obstetric radiology. Letter to the editor. Lancet 2:1151, 1971.
24. Osborn SB: The implications of the reports of the Committee on Radiology Hazards to Patients (Adrian Committee). A symposium given at the Annual Congress of the British Institute of Radiology, April 27, 1962. I. Variations in the radiation dose received by the patient in diagnostic radiology. Br J Radiol 36:230, 1963.
25. Oxorn H: Human Labor and Birth, 5th Ed. Norwalk, Appleton-Century-Crofts 1986, pp 23–33.
26. Powell MC, Buckley J, Price H, et al: Magnetic resonance imaging and placenta previa. Am J Obstet Gynecol 154:565, 1986.
27. Powell MC, Buckley J, Worthington BS, Symonds EM: Magnetic resonance imaging and hydatidiform mole. Br J Radiol 59:561, 1986.
28. Powell MC, Worthington BS: MRI a new milestone in modern Ob care. Diagnostic Imaging April 1986, p 86.
29. Pritchard J, MacDonald P, Gent N: Williams Obstetrics, 17th Ed. Norwalk, Appleton-Century-Crofts 1985, pp 221–223.
30. Reekie D, Davison M, Davidson JK: The radiation hazard in radiography of the female abdomen and pelvis. Br J Radiol 40:849, 1967.
31. Reid A, Smith PW, Hutchinson MJS: Nuclear magnetic resonance imaging and its safety implications: Follow-up of 181 patients. Br J Radiol 55:784, 1982.
32. Revised guidance on acceptable limits of exposure during nuclear magnetic resonance imaging. Br J Radiol 56:974, 1983.
33. Schwartz JL, Cooks LE: NMR imaging produces no observable mutations or cytotoxicity in mammalian cells. AJR 139:583, 1982.
34. Sholl JS, Sabbagh RE: Ultrasound detection. In Lin CC, Evans MI (eds): Intrauterine Growth Retardation. New York, McGraw-Hill, 1984, pp 225–254.
35. Siegel HA, Seltzer SE, Miller S: Prenatal computed tomography: Are there indications? J Comput Assist Tomogr 8:871, 1984.
36. Smith FW, Adam AH, Phillips WDP: NMR imaging in pregnancy. (Letter.) Lancet 1:61, 1984.
37. Smith FW, MacLennan F, Abramovich DR, et al: NMR imaging in human pregnancy: A preliminary study. Magn Reson Imaging 2:57, 1984.
38. Stark DD, McCarthy SM, Filly RA, et al: Pelvimetry by magnetic resonance imaging. AJR 144:947, 1985.
39. Stark DD, McCarthy SM, Filly RA, et al: Evaluation of intrauterine growth retardation by magnetic resonance imaging. Radiology 155:425, 1985.
40. Stewart A, Kneale GW: Radiation dose effects in relation to obstetric x-rays and childhood cancers. Lancet 1:1185, 1970.
41. Thickman D, Mintz M, Mennuti M, Kressel HY: MR imaging of cerebral abnormalities in utero. J Comput Assist Tomogr 8:1058, 1984.
42. Thomas A, Morris PG: The effects of NMR exposure on living organisms. I. A microbial assay. Br J Radiol 54:615, 1981.
43. Varner MW, Cruikshank DP, Lanke DW: X-ray pelvimetry in clinical obstetrics. Obstet Gynecol 56:296, 1980.

44. Withers HR, Mason KA, Davis CA: MR effect on murine spermatogenesis. Radiology 156:741, 1985.
45. Wolff S, Crooks LE, Brown P, et al: Tests for DNA and chromosomal damage induced by nuclear magnetic resonance imaging. Radiology 136:707, 1980.
46. Weinreb JC, Brown C, Cohen JM, Erdman WA: Obstetrical MRI: Experience with 65 pregnant women. Soc Magn Reson Med, Montreal 4:1253, 1986.
47. Weinreb JC, Brown CE, Lowe TW, et al: Pelvic masses in pregnancy patients: MR and US imaging. Radiology 159:717, 1986.
48. Weinreb JC, Lowe TW, Santos-Ramos R, et al: Magnetic resonance imaging in obstetric diagnosis. Radiology 154:157, 1985.
49. Weinreb JC, Lowe T, Cohen JM, Kutler M: Human fetal anatomy: MR imaging. Radiology 157:715, 1985.

17

THE PRENATAL MANAGEMENT OF THE FETUS WITH A CORRECTABLE DEFECT

Michael R. Harrison, M.D.
N. Scott Adzick, M.D.
Alan W. Flake, M.D.

The diagnosis and treatment of human fetal defects have evolved rapidly over the last decade owing to improved fetal imaging techniques and better understanding of fetal pathophysiology derived from animal models.[21] Although some fetal malformations with a known pattern of inheritance may be specifically sought, many are identified serendipitously during obstetric ultrasonography. Until recently, the only question raised by the prenatal diagnosis of a fetal malformation was whether the fetus should be aborted, but other therapeutic alternatives are becoming available. The detection of a fetal abnormality may now lead to a change in the timing of delivery, a change in the mode of delivery, and even prenatal treatment.

Since most diagnostic and therapeutic maneuvers involve some risk to the fetus and mother, there must be a reasonable expectation that a procedure is feasible, safe, and effective before it can be attempted in humans.[28] This requires reliable information about the pathophysiology and natural history of the disease process, the efficacy of

intervention in ameliorating the disease, and the feasibility and safety of the proposed intervention. The authors have tentatively outlined the diagnostic and therapeutic alternatives for the management of specific fetal malformations that can be recognized in utero.[15, 27]

MALFORMATIONS BEST TREATED AFTER TERM DELIVERY

Most correctable malformations that can be diagnosed in utero are best managed by appropriate medical and surgical therapy after delivery at term. The term infant is a better anesthetic and surgical risk than the preterm infant. Examples of such malformations that have been diagnosed in utero are given in Table 17–1. Although this list is not exhaustive, most neonatal surgical disorders fall into this category. Knowledge that a fetus has one of these anomalies may improve perinatal management by allowing preparation for appropriate postnatal care.

364

Table 17–1. MALFORMATIONS DETECTABLE IN UTERO BUT BEST CORRECTED AFTER DELIVERY AT TERM

Esophageal, duodenal, jejunoileal, and anorectal atresias
Meconium ileus (cystic fibrosis)
Enteric cysts and duplications
Small intact omphalocele
Small intact meningocele, myelomeningocele, and spina bifida
Unilateral multicystic dysplastic kidney
Craniofacial, extremity, and chest wall deformities
Cystic hygroma
Small sacrococcygeal teratoma
Ovarian cysts

Therapy for polyhydramnios and premature labor may be desirable to allow the fetus to remain in utero as long as possible. The delivery can be planned so that appropriate personnel (neonatologist, anesthesiologist, pediatric surgeon) are available. When the neonate will require highly specialized services, transporting the fetus in situ (maternal transport) may be preferable to postnatal transport of the fragile newborn.

MALFORMATIONS USUALLY MANAGED BY SELECTIVE ABORTION

When serious malformations incompatible with normal postnatal life are diagnosed early enough, the mother has the option of terminating the pregnancy. When these malformations are recognized too late for safe termination, the mother can be counseled and appropriate postnatal management arranged. Table 17–2 list examples of severe anatomic malformations that are considered indications for selective termination. These anatomic abnormalities join a long list of inherited chromosomal and metabolic disorders that can be diagnosed in utero and may lead to selective termination.

PRENATAL DIAGNOSIS LEADING TO EARLY DELIVERY

Early delivery may be indicated for certain fetal anomalies that require correction as soon as possible after diagnosis (Table 17–3). In each of these cases, the risk of premature delivery must be weighed against the risk of continued gestation. This approach has already proven beneficial in managing the fetus with hydrops fetalis and intrauterine growth retardation. Advances in stimulating fetal surfactant production with corticosteroids and in ventilating small babies have greatly improved the outcome for premature infants with respiratory distress syndrome.

The rationale for early correction is unique to each anomaly, but the principle remains the same: continued gestation would have a progressive ill effect on the fetus. In some cases, the function of a specific organ system is compromised by the lesion and will continue to deteriorate until it is corrected. In congenital hydronephrosis, unrelieved urinary tract obstruction results in progressive deterioration of renal function. Preterm delivery for early decompression of the urinary tract should reverse the renal maldevelopment at the earliest possible time, maximizing subsequent renal growth and development.[16] In obstructive hydrocephalus, high intraventricular pressure compresses the developing brain. Early delivery for ventricular decompression should maximize the opportunity for subsequent brain development and may avoid the difficult obstetric problem of delivering a baby with an abnormally large head.

Table 17–2. MALFORMATIONS USUALLY MANAGED BY SELECTIVE ABORTION

Anencephaly, porencephaly, encephalocele, and giant hydrocephalus
Severe anomalies associated with chromosomal abnormalities (Trisomy 13, Trisomy 18, and similar conditions)
Renal agenesis or bilateral polycystic kidney disease
Inherited chromosomal, metabolic, and hematologic abnormalities (hemoglobinopathies, Tay-Sachs disease, and similar conditions)

Table 17–3. MALFORMATIONS THAT MAY REQUIRE INDUCED PRETERM DELIVERY FOR EARLY CORRECTION EX UTERO

Obstructive hydronephrosis
Obstructive hydrocephalus
Amniotic band malformation complex
Gastroschisis or ruptured omphalocele
Intestinal ischemia/necrosis secondary to volvulus, meconium ileus, and similar conditions
Hydrops fetalis
Intrauterine growth retardation

Anomalies associated with progressive organ ischemia should be corrected as soon as possible. Volvulus associated with intestinal malrotation or meconium ileus may lead to intestinal gangrene, perforation, and meconium peritonitis. Early delivery for correction of this type of bowel lesion would be aimed at minimizing the amount of bowel lost to the ischemic process. In some malformations, the progressive ill effects on the fetus result directly from being in utero. In the amniotic band complex, a fetal part is compressed or strangulated by herniation through a defect in the fetal membranes, resulting in amputation or deformity. This simple mechanical restriction to growth and development should be relieved at the earliest possible time to prevent further deformity. In ruptured omphalocele or gastroschisis, the bowel exposed to amniotic fluid becomes coated with a thick fibrous inflammatory peel that may hinder repair and delay resumption of function. Early delivery should minimize the damage by shortening the time the bowel is exposed to the amniotic fluid.[36]

PRENATAL DIAGNOSIS LEADING TO CESAREAN DELIVERY

Elective cesarean delivery rather than a trial at vaginal delivery may be indicated for the fetal malformations listed in Table 17–4. In most cases, this is because the malformation would cause dystocia. Another indication for elective cesarean delivery is a malformation requiring immediate surgical correction best performed in a sterile environment. A good example is an uncovered meningomyelocele. In this circumstance, the baby can be resuscitated in an adjacent sterile operating room and undergo immediate surgical correction. Finally, a cesarean delivery may be required if preterm delivery of an affected fetus is elected but labor is inadequate or if the fetus does not tolerate labor as determined by fetal monitoring.

PRENATAL DIAGNOSIS LEADING TO INTERVENTION BEFORE BIRTH

Fetal Deficiencies

Some fetal deficiency states may be alleviated by treatment before birth (Table 17–5). In respiratory distress syndrome, glucocorticoids given to the mother increase deficient fetal pulmonary surfactant and alleviate the disease. Fetal anemia secondary to isoimmunization-induced hemolysis can be treated by transfusing red blood cells into the fetal peritoneal cavity. The authors have treated severe hydrops by administering digitalis and diuretics along with the blood. A fetus with vitamin B_{12}–responsive methylmalonic acidemia has been treated in utero by giving massive doses of B_{12} to the mother. A fetus with biotin-dependent multiple carboxylase deficiency has been treated by giving the mother pharmacologic doses of biotin during the last half of pregnancy.

Medications and nutrients injected into the amniotic fluid are swallowed and absorbed by the fetus. Intra-amniotic thyroid hormone can be used to treat congenital hypothyroidism and goiter and to help mature the fetal lung. The intrauterine growth-retarded fetus might be fed orally by instilling nutrients into the amniotic fluid.[29] In the future, it is possible that deficiencies in cellular function will be corrected by providing the appropriate stem cell graft.[9]

Anatomic Malformations

Correcting an anatomic malformation in utero is more difficult than providing a missing substrate, hormone, or medication to the fetus. The only anatomic malformations that warrant consideration are those that interfere with fetal organ development and that, if alleviated, would allow normal fetal development to proceed. At present, only three anatomic malformations deserve consideration (Table 17–6). A few others, such as cystic adenomatoid malformation of the

Table 17–4. MALFORMATIONS THAT MAY REQUIRE CESAREAN DELIVERY

Conjoined twins
Giant omphalocele
Large hydrocephalus
Large sacrococcygeal teratoma
Large cystic hygroma
Large or ruptured meningomyelocele
Malformations requiring preterm delivery in the presence of inadequate labor or fetal distress

Table 17–5. FETAL CONDITIONS THAT MAY REQUIRE MEDICAL TREATMENT BEFORE BIRTH

Disorder		Treatment
Erythroblastosis fetalis (RBC deficiency)		Red blood cells—intraperitoneal or intravenous
Pulmonary immaturity (surfactant deficiency)		Glucocorticoids—transplacental
Metabolic block	e.g., Methylmalonic acidemia	B_{12}—transplacental
	e.g., Multiple carboxylase deficiency	Biotin—transplacental
Cardiac arrhythmia	e.g., Supraventricular tachycardia	Digitalis, propranolol, procainamide— transplacental
Endocrine deficiency	e.g., Hypothyroidism	Thyroid—transamniotic
	e.g., Adrenal hyperplasia	Corticosteroids—transplacental
Nutritional deficiency	e.g., Intrauterine growth retardation	? Protein-calories—transamniotic or intravenous
Cellular deficiency	e.g., Severe combined immunodeficiency	? Stem cell reconstitution

lung,[4] may become candidates as their pathophysiology is unraveled.

CONGENITAL HYDRONEPHROSIS. Congenital hydronephrosis secondary to urethral obstruction is an excellent example of an anatomically simple lesion having devastating consequences on the developing fetus that may be prevented by correction before birth. Fetal hydronephrosis is being recognized with increasing frequency because fluid-filled masses are particularly easy to detect by sonography and because associated oligohydramnios is a common obstetric indication for sonography. The authors have managed more than 80 fetuses with urinary tract malformations and have developed an approach based on the predictable pathophysiologic consequences of obstruction on renal and pulmonary development.[12, 16, 30] The algorithm is presented in Figure 17–1.

The fetus with unilateral hydronephrosis or mild bilateral hydronephrosis with evidence of continuing good renal function does not require prenatal intervention but will benefit from early recognition and prompt postnatal treatment. Conversely, the fetus with severe irreversible renal damage, as evidenced by oligohydramnios or severe renal dysplasia before 20 weeks, probably cannot be salvaged.[30]

Table 17–6. ANATOMIC DEFECTS THAT INTERFERE WITH DEVELOPMENT AND MAY REQUIRE EARLY SURGICAL RELIEF

Malformation	Effect on Development	
Urethral obstruction	Hydronephrosis/ lung hypoplasia	Renal/respiratory failure
Diaphragmatic hernia	Lung hypoplasia	Respiratory failure
Aqueductal stenosis	Hydrocephalus	Brain damage

The fetus with bilateral hydronephrosis secondary to urethral obstruction who develops oligohydramnios after 20 weeks may benefit from early decompression to halt the ongoing damage to the developing kidneys and lungs. The fetus older than 32 weeks can be delivered early and decompressed ex utero. For the younger fetus, decompression in utero may be necessary.

Selecting appropriate management for the fetus with obstructive uropathy depends on the ability to accurately assess the severity of existing renal damage and to predict the potential for recovery of renal function if the obstruction is relieved. Clinical assessment of the functional potential of the obstructed fetal urinary tract has proved to be difficult. Evaluative tests using either urine reaccumulation after bladder aspiration[5] or furosemide (Lasix) stimulation of urine output[41] are unreliable. Amniotic fluid status is predictive only in the extremes, i.e., normal volume late in gestation suggests adequate function whereas severe oligohydramnios early in gestation suggests poor function.[30] Similarly, the ultrasonographic appearance of the fetal kidneys lacks the sensitivity and specificity to be used as the sole predictor of function.[35] Clinical use of diagnostic fetal bladder catheterization to assess urine sodium and chloride concentration and hourly urine output has proved to be extremely helpful (Figs. 17–2, 17–3). Normal fetal urine is hypotonic,[34] whereas the authors' clinical work has demonstrated that human fetuses with obstructive uropathy and renal dysplasia produce minimal amounts of nearly isotonic urine.[12] Finally, laboratory studies suggest that fetal creatinine clearance will allow a simple, quantitative estimate of fetal renal function.[2] Since maternal and fetal serum creatinine levels are

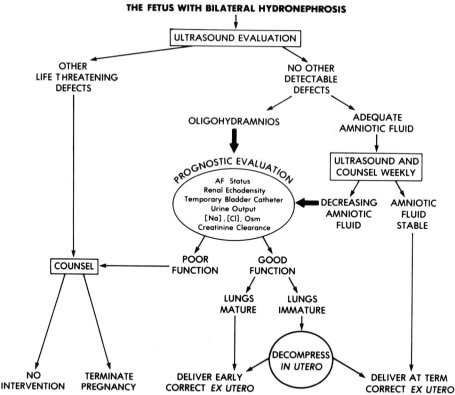

Figure 17–1. Management scheme for the fetus with bilateral hydronephrosis. (*From* Adzick NS, Flake AW, Harrison MR: Recent advances in prenatal diagnosis and treatment. Pediatr Clin North Am 32:1103, 1985.)

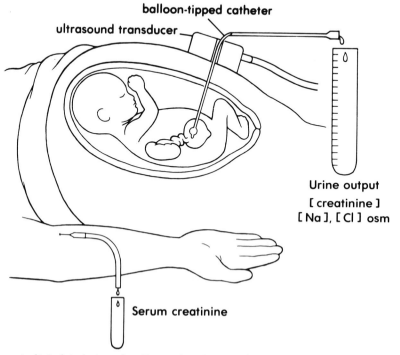

Figure 17–2. Current clinical technique for diagnostic urinary catheterization. A No. 4 French balloon-tipped catheter is placed into the distended fetal bladder. Fetal urine output, urinary electrolytes, and creatinine clearance can be determined with this method. (*From* Adzick NS, Flake AW, Harrison MR: Recent advances in prenatal diagnosis and treatment. Pediatr Clin North Am 32:1103, 1985.)

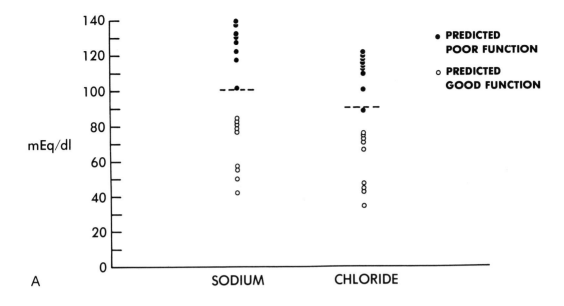

Predicted Function	Amniotic Fluid Status At the Time of Initial Presentation	Sonographic Appearance of Kidneys	Fetal Urine			
			Sodium (mEq/mL)	Chloride (mEq/mL)	Osmolarity (mosm)	Output (mL/H)
Poor	Moderate to severely decreased	Echogenic to cystic	> 100	> 90	> 210	< 2
Good	Normal to moderately decreased	Normal to echogenic	< 100	< 90	< 210	> 2

B

Figure 17–3. *A,* Graph of fetal urinary sodium and chloride concentrations in fetuses with good and poor function. Fetuses with poor renal function have "salt wasting" and urinary sodium levels >100 mEq/dl. *B,* Prognostic criteria for the fetus with bilateral obstructive uropathy. (*From* Glick PL, Harrison MR, Golbus MS, et al: Management of the fetus with congenital hydronephrosis II: Prognostic criteria and selection for treatment. J Pediatr Surg 20:376, 1985.)

equal,[31–33] fetal creatinine clearance can be determined by fetal urine collection and maternal blood sampling alone, obviating the need for simultaneous fetal blood sampling.

Experimentally, prenatal decompression arrests the adverse effects on renal development and reverses otherwise lethal pulmonary hypoplasia.[10, 11, 23, 24] Prenatal intervention is safe and feasible in a rigorous primate model.[3, 20, 38] The authors have developed techniques for sonographically guided percutaneous placement of fetal shunt catheters (Fig. 17–4) and for surgical exteriorization of the fetal urinary tract, and have begun to apply these techniques in highly selected cases.[12, 22, 30] Although percutaneous drainage has been successful, all catheters are prone

to obstruction and migration, necessitating close observation and frequent catheter replacement. The authors favor surgical decompression by bladder marsupialization or bilateral ureterostomies for the singleton fetus with bilateral hydronephrosis who has evidence of compromised renal function and is too immature to be delivered for postnatal decompression.[12]

Congenital Diaphragmatic Hernia. Congenital diaphragmatic hernia (CDH) is an anatomically simple defect that is easily correctable after birth by removing the herniated viscera from the chest and closing the diaphragm. However, 50 to 80 percent of all infants with CDH die of pulmonary insufficiency despite optimal postnatal care because their lungs are too hypoplastic to sup-

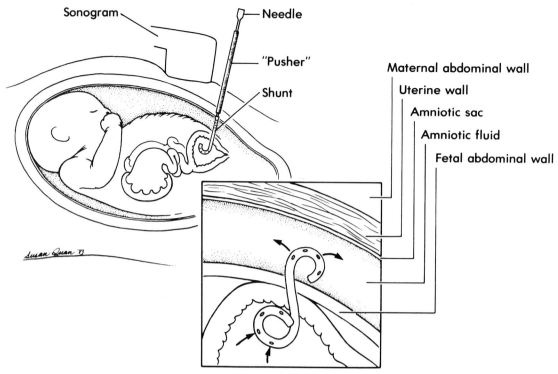

Figure 17–4. Placement of a fetal bladder shunt depicted schematically. The double pigtail catheter is pushed off the needle so that one end is in the bladder and the other end is in the amniotic space. (*From Adzick NS, Flake AW, Harrison MR: Recent advances in prenatal diagnosis and treatment. Pediatr Clin North Am 32:1103, 1985.*)

port extrauterine life even at term.[25, 26] Since the pulmonary hypoplasia appears to be a developmental consequence of compression by the herniated viscera, removal of this space-occupying lesion in utero should allow pulmonary development to proceed so that pulmonary function will be adequate to support life at birth.

The authors have demonstrated in fetal lambs that compression of the lung during the last trimester results in fatal pulmonary hypoplasia, and that removal of the compressing lesion allows the lung to grow and develop sufficiently to reverse the fatal pulmonary hypoplasia and allow survival at birth.[17, 18] Congenital diaphragmatic hernia can be diagnosed in utero, and a technique for successful surgical correction in utero has been developed experimentally.[19] This is illustrated in Figure 17–5.

The authors have studied the prenatal diagnosis and natural history of human fetal diaphragmatic hernia in 94 cases.[1] Prenatal diagnosis of CDH is accurate, and current techniques can detect lethal nonpulmonary anomalies and prevent diagnostic errors. Despite optimal conventional therapy, most

fetuses with detectable CDH will die in the neonatal period (80 percent mortality). Polyhydramnios is both a common prenatal marker for CDH (present in 76 percent of fetuses studied) and a predictor for poor clinical outcome (only 11 percent survived). Fetal CDH is a dynamic process—nonsurvivors have larger defects and may have more viscera displaced into the chest at an earlier stage of development. It appears that surgical intervention before birth may be necessary to improve survival rates of fetuses with CDH and polyhydramnios.

Prenatal diagnosis may permit surgical intervention before birth. Six years of experimental and clinical investigation suggest that prenatal repair offers great hope for the fetus with CDH. The optimal time for intervention appears to be between 22 and 28 weeks of gestation. However, prenatal intervention carries considerable risk for both the fetus and the mother, and the authors remain convinced that it should not be attempted until (1) the physiologic rationale, efficacy, and feasibility are demonstrated experimentally;[17, 19, 40] (2) the prenatal diagnosis of CDH is shown to be accurate, capable of excluding

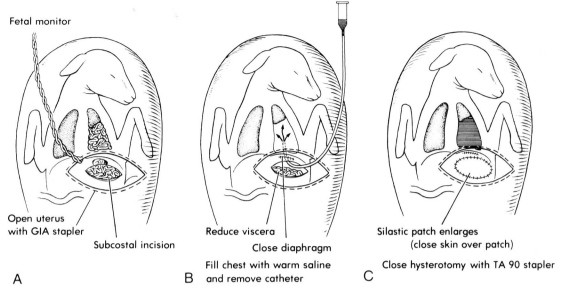

Fiture 17–5. Technique developed in lambs for correction of congenital diaphragmatic hernia (CDH) in utero. *A*, Surgical exposure through a stapled hysterotomy. A screw-in fetal scalp electrode monitors heart rate and variability during surgery. *B*, The herniated viscera are reduced, the air in the chest is replaced with warm Ringer's lactate, and the diaphragm is closed with a single layer of nonabsorbable sutures. *C*, The abdomen is enlarged by Silastic abdominoplasty, and the uterus is closed with staples. Fetal operating time is less than 30 minutes. (*From* Harrison MR, Ross NA, de Lorimier AA: Correction of congenital diaphragmatic hernia in utero. III. Development of a successful surgical technique using abdominoplasty to avoid compromise of umbilical blood flow. J Pediatr Surg 16:934, 1981.)

other anomalies, and able to predict which fetuses have sufficiently bad prognosis to justify in utero intervention;[1] (3) the natural history and outcome of CDH in the untreated human fetus is defined by serial observations;[1, 39] and (4) the safety of hysterotomy and control of preterm labor are established in the nonhuman primate.[3, 20, 38] Although these criteria can now be satisfied, the repair of human fetal CDH remains a formidable challenge that should not be attempted under any but the most rigorous conditions. Diaphragmatic hernia remains the best studied and most compelling example of a defect requiring correction before birth.

CONGENITAL OBSTRUCTIVE HYDROCEPHALUS. Another simple obstructive lesion with severe developmental consequences is obstructive hydrocephalus secondary to stenosis of the aqueduct of Sylvius. Here, obstruction of the flow of cerebrospinal fluid (CSF) produces back pressure that dilates the ventricles, compresses the developing brain, and eventually destroys neurologic function. Decompressing the ventricles may reverse the adverse effects of high-pressure hydrocephalus and allow development to proceed normally.

Fetal ventriculomegaly can be detected by 15 to 18 weeks of gestation.[8] The authors have evaluated the course and outcome of 24 fetuses with ventriculomegaly and have developed some guidelines for prenatal diagnosis and management (Fig. 17–6).[14]

The fetus with ventriculomegaly who on complete evaluation is *otherwise normal* should have serial sonographic evaluation to assess the severity and progression of the disease. Most cases do not progress and will not require intervention. A few fetuses with progressive disease may have CSF repeatedly aspirated or drained into the amniotic fluid by means of a catheter shunt.[6, 7] Although the pathophysiology of fetal hydrocephalus and its correction are being studied experimentally,[13, 37] there are significant unsolved problems with their clinical application.[8] The authors continue to manage fetal ventriculomegaly conservatively.

ABDOMINAL WALL DEFECT. Optimal perinatal management of abdominal wall defects depends on distinguishing before birth those lesions with a good prognosis (gastroschisis and small omphalocele or hernia of the cord) from those lesions causing a high perinatal morbidity and mortality (large omphalocele

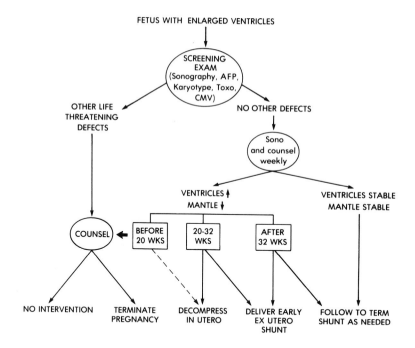

Figure 17–6. Management of the fetus with ventriculomegaly. Severe ventriculomegaly associated with some other malfunction or infection usually leads to termination of the pregnancy. Isolated obstructive ventriculomegaly requires serial assessment. Most cases do not progress. If obstruction produces progressive dilation and cortical thinning, early cerebrospinal fluid decompression may ameliorate further neurologic impairment. Sono, obstetric ultrasound; AFP, alpha-fetoprotein; Toxo, toxoplasmosis; CMV, cytomegalovirus. (*From* Glick PL, Harrison MR, Nakayama DK, et al: Management of ventriculomegaly in the fetus. J Pediatr Surg 105:97, 1984).

with associated anomalies and syndrome-related omphalocele). From experience managing 15 fetal cases, the authors have developed the approach to diagnosis and management outlined in Figure 17–7.[36]

If the liver is out, the abdominal wall defect is usually a large omphalocele, and management depends on the associated anomalies. A chromosomal defect or other severe malformations may lead to termination. A small omphalocele or hernia of the cord (liver in, sac intact) has an excellent prognosis with standard care. In cases of gastroschisis, a sac is not present, and bowel is

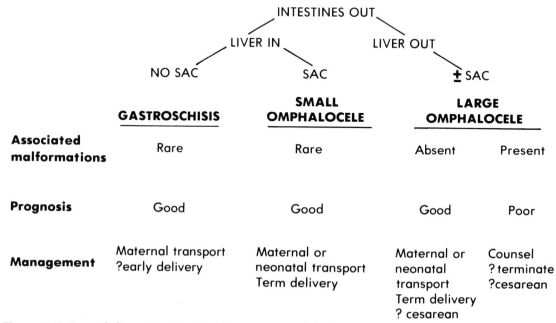

Figure 17–7. Prenatal diagnosis and perinatal management of the fetus with an abdominal wall defect. (*From* Nakayama DK, Harrison MR, Gross BH: Management of the fetus with an abdominal wall defect. J Pediatr Surg 19:408, 1984.)

exposed to amniotic fluid. Elective preterm delivery may minimize the inflammatory thickening of the bowel that compromises functional recovery. Despite some theoretic advantages (sterility and avoiding visceral injury), cesarean delivery has little advantage over vaginal delivery in managing most fetal abdominal wall defects.[36]

THE FUTURE OF FETAL TREATMENT

Prenatal diagnosis offers new hope for improved management of the fetus with a congenital defect, but the more invasive diagnostic and therapeutic procedures involve significant risks for both fetus and mother, raising difficult ethical questions about risks versus benefits and about the rights of the fetus and mother. A great deal of clinical and laboratory experience will be required to establish which procedures are truly safe and feasible. In the meantime, it is important to maintain a healthy skepticism about fetal treatment. Because a procedure can be done does not mean that it should be.

At this very early stage, fetal intervention should be pursued only in centers committed to research and development as well as (and before) responsible clinical application. The minimum requirements for fetal intervention include the cooperative efforts of an obstetrician experienced in prenatal intervention, a sonographer experienced and skilled in fetal diagnosis, a surgeon experienced in operating on tiny preterm infants and in performing fetal procedures in the laboratory, a perinatologist working in a high-risk obstetric unit associated with a tertiary intensive care nursery, a reasonable and compassionate bioethicist, and uninvolved professional colleagues who will monitor such innovative therapy (i.e., a committee on human research). Since there is considerable potential for doing harm, a fetal abnormality of any type should never be treated simply "because it is there" and never by someone unprepared for this fearsome responsibility. The responsibility of those undertaking fetal therapy includes an obligation to report to the medical profession all results, good or bad, so that the merits and liabilities of fetal treatment can be established as soon as possible.

The ability to diagnose fetal birth defects has achieved considerable sophistication. Treatment of several fetal disorders has proved feasible, and treatment of more complicated lesions will undoubtedly expand as techniques for fetal intervention improve.

References

1. Adzick NS, Harrison MR, et al: Diaphragmatic hernia in the fetus: Prenatal diagnosis and outcome in 94 cases. J Pediatr Surg 20:357, 1985.
2. Adzick NS, Harrison MR, Flake AW, et al: Development of a fetal renal function test using endogenous creatinine clearance. J Pediatr Surg 20:602, 1985.
3. Adzick NS, Harrison MR, et al: Fetal surgery in the primate III: Maternal outcome after fetal surgery. J Pediatr Surg 21:477, 1986.
4. Adzick NS, Harrison MR, Glick PL, et al: Fetal cystic adenomatoid malformation: Prenatal diagnosis and natural history. J Pediatr Surg 20:483, 1985.
5. Bellinger MF, Comstock C, Grosso D, et al: Fetal posterior urethral valves and renal dysplasia at 15 weeks gestational age. J Urol 129:1238, 1983.
6. Birnholtz JC, Frigoletto FD: Antenatal treatment for hydrocephalus. N Engl J Med 304:1021, 1981.
7. Clewell WH, Johnson ML, Meier PR, et al: A surgical approach to the treatment of fetal hydrocephalus. N Engl J Med 306:1320, 1982.
8. Fiske CE, Filly RA: Ultrasound of the normal and abnormal fetal neural axis. Rad Clin N Am 20:285, 1982.
9. Fleischman RA, Mintz B: Prevention of genetic anemias in mice by microinjection of normal hematopoietic stem cells into the fetal placenta. Proc Natl Acad Sci USA 76:5736, 1979.
10. Glick PL, Harrison MR, Noall R, et al: Correction of congenital hydronephrosis in utero III. Early mid-trimester ureteral obstruction produces renal dysplasia. J Pediatr Surg 18:681, 1983.
11. Glick PL, Harrison MR, Adzick NS, et al: Correction of congenital hydronephrosis in utero IV: In utero decompression prevents renal dysplasia. J Pediatr Surg 19:649, 1984.
12. Glick PL, Harrison MR, Golbus MS, et al: Management of the fetus with congenital hydronephrosis II: Prognostic criteria and selection for treatment. J Pediatr Surg 20:376, 1985.
13. Glick PL, Harrison MR, Halks-Miller M, et al: Correction of congenital hydrocephalus in utero II. Efficacy of in utero shunting. J Pediatr Surg 19:851, 1984.
14. Glick PL, Harrison MR, Nakayama DK, et al: Management of ventriculomegaly in the fetus. J Pediatr 105:97, 1984.
15. Harrison MR, Golbus MS, Filly RA: Management of the fetus with a correctable congenital defect. JAMA 246:774, 1981.
16. Harrison MR, Filly RA, Parer JT: Management of the fetus with a urinary tract malformation. JAMA 246:635, 1981.
17. Harrison MR, Jester JA, Ross NA: Correction of congenital diaphragmatic hernia in utero. I. The model: Intrathoracic balloon produced fetal pulmonary hypoplasia. Surgery 88:174, 1980.

18. Harrison MR, Bressack MA, Churg AM: Correction of congenital diaphragmatic hernia in utero. II. Simulated correction permits fetal lung growth with survival at birth. Surgery 88:260, 1980.

19. Harrison MR, Ross NA, deLorimier AA: Correction of congenital diaphragmatic hernia in utero. III. Development of a successful surgical technique using abdominoplasty to avoid compromise of umbilical blood flow. J Pediatr Surg 16:934, 1981.

20. Harrison MR, Anderson J, Rosen MA, et al: Fetal surgery in the primate I. Anesthetic, surgical, and tocolytic management to maximize fetal-neonatal survival. J Pediatr Surg; 17:115, 1982.

21. Harrison MR, Golbus MS, Filly RA: The Unborn Patient. Orlando, Grune & Stratton, 1984.

22. Harrison MR, Golbus MS, Filly RA, et al: Fetal surgery for congenital hydronephrosis. N Engl J Med 306:591, 1982.

23. Harrison MR, Ross N, Noall R, et al: Correction of congenital hydronephrosis in utero I. The model: Fetal urethral obstruction produces hydronephrosis and pulmonary hypoplasia in fetal lambs. J Pediatr Surg 18:247, 1983.

24. Harrison MR, Nakayama DK, Noall R, et al: Correction of congenital hydronephrosis in utero II. Decompression reverses the effects of obstruction on the fetal lung and urinary tract. J Pediatr Surg 17:965, 1982.

25. Harrison MR, Bjordal RI, Landmark F, et al: Congenital diaphragmatic hernia. The hidden mortality. J Pediatr Surg 13:227, 1979.

26. Harrison MR, deLorimier AA: Congenital diaphragmatic hernia. Surg Clin North Am 61:1023, 1981.

27. Harrison MR, Golbus MS, Filly RA: Fetal surgical treatment. Pediatr Ann 11:896, 1982.

28. Harrison MR, Golbus MS, Filly RA, et al: Fetal treatment 1982. N Engl J Med 307:1651, 1982.

29. Harrison MR, Villa RL: Trans-amniotic fetal feeding I. Development of an animal model: Continuous amniotic infusion in rabbits. J Pediatr Surg 178:376, 1982.

30. Harrison MR, Golbus MS, Filly RA, et al: Management of the fetus with congenital hydronephrosis. J Pediatr Surg 17:728, 1982.

31. Hodari AA, Mariona FG, Houlihan RT, et al: Creatinine transport in the maternal-fetal complex. Obstet Gynecol 41:55, 1973.

32. Hutchinson DL, Bashore RA, Will DW: Creatinine equilibrium between mother and nephrectomized primate fetus. Proc Soc Exp Biol Med 110:395, 1962.

33. McGaughey HS, Corey EL, Scoggin WA, et al: Creatinine transport between baby and mother at term. Am J Obstet Gynecol 80:108, 1960.

34. McGrory WW: Development of renal function in utero. In Developmental Nephrology. Cambridge, Harvard University Press, 1972, pp 51–78.

35. Mahony BS, Filly RA, Callen PW, et al: Sonographic evaluation of fetal renal dysplasia. Radiology 152:143, 1984.

36. Nakayama DK, Harrison MR, Gross BH: Management of the fetus with an abdominal wall defect. J Pediatr Surg 19:408, 1984.

37. Nakayama DK, Harrison MR, Berger MS, et al: Correction of congenital hydrocephalus in utero I. The model: Intracisternal kaolin produces hydrocephalus in fetal lambs and rhesus monkeys. J Pediatr Surg 18:331, 1983.

38. Nakayama DK, Harrison MR, Seron-Ferre M, Villa RL: Fetal surgery in the primate II. Uterine electromyographic response to operative procedures and pharmacologic agents. J Pediatr Surg 19:333, 1984.

39. Nakayama DK, Harrison MR, Chinn DH, et al: Prenatal diagnosis and natural history of the fetus with a congenital diaphragmatic hernia: Initial clinical experience. J Pediatr Surg 20:118, 1985.

40. Pringle KC: Fetal lamb and fetal lamb lung growth following creation and repair of a diaphragmatic hernia. In Nathanielsz PW (ed): Animal Models in Fetal Medicine. Ithaca, NY, Perinatology Press, 1984.

41. Wladimiroff JW: Effect of furosemide on fetal urine production. Br J Obstet Gynaecol 82:221, 1975.

NORMAL ANATOMY OF THE FEMALE PELVIS

Clifford S. Levi, M.D.
Edward A. Lyons, M.D.
Daniel J. Lindsay, M.D.
Geraldine Ballard, R.D.M.S.

The anatomy of the normal female pelvis is dynamic. Nowhere else in the body are age-related and hormonally stimulated changes as profound. The anatomy pertinent to the practice of obstetric and gynecologic sonography will be discussed in this chapter. Chapter 19 (Ultrasound Evaluation of the Uterus) and Chapter 21 (Ultrasound Evaluation of the Ovary) will discuss the physiologic changes of these organs.

The traditional method of sonographic evaluation of the female pelvis is through the distended urinary bladder (Fig. 18–1). This method is referred to as transabdominal sonography (TAS). The full urinary bladder is used to displace small bowel out of the true pelvis into the false pelvis (see below) and to provide a "sonic window" to view the pelvic contents.[1–3]

The pelvis is arbitrarily divided into two structurally continuous compartments: the true and false pelves. The division is defined by the sacral promontory and the lineae terminales.[4] The lineae terminales are the arcuate line of the ilium, the iliopectineal line, and the crest of the pubis. The false pelvis is bounded by the flanged portions of the iliac bones, the base of the sacrum posteriorly, and the abdominal wall anteriorly and laterally. The true pelvis is bounded anteriorly by the pubis and rami, posteriorly by the sacrum and coccyx, and laterally by the fused ilium and ischium. With the muscles of the pelvic floor in place, the true pelvis forms a basin.

On TAS, visualization of the pelvic organs is limited by body habitus owing to sonic attenuation of the intervening anterior abdominal wall, subcutaneous and properitoneal fat, and fat in the mesentery and omentum. As a result of this attenuation and the distance of the area of interest from the anterior abdominal wall, it is often not possible to use high-frequency transducers and benefit from their inherent enhanced axial and lateral resolution. In the authors' practice, although a 5.0 MHz transducer is used whenever possible, most transvesical examinations are performed with a 3.5 MHz transducer.

More recently, endovaginal sonography (EVS) has become available and is gaining widespread acceptance. Because of the proximity of the vaginal fornices to the uterus and adnexa, the problem of sonic attenuation is much less significant with EVS in the evaluation of the viscera of the true pelvis. As a result, higher frequency transducers

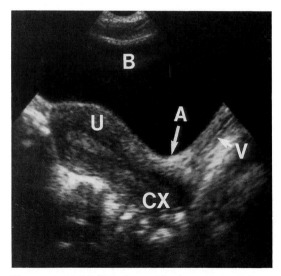

Figure 18–1. Midline longitudinal (median sagittal) scan through the distended urinary bladder (B), demonstrating the uterus (U) and vagina (V). The cervix (CX) is posterior to the angle of the bladder (A).

can be used in EVS. All the endovaginal scans shown in this chapter were performed with a 6.5 MHz transducer. The normal and pathologic anatomy of the uterus, ovaries, and uterine tubes, if within the field of view of the transducer, is demonstrated to better advantage using the endovaginal rather than the transvesical approach. In our experience,

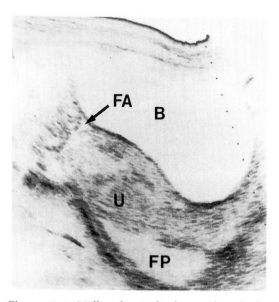

Figure 18–2. Midline longitudinal scan through the distended urinary bladder (B) and uterus (U) in a patient with a ruptured ectopic pregnancy. Free intraperitoneal fluid is present in the posterior (FP) and anterior (FA) cul-de-sac.

patient acceptance of EVS is actually better than for the transvesical approach because EVS obviates the need for a full bladder.

The disadvantages of EVS when compared with TAS include a limited field of view and an inability to examine the false pelvis adequately. The full urinary bladder in TAS provides a window to examine the true pelvis by displacement of bowel but may also inadvertently displace pathologic structures into the false pelvis (Fig. 18–2).[5, 6] A quick scan of the true and false pelves at the end of the study after the patient has voided is part of a routine examination. It will allow one readily to detect large masses that have been displaced by the full bladder and masses that mimic a full bladder. On the postvoid examination, it is often necessary to use compression to displace gas in loops of small bowel and colon, especially when searching for a small mass in the false pelvis.

THE PELVIC MUSCULATURE AND FASCIAL PLANES

The superficial or subcutaneous fascia is areolar in texture and contains varying amounts of fat. The subcutaneous fascia is continuous with the superficial fascia of the thigh, labia majora, and perineum. The anterior and lateral walls of the false pelvis are the anterior and lateral muscles of the abdominal wall. Laterally, these muscles include the external and internal obliques and the transversus abdominis (innermost).[7, 8] The rectus abdominis muscles are paired paramedian muscles oriented longitudinally on either side of the linea alba. The pelvic attachment of the rectus abdominis muscles is to the crest of the pubis. The aponeuroses of the external and internal obliques and transversus muscles fuse with the anterior rectus abdominis fascia to form the linea alba in the midline. It should be noted that the anatomy of the rectus sheath is different above and below the arcuate line (Fig. 18–3).[7] Below the arcuate line, a rectus sheath hematoma may extend across the midline and displace the bladder posteriorly.[9] Above the arcuate line, however, a hematoma will be confined and not cross the midline. Without careful evaluation of the abdominal wall and the epicenter of the mass, a hematoma of the rectus sheath may be mistaken for a mass of pelvic origin.

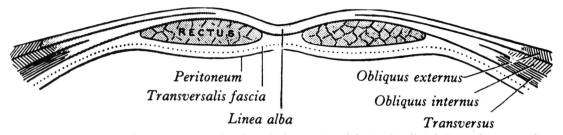

Figure 18–3. A diagram of a transverse section through the anterior abdominal wall, inferior to the arcuate line. (*From* Williams PL: Myology. *In* Gray's Anatomy, 36th Ed. Harlow, Essex, England, Longman Group, 1980.)

Masses in the space of Retzius (also known as the prevesical or retropubic space) may also be confused with masses arising from the pelvic viscera. The space of Retzius is situated between the transversalis fascia and the extraperitoneal fascia. The transversalis fascia is a thin layer of connective tissue separating the transversus abdominis from the extraperitoneal fascia.[7, 8] Below the umbilicus, the extraperitoneal fascia presents two well-defined layers. The umbilical vesical fascia is the deeper of the two and is continuous with the vesical fascia. The umbilical prevesical fascia lies between the transversalis and umbilical vesical fasciae and is fused to the latter. It is also fused to the transversalis fascia along the medial umbilical ligaments and at the umbilicus. The resultant space between the transversalis fascia and the umbilical prevesical fascia is the space of Retzius.[8] Sonographically, masses in the space of Retzius (usually hematomas or abscesses) displace the bladder posteriorly (Fig. 18–4) and can be differentiated from pelvic or abdominal masses that displace the bladder inferiorly or anteriorly.[10]

Muscles of the pelvis include those of:

1. The lower limb: psoas major, iliacus, piriformis, obturator internus.

2. The pelvic diaphragm: levator ani, coccygeus.[8, 11]

The psoas major is a large triangular-shaped muscle that arises from the lumbar transverse processes and the bodies and discs of T12 to L2. It descends through the false pelvis on the pelvic sidewall anteriorly and exits posterior to the inguinal ligament. It converges with the iliacus to form a tendon that inserts on the lesser trochanter of the femur. The iliacus arises from the concavity of the upper two-thirds of the iliac fossa.

Sonographically, the psoas is seen in the lower abdomen in a paravertebral position.[1–3] In the transverse plane of the lower abdomen, the psoas is rounded in shape and hypoechoic. As the transducer is angled inferiorly, the psoas muscles diverge laterally and, in the false pelvis, assume a position medial and slightly anterior to the iliacus muscle (Figs. 18–5, 18–6). In the false pelvis, the iliac wings are identified as brightly echogenic linear structures with loss of distal sonic information. More inferiorly, within the true pelvis, the iliacus/psoas muscle is seen as a hypoechoic, discretely marginated muscle with its two component muscles separated by a brightly echogenic line, which represents interposed fascia continuous with the psoas tendon (Fig. 18–7). The psoas may be demonstrated in its long axis by scanning in a longitudinal oblique plane (Fig. 18–8). In thin patients, the fasciculi of the psoas muscle may be identified (Fig. 18–8). Movement of the normal psoas muscle may be seen with flexion of the hip.

The piriformis muscle arises from the sacrum between the pelvic sacral foramina, and from the gluteal surface of the ilium (Fig.

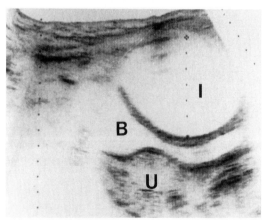

Figure 18–4. Midline longitudinal scan after renal transplant. The bladder (B) is displayed posteriorly by a lymphocele (l) in the space of Retzius. U, uterus.

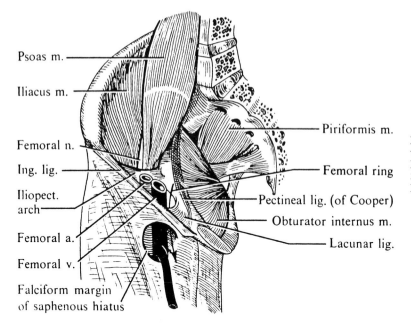

Psoas m.

Iliacus m.

Femoral n.

Ing. lig.

Iliopect. arch

Femoral a.

Femoral v.

Falciform margin of saphenous hiatus

Piriformis m.

Femoral ring

Pectineal lig. (of Cooper)

Obturator internus m.

Lacunar lig.

Figure 18–5. Diagram of the pelvic musculature. (*From* Pansky B: *In* Review of Gross Anatomy, 5th Ed. New York, Macmillan Publishing Co, 1987, p 499.)

18–9).[8, 11] On pelvic sonography, the piriformis can be identified posteriorly within the pelvis until it passes through the greater sciatic notch (Fig. 18–10) to insert onto the greater trochanter of the femur. The obturator internus muscle arises from the anterolateral pelvic wall surrounding the obturator foramen and passes through the lesser sciatic foramen to insert on the greater trochanter

of the femur (Fig. 18–11). The levator ani and coccygeus muscles of the pelvic floor can be routinely identified on TAS when the transducer is angled inferiorly (Fig. 18–12).

VASCULAR ANATOMY

The common iliac arteries course anteriorly and medially to the psoas muscles

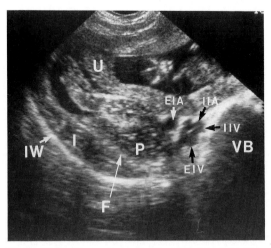

Figure 18–6. Transverse scan through the right iliac fossa, using the gravid uterus (U) as a sonic window, showing the relative positions of the iliacus (I) and psoas major (P) muscles separated by a fascial plane (F) in the false pelvis. The iliac vessels are medial to the psoas. EIA, external iliac artery; IIA, internal iliac artery; EIV, external iliac vein; IIV, internal iliac vein. VB, vertebral body; IW, iliac wing.

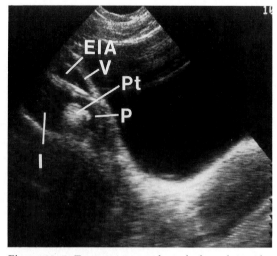

Figure 18–7. Transverse scan through the pelvic sidewall, angled to the right to visualize the psoas major (P), the iliacus (I), and the psoas tendon (Pt). The external iliac artery (EIA) and vein (V) are anterior to the iliopsoas muscle bundle.

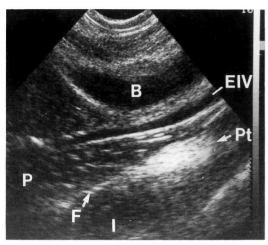

Figure 18–8. Coronal scan through the distended urinary bladder (B), with the transducer situated medially and angled laterally to visualize the psoas major (P) and the iliacus (I) muscles in their long axes. F, iliopsoas fascial plane; Pt, psoas tendon; EIV, external iliac vein.

(Fig. 18–13).[8, 12, 13] The right common iliac vein ascends posteriorly and then laterally to the right common iliac artery. The left common iliac vein ascends medially and then posteriorly to the left common iliac artery. The common iliac arteries bifurcate to form the external and internal iliac arteries. The external iliac arteries supply most of the lower limbs. The internal iliac arteries supply the viscera, walls of the pelvis, perineum, and gluteal regions (Fig. 18–14).

The external iliac arteries course through the false pelvis without entering the true pelvis. In the nongravid state, the caliber of the external iliac arteries is greater than that of the internal iliac arteries. The external iliac arteries assume a course adjacent to the medial psoas border and exit the pelvis through the femoral canals at the level of the inguinal ligaments (Figs. 18–6, 18–7, 18–15). The right external iliac vein ascends medially and then posteriorly to the right

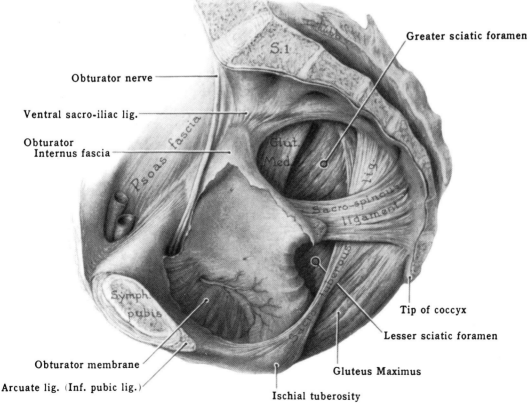

Figure 18–9. The muscles and ligaments of the lateral pelvic wall as viewed from the pelvis. (*Reproduced by permission from* Grant JCB: Grant's Atlas of Anatomy, 5th Ed. Baltimore, Williams & Wilkins Co, 1962, p 217. Copyright 1962, The Williams & Wilkins Company.)

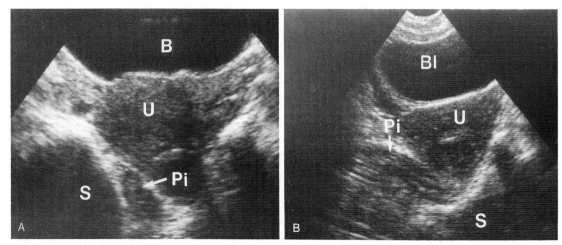

Figure 18–10. *A,* Longitudinal scan to the right of the midline, through the bladder (B), showing the right piriformis muscle (Pi) in cross section. *B,* Transverse scan through the bladder (Bl), angled to the right, showing the right piriformis muscle (Pi) in its length. U, uterus; S, sacrum.

external iliac artery. The left external iliac vein is medial to the left external iliac artery.[8, 12, 13] The internal iliac arteries arise at the bifurcation of the common iliac arteries at the level of the L_5/S_1 disc immediately anterior to the sacroiliac joints. They course approximately 4 cm posteriorly to the superior margin of the greater sciatic foramen. The internal iliac arteries divide into anterior and posterior trunks, which pass posteriorly into the greater sciatic foramina. Anterior to the internal iliac arteries are the ureters, ovaries, and fimbriated ends of the uterine tubes (Fig. 18–16). The internal iliac veins are posterior to their respective arteries. The proximal portion of the posterior trunk, as well as the anterior trunk and some

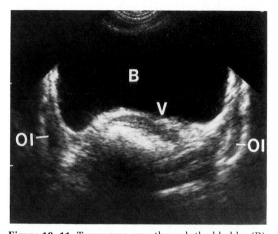

Figure 18–11. Transverse scan through the bladder (B), at the level of the vagina (V), showing the obturator internus muscles (OI) bilaterally.

of its major branches, can be identified on EVS (Fig. 18–17).

The uterine artery, an important branch of the anterior trunk, runs medially on the levator ani to the cervix. Approximately 2 cm from the cervix, it crosses superiorly and anteriorly to the ureter (Fig. 18–18). The uterine artery ascends lateral to the uterus in the broad ligament to the junction of the fallopian tube and the uterus. From the cornua of the uterus, the uterine artery courses laterally to reach the hilum of the ovary, and it ends by joining with the ovarian artery. The uterine arteries anastomose extensively with each other across the midline through anterior and posterior arcuate arteries.[8, 12] The arcuate arteries run within the broad ligament and then enter the myometrium.

The uterine plexus of veins accompanies the arcuate arteries, passing circumferentially within the myometrium.[8, 13] The arcuate vessels lie between the intermediate and external layers of the myometrium. The venous plexus is larger than the associated arterial channels and is frequently identified sonographically by both the transabdominal and endovaginal approaches (Figs. 18–18, 18–19, 18–20).

The ovarian arteries arise from the lateral margin of the aorta at a level slightly inferior to the renal arteries. At the pelvic brim, they cross the external iliac artery and vein and course medially within the suspensory ligament of the ovary (Figs. 18–18, 18–21). The ovarian artery passes posteriorly in the me-

Text continued on page 385

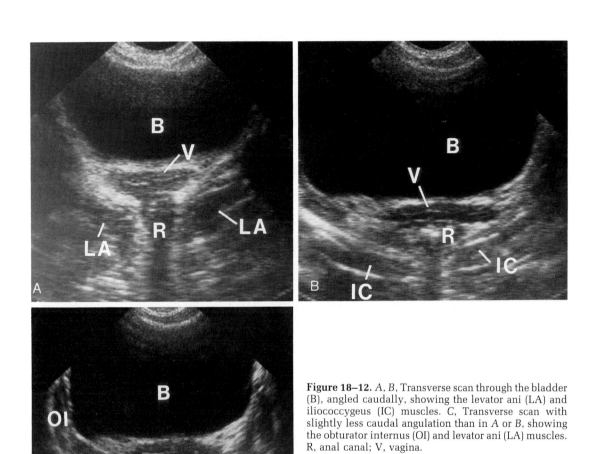

Figure 18–12. *A*, *B*, Transverse scan through the bladder (B), angled caudally, showing the levator ani (LA) and iliococcygeus (IC) muscles. *C*, Transverse scan with slightly less caudal angulation than in *A* or *B*, showing the obturator internus (OI) and levator ani (LA) muscles. R, anal canal; V, vagina.

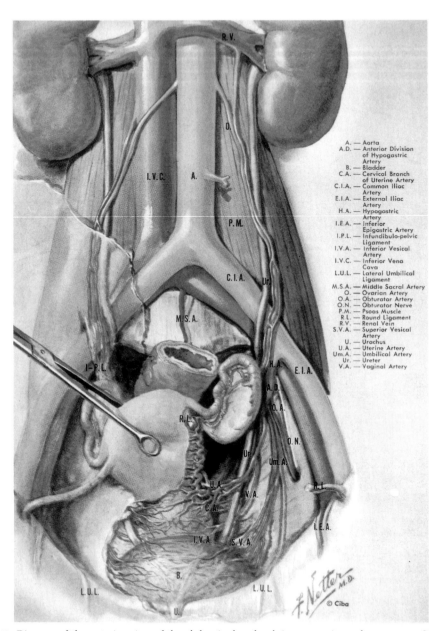

A. — Aorta
A.D. — Anterior Division of Hypogastric Artery
B. — Bladder
C.A. — Cervical Branch of Uterine Artery
C.I.A. — Common Iliac Artery
E.I.A. — External Iliac Artery
H.A. — Hypogastric Artery
I.E.A. — Inferior Epigastric Artery
I.P.L. — Infundibulo-pelvic Ligament
I.V.A. — Inferior Vesical Artery
I.V.C. — Inferior Vena Cava
L.U.L. — Lateral Umbilical Ligament
M.S.A. — Middle Sacral Artery
O. — Ovarian Artery
O.A. — Obturator Artery
O.N. — Obturator Nerve
P.M. — Psoas Muscle
R.L. — Round Ligament
R.V. — Renal Vein
S.V.A. — Superior Vesical Artery
U. — Urachus
U.A. — Uterine Artery
Um.A. — Umbilical Artery
Ur. — Ureter
V.A. — Vaginal Artery

Figure 18–13. Diagram of the anterior view of the abdominal and pelvic retroperitoneal structures. See color plate, p xv. (*From* Netter FH: Medical Illustrations: Reproductive System, Vol 2. West Caldwell, New Jersey, CIBA-Geigy Corp, 1954, p 97. ©*Copyright* 1954. CIBA-Geigy Corporation. *Reproduced with permission from* THE CIBA COLLECTION OF MEDICAL ILLUSTRATIONS by Frank H. Netter, MD. All rights reserved.)

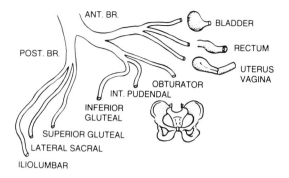

Figure 18–14. Schematic diagram of the branches of the internal iliac arteries and the pelvic viscera, which they supply.

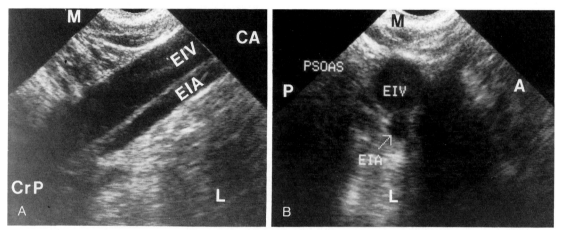

Figure 18–15. *A,* Endovaginal scan of the external iliac vessels. The transducer was initially in the sagittal plane and was then angled to the right to obtain this image. CA, caudad–anterior; CrP, cranial–posterior; M, medial; L, lateral. (For a schematic diagram see Fig. 18–22B.) *B,* Endovaginal scan in the coronal plane, with the transducer angled to the right. M, medial; L, lateral; A, anterior; P, posterior. EIA, external iliac artery; EIV, external iliac vein.

Figure 18–16. *A,* Transverse scan angled to the right through the bladder, showing the right ovary (O) immediately anterior to the right internal iliac artery (IIA). *B,* Longitudinal scan to the right of the midline, showing the relationship of the right ovary to the right internal iliac artery.

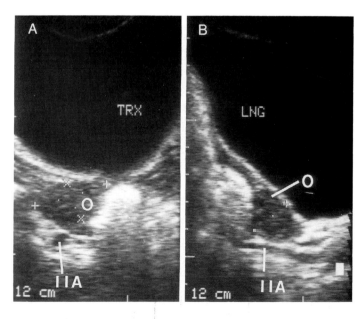

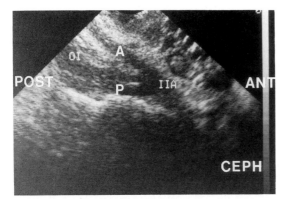

Figure 18–17. Endovaginal scan of the internal iliac artery and branches. The transducer was initially in the sagittal plane and was then angled to the right to obtain this image. IIA, internal iliac artery; anterior (A) and posterior (P) branches of the internal iliac artery; OI, obturator internus. Orientation: posterior (POST), anterior (ANT), Cephalad (CEPH). (For a schematic diagram see Fig. 18–22B).

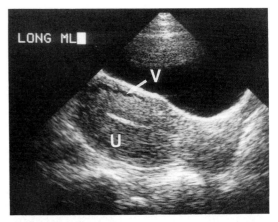

Figure 18–19. Longitudinal midline scan of the uterus (U) through the bladder, demonstrating the uterine plexus of veins (V) within the myometrium, between the intermediate and external layers.

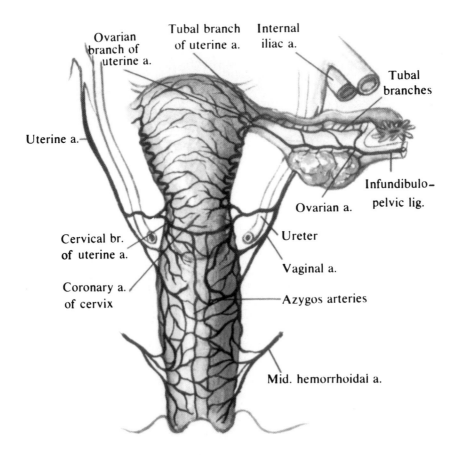

Figure 18–18. Diagram of the ovarian, uterine, and vaginal arteries and the ipsilateral ureter. (*From Healey JE: A Synopsis of Clinical Anatomy. Philadelphia, WB Saunders Co, 1969, p 231.*)

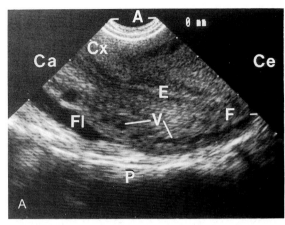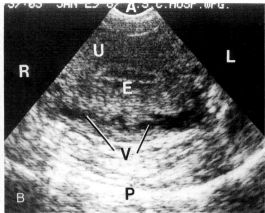

Figure 18–20. *A,* Endovaginal scan in the sagittal plane, through the anterior fornix of the vagina. The normally positioned uterine fundus (F) is displayed to the right of the image, and the cervix (Cx) is displayed to the left. The uterine plexus of veins (V) is visualized with the myometrium. A small amount of fluid (Fl) is present in the posterior cul-de-sac. E, endometrium. Orientation: anterior (A), posterior (P), cephalad (Ce), caudad (Ca). *B,* Endovaginal scan in the coronal plane, showing the uterine plexus of the veins (V). U, uterus; E, endometrium. Orientation: anterior (A), posterior (P), right (R), left (L).

sovarium and breaks up into branches.[12] The right ovarian vein empties into the inferior vena cava just below the renal vein. The left ovarian vein empties into the left renal vein.

The lymph nodes and lymphatic channels are not normally visualized by sonography. However, knowledge of the location of the major lymph node groups is important in order to recognize them when they are pathologically enlarged. The main groups are:

1. The common iliac lymph nodes that accompany the common iliac artery.

2. The external iliac lymph nodes that are

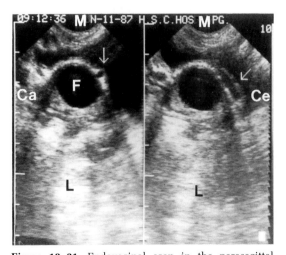

Figure 18–21. Endovaginal scan in the parasagittal plane, angled to the left. The ovarian artery *(arrow)* is identified entering the superior surface of the ovary. F, ovarian follicle. Orientation: medial (M), lateral (L), cephalad (Ce), caudad (Ca).

situated in the false pelvis and pelvic sidewall lateral to the bladder and are associated with the external iliac artery and vein.

3. The internal iliac lymph nodes that surround the internal iliac vessels. Outlying groups include the sacral and obturator nodes.

The lymphatic drainage of the pelvic viscera is variable. The following is a general guideline to drainage of specific viscera, which is important in assessing nodal spread in neoplasia:

1. Ovaries: The lymphatic channels ascend along the ovarian arteries to the lateral aortic and preaortic nodes at the level of the renal hila.

2. Cervix: The lymphatic channels course lateral in the parametrium to the external iliac nodes, posterolateral to the internal iliac nodes, and posterior to the rectal or sacral nodes.

3. Uterus, lower corpus: The lymphatics course lateral to the external iliacs through the parametrium.

4. Uterus, upper corpus, fundus, and tube: The lymphatics accompany the ovarian channels.

5. Vagina: The lymphatics of the upper vagina accompany the uterine artery to the internal and external iliac lymph nodes, whereas those of the midvagina accompany the vaginal artery to the internal iliac lymph nodes. The vagina external to the hymen drains to the superficial inguinal nodes.[14] This reflects the embryologic origin of the

vagina, where the fibromuscular wall of the upper two-thirds of the vagina arises from the paramesonephric (müllerian) duct, which also gives rise to the uterus and fallopian tubes. The lower one-third of the vagina arises from the urogenital sinus and therefore shares the lymphatic drainage with the external genitalia.

THE OVARIES

The ovaries are ellipsoid in shape, with the long axis usually oriented vertically when the bladder is empty. Ovarian location is variable, especially in women who have been pregnant. In the nulliparous female, the ovaries are situated in the ovarian fossa (also known as the fossa of Waldeyer (Fig. 18–22).[8, 15, 16] The ovarian fossa is situated on the lateral pelvic wall and is bounded by the obliterated umbilical artery anteriorly, the ureter and internal iliac artery posteriorly, and the external iliac vein superiorly. On the superior surface of the ovary are attached the ovarian fimbria of the uterine tube and the suspensory ligament of the ovary (Fig. 18–23). The suspensory ligament of the ovary is a fold of peritoneum that arises from the pelvic sidewall and contains the ovarian vessels and nerves. The ovarian

ligament extends between the medial pole of the ovary and the ipsilateral uterine cornua.

THE FALLOPIAN (UTERINE) TUBE

The fallopian tube is approximately 10 cm in length and lies in the superior part of the broad ligament. The fimbriated end is open to the peritoneal cavity and has an ostium measuring approximately 3 mm in diameter. The medial third is referred to as the isthmus, which is round and cordlike. The intramural portion of the fallopian tube is approximately 1 cm in length.[15] The normal tube is not seen on TAS but may be identified frequently by the endovaginal approach (Fig. 18–24).

THE UTERUS AND VAGINA

The uterus is located in the true pelvis, between the urinary bladder anteriorly and the rectosigmoid posteriorly. Uterine position is highly variable and changes with varying degrees of bladder and rectal distention. Sonographically, the uterus is a hypoechoic mass of uniform echogenicity. The endometrial echo complex is variable in

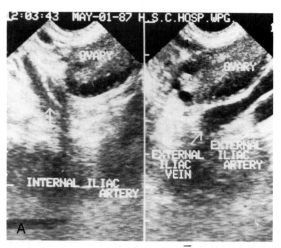

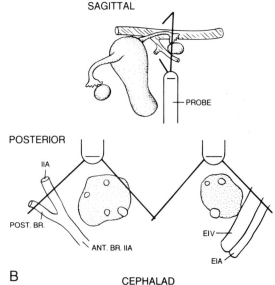

Figure 18–22. *A,* Endovaginal scan of the fossa of Waldeyer, showing the ovary, internal iliac artery, and the external iliac artery and vein. *B,* A schematic diagram of the scan plane of *A.* The transducer was initially in the sagittal plane and angled to the right to obtain the image of the fossa of Waldeyer and the surrounding vessels. IIA, internal iliac artery; EIV, external iliac vein; EIA, external iliac artery.

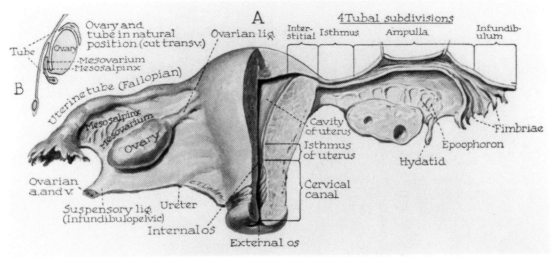

Figure 18–23. Diagram of the ovary, uterus, and adjacent peritoneal reflections and ligaments. (*From* Thorek P: Pelvic viscera. *In* Anatomy in Surgery, 2nd Ed. Philadelphia, JB Lippincott Co, 1962, pp 537–565.)

thickness and echogenicity related to the phase of the menstrual cycle as well as the level of ovarian activity (premenarchal, reproductive, postmenopausal). As noted previously, venous channels are often identified within the myometrium (Figs. 18–19, 18–20).

The vagina is seen as a hypoechoic tubular structure with an echogenic lumen that curves inferiorly over the muscular perineal body at the introitus. The bladder, trigone, and urethra are anterior to the vagina, and the rectum is posterior. The distal ureters are lateral to the upper vagina and pass anteriorly to enter the bladder.[15, 17] The posterior fornix of the vagina is closely related

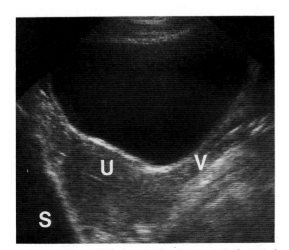

Figure 18–24. Midline longitudinal transvesical scan of the uterus (U) and vagina (V). The vagina curves inferiorly over the perineum. S, sacrum.

to the rectouterine recess of the peritoneal cavity (posterior cul-de-sac)[15] and is separated by the thickness of the vaginal wall and peritoneal membrane (Figs. 18–2, 18–20, 18–25).

The cervix projects through the anterior vaginal wall, separating the vagina into the anterior, posterior, and two lateral fornices. The cervix can be identified sonographically in the sagittal plane as that portion of the uterus immediately posterior to the angle of the bladder (Fig. 18–1). The cervix is anchored at the angle of the bladder by the parametrium and is less freely movable than the corpus or fundus of the uterus. When the bladder is empty, the cervix and the vagina form a 90° angle, a condition referred to as anteversion. The more movable corpus is usually flexed anteriorly on the cervix (anteflexed). Filling of the bladder usually straightens out the uterus so that on TAS the uterus does not appear anteflexed and the angle between the cervix and vagina is greater than 90°. Retroversion of the uterus or tilting of the uterus to the right or left are considered to be normal variants in position.[15] Retroversion of the uterus can result in poor visualization of the endometrial canal on TAS and widening of the adnexa due to visualization of the broad ligaments. In addition, owing to attenuation of sound by the uterus, the fundus of a retroverted uterus may be echo-poor in appearance (Fig. 18–26). This "dropout" phenomenon may simulate the appearance of a fundal fibroid. The differentiation between a fundal fibroid

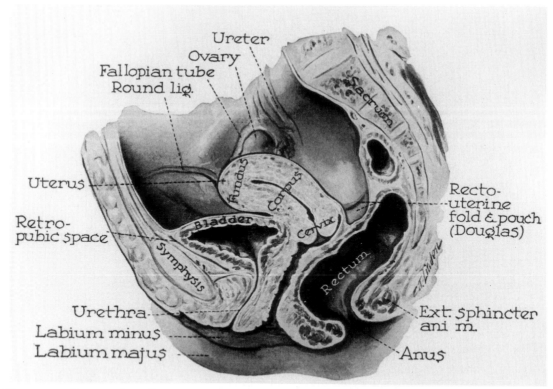

Figure 18–25. Diagram of a midline sagittal section through the pelvis, showing the peritoneal reflections, including the anterior cul-de-sac (vesicouterine recess) and the posterior cul-de-sac (rectouterine recess). The posterior cul-de-sac is closely related to the posterior fornix of the vagina. (*From* Thorek P: Pelvic viscera. *In* Anatomy in Surgery, 2nd Ed. Philadelphia, JB Lippincott Co, 1962, pp 537–565.)

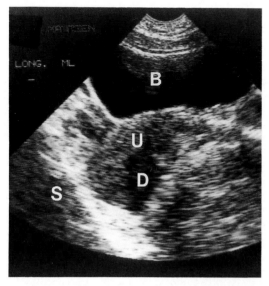

Figure 18–26. Longitudinal transabdominal scan of a retroverted uterus (U) demonstrating "dropout" (D) artifact in the uterine fundus. S, sacrum; B, bladder.

and dropout of sound may be made by the lack of displacement of the endometrial canal and the lack of a contour abnormality of the latter. Alternatively, dropout in the fundus of a retroverted uterus is usually not a problem in EVS (Fig. 18–27). The endovaginal approach may be used to assess the presence or absence of a fibroid when the fundus of a retroverted uterus is echo-poor on TAS.

The anterior surface of the uterus is covered with peritoneum to the level of the junction between the uterine corpus and cervix.[15] The peritoneal space anterior to the uterus is the vesicouterine pouch or anterior cul-de-sac (Fig. 18–25). This space is usually empty but may contain loops of small bowel. Posteriorly, the peritoneal reflection extends to the posterior fornix of the vagina, forming the posterior cul-de-sac. Laterally, the peritoneal membrane reflects to form the broad ligaments.

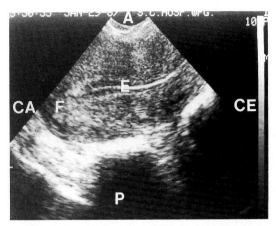

Figure 18–27. Endovaginal scan in the sagittal plane of a retroverted uterus. The fundus (F) is directed caudally and displayed on the left of the image. E, endometrium. Orientation: anterior (A), posterior (P), cephalad (CE), caudad (CA).

THE URETERS

The ureters are muscular tubes, measuring 25 to 30 cm in length in the adult. In the pelvis, the ureters course within the extraperitoneal areolar tissue. In the true pelvis, the ureter begins anterior to the internal iliac artery and posterior to the ovary (Fig. 18–28). From there it courses anteriorly and medially to lie within the inferior medial portion of the broad ligament, where it is in close proximity to the uterine artery. The ureter then runs anterior, situated in front of the lateral fornices of the vagina, about 2

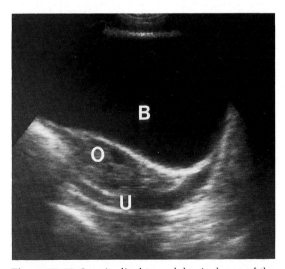

Figure 18–28. Longitudinal transabdominal scan of the right ovary (O) with a dilated ureter (U) demonstrated immediately posterior. B, bladder.

cm lateral to the supravaginal cervix, and then passes medially to enter the trigone of the bladder anterior to the vagina (Fig. 18–29).[17] The relationships of the ureter to the ovary, cervix, uterine artery, and vagina are of clinical importance because pelvic pathology may result in secondary hydronephrosis due to ureteric obstruction (Fig. 18–30). As a result, the authors routinely evaluate the kidneys after the postvoid examination during gynecologic sonography. This is done to confirm the presence of two kidneys, to assess their position, and to identify any degree of obstructive uropathy.

THE URINARY BLADDER

The bladder is a distensible reservoir for urine. Its shape depends on the degree of distention of itself and neighboring viscera. The bladder is fixed inferiorly at the urethral orifice, base, and angle, and as the bladder fills, the remainder of the walls displace movable viscera and conform to the space available within the confines of the true pelvis.[17] A transverse scan through the bladder superiorly gives it a rounded appearance. More inferiorly, the pelvic musculature and bones cause the bladder to appear square in the transverse plane. In the longitudinal plane, it is triangular in shape.[3]

The ureteric and urethral orifices are visualized at the base and neck of the bladder, respectively.

On occasion, centrally located cysts or large bladder diverticula may mimic the bladder in both appearance and position. The potential pitfall of mistaking a cyst for the urinary bladder can be avoided easily with the use of the postvoid examination.[5]

THE LIGAMENTS

The broad ligaments extend from the lateral aspect of the uterus to the lateral pelvic sidewalls (Fig. 18–23). The free border of the broad ligament contains the uterine tube. The broad ligaments may be identified sonographically when they are outlined by free intraperitoneal fluid (Fig. 18–31) or when the uterus is retroverted. The portion of the broad ligament between the fallopian tube and the ligament of the ovary and mesovarium is the mesosalpinx. The ovary is at-

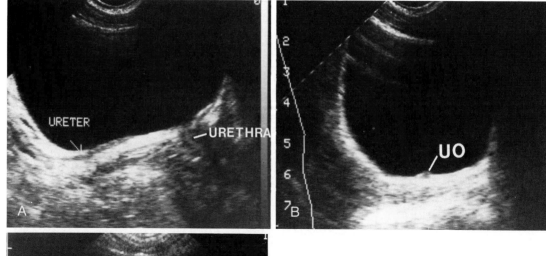

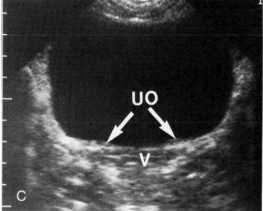

Figure 18–29. *A*, Longitudinal transabdominal scan of the right ureter and the urethra. *B*, Longitudinal transabdominal scan of the right ureteric orifice (UO). *C*, Transverse transabdominal scan of both ureteric orifices (UO). V, vagina.

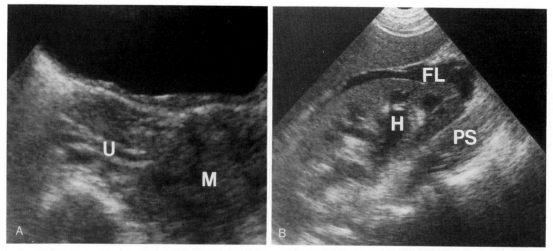

Figure 18–30. *A*, Longitudinal transabdominal scan of the distal right ureter (U). A mass (M) is noted encasing and obstructing the distal ureter in this patient with cervical carcinoma extending locally. *B*, Coronal scan of the right kidney. There is hydronephrosis (H) secondary to the distal ureteric obstruction. A urinoma (FL) is present within the perirenal space. PS, psoas major.

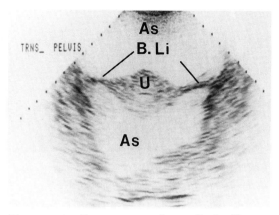

Figure 18–31. Transverse scan in a patient with gross ascites (As). The broad ligaments (B. Li) are well visualized. U, uterus.

tached to the posterior layer of the broad ligament by the mesovarium.[8, 15]

The portion of the ligament that extends from the infundibulum of the tube and upper pole of the ovary to the pelvic sidewall is referred to as the suspensory ligament of the ovary. In it course the ovarian vessels and nerves.

The round ligaments arise in the uterine cornua, anterior to the fallopian tubes in the broad ligaments, and extend anterolaterally to run beneath the inguinal ligament and insert into the fascia of the labia majora. The mesovarium, mesosalpinx, and round ligaments are not identified sonographically. The suspensory ligament of the ovary is usually not seen; however, the ovarian artery within the ligament may be identified occasionally by TAS or EVS.

THE RECTOSIGMOID COLON

The sigmoid colon begins at the inlet to the true pelvis and is extremely variable in length. It has a mesentery, and its course is variable, looping either to the left or right before ascending on the left to join the descending colon. The rectum begins at the third sacral vertebra and is fixed in position.[8]

The rectosigmoid colon usually contains gas and fecal material that cast an acoustic shadow and may make identification or differentiation from pelvic masses difficult. Often, the differentiation between a pelvic mass and the rectosigmoid colon can be made by real-time imaging if peristalsis can

be visualized. Occasionally, digital rectal, digital vaginal, or water enema combined with TAS may be necessary to distinguish between bowel contents and a mass.[18] Owing to the improved resolution afforded by EVS and the proximity of the transducer, differentiation between bowel contents and a mass is not usually a problem if the endovaginal approach is used.

References

1. Hagen-Ansert SL, Ezo MG, Kurtz AB: Techniques of ultrasound pelvic examination. Semin Ultrasound 1:10, 1980.
2. Deutsch AL, Gosink BB: Normal female pelvic anatomy. Semin Roentgenol 17:241, 1982.
3. Kurtz AB, Rifkin MD: Normal anatomy of the female pelvis. *In* Callen PW (ed): Ultrasonography in Obstetrics and Gynecology. Philadelphia, WB Saunders Co, 1983, pp 193–208.
4. Osteology: Skeleton of lower limb. *In* Williams PM, Warwick R (eds): Gray's Anatomy, 36th Ed. Edinburgh, Churchill Livingstone, 1980, pp 378–390.
5. Fiske CE, Callen PW: Fluid collections ultrasonically simulating urinary bladder. J Can Assoc Radiol 31:254, 1980.
6. Levi CS, Lyons EA, Schollenberg J, Bristowe JRB: The value of post void scans in the diagnosis of ruptured ectopic pregnancy. J Ultrasound Med 1:253, 1982.
7. Myology: Fasciae and muscles of the trunk. *In* Williams PM, Warwick R (eds): Gray's Anatomy, 36th Ed. Edinburgh, Churchill Livingstone, 1980, pp 551–564.
8. Gardner E, Gray DJ, O'Rahilly R: The pelvis. *In* Anatomy: A Regional Study of Human Structure, 5th Ed. Philadelphia, WB Saunders Co, 1986, pp 445–512.
9. Benson M: Rectus sheath haematomas simulating pelvic pathology: The ultrasound appearances. Clin Radiol 33:651, 1982.
10. Spring DB, Deshon GE Jr, Babu S: The sonographic appearance of fluid in the prevesical space. Radiology 147:205, 1983.
11. Myology: Fasciae and muscles of the lower limb. *In* Williams PM, Warwick R (eds): Gray's Anatomy, 36th Ed. Edinburgh, Churchill Livingstone, 1980, pp 593–595.
12. Angiology: Iliac arterial system. *In* Williams PM, Warwick R (eds): Gray's Anatomy, 36th Ed. Edinburgh, Churchill Livingstone, 1980, pp 719–724.
13. Angiology: Veins of the abdomen and pelvis. *In* Williams PM, Warwick R (eds): Gray's Anatomy, 36th Ed. Edinburgh, Churchill Livingstone, 1980, pp 759–765.
14. Angiology: The lymphatic drainage of the abdomen and pelvis. *In* Williams PM, Warwick R (eds): Gray's Anatomy, 36th Ed. Edinburgh, Churchill Livingstone, 1980, pp 793–798.
15. Splanchnology: Reproductive organs of the female. *In* Williams PM, Warwick R (eds): Gray's Anatomy,

36th Ed. Edinburgh. Churchill Livingstone, 1980, pp 1423–1433.

16. Hall DH: Sonographic appearance of the normal ovary, of polycystic ovary disease, and of functional ovarian cysts. Semin Ultrasound 4:149, 1983.

17. Splanchnology: The urinary organs. *In* Williams PM, Warwick R, (eds): Gray's Anatomy, 36th Ed. Edinburgh, Churchill Livingstone, 1980, 1387–1423.

18. Bluth EJ, Ferrari BT, Sullivan MA: Real-time pelvic ultrasonography as an adjunct to digital examination. Radiology 153:789, 1984.

19

ULTRASOUND EVALUATION OF THE UTERUS

Peter L. Cooperberg, M.D.
Maria R. Kidney, M.B.

The accuracy of ultrasound in diagnosing uterine abnormalities has been well established.[3, 9, 22, 24, 46] Ultrasound is particularly well suited to examine the uterus. The filled urinary bladder can displace bowel gas and provides an excellent acoustic window to visualize the more deeply seated uterus and adnexal structures. As the uterus is a relatively homogeneous organ, ultrasound can easily detect focal areas of inhomogeneity, as well as abnormalities of size and shape. In addition to transabdominal sonography, endovaginal scanning is now becoming a useful adjunct in the evaluation of the uterus and adnexal structures. Rarely, hysterosalpingography, or even computed tomography and magnetic resonance imaging, can be performed for further evaluation, but most of the time, ultrasound suffices for a definitive diagnosis.

In this chapter, the ultrasonographic examination of the uterus is reviewed. Ultrasonography of the normal uterus, developmental anomalies, and benign and malignant disease processes of the uterus are discussed. Pregnancy and its complications are discussed elsewhere in this text, as is gestational trophoblastic disease.

METHOD

In preparation, the patient requires a distended urinary bladder. An empty bladder and gas in the sigmoid colon or small bowel completely obscure the underlying pelvic structures. In addition, the uterus would be anteflexed, and the sound beam would have to travel from the fundus to the cervix.

With a filled urinary bladder, not only is the bowel displaced, but the uterus is displaced posteriorly so that it can be viewed from the anterior through to the posterior surface. As the uterus is displaced approximately 5 to 10 cm from the abdominal wall, it lies in an appropriate focal zone for most real-time transducers. Usually, a 3.5 MHz transducer has the appropriate focal zone. Although the urine-filled bladder can be penetrated by a 5 MHz transducer, these commonly have a shorter focal zone than is necessary to see the deeper structures. The pelvis is examined in a sagittal plane of section to visualize the long axis of the uterus (Fig. 19–1A). It may be necessary to angle the plane of section obliquely somewhat to the right or the left in order to line up the fundus with the cervix. The central

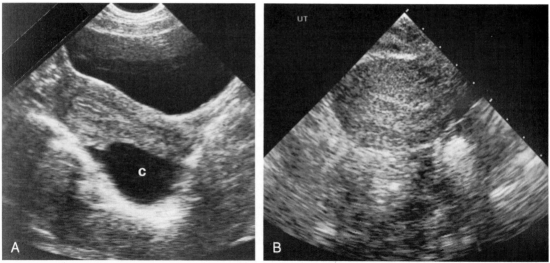

Figure 19–1. *A*, Sagittal transabdominal scan of a normal uterus with fluid in the cul-de-sac (c), showing one example of the endometrial echo complex: echogenic line *(arrow)*, echo-poor halo, echogenic oval, and slightly echo-poor halo around that. *B*, Endovaginal scan showing a normal uterine corpus with the endometrial echo complex as a single echogenic line *(arrow)*.

uterine cavity echo should be carefully sought. The plane of section is then swept from side to side to visualize the entire volume of the uterus. The transducer is then rotated into a transverse direction to thoroughly examine the short axis of the uterus from the fundus to the cervix and back.

For endovaginal scanning, a full bladder is not required. On the contrary, an empty bladder is preferable so that the uterus resumes its normal anteverted position. Dedicated real-time transducers, either phased-array or mechanical sector scanners, attached to a long handle are now available. With a protective sheath over the transducer, it is introduced through the introitus approximately 6 to 10 cm into the vagina. The best view of the uterus is obtained when the transducer is more superficial and not advanced into the posterior fornix of the vagina. On the sagittal view, the fundus of the uterus lies just under the abdominal wall, which is displayed toward the left side of the screen (Fig. 19–1*B*). By turning the transducer 90° in a counterclockwise fashion, coronal sections are obtained. Since the uterus is anteverted, the fundus and body lie in an anteroposterior plane. Therefore, the coronal sections give images equivalent to the transverse scans of transabdominal sonography.

THE NORMAL UTERUS AND ITS ULTRASONOGRAPHIC APPEARANCE

Position

On transabdominal scanning, the uterus lies between the distended bladder anteriorly and the rectum posteriorly. The cervix generally lies in the midline, but the fundus of the uterus commonly lies obliquely to the right or left of the midline, even in the absence of pelvic disease.[39]

Size

Although the size of the uterus varies widely, especially dependent upon the parity of the patient, the usual maximal postpubertal size is approximately 7 by 4 by 5 cm.[4, 25, 31, 39] It is said that multiparity increases the normal size by 1 to 2 cm in all directions.[31] The prepubertal uterus is significantly smaller, measuring approximately 3 cm in length by 1 cm in width and depth.[25, 29] Postmenopausally, the uterus atrophies with a range of 1 to 2 cm in thickness and 3 to 7 cm in length.[31]

The most common postpubertal causes of enlarged uterus are pregnancy and uterine leiomyomas.[14]

Shape

Prior to puberty, the body of the uterus accounts for only one-third of the length, with the cervix accounting for the other two-thirds.[39] Subsequently, post puberty, the fundus lengthens out of proportion to the cervix and reverses this ratio.

Version and Flexion

With an empty bladder, the uterus is anteverted so that the fundus lies almost directly anterior or even anteroinferior to the cervix (Fig. 19–2A). With the distended bladder, the uterus is in varying degrees of slight anteversion. Similarly, the uterus that is retroverted on palpation with an empty bladder can be pulled by the round liga-

ments into a more normal position with a full bladder (Fig. 19–2B, C). Less commonly, the fundus of the uterus may be retropositioned even with a full bladder (Fig. 19–3).

There are two types of uterine retroposition. If the entire uterus is tilted backward from a fulcrum at the cervix, it is *retroverted*. In *retroflexion*, only the body and fundus of the uterus are flexed posteriorly. Although the two are often indistinguishable sonographically, sometimes retroflexion can be diagnosed when a "fold" is seen between the cervix and the fundus along the posterior aspect (Fig. 19–2B).[23] Retroverted or retroflexed gravid uteri typically become anteverted during the third month of pregnancy. Adhesions may prevent spontaneous reduction, and if manual repositioning is not performed, abortion or even uterine rupture may occasionally result.[19] Because the fun-

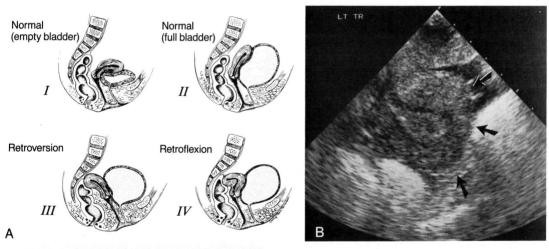

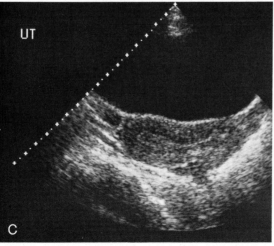

Figure 19–2. *A,* Alterations in uterine position. The normal position (I) of the uterus in 80 percent of women is anteverted with a mild degree of anteflexion (II). In retroversion, the long axis of the uterus and cervix points more posteriorly than the long axis of the vagina (III). In retroflexion, the body of the uterus is angled posteriorly relative to the cervix (IV). *B,* Endovaginal scan showing retroflexion of the uterus. Note that the fundus of the uterus *(arrows)* is pointing posteriorly with the empty bladder. There is a small amount of fluid in the cul-de-sac in the fold between the corpus and the cervix. *C,* Transabdominal scan with a full bladder, showing that the uterus is no longer retroverted, presumably because of the tension on the round ligaments by the filled urinary bladder.

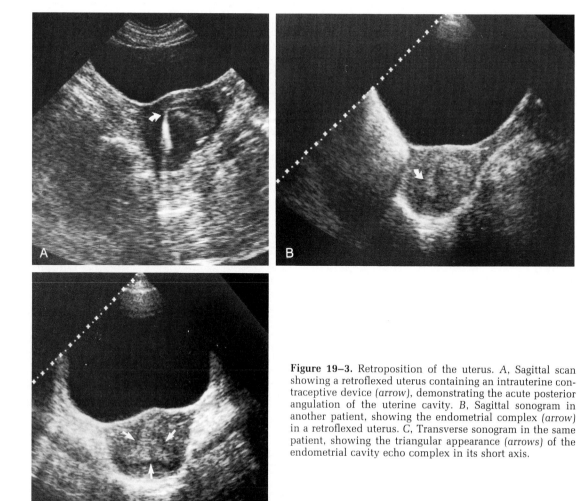

Figure 19–3. Retroposition of the uterus. *A*, Sagittal scan showing a retroflexed uterus containing an intrauterine contraceptive device *(arrow)*, demonstrating the acute posterior angulation of the uterine cavity. *B*, Sagittal sonogram in another patient, showing the endometrial complex *(arrow)* in a retroflexed uterus. *C*, Transverse sonogram in the same patient, showing the triangular appearance *(arrows)* of the endometrial cavity echo complex in its short axis.

dus of the uterus is situated farther from the transducer and may be partially shadowed by the remainder of the uterus, it can simulate uterine fibroids. On the other hand, leiomyomas may distort the uterine shape and simulate a retroverted uterus. Alterations in shape also occur with various congenital uterine anomalies.

Texture

The myometrium is normally homogeneous with low- to moderate-level echogenicity (Fig. 19–1*A*, *B*). Focal echo-poor areas may be noted, which can be due to leiomy-

omas. Occasionally, small fibroids may be more echogenic or even calcified in the myometrium. There are various types of shadowing that can interfere with the normal homogeneity of the myometrial echoes. Frequently, the sound traversing the oblique bladder–uterine interface can cause a broad refractive shadow through the lower portion of the uterus. Also, as mentioned above, the fundus of a retroverted uterus may appear more echo-poor. Focal cystic areas in the periphery can be due to uterine varices (Fig. 19–4).[12] Chronic inflammation of the cervix may result in trapping of mucous secretions and the formation of nabothian retention cysts (Fig. 19–5).[11]

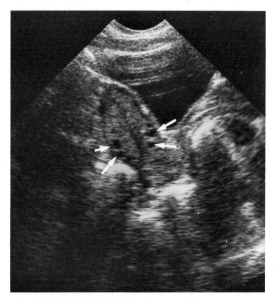

Figure 19–4. Sagittal scan of a normal uterus showing cystic areas in the periphery *(arrows)*. These interconnected, and Doppler examination confirmed that they were venous structures. They are referred to as uterine varices but are not necessarily abnormal.

Central Endometrial Echo Complex

ENDOMETRIAL CAVITY. The normal central uterine cavity is seen as a moderate- to high-amplitude thin echogenic line. This should be seen in virtually all normal women provided there is no intrauterine gestation and the uterus is slightly anteverted. The high amplitude of the echo is due to the specular reflection from the large perpendicular surfaces of the endometrial cavity. If the long axis of the uterus is rotated to the right or left, the endometrial cavity echo will only be seen if the plane of section is appropriately angled. Similarly, it is not always seen with a retroverted or retroflexed uterus since the endometrial cavity may be almost parallel to the sound beam.[2]

ENDOMETRIUM. The zone surrounding the central uterine cavity echo is now known to correspond histologically to the endometrium (Fig. 19–6).[10] The thickness of the endometrium is normally 2 to 4 mm in the proliferative phase and approximately 5 to 6 mm in the secretory phase.[8]

In postmenopausal patients in the absence of estrogen replacement treatment, the endometrium, when visualized, is thinner, measuring 1 to 3 mm.[10] An endometrial echo of greater than 5 mm should be considered abnormal, and further investigation, such as dilatation and curettage, is warranted in the postmenopausal patient. An irregular outline to an enlarged endometrial echo also suggests abnormality. Endometrial carcinoma and hyperplasia are common causes of this finding.[16]

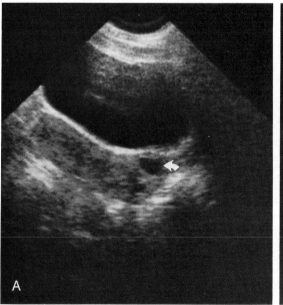

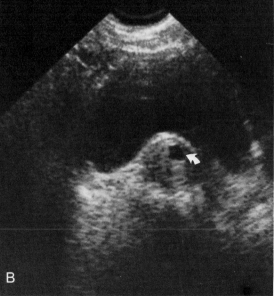

Figure 19–5. Sagittal *(A)* and transverse *(B)* scans showing a small nabothian cyst *(arrow)* in the anterior lip of the cervix.

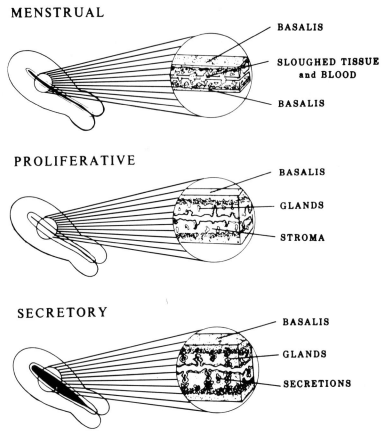

Figure 19–6. Diagram of the major phases of endometrial development. In the menstrual phase, the endometrium appears as a thin, irregular interface. In the proliferative phase, the endometrium is relatively hypoechoic, probably because of the straight and orderly arrangement of glandular elements. In the secretory phase, the endometrium achieves its maximal thickness and echogenicity. This appearance probably arises from the distended and tortuous glands that contain echogenic secretions. (*Reprinted with permission from* Fleisher AC, Entman SS, Kalemeris GE: Ultrasound Med Biol 12:271, copyright 1986, Pergamon Journals, Ltd.)

ECHO-POOR HALO. In the premenopausal patient, an echo-poor halo is often seen surrounding the endometrium. Although this was previously thought to represent the endometrium, correlation with histopathology indicates that this "halo" most likely represents a network of capillaries and veins around the muscle fibers in the inner, relatively compact, layer of the myometrium.[6] This is most commonly seen in postovulatory and premenstrual portions of the cycle.[35]

The endometrial echo complex should be seen in most patients and helps to identify the sites of early pregnancy, decidual reaction, or endometrial abnormalities. Furthermore, the identification of the endometrial cavity echo complex helps one to differentiate the uterus definitively from any adnexal masses that may occasionally simulate the uterus. Usually, adnexal lesions are clearly separate from the uterus. However, occasionally it is difficult to differentiate an adnexal mass from a mass of uterine origin. The identification of the relationship of the endometrial cavity echo to the mass can help in this determination. For example, a pelvic mass that touches the endometrial echo must be uterine in origin.

The endometrial cavity echo is normally central within the uterus. Any deviation of this line suggests the presence of leiomyomas, adenomyosis, or other masses.

DEVELOPMENTAL VARIANTS

The uterus is derived from the paired müllerian ducts. The cranial ends of the ducts form the ostia of the fallopian tubes;

the caudal ends fuse to form the uterus.[18] The overall incidence of congenital uterine abnormalities is less than 1 percent. A higher incidence has been reported in women undergoing hysterosalpingography.[28, 48]

Uterine malformations can be classified according to the development of the müllerian ducts:

1. Arrested development of the müllerian ducts.
   a. Uterine aplasia—bilateral arrested development.
   b. Uterus unicornis unicollis—unilateral arrested development.
2. Failure of fusion of the müllerian ducts.
   a. Uterus didelphys—total failure of fusion (two vaginas, two cervices, two uterine bodies).
   b. Uterus bicornis bicollis—partial fusion (one vagina, two cervices, two uterine bodies).
   c. Uterus bicornis unicollis—partial fusion (one vagina, one cervix, two uterine horns).

d. Uterus arcuatus—near complete fusion.
3. Incomplete resorption of the sagittal septum.
   a. Uterus septus—nonresorption of the septum.
   b. Uterus subseptus—partial resorption of the septum.
4. Miscellaneous defects, including various anomalies of shape.

Some of these malformations are illustrated in Figure 19–7.

Uterine anomalies may be associated with sterility or increased incidence of spontaneous abortion. Renal agenesis occurs throughout the range of uterine malformations. This is virtually always ipsilateral.[17] All patients with uterine anomalies should undergo sonographic examination of the kidneys and vice versa.

Anomalies of the nongravid uterus are occasionally detected on ultrasound.[26, 33] This is easiest if two endometrial cavity echo complexes can be seen (Fig. 19–8). Most

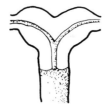

Uterus didelphys bicollis

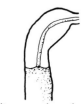

Uterus bicornis bicollis

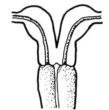

Uterus bicornis unicollis

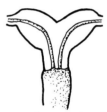

Uterus unicornis

Figure 19–7. Diagram of the more commonly diagnosed uterine anomalies.

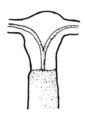

Uterus subseptus

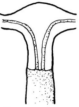

Uterus septus

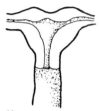

Uterus arcuatus

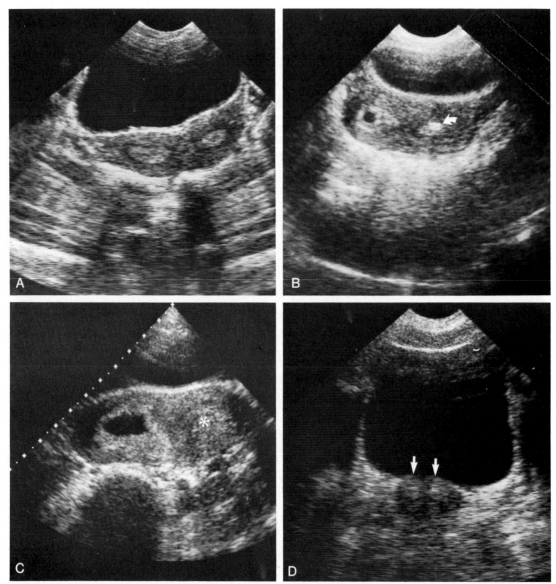

Figure 19–8. Bicornuate uterus. *A,* Transverse scan showing double prominent endometrial echo complexes. *B,* Transverse scan showing an early gestational sac in the right horn and an intrauterine contraceptive device in the left horn *(arrow).* *C,* Transverse scan showing a nonviable early gestation in the right horn. In this case, the left horn *(asterisk)* could be confused with a fibroid. *D,* Transverse scan showing an artifactual double cervix *(arrows)* caused by the rectus muscle refraction. (*From* Müller NL, Cooperberg PL, Rowley VA, et al: Utrasonic reflection by the rectus abdominis muscles: The double image artifact. J Ultrasound Med 3:515, 1984.)

Figure 19–9. *A,* Sagittal transabdominal scan showing an echo-poor fibroid *(arrow),* 1 cm in diameter, in the posterior myometrium. *B,* Endovaginal scan showing a 1 cm posterior echo-poor subserous fibroid *(arrows).* *C,* Echo-poor fibroid arising from the posterior aspect of the lower uterus. *D,* Echo-poor fibroid, with considerable sound attenuation (shadowing), causing bladder indentation. *E,* Subserous fibroid with peripheral calcification *(arrows).* Note that the fibroid extends almost to the endometrial cavity echo *(curved arrow).* *F,* Pedunculated fibroid with peripheral calcification arising anteriorly and displacing the fundus *(arrows)* posteriorly.

Illustration continued on page 402

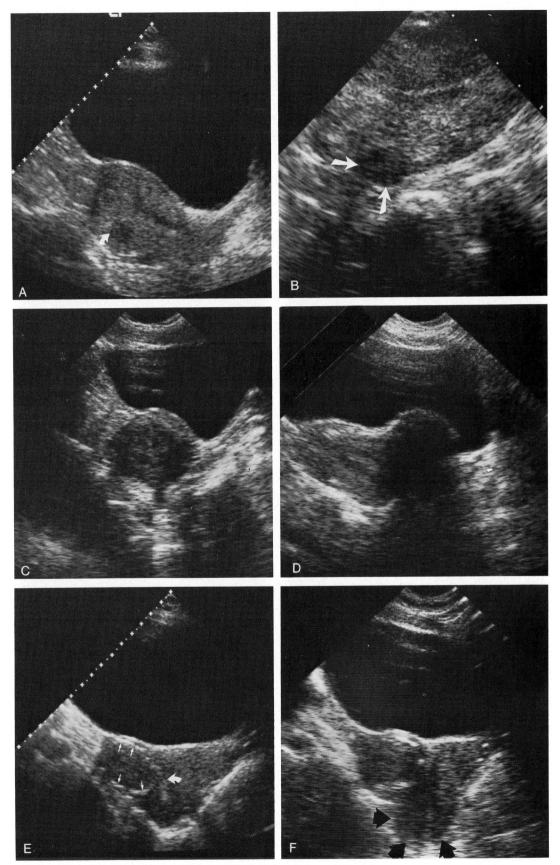

Figure 19–9 See legend on opposite page

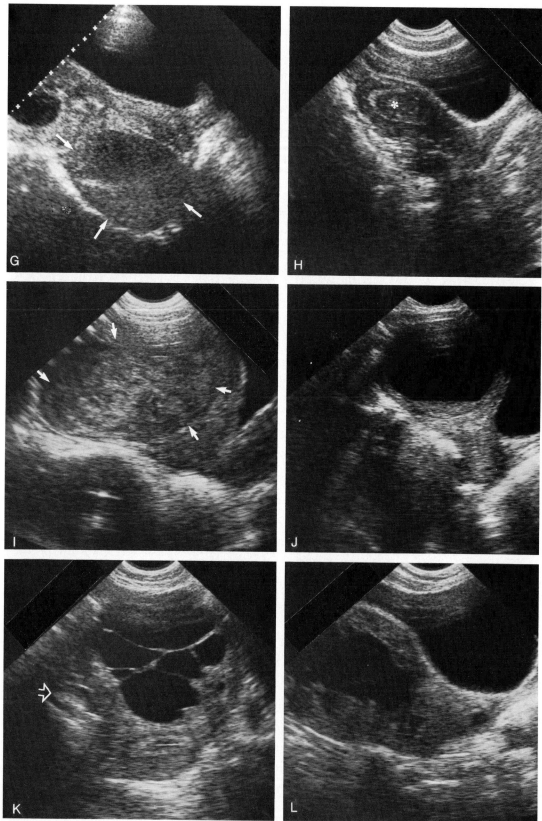

Figure 19–9 *Continued G,* Large echo-poor pedunculated fibroid *(arrows)* presenting as a retrocervical mass in a pregnant patient. *H,* Submucous fibroid *(asterisk)* arising from the anterior myometrium and splaying the endometrial cavity complex around it (mimicking an endometrial polyp). *I,* Large echogenic submucous fibroid *(arrows). J,* Fundal fibroid with cystic degeneration and dependent layering of debris. *K,* Cystic degeneration with septations in a fundal fibroid. Note the endometrial echo complex *(arrow)* deep to the lesion. *L,* Cystic degeneration in a fibroid mimicking hematometra.

commonly, these anomalies are first appreciated in early pregnancy when a gestational sac can be seen in one horn and a decidual reaction in the other.[28] It is important not to confuse a bicornuate uterus with a fibroid, an adnexal mass, or an ectopic pregnancy. A very rare mimic of an adnexal cystic structure would be a didelphic uterus with an obstructed hydrometra on one side.

It is important to be aware of a double uterus if an IUD is going to be used for contraception since two will be necessary (a Copper-14).

Occasionally, a refractive artifact can simulate a double cervix (Fig. 19–8D).[32]

ACQUIRED UTERINE DISORDERS

Neoplasms

LEIOMYOMA. Leiomyoma (Fig. 19–9) is a common benign neoplasm of the uterus, occurring in approximately 40 percent of women over 35 years of age.[13] Leiomyomas are usually multiple and most commonly asymptomatic.[27] The most frequent symptoms are pain and uterine bleeding. Although myomas may impair fertility or pregnancy, they more commonly do not interfere with the normal course of pregnancy.[18] Myomas are classified as submucosal (submucous), intramural, and subserosal (subserous). Submucosal fibroids are least common but are the most likely to produce symptoms,[44] to become infected, and to undergo sarcomatous change.[18] Intramural fibroids are the most common type. Subserosal fibroids are frequently pedunculated and may simulate adnexal masses.[13] Broad ligament myomas may also simulate adnexal masses. Cervical myomas are rare (Fig. 19–9G).

Myomas undergo a spectrum of secondary changes that include hyaline degeneration, fatty degeneration, calcification, hemorrhage, and necrosis. The sonographic appearance of a myoma depends on its location, the presence or absence of secondary change, and also the relative amounts of its stromal and muscular constituents.[44] It is not surprising, therefore, that fibroids can have a wide variety of appearances sonographically. Classically, a myoma is hypoechoic, with relatively poor sound through transmission (Fig. 19–9A, B, C, D). However,

it is most commonly identified by a deformation of the contour (Fig. 19–9C, D). The uterus may be markedly increased in size, with an inhomogeneous texture (Fig. 19–9I). Focal areas of increased echogenicity, particularly with shadows, indicate calcification, which is common in fibroids in older women (Fig. 19–9E). Alternatively, degeneration and necrosis may result in decreased echogenicity and increased through transmission,[15] progressing to a frankly cystic center (Fig. 19–9J, K, L).[21] The fundus of a retroverted uterus typically appears hypoechoic, and a lobular contour is common, so that myomas are more difficult to diagnose in these patients (Fig. 19–9F).

Although the etiology of myomas is not established, they are clearly stimulated by estrogens.[13] Myomas may grow rapidly during anovulatory menstrual cycles,[43] and most myomas increase in size during pregnancy.[15] "Young" fibroids are composed homogeneously of fibrous and smooth muscle cells, giving them a relatively hypoechoic and attenuating sonographic appearance. When they start to degenerate, tiny cystic areas appear within them that cause increased echogenicity with increased through transmission. This may occur during pregnancy. Large lower uterine or cervical myomas may mechanically block vaginal delivery.[18] Otherwise, even very large myomas may be compatible with uncomplicated pregnancy and normal vaginal delivery.

Myomas rarely develop in postmenopausal patients. Most tumors typically stabilize or diminish in size after menopause.[18] Occasionally, the degeneration results in large clumps of calcification that can be easily seen, even on a plain radiograph of the pelvis. Postmenopausal increase in size of the uterus may result from secondary changes but should always cause one to suspect sarcomatous degeneration.[27] This is very rare.

ENDOMETRIAL POLYPS. The common endometrial polyp (Fig. 19–10) is composed of hyperplastic or adenomatous endometrial tissue that is unresponsive to progesterone. Although most polyps are asymptomatic, the usual symptom is uterine bleeding. In rare cases, a polyp will have a pedicle long enough to allow it to protrude beyond the cervix or even the vagina. Polyps may occur at any age but are somewhat more common at or near menopause. Although they rarely

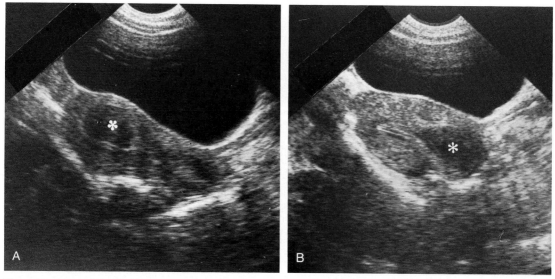

Figure 19–10. *A, B,* Sagittal scans, three months apart, in a woman diagnosed originally as having an echo-poor submucous fibroid *(asterisk).* In the follow-up examination *(B),* this structure was clearly seen to move, indicating it to be an endometrial polyp.

undergo malignant degeneration,[18] endometrial cancers may be polypoid. Submucosal leiomyomas may also be pedunculated and present as polypoid lesions. Sonographically, polyps usually cause a prominent endometrial echo complex. Occasionally, they may actually be seen as a discrete mass within the endometrial cavity and may even cause uterine enlargement.

ENDOMETRIAL CARCINOMA. Carcinoma of the endometrium (Fig. 19–11) most commonly presents with postmenopausal bleeding. The etiology is unknown, but the tumor seems to be associated with estrogen stimulation that occurs with nulliparity, failure of ovulation, late menopause, and obesity.[13] If the postmenopausal bleeding occurs early in the course of the endometrial carcinoma, only a prominent endometrial echo complex may be seen.[36] This should arouse more suspicion in a postmenopausal patient than would the similar-appearing luteal phase endometrium in a premenopausal woman. Occasionally, local invasion can be demonstrated.[7, 10] At a later stage, endometrial carcinoma may be seen as an enlarged uterus with irregular areas of low-level echoes and, occasionally, focal areas of high-intensity echoes (Fig. 19–11*A, B, C*). This appearance may simulate leiomyomas. Indeed, a significant percentage of patients with endometrial carcinomas have concomitant leiomyomas, making the distinction difficult sonographically.

Nevertheless, ultrasound has a role in the assessment of endometrial carcinoma by helping to separate carcinoma limited to the uterus (Stages I and II) from carcinoma extending beyond the uterus (Stages III and IV). Endometrial carcinoma may obstruct the endometrial cavity, resulting in hydrometra, pyometra, or hematometra.[36, 41] However, it should be noted that patients with endometrial carcinoma may even have a normal pelvic sonogram.[36]

LEIOMYOSARCOMA. This is a rare condition, accounting for only 3 percent of uterine tumors.[44] Most leiomyosarcomas are believed to arise from pre-existing leiomyomas. Uterine bleeding is the usual symptom, but, often, patients are asymptomatic. Sonographically, these tumors commonly have areas of cystic degeneration; however, in the absence of local invasion or distant metastases, they are indistinguishable from myomas. Leiomyosarcoma is rarely diagnosed preoperatively.[18]

CERVICAL CARCINOMA. Formerly, cervical carcinoma was the most common invasive gynecologic neoplasm. Thanks to widespread screening of exfoliative cytology (the Pap smear and the diagnostic and therapeutic cone biopsy), this disease has greatly decreased in incidence. When it is not detected earlier, as carcinoma in situ, it presents in the perimenopausal age group. The etiology is unknown but is thought to be multifactorial. Sonographically, one may see

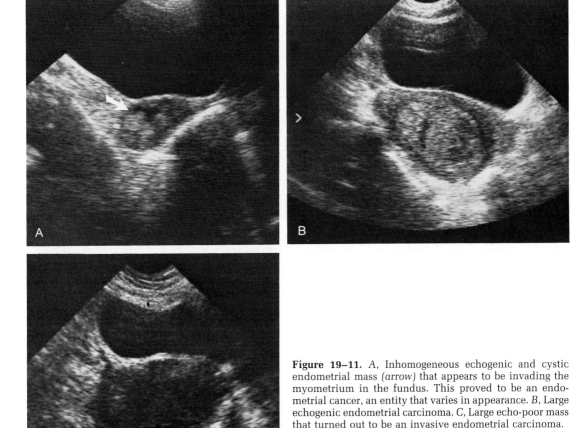

Figure 19–11. A, Inhomogeneous echogenic and cystic endometrial mass *(arrow)* that appears to be invading the myometrium in the fundus. This proved to be an endometrial cancer, an entity that varies in appearance. B, Large echogenic endometrial carcinoma. C, Large echo-poor mass that turned out to be an invasive endometrial carcinoma.

a solid retrovesical mass that is indistinguishable from a cervical myoma.[45] Patients are infrequently referred for sonographic examination when a cervical lesion is suspected on speculum examination. Ultrasound may be useful for staging cervical carcinoma by the detection of involvement of the pelvic sidewalls or extension into the bladder.[14] However, computed tomography is preferable for staging.[44] Magnetic resonance imaging may also be useful. Cervical carcinoma may also cause hematometra. Rarely, other lesions may arise in the cervix (Fig. 19–12).

Non-neoplastic Disorders

ENDOMETRIAL HYPERPLASIA. Endometrial hyperplasia (Fig. 19–13) is caused by unopposed estrogen stimulation and is the most common cause of uterine bleeding. It occurs during the menstrual years as well as in postmenopausal women. On curettage in most patients, the microscopic pattern is frankly benign. Adenomatous hyperplasia, characterized by glandular proliferation, occurs in a small percentage of patients. When there is associated cellular atypia, the his-

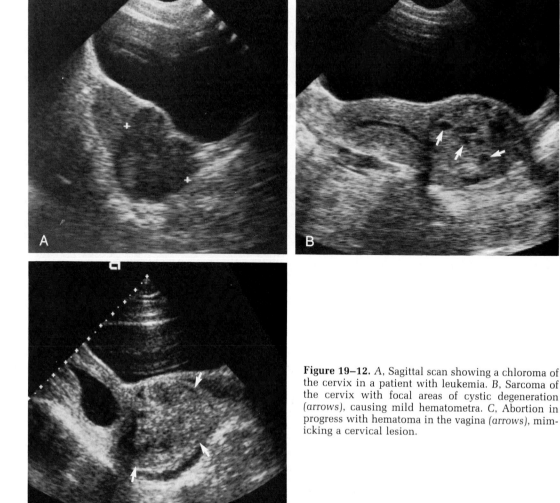

Figure 19–12. *A*, Sagittal scan showing a chloroma of the cervix in a patient with leukemia. *B*, Sarcoma of the cervix with focal areas of cystic degeneration (*arrows*), causing mild hematometra. *C*, Abortion in progress with hematoma in the vagina (*arrows*), mimicking a cervical lesion.

tologic appearance may be difficult to separate from endometrial carcinoma.[18]

Sonographically, endometrial hyperplasia presents with the same prominent central uterine cavity echo complex that can be seen with an endometrial polyp or endometrial carcinoma.[16]

ADENOMYOSIS. Adenomyosis refers to a form of endometriosis wherein glandular tissue or stroma from the basal layer of the endometrium invades the myometrium.[37] Most commonly, this invasion by nests of endometrial tissue results in diffuse uterine enlargement, with a normal central cavity echo complex, normal echo texture of the myometrium, and normal uterine contour.

Only occasionally is adenomyosis focal. In these cases, contour abnormality with preservation of the endometrial echo complex is seen.[5] However, it is is not always possible to differentiate these from leiomyomas. Indeed, leiomyomas, endometriosis, or endometrial hyperplasia commonly are coexistent. In patients with accompanying leiomyomas, the concurrent adenomyosis is usually masked sonographically.[42]

The exact significance of adenomyosis is dubious, and it is likely that the symptoms (such as dysfunctional uterine bleeding, dysmenorrhea, and similar conditions) may be attributable to other coexisting entities.[34]

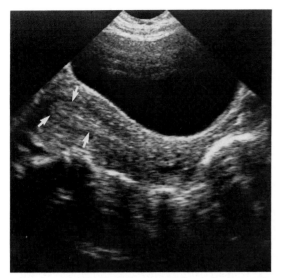

Figure 19–13. Endometrial hyperplasia. Note the prominent endometrial echo complex *(arrows)*. This patient was postmenopausal. In a menstruating female, a luteal phase endometrium can appear identical.

HYDROMETRA, PYOMETRA, AND HEMATOMETRA. Obstruction of the genital tract by an imperforate hymen causes accumulation of secretions in the vagina and uterus, which is called hydrometrocolpos (Fig. 19–14*A*).[47] If the obstruction is at the level of the cervix, there will be fluid distention of the uterus, called hydrometra. Superimposed infection is called pyometra (Fig. 19–14*B*). After puberty, menstruation results in hematometra. In the young patient, the usual cause is an intact hymen, vaginal membrane, or vaginal atresia.[47] In the older age group, hematometra usually results from uterine or cervical malignant disease or from radiation-induced cervical stenosis. Sonographically, there is cystic distention of the endometrial cavity. There may be layering of echogenic material. Occasionally, the fluid may be so echogenic as to be indistinguishable from an endometrial polyp or endometrial cancer (Fig. 19–14*C, D, E*).[38] Retained products of concep-

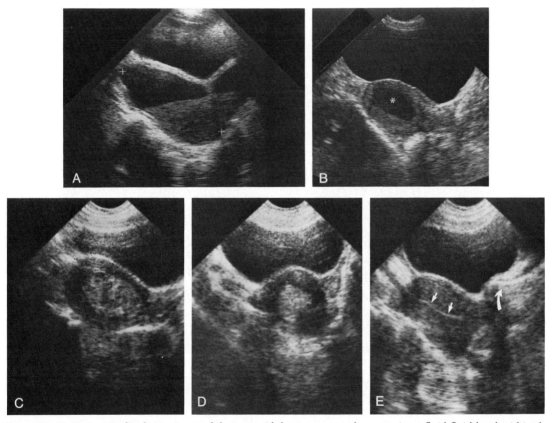

Figure 19–14. *A*, Longitudinal scan in an adolescent with hematometrocolpos causing a fluid-fluid level within the vagina and uterus. *B*, Sagittal scan in a patient with pyometra *(asterisk)* secondary to cervical carcinoma, which was not identified during this scan or even on dilatation and curettage (D&C). It was diagnosed on hysterectomy specimen. *C, D, E*, Hematometra with cervical stenosis, showing very echogenic blood longitudinally *(C)* and transversely *(D)*. At D&C, only cervical stenosis was found. Postoperatively, only a thin endometrial echo *(arrows)* was identified *(E)*. Note, incidentally, the tampon in the vagina *(curved arrow)*.

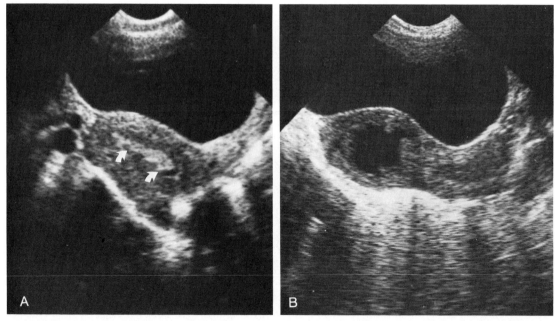

Figure 19–15. Retained products of conception. *A,* Longitudinal scan showing echogenic material and a small amount of fluid *(arrows)* in the uterus after therapeutic abortion. *B,* Sagittal scan showing a large collection of fluid in the uterus after spontaneous abortion.

tion after delivery, or, more commonly, after spontaneous or therapeutic abortion, may be seen as echogenic material in the endometrial cavity (Fig. 19–15A), or it may mimic hematometra (Fig. 19–15B). Calcification can occasionally be found in the endometrial cavity in Asherman's syndrome (Fig. 19–16).

INCOMPETENT CERVIX. Incompetent cervix is a premature dilatation of the endocervical canal in pregnancy before the onset of labor.[20] Causes include previous obstetric trauma, previous dilatation and curettage or cone biopsy, and anatomic variations leading to defective structure of the cervical

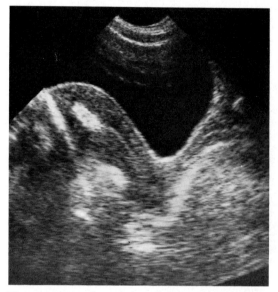

Figure 19–16. Asherman's syndrome. Large echogenic calcified collection in the uterus of a patient with a history of three therapeutic abortions.

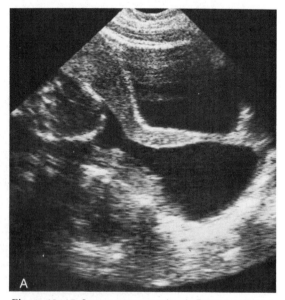

Figure 19–17. Incompetent cervix. *A,* Pregnant patient with the amniotic membrane and fluid projecting through the endocervical canal into the vagina.

Illustration continued on opposite page

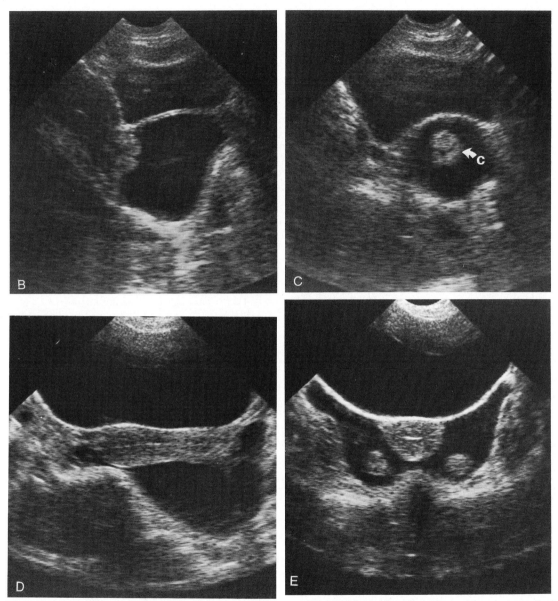

Figure 19–17 *Continued*. Sagittal *(B)* and transverse *(C)* scans of fluid in the vagina of a patient with a vesicovaginal fistula and well-developed vaginal muscles to provide relative urinary continence. C, cervix. Sagittal *(D)* and transverse *(E)* scans showing a normal uterus with a large collection of fluid in the cul-de-sac extending into the retrovaginal area. Cases *B* through *E* should not be confused with amniotic fluid prolapse.

ring.[40] The incompetent cervix may cause mid-trimester spontaneous abortion[29] or result in preterm delivery.[30] If the diagnosis can be established early, cervical cerclage may save the pregnancy.[40]

Detection of the incompetent cervix by ultrasound is based on the demonstration of a shortened (< 3 cm) cervix,[1] sometimes with fluid or fetal parts in the endocervical canal.[20] It is important to scan the patient with an incompletely filled bladder, since an overly distended bladder may compress the opposing walls of the lower uterine segment, simulating a long cervix. When incompetent cervix is a clinical consideration, scans after partial emptying of the bladder must be obtained. Definite evidence of an incompetent cervix is the appearance of fluid-containing membranes protruding through the endocervical canal (Fig. 19–17).[30] This may be a separate entity representing the sonographic picture of abortion in progress.[29]

In conclusion, ultrasound has proved particularly useful in the diagnosis and evaluation of a wide variety of uterine abnormalities. As in other areas of the body, ultrasound is not necessarily specific and frequently cannot differentiate benign from malignant neoplasms. There is a definite but limited role for ultrasound in the staging of uterine malignancies.

References

1. Bernstine RL, Lee SH, Crawford WL, et al: Sonographic evaluation of the incompetent cervix. JCU 9:417, 1981.
2. Callen PW, DeMartini WJ, Filly RA: The central uterine cavity echo: A useful anatomic sign in the ultrasonographic evaluation of the female pelvis. Radiology 131:187, 1979.
3. Cochrane WJ, Thomas MA: Ultrasound diagnosis of gynecologic pelvic masses. Radiology 110:649, 1974.
4. Callen PW: Ultrasonographic evaluation of pelvic disease. In Goldberg HI (ed): Interventional Radiology and Diagnostic Imaging Modalities. Department of Radiology, University of California, San Francisco, 1982, pp 209–214.
5. de Mendonça LK, Fernandes MT, Dos Reis Barbierei CM: Diagnostica ecografico da adenomiose. Rev Imagem 7:91, 1985.
6. Farrer-Brown G, Beilby J: The blood supply of the uterus. II. Venous pattern. J Obstet Gynaecol Br Commonw 77:682, 1970.
7. Fleischer AC, Dudley BS, Entman SS, et al: My-

8. Fleischer AC, Entman SS, Kalemeris GE: Sonographic depiction of normal cyclical changes of endometrium. Ultrasound Med Biol 12:271, 1986.
9. Fleischer AC, James AE Jr, Millis JB, et al: Differential diagnosis of pelvic masses by gray scale sonography. Am J Roentgenol 131, 469, 1978.
10. Fleischer AC, Kalemeris GE, Jachin JE, et al: Sonographic depiction of normal and abnormal endometrium with histopathologic correlation. J Ultrasound Med 5:445, 1986.
11. Fogel SR, Slasley BS: Sonography of nabothian cysts. Am J Roentgenol 138:927, 1982.
12. Frede TE: Ultrasonic visualization of varicosities in the female genital tract. J Ultrasound Med 3:365, 1984.
13. Gompel C, Silverberg SG: Pathology in Gynecology and Obstetrics, 3rd Ed. Philadelphia, JB Lippincott Co, 1985.
14. Gottesfeld KR: The role of ultrasound in gynecologic diagnosis. Clin Diagn Ultrasound 2:207, 1979.
15. Hassani S, Bard R: Ultrasonic changes of uterine fibroids in pregnancy. Abstract presented at the annual meeting of the American Institute of Ultrasound in Medicine, San Francisco, California, 1979.
16. Johnson MA, Graham MF, Cooperberg PL: Abnormal endometrial echoes: Sonographic spectrum of endometrial pathology. J Ultrasound Med 1:161, 1982.
17. Jones TB, Fleischer AC, Daniell JF, et al: Sonographic characteristics of congenital uterine abnormalities and associated pregnancy. JCU 8:435, 1980.
18. Jones HW Jr, Jones GS: Novak's Textbook of Gynecology. Baltimore, Williams & Wilkins, 1981.
19. Laing FC: Sonography of a persistently retroverted gravid uterus. Am J Roentgenol 136:413, 1981.
20. Laing FC: Diagnostic dilemmas in obstetrical and gynecologic ultrasound. Syllabus for the Categorical Course in Ultrasonography, presented at the annual meeting of the American Roentgen Ray Society, San Francisco, California, March 22–27, 1981, pp 229–251.
21. Laing FC, Filly RA, Marks WM, et al: Ultrasonic demonstration of endometrial fluid collections unassociated with pregnancy. Radiology 137:471, 1980.
22. Lawson TL, Albarelli JN: Diagnosis of gynecologic pelvic masses by gray scale ultrasonography: Analysis of specificity and accuracy. Am J Roentgenol 128:1003, 1977.
23. Lewandowski B: Personal communication, 1987.
24. Levi S, Delval R: Value of ultrasonic diagnosis of gynecological tumors in 370 surgical cases. Acta Obstet Gynecol Scand 55:261, 1976.
25. Lippe BM, Sample WF: Pelvic ultrasonography in pediatric and adolescent endocrine disorders. J Pediatr 92:897, 1978.
26. Malini S, Valdes C, Malinak LR: Sonographic changes and classification of the female genital tract. J Ultrasound Med 3:397, 1984.
27. Mattingly RF: TeLinde's Operative Gynecology, 5th Ed. Philadelphia, JB Lippincott Co, 1977.
28. McArdle CR, Berezin AF: Ultrasound demonstration of uterus subseptus. JCU 8:139, 1980.
29. McGahan JP, Phillips HE, Bowen MS: Prolapse of the amniotic sac ("hourglass membranes"): Ultrasound appearance. Radiology 140:463, 1981.

30. Michaels WH, Montgomery C, Karo J, et al: Ultrasound differentiation of the competent from the incompetent cervix. Prevention of preterm delivery. Am J Obstet Gynecol 154:537, 1986.
31. Miller EI, Thomas RH, Lines P: The atrophic post-menopausal uterus. JCU 5:261, 1977.
32. Müller NL, Cooperberg PL, Rowley VA, et al: Ultrasonic refraction by the rectus abdominis muscles: The double image artifact. J Ultrasound Med 3:515, 1984.
33. Nicolini U, Belotti M, Bonazzi B, et al: Can ultrasound be used to screen uterine malformations? Fertil Steril 47:89, 1987.
34. Nikkanen V, Punnonen R: Clinical significance of adenomyosis. Ann Chir Gynaecol 69:278, 1980.
35. Pupols A, Wilson S: Ultrasonographic interpretation of physiological changes in the female pelvis. J Can Assoc Radiol 35:34, 1984.
36. Requard CK, Wicks JD, Mettler FA Jr: Ultrasonography in the staging of endometrial adenocarcinoma. Radiology 140:781, 1981.
37. Robbins SL, Cotran RS, Kumar V: Pathologic Basis of Disease, 3rd Ed. Philadelphia, WB Saunders Co, 1984, p 1130.
38. Rubin D, Graham MF, Cronhelm C, Cooperberg PL: Echogenic hematometria mimicking endometrial carcinoma. J Ultrasound Med 4:47, 1985.
39. Sample WF, Lippe BM, Gyepes MT: Gray-scale ultrasonography of the normal female pelvis. Radiology 125:477, 1977.
40. Sarti DA, Sample WF, Hobel CJ, et al: Ultrasonic visualization of a dilated cervix during pregnancy. Radiology 130:417, 1979.
41. Scott WW Jr, Rosenshein NB, Siegelman SS, et al: The obstructed uterus. Radiology 141:767, 1981.
42. Siedler D, Laing FC, Jeffrey RB, Wing VW: Uterine adenomyosis: A difficult sonographic diagnosis. J Ultrasound Med 6:345, 1987.
43. Smith JP, Weiser EB, Karnei RF Jr, et al: Ultrasonography of rapidly growing uterine leiomyomata associated with anovulatory cycles. Radiology 134:713, 1980.
44. Walsh JW, Brewer WH, Schneider V: Ultrasound diagnosis in diseases of the uterine corpus and cervix. Semin Ultrasound 1:30, 1980.
45. Walsh JW, Rosenfield AT, Jaffe CC, et al: Prospective comparison of ultrasound and computed tomography in the evaluation of gynecologic pelvic masses. Am J Roentgenol 131:955, 1978.
46. Walsh JW, Taylor KJW, Wasson JFM, et al: Gray-scale ultrasound in 204 proved gynecologic masses: Accuracy and specific diagnostic criteria. Radiology 130:391, 1979.
47. Wilson DA, Stacy TM, Smith EI: Ultrasound diagnosis of hydrocolpos and hydrometrocolpos. Radiology 128:451, 1978.
48. Zanetti E, Ferrari LR, Rossi G: Classification and radiographic features of uterine malformations: Hysterosalpingographic study. Br J Radiol 51:161, 1978.

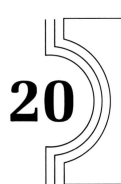

20

ULTRASOUND EVALUATION OF GESTATIONAL TROPHOBLASTIC DISEASE

Peter W. Callen, M.D.

Although gestational trophoblastic disease (GTD) is one of the more potentially confusing diseases, it is also, fortunately, one of the most favorable gynecologic neoplasms. The confusion is due to the varied terminology used to describe this disease and also to the existence of a number of conditions that mimic GTD. The favorable nature of this neoplasm is based upon the fact that even in patients with high-risk metastatic disease, cure rates of 80 to 90 percent have been achieved.[1, 2]

Terminology

Most practitioners are aware of the entity hydatidiform mole, but this is just one of the manifestations of GTD. Gestational trophoblastic disease is a proliferative disease of the trophoblast that may present as a relatively benign form, hydatidiform mole, or, in contrast, as the more malignant forms, invasive mole or choriocarcinoma.

Although in one sense the division of this disease entity into these three categories is useful for understanding the various manifestations and progression of the disease, it should be recognized that since the advent

of an accurate immunologic biologic marker for this disease, specifically the beta subunit of human chorionic gonadotropin (β-hCG), this division has less clinical utility.

HYDATIDIFORM MOLE

Epidemiology

Hydatidiform mole is the most benign and most common form of trophoblastic disease. Its incidence varies geographically. In the United States, the incidence is approximately one in 1200 to 2000 pregnancies; in France, the incidence has been reported to be one in 500; and the greatest frequency is in the Far East, with a reported incidence of more than one in 100 in some Indonesian hospitals.[3, 4] Age also appears to influence the risk of women developing a hydatidiform mole. Those women who are at the end of their reproductive years have an increased incidence of trophoblastic disease, despite race or geography.[5, 6]

Women who have had a previous hydatidiform mole have an increased risk of having another,[5, 6–8] ranging from 20 to 40 times that for the general population.[5, 6, 9] This risk may be less if one or more normal pregnancies have intervened.[5]

Genetics

There are at least two different genetic types of hydatidiform mole, each with a different etiology.[5, 10–12] A complete or "classic" mole usually has a chromosomal make-up of 46 XX, which is derived entirely from the father.[5] This event likely results from an egg with an absent or inactivated nucleus in which there is fertilization by a haploid sperm that then duplicates to the normal diploid number.[5] The other genetic type of hydatidiform mole is one in which there is a 46 XY chromosomal complement. This is thought to result from fertilization of an egg with an absent nucleus by two different haploid sperm.[5, 13, 14] This likely occurs in only a small percentage of cases. In either case, the genetic origin of the nuclear DNA is paternal.

Pathophysiology

The standard explanation for the pathophysiology of a hydatidiform mole is that the chorionic villi of a blighted ovum in a missed abortion persist and continue to undergo hydatid swelling. This accounts for the characteristic vesicular appearance of the swollen chorionic villi but not for the primary pathologic feature of this disease, trophoblastic proliferation. Thus, some investigators have postulated that the primary event may well be abnormal proliferation of the trophoblast, the hydropic change being a secondary phenomenon.

Pathology

The pathologic characteristics of hydatidiform mole are (1) marked edema and enlargement of the chorionic villi, (2) disappearance of the villus blood vessels, (3) proliferation of the lining trophoblast of the chorionic villi, and (4) absence of fetal tissue. As stated earlier, perhaps the most important characteristic that separates hydatidiform mole from other nontrophoblastic diseases is the proliferation of the lining trophoblast of the chorionic villi. One sees

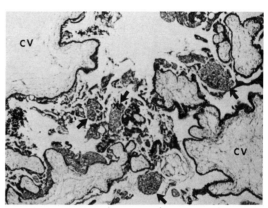

Figure 20–1. Photomicrograph from a patient with a hydatidiform mole. Abnormal nests of trophoblastic cells *(arrows)* are seen scattered among markedly swollen chorionic villi (CV). The degree of hydropic change of the chorionic villus, in addition to the presence of trophoblastic proliferation, distinguishes this from hydropic degeneration occurring in otherwise normal pregnancies. See color plate, p xvi.

small islands of chorionic villus in the normal placenta, the trophoblastic elements forming a thin "limiting border." With a hydatidiform mole, the chorionic villus becomes markedly swollen with proliferating nests of trophoblastic cells scattered throughout (Fig. 20–1).

Ultrasonographic Appearance

Characteristically, a hydatidiform mole appears as a large, moderately echogenic, soft tissue mass filling the uterine cavity. Numerous small cystic fluid-containing spaces are scattered throughout (Fig. 20–2A). When the tumor volume is small, the myometrium may be perceived as less echogenic soft tissue surrounding the more echogenic mass filling the uterine cavity (Fig. 20–2B).

Although these features have come to be recognized as typical of a hydatidiform mole, this appearance is only specific for a second trimester mole.[15] Cases of first trimester molar pregnancies have been reported in the literature widely and have a variable appearance. First trimester moles, in some cases, may have an appearance simulating a blighted ovum or a threatened abortion; others may show a small echogenic mass filling the uterine cavity without the characteristic vesicular appearance (Fig. 20–3).[16] In these cases, only a high index of suspicion in addition to correlation with the level of hCG

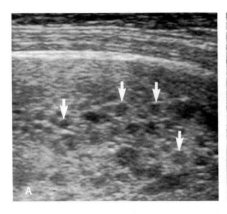
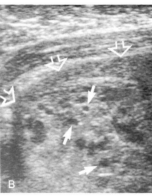

Figure 20–2. A, Longitudinal ultrasonogram from a patient with a second trimester hydatidiform mole. A large, moderately echogenic mass with numerous small cystic spaces (arrows) is seen filling the central uterine cavity. The cystic spaces undoubtedly represent the markedly hydropic chorionic villi. B, Sonogram from a patient with an early second trimester hydatidiform mole. Numerous vesicles (arrows) and echogenic tissue are seen filling the uterine cavity. The adjacent, less echogenic myometrium is well seen (open arrows).

will allow the sonographer to suggest the correct diagnosis.

COMPLICATIONS OF TROPHOBLASTIC DISEASE

Hemorrhage

Perhaps one of the most common complications of trophoblastic disease, which can be readily identified on the ultrasonogram, is a hemorrhage within this lesion or within adjacent tissues. The areas of hemorrhage usually appear as crescentic anechoic regions surrounding the tumor (Fig. 20–4).

Theca-Lutein Cysts

The other feature frequently associated with hydatidiform mole and trophoblastic disease is theca-lutein cysts. The incidence of theca-lutein cysts in patients with trophoblastic disease is approximately 20 to 50 percent. The number detected using ultrasonography is usually higher than that with clinical examination. This difference is probably due to the fact that with excessive uterine enlargement, the ovaries may be difficult to palpate, since they are displaced in a cephalic direction out of the true pelvis.

Theca-lutein cysts are thought to be secondary to a markedly elevated circulating

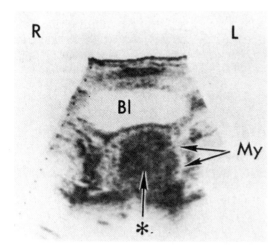

Figure 20–3. Transverse ultrasonogram from a patient with a first trimester hydatidiform mole. In this case, an echogenic mass (asterisk) is seen filling the central uterine cavity. Noticeably absent are the multiple small cystic spaces that are characteristically seen in more advanced molar pregnancies. Bl, urinary bladder; My, myometrium. (From Munyer TP, Callen PW, Filly RA, et al: Further observations on the sonographic spectrum of gestational trophoblastic disease. J Clin Ultrasound 9:349, 1981.).

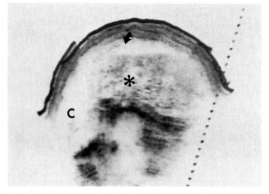

Figure 20–4. Transverse ultrasonogram from a patient with a second trimester hydatidiform mole. A moderately echogenic mass (asterisk) is filling the uterine cavity. A crescentic anechoic region (arrow) is seen anteriorly adjacent to the anterior abdominal wall, probably representing hemorrhage. In addition, evidence of a theca-lutein cyst (C) is seen on the right side.

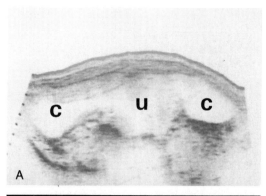

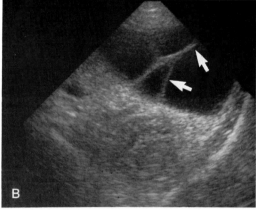

Figure 20–5. *A*, Transverse ultrasonogram from a patient with a second trimester hydatidiform mole. Large theca-lutein cysts (c) are seen bilaterally. U, uterus. *B*, The characteristic multiseptated *(arrows)* appearance is readily demonstrated.

level of hCG. Analysis of the cysts shows them to be multilocular, containing amber-colored or serosanguineous fluid.[17] The ultrasonogram accurately depicts this pathologic description: multiseptated cysts are the most common presentation (Fig. 20–5). The ultrasonographer should remember that it may take approximately two to four months for these cysts to regress after molar evacuation; thus, they cannot be used as evidence of persistent or recurrent disease.[18]

DISEASES SIMULATING HYDATIDIFORM MOLE

The older literature about trophoblastic disease tended to be confusing since several diseases that were not truly hydatidiform moles, such as hydropic degeneration or partial moles, were included in this classification. If one adheres strictly to the pathologic criterion stated earlier for hydatidi-

form mole, one will be less prone to overestimate the prevalence of this disease. One entity that has been frequently included with hydatidiform mole and should remain separate is *hydropic degeneration of the placenta.*

Hydropic changes of the placenta may occur in approximately 1 to 3 percent of pregnancies.[19] Although the chorionic villi may be engorged, a specific feature of trophoblastic disease, proliferation of the lining trophoblast of the chorionic villi, is not seen. The ultrasonographer may find it extremely difficult to distinguish between a missed abortion, in which there is hydropic degeneration, and a molar pregnancy (Fig. 20–6). In these cases, determination of the levels of serum hCG as well as pathologic evaluation of the specimen will be needed to make this distinction.[20]

Although leiomyomas involving the uterus do not usually present a diagnostic dilemma, occasionally a leiomyoma with cystic degeneration may simulate the appearance of a hydatidiform mole (Fig. 20–7). In these cases, careful evaluation of the highly attenuating nature of myomatous disease may help distinguish it from trophoblastic disease.

FOLLOW-UP EVALUATION AND TREATMENT

The treatment and follow-up of trophoblastic disease are beyond the scope of this

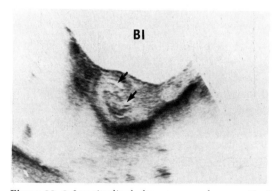

Figure 20–6. Longitudinal ultrasonogram from a patient with vaginal bleeding and a positive pregnancy test. Irregular cystic spaces *(arrows)* can be seen within the uterus. While the appearance is certainly not specific, this case of hydropic degeneration with fetal demise may be very difficult to differentiate from a first trimester molar pregnancy. Bl, maternal urinary bladder.

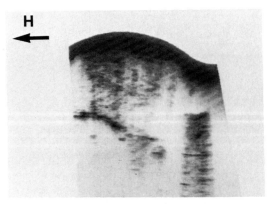

Figure 20–7. Longitudinal ultrasonogram from a patient with vaginal bleeding and a large pelvic mass. While the poorly echogenic areas may simulate a molar pregnancy, the attenuation of sound and absence of numerous well-defined cystic spaces would make this atypical for a second trimester mole. The serum β-hCG tested negative and may be useful in making the distinction between this leiomyoma with cystic degeneration and a molar pregnancy. H, head.

discussion, but some general points will be mentioned. Once hydatidiform mole has been diagnosed, suction evacuation of the uterus is usually performed, followed by curettage of the endometrium to determine if there is myometrial invasion. A baseline chest radiograph is used to examine for evidence of metastatic disease. Declining serum levels of β-hCG may then be followed until normal. Normally, the serum β-hCG level falls toward zero approximately 10 to 12 weeks after evacuation of the molar pregnancy (Fig. 20–8).[18]

VARIATIONS OF MOLAR PREGNANCY

Coexistent Mole and Fetus

Several reports in the literature have noted that a living fetus was associated with a molar pregnancy.[21–23] Unfortunately, many patients were included in this category in whom there was hydropic degeneration or an incomplete mole rather than a true hydatidiform mole. Nevertheless, several well-documented cases of coexistent fetus and mole have been seen. Because absence of fetal structure is one of the pathologic requirements for a true hydatidiform mole, the presumed mechanism for coexistence of a true mole and normal fetus is molar transformation of one binovular twin placenta

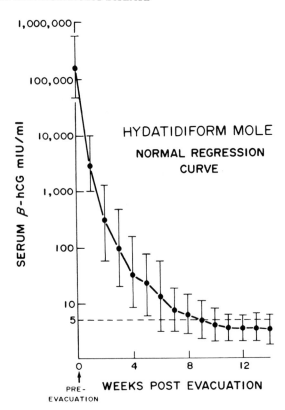

Figure 20–8. Normal regression curve after evacuation for patients with a hydatidiform mole. By 12 weeks after evacuation, the β-hCG level should have returned to near zero.

(Fig. 20–9). Although the diagnosis may be suggested and made with a high degree of certainty on the ultrasonogram, it should be confirmed pathologically, since these lesions

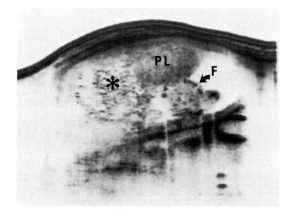

Figure 20–9. Longitudinal ultrasonogram from a patient with a true hydatidiform mole coexisting with a normal fetus. The fetus (F) was living at the time of the examination, and the placenta (PL) was normal in appearance. The more characteristically appearing molar pregnancy can be seen (*asterisk*) superior and adjacent to the normal pregnancy.

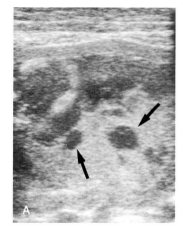
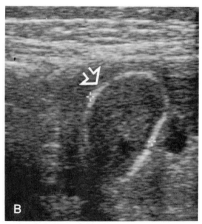

Figure 20–10. A, Partial hydatidiform mole. Scans of the placenta demonstrate numerous cystic spaces (arrows). B, The fetus was severely growth retarded and dysmorphic, with a deformed skull (open arrow).

must be considered as having the same malignant potential as a more classically appearing molar pregnancy.

Incomplete or Partial Mole (Triploidy)

Several entities, including hydropic degeneration, have been placed in this category. The following pathologic findings for incomplete or partial moles are well presented in a review by Szulman and Surti: (1) identifiable fetal tissues, (2) edematous chorionic villi with little or no trophoblastic proliferation, and (3) multiple congenital anomalies in which a chromosomal analysis usually reveals a triploid chromosomal complement (Fig. 20–10).[24]

For the sonographer, the goal is to differentiate a partial or incomplete molar pregnancy from a true hydatidiform mole or a normal pregnancy with avillous areas within the placenta. Patients with a partial mole demonstrate a pregnancy with a "formed" placenta in which there are numerous cystic spaces. (This is quite different from a hydatidiform mole in which a globular echogenic mass, rather than a formed placenta, is seen within the uterus.) In addition, in nearly all cases of partial mole, the fetus is growth retarded or dysmorphic.[25] If necessary, amniocentesis is helpful in demonstrating a triploid chromosomal complement.

In addition to identifying an abnormal fetus in these pregnancies, it is important to make the diagnosis for further follow-up. There have been at least two cases of partial hydatidiform mole in which persistent trophoblastic disease requiring chemotherapy has developed after evacuation.[8, 25, 26]

Invasive Mole

In approximately 80 percent of patients initially diagnosed as having hydatidiform mole, the disease will follow a benign course, with resolution after evacuation (Fig. 20–11). However, in approximately 12 to 15 percent of patients, invasive mole develops, and in 5 to 8 percent, metastatic choriocarcinoma develops.

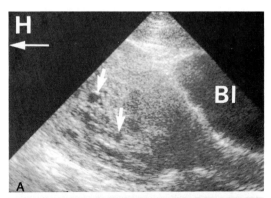
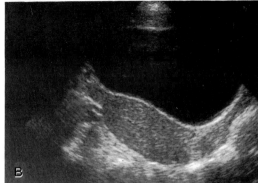

Figure 20–11. A, Uterine enlargement due to a hydatidiform mole. Cystic spaces are readily seen (arrows). Bl, bladder; H, head. B, Six weeks after evacuation, the uterus has returned to normal size.

The pathologic features of invasive mole are: (1) extensive local invasion, (2) excessive trophoblastic proliferation, and (3) preservation of the villous pattern. The differentiating feature between invasive mole and choriocarcinoma is preservation of the villous pattern in invasive molar disease. Examination of a specimen from a patient with an invasive mole reveals that the characteristic elements seen with hydatidiform mole—nests of trophoblastic cells as well as swollen chorionic villi—rather than being within the central cavity of the uterus, are found within the myometrium.

Invasive mole is infrequently diagnosed without hysterectomy, since it is uncommon to obtain myometrium during curettage. And since hysterectomies are not commonly performed for any form of trophoblastic disease, the diagnosis may not be suggested by the clinician. The morbidity and mortality caused by invasive mole result from the penetration of the tumor through the myometrium and pelvic vessels, producing hemorrhage.[17, 27] Although the ultrasonographer may have a difficult time diagnosing this more aggressive form of the disease, hemorrhagic necrosis involving the myometrium and extending into the parametrial areas should make one suspect this entity (Fig. 20–12).

Choriocarcinoma

This most malignant form of trophoblastic disease has an incidence of approximately one in 40,000 pregnancies in the US. Approximately 50 percent of the cases of choriocarcinoma are preceded by a molar pregnancy; however, only 3 to 5 percent of all molar pregnancies result in choriocarcinoma. Approximately one-half of cases of choriocarcinoma occur in association with a molar pregnancy, 25 percent occur after an abortion, 22 percent occur after normal pregnancy, and approximately 3 percent may occur after an ectopic pregnancy (Fig. 20–13).

Pathology

Gross examination of the uterus in a patient with choriocarcinoma will reveal a dark hemorrhagic mass on the uterine wall, cervix, or vagina, which may show extensive ulceration and penetration of the tumor into the musculature (Fig. 20–14). Microscopically, the villous pattern is completely blotted out by the proliferating trophoblast (Fig. 20–15). This feature separates this disease entity from the less benign forms of trophoblastic disease.[17, 27] Choriocarcinoma is known to metastasize to the lung, brain, liver, bone, gastrointestinal tract, and skin. As such, the ultrasonographer may help in evaluating the extent of the disease, particularly in the liver (Fig. 20–16).

PROGRESSION OF DISEASE

As stated earlier, most patients originally diagnosed as having trophoblastic disease (i.e., hydatidiform mole) have resolution of their disease after evacuation of the molar pregnancy. There are those patients, how-

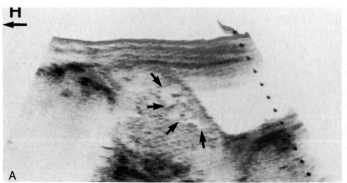
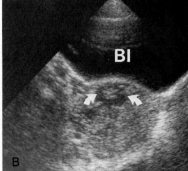

Figure 20–12. A, B, Extension of an invasive mole (arrows) into the myometrium in two patients with markedly elevated hCG levels. H, head; Bl, bladder.

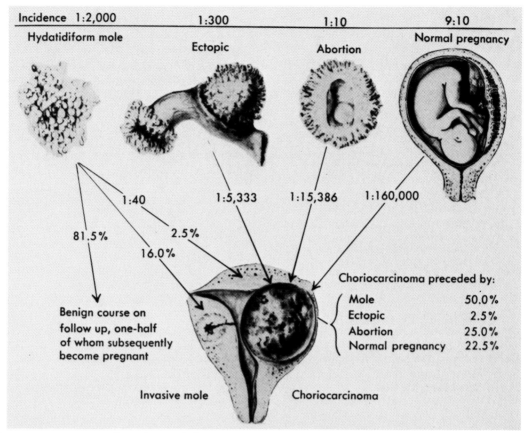

Figure 20–13. Origin and incidence of choriocarcinoma. (*From* Rosai J: Female reproductive system/placenta. Ackerman's Surgical Pathology, 6th Ed. St. Louis, CV Mosby Co, 1981, p 1079.)

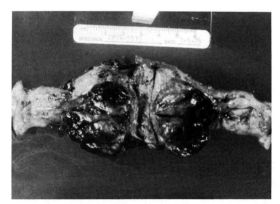

Figure 20–14. Pathologic specimen from a patient with choriocarcinoma. The bivalved uterus demonstrates a large, hemorrhagic necrotic mass involving the body of the uterus. See color plate, p xvi.

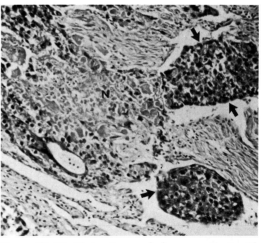

Figure 20–15. Photomicrograph from a patient with choriocarcinoma. Multiple cords (*arrows*) of malignant trophoblastic tissue infiltrate the uterine stroma. The absence of villi and the necrosis (N) of the tumor differentiate this process from invasive trophoblastic disease and a hydatidiform mole. See color plate, p xvi.

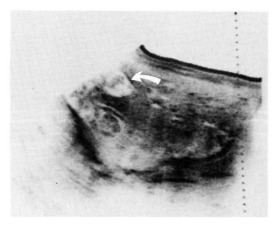

Figure 20–16. Longitudinal ultrasonogram from a patient with metastatic choriocarcinoma. There is evidence of metastatic disease involving the liver, in which a necrotic metastasis with hemorrhage *(arrow)* is seen. The patient died of a massive hemoperitoneum from bleeding hepatic metastases.

ever, who may present initially with choriocarcinoma or develop persistent disease after a preceding pregnancy.

During the past 30 years, it has been recognized that trophoblastic disease is uniquely sensitive to systemic chemotherapy, and thus potentially curable. As with other malignancies, it has become important to define subgroups of these patients to determine adequate treatment regimens. Thus, patients are divided into those groups with nonmetastatic and metastatic trophoblastic disease. The group with metastatic disease

is subdivided into low-, intermediate-, and high-risk groups (Table 20–1).[28–31]

The ultrasonographer or radiologist has two major goals in evaluating the patient suspected of having persistent trophoblastic diseased: (1) to determine if the rise of hCG is due to a normal pregnancy rather than persistent disease, and (2) to determine the sites of metastatic disease.

The major pathologic feature of trophoblastic disease is abnormal proliferation of trophoblastic tissue after a gestational event. Although pathologic confirmation of choriocarcinoma is difficult because hysterectomies are now infrequently performed for this disease, correlation of the appearance of the uterus with an evaluation of known metastatic surveys as well as the level of serum β-hCG has proved interesting in assessing local involvement.[15] Patients with persistent trophoblastic disease may have focal areas of increased echogenicity within the myometrium as the only imaged evidence of disease (Fig. 20–17). The author hypothesizes that trophoblastic disease appears on the ultrasonogram as highly echogenic tissue within the uterus in which visualization depends on the amount of tissue present as well as secondary changes. If molar pregnancy is detected early, in a first trimester mole or in cases of early detection of persistent or locally invasive disease, the vesicles that give hydatidiform mole its characteristic and easily recognizable appearance

Table 20–1. MODIFIED NIH CLASSIFICATION OF GESTATIONAL TROPHOBLASTIC DISEASE

Nonmetastatic Trophoblastic Disease
  Hydatidiform mole
    Undelivered
    Delivered (> 8 wk)
  Persistent mole (>8 wk)
  Invasive mole or choriocarcinoma confined to the
    uterus
Metastatic Trophoblastic Disease
  Low risk
    Short duration (≤4 mo)
    Low hCG titer (≤100,000 mIU/24 hr)
    Lung or vaginal metastasis
  Intermediate risk
    Long duration (>4 mo)
    High hCG titer (>100,000 mIU/24 hr)
    Metastasis other than to CNS or liver
  High risk
    CNS metastasis
    Liver metastasis

From Hilgers RA: Improving the outcome of high-risk gestational trophoblastic neoplasia. Contemp Obstet Gynecol 73:92, 1987.

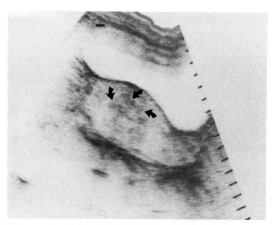

Figure 20–17. Longitudinal ultrasonogram from a patient with persistent trophoblastic disease. Despite a markedly elevated serum β-hCG level, the results of a metastic work-up were negative. There was, however, a focus of increased echogenic tissue *(arrows)* adjacent to the central uterine cavity, which most likely represents persistent trophoblastic tissue.

either may not be present or may be too small to be seen. Therefore, first trimester molar pregnancies may often be misdiagnosed as a missed abortion, or persistent disease may not be readily apparent on the ultrasonogram. As the molar pregnancy progresses into the second trimester, the pathognomonic vesicles and theca-lutein cysts become evident. This progression is supported by studies of Szulman and Surti, who have established a roughly linear relationship between gestational age of the molar pregnancy and the microscopic size of the swollen chorionic villi.[32] For example, their earliest hydatidiform mole, with a gestational age of 8½ gestational weeks, yielded vesicles with a maximum diameter of 2 mm. This result contrasts with their most advanced case of 18½ gestational weeks, yielding vesicles with a maximum diameter of 10 mm. As stated previously, in cases of first trimester molar pregnancy or in cases of persistent or locally invasive disease when recurrence is detected by serial determinations of hCG levels, the characteristic vesicles may be too small to be imaged by ultrasound.

In addition to evaluation of the uterus, ultrasound is able to determine if there is evidence of parametrial extension of disease or hepatic metastases. During the past several years, the newer imaging modalities of computed tomography and magnetic resonance imaging have shown the ability to detect metastatic disease that was not seen by conventional imaging methods.[33-35]

Knowledge of the various manifestations of trophoblastic disease as well as the complications that can be seen on the ultrasonogram will aid the clinician in managing the disease. Differentiation between trophoblastic disease and a normal intrauterine pregnancy, as well as following the extent of spread of disease or response to therapy in advanced cases, may all be accomplished using ultrasonography.

References

1. Lurain JR, Brewer JI, Torak EE, et al: Gestational trophoblastic disease: Treatment results at the Brewer Trophoblastic Disease Center. Obstet Gynecol 60:354, 1982.
2. Hammond CB, Weed JC, Currie JC: The role of operation in the current therapy of gestational trophoblastic disease. Am J Obstet Gynecol 136:844, 1980.
3. Sand PK, Lurain JR, Brewer JI: Repeat gestational trophoblastic disease. Obstet Gynecol 63:140, 1984.
4. Poen HJT, Djojopranoto M: The possible etiologic factors of hydatidiform mole and choriocarcinoma. Am J Obstet Gynecol 92:510, 1965.
5. Grimes DA: Epidemiology of gestational trophoblastic disease. Am J Obstet Gynecol 150:309, 1984.
6. Yen S, MacMahan B: Epidemiologic features of trophoblastic disease. Am J Obstet Gynecol 101:126, 1968.
7. MacGregor C, Ontiveros E, Vargas E, Valenzuela S: Hydatidiform mole. Obstet Gynecol 33:343, 1969.
8. Berkowitz RS, Goldstein DP: Pathogenesis of gestational trophoblastic neoplasms. Pathobiol Annu 11:391, 1981.
9. Rolan PA, deLopez BH. Epidemiologic aspects of hydatidiform mole in the Republic of Paraguay (South America). Br J Obstet Gynaecol 84:862, 1977.
10. Vassilahos P, Protton G, Kaju T: Hydatidiform mole: Two entities. Am J Obstet Gynecol 127:167, 1977.
11. Kaju T, Ohama K: Androgenetic origin of hydatidiform mole. Nature 268:633, 1977.
12. Szulman AE, Surti U: The syndromes of hydatidiform mole. Am J Obstet Gynecol 131:665, 1978.
13. Surti U, Szulman AE, O'Brien S: Complete (classic) hydatidiform mole with 46 XY karyotype of paternal origin. Hum Genet 51:153, 1979.
14. Ohami K, Kaju T, Ohamoto K, et al: Dispermic origin of XY hydatidiform moles. Nature 292:551, 1981.
15. Munyer TP, Callen PW, Filly RA, et al: Further observations on the sonographic spectrum of gestational trophoblastic disease. JCU 9:349, 1981.
16. Woodward RM, Filly RA, Callen PW: First trimester molar pregnancy: Nonspecific ultrasonographic appearance. Obstet Gynecol 55:315, 1980.
17. Kraus FT: Female genitalia. In Anderson WAD, Kissane JR (eds): Pathology, 7th Ed. St Louis, CV Mosby Co, 1977.
18. Goldstein DP, Berkowitz RJ, Cohen SM: The current management of molar pregnancy. Curr Probl Obstet Gynecol 3:1, 1979.
19. Hertig AT: Human Trophoblast. Springfield, Illinois, Charles C Thomas, 1968, pp 228–237.
20. Romero R, Horgan JG, Kohorn EF, et al: New criteria for the diagnosis of gestational trophoblastic disease. Obstet Gynecol 66:553, 1985.
21. Bree RL, Silver TM, Wichs JD, et al: Trophoblastic disease with coexistent fetus: A sonographic and clinical spectrum. JCU 6:310, 1978.
22. Fleisher AC, James AD, Krause DA, et al: Sonographic patterns in trophoblastic diseases. Radiology 126:215, 1978.
23. Sauerbrei EE, Salem S, Fayle B: Coexistent hydatidiform mole and live fetus in the second trimester. Radiology 135:415, 1980.
24. Szulman AE, Surti U: The syndromes of hydatidiform mole. I. Cytogenic and morphologic correlations. Am J Obstet Gynecol 13:655, 1978.
25. Crane JP, Beaver HA, Cheung SW: Antenatal ultrasound finding in fetal triploidy syndrome. J Ultrasound Med 4:519, 1985.
26. Szulman AE, Ma HK, Wong LC, Hsu C: Residual trophoblastic disease in association with partial hydatidiform mole. Obstet Gynecol 57:392, 1981.
27. Jones HW III: Gestational trophoblastic disease. In Jones H, Jones GS (eds): Novak's Textbook of Gynecology, 10th Ed. Baltimore, Williams & Wilkins, 1981.

28. Hilgers RD: Improving the outcome of high-risk gestational trophoblastic neoplasia. Contemp Obstet Gynecol 73:92, 1987.
29. Hilgers RD, Lewis JL Jr: Gestational trophoblastic disease. In Danforth DN (ed): Obstetrics and Gynecology, 4th Ed. Hagerstown, Maryland, Harper & Row, 1982, pp 393–406.
30. Bagshawe KD: Risk and prognostic factors in trophoblastic neoplasia. Cancer 38:1373, 1976.
31. World Health Organization Scientific Group, Gestational Trophoblastic Diseases. WHO Technical Report Series 692. Geneva, Switzerland, 1983.
32. Szulman AE, Surti U: The syndromes of hydatidiform mole. II. Morphologic evolution of the complete and partial mole. Am J Obstet Gynecol 132:20, 1978.
33. Sanders C, Rubin E: Malignant gestational trophoblastic disease: CT findings. Am J Roentgenol 148:165, 1987.
34. Mutch DG, Soper JT, Baker ME, et al: Role of computed axial tomography of the chest in staging patients with nonmetastatic gestational trophoblastic disease. Obstet Gynecol 68:348, 1986.
35. Hricak H, Demas BE, Broga CA, et al: Gestational trophoblastic neoplasm of the uterus: MR assessment. Radiology 161:11, 1986.

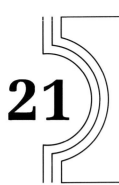

21

ULTRASOUND EVALUATION OF THE OVARY

Harvey L. Neiman, M.D.
Ellen B. Mendelson, M.D.

The ovary is one of the body's most dynamic organs, changing with age, hormonal environment, and reproductive status. Ultrasound has proved to be an accurate and consistent method of imaging the normal ovary with its associated physiologic changes and of identifying abnormalities in the ovary and adjacent adnexal structures. Recent improvements in instrumentation, such as phased-array and annular array transducers and, most recently, transvaginal probes, have provided powerful sonographic tools. Doppler techniques[54] and transrectal scanning may also aid in evaluation.

TECHNIQUE

The authors' routine technique for evaluation of the ovary and adnexa uses real-time equipment and a transabdominal suprapubic approach. A fully distended urinary bladder is necessary to visualize the pelvis optimally. The full bladder displaces bowel loops cephalad and serves as an acoustic window. The highest frequency transducer that will provide adequate penetration is used, most often a 5 MHz medium- or, occasionally, long-focus probe. The authors no longer employ static image articulated-arm scans. Meticulous technique must be used to ensure that the entire volume of the pelvis has been studied. Transverse and longitudinal sections are routinely obtained. Angling the probe obliquely through the urinary bladder to the contralateral ovary may occasionally permit better visualization than scanning directly over an ovary that may be hidden by bowel.

The position of the ovary can be somewhat variable, and on occasion it may be found behind the uterus in the cul-de-sac or adjacent to the apex of the urinary bladder as it rises out of the pelvis. If the ovary is not identified with routine views, a careful search must be made throughout the pelvis. Occasionally, a water enema[45] can be useful for differentiating an adnexal mass from normal bowel loops.

Transvaginal ultrasound may be helpful in locating an elusive ovary, and the intravaginal probe, if available, should be used in this situation. Ovaries adjacent to the uterus and those surrounded by bowel loops may be identified and well-characterized transvaginally. In the authors' experience, the internal architecture of adnexal masses is much better imaged transvaginally than by standard full-bladder techniques. Enhanced diagnostic confidence afforded by this technique most likely derives from the improved geometry of the intravaginal probe, in close proximity to the pelvic organs.[28]

Transvaginal sonography may be rapidly performed. The probe is sheathed with a condom containing coupling gel. Additional coupling gel is then applied to the external surface of the condom. When the study is performed to assess follicular maturity, external coupling may be carried out with water since many commonly available gels may retard sperm motility.

Intravaginal transducers currently available or being developed range in frequency from 3.5 to 7.5 MHz. They are end-firing probes of either straight or angulated configuration. The authors have most frequently used a 5 MHz club-shaped transducer with a 28 mm diameter footprint that encompasses a sector angle of 90°.

The patient, who should empty her bladder at the outset, is studied in supine position, knees gently flexed. The transducer may be inserted by the patient, the technologist, or the physician, according to preference. The probe rests in the vaginal vault, and slight angulation in appropriate directions will permit visualization of the uterus and adnexa. In over 90 percent of cases, the ovaries will be well imaged. Coronal and sagittal views of each organ are obtained. Initially, orientation to these planes of section is difficult, but one soon becomes accustomed to transvaginal pelvic anatomy. Patient acceptance is excellent, and many patients have noted that they prefer the transvaginal study because they do not have to endure the discomfort of a full urinary bladder.

For most pre- and perimenopausal patients, routine examination includes both transvaginal and full-bladder transabdominal studies. The standard transabdominal approach provides a global overview of the pelvis and is important for anatomic orientation.

Some elderly women have been difficult to study transvaginally because of the size of presently available probes. Transvaginal probes of smaller diameter are being developed, and transvaginal examination of postmenopausal women may prove to be an effective screening method for ovarian carcinoma.

NORMAL ANATOMY

The adnexa consists of ovaries, fallopian tubes, and various ligaments that attach the ovaries to the uterus and to the pelvic sidewalls. The ovaries are intraperitoneal.

The ovaries lie against the lateral pelvic walls, each enclosed within the mesovarium of the broad ligament. Each rests in the ovarian fossa, a shallow depression of parietal peritoneum bounded posteroinferiorly by the ureter, superiorly by the external iliac vessels, and anteriorly by the pelvic attachment of the broad ligament.

When the uterus is in its common anteflexed midline position, the ovaries are usually directly lateral (Fig. 21–1A, B) or posterolateral to it. The ovaries are frequently lateral and superior to a retroverted uterus, near the uterine fundus. When the uterus is deviated to one side, the ipsilateral ovary is often superior to the uterine fundus.

The ovaries are ovoid structures with their craniocaudad axes parallel to the internal iliac arteries and veins. Ovarian vessels within the infundibulopelvic ligament may or may not be visualized at the superior aspect of the ovary (Fig. 21–1C). Ovarian appearance changes with age and with the stage of the menstrual cycle (Figs. 21–2, 21–3).[18, 31, 46] The normal ovary may be variable in shape; therefore, volume is a better determinant of ovarian size than any one of two measurements. Volume may be based on a simplified formula for a prolate ellipse (length × width × height divided by 2).

In the child under 5 years of age, ovarian volume is less than 1 cc.[22, 33] The ovary then increases in size until menarche, when it is 4.18 ± 2.3 cc.[33] It is now appreciated, however, that the ovary in teenagers and young adults can be significantly larger than the mean of 6 cc (approximately 2 cm × 2 cm × 3 cm), formerly used as the standard.[46] The maximum volume in this group can be as high as 14 cc.[31, 32] For postmenopausal women, ovarian volumes should be 2.5 cc or less.[18]

In premenopausal women, free fluid in the pelvis can be noted during all phases of the menstrual cycle. Blood or fluid produced by follicular rupture, estrogen-induced increased capillary permeability of the ovarian surface, and blood secondary to retrograde

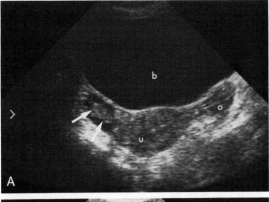

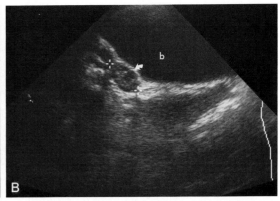

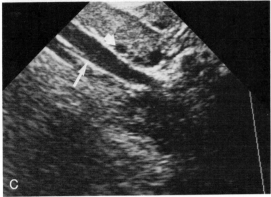

Figure 21–1. Normal ovaries. *A*, Transverse scan in a 22 year old patient. The corticomedullary junction is well defined in the right ovary *(arrows)*. O, left ovary; u, uterus; b, bladder. *B*, Longitudinal view of a normal ovary *(cursors)* in the same patient. *C*, Longitudinal view of the ovary and infundibulopelvic ligament. The ovarian vessels are seen posteriorly *(arrow)*. *Wide arrow,* ovarian follicles.

menstruation have all been implicated as causes of fluid during the menstrual cycle.[8]

The normal ovary demonstrates a mid-level, fine, homogeneous echoarchitecture. Its echogenicity is greater than that of the adjacent uterus and somewhat more homo-geneous. With transvaginal scanning, one can frequently differentiate the central, more echogenic ovarian medulla from the sur-rounding cortex (Fig. 21–4). In the postpub-ertal premenopausal period, multiple folli-cles can be seen developing during each

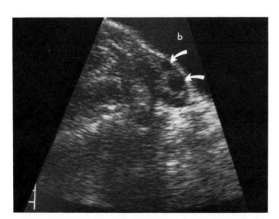

Figure 21–2. Two small follicles *(arrows)* are seen in this magnified longitudinal view of a normal ovary in a 35 year old woman. B, bladder. This is Day 11 of a 28 day cycle.

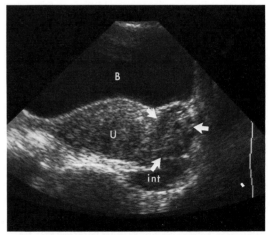

Figure 21–3. This transverse transabdominal view shows the uterus (U) and normal left ovary *(arrows)* tucked next to the bladder (B) in this 45 year old woman. A loop of bowel (int) is posterior to the ovary.

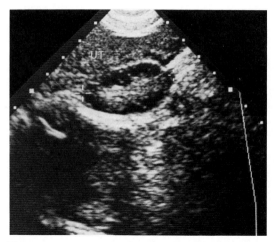

Figure 21–4. Transvaginal scan of a normal ovary. This sagittal view in a 27 year old patient shows a portion of the uterus (UT) and an adjacent ovary *(cursors)* with a hypoechoic cortex, well differentiated from the central, more echogenic medulla.

menstrual cycle along the periphery of the ovarian cortex (Fig. 21–5). These follicles do not exceed 25 mm in diameter and are round or ovoid, sharply marginated, and anechoic. If larger, a physiologic cyst or other abnormality must be considered.

Adnexal components other than the ovary are infrequently identified as discrete structures. Normal fallopian tubes are not imaged except in cases of considerable ascites. The broad ligaments may be seen as beaklike extensions from the lateral aspect of the uterus.[46] The ligaments are otherwise not visualized.

Three major muscle groups can be identified forming the boundaries of the true pel-vis. These include the piriform muscles posterolaterally, the internal obturator muscles laterally, and the iliopsoas muscles anterolaterally. These muscles may have an echogenicity and morphology similar to that of the ovary, and they can be mistaken for ovarian tissue.

The piriform muscles are triangular in shape and are most frequently mistaken for ovaries. They are best seen on transverse scans angled 10 to 15° cephalad. Laterally, the fan-shaped internal obturator muscles are noted on more caudal transverse scans and are accentuated by angling the transducer 10 to 15° caudad.[46]

The iliopsoas muscles can be demonstrated by their course extending cranially on either side of the lumbar spine and by the central area of echogenicity created by the fascial sheath separating the iliac from the psoas muscle.

OVARIAN PHYSIOLOGY

During fetal development, the ovaries contain over 7 million germ cells. Most undergo atresia antenatally, and at birth there are 2 million ova. Atresia continues through childhood, and, by the time of puberty, there are fewer than 300,000 ova. Under estrogenic stimulation, only one of these ova per spontaneous cycle (or about 500 in the course of a normal reproductive life) will arrive at maturity. This ovum is contained within a maturing (graafian) follicle (Fig. 21–6). At about the 14th day of the cycle, ovulation

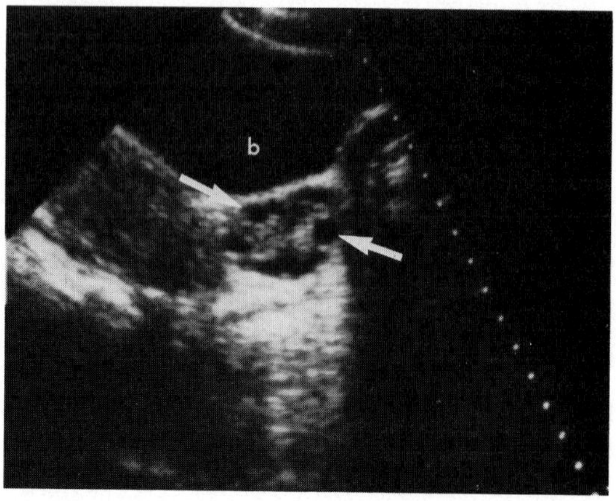

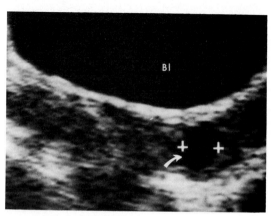

Figure 21–5. In a 29 year old patient, the normal left ovary *(arrows)* is seen in this transverse view. Many small follicles are present. B, bladder.

Figure 21–6. Single dominant graafian follicle *(arrow)* measuring 18 mm in diameter in a normal spontaneous menstrual cycle. Bl, bladder.

occurs, the ovum extruded from the distended follicle into the abdominal cavity. The graafian follicle that ruptures at the time of ovulation collapses in upon itself and fills with blood, forming a corpus hemorrhagicum. Granulosa and theca cells lining the follicle begin to proliferate, and the clotted blood is rapidly replaced with the yellowish lipid-rich luteal cells compromising the corpus luteum. If pregnancy occurs, the corpus luteum, which produces progesterone and other corticosteroids, persists. Menstruation does not occur again until after delivery. If there is no pregnancy, the corpus luteum begins to degenerate about four days before the next menses (i.e., the 24th day of the cycle). Scar tissue, the corpus albicans, marks the site of the corpus luteum.[13]

INFERTILITY

Ultrasound is important in the evaluation and treatment of female infertility related to the ovary. First, sonography can establish that anatomically normal ovaries are present and that they manifest expected physiologic changes—i.e., development of an ordinarily single, dominant follicle during a spontaneous menstrual cycle. Second, sonography can confirm ovarian response to the various pharmaceutical regimens for induction. Third, sonography aids in the recognition of imminence of ovulation. Reasons for precise timing of this process include optimizing the harvesting of ova for in vitro fertilization and embryo transfer programs, deciding whether to administer human chorionic gonadotropin (hCG) to the stimulated ovary, and scheduling husband or donor insemination. Fourth, ultrasound can suggest that ovulation has occurred. Fifth, sonography can identify the hyperstimulated ovary to avert medical complications.

In the normal ovary, follicles may be first identified when they are 4 to 5 mm in diameter. Ordinarily, only one follicle reaches maturity (Fig. 21–6), but in ovaries stimulated by clomiphene citrate or human menopausal gonadotropin, multiple developing follicles may be observed. In the spontaneous cycle, the follicle will grow at approximately 2 to 3 mm per day from day 9 or 10 until ovulation. The average size of a dominant follicle at ovulation is approximately 21 mm (with a range of 17 to 24 mm).[5, 10, 21, 29]

With conventional equipment, the cumulus oophorus, which contains the oocyte surrounded by a cluster of granulosa cells, can be seen in 15 to 80 percent of cases, according to various reports.[26, 43] The cumulus oophorus is a 1 mm echogenic mural projection into the antrum of the follicle.

Ovulatory dysfunction is present in 15 to 25 percent of infertile women.[43] Several pharmaceutical regimens have been designed for inducing follicular growth and ovulation. Most commonly, clomiphene citrate (Clomid) and human menopausal gonadotropin (Pergonal) are used. Human chorionic gonadotropin is frequently administered with these drugs to stimulate ovulation. Hypothalamic gonadotropin-releasing factor has also been used.[62]

Patients receiving clomiphene citrate or clomiphene plus hCG should have scans begun at approximately Day 10 or 11 of a 28 day cycle, and studies should be performed every day until ovulation. Those patients receiving human menopausal gonadotropin alone or with other agents should have studies begun on Day 9 of a 28 day cycle and then should be scanned daily or every other day (Fig. 21–7).

Sonographic examination of patients in an in vitro fertilization and embryo transfer program should commence on approximately Day 9, with sequential studies performed daily until the anticipated day of ovulation, when harvesting of the oocyte

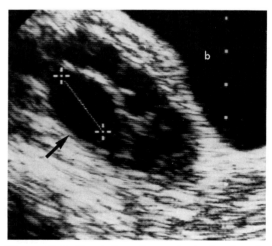

Figure 21–7. Day 9 in a Pergonal-stimulated cycle: multiple small follicles in the ovarian periphery surround a larger follicle (*arrow*). b, bladder.

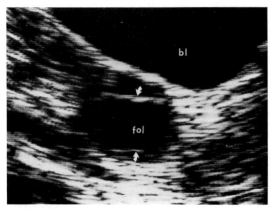

Figure 21–8. Spontaneous cycle in a 22 year old woman. This highly magnified view of the left ovary shows a dominant follicle (fol) with infolding of its walls (arrows), crenation, which is occasionally seen and signifies imminent ovulation. bl, bladder.

occurs. As there may be great variability in the number of follicles within the ovary, with small daily changes, every attempt should be made for the same sonographer and sonologist to scan the patient throughout a particular cycle to minimize interobserver error.[37]

Numerous sonographic manifestations of follicular maturity have been proposed; these include follicular size, fluid in the cul-de-sac, the presence of a cumulus oophorus, internal echogenicity, irregularity of the wall (crenation) (Fig. 21–8), ovarian hyperstimulation (large, multiple, tightly packed follicles), and thickness of follicular walls and septations.[29]

Although mean diameter and mean vol-ume can be determined, and thus the possibility of ovulation can be suggested, the sizes of mature follicles immediately before ovulation range widely (18 to 25 mm). The usefulness of follicular size as an absolute predictor of the moment of ovulation is, therefore, limited.[38]

The presence of a cumulus oophorus confirms a mature, oocyte-containing follicle, with ovulation expected within 36 hours (Fig. 21–9).[43] However, the cumulus is often not visualized; thus, the inability to image this mural focus cannot be used to exclude impending ovulation.

Development of intrafollicular echogenicity (Fig. 21–10), possibly representing the periovulatory detachment of the cumulus from the follicular wall, has been suggested as a useful sign of imminent ovulation, and as having a positive predictive value for ultimate conception. It, too, is seen only in a limited number of cases, however.[29]

The presence of large ovaries, greater than 5 cm in length, with the normal echogenic tissue replaced by multiple septated cystic structures indicates ovarian hyperstimulation (Fig. 21–11). This condition is associated with an increased likelihood of pregnancy, including multiple gestations.[38, 43] Diagnosis of this sonographic abnormality should also alert one to the possibility of progression to ovarian hyperstimulation syndrome, which can be life threatening if severe, because of electrolyte imbalances and potential ovarian rupture.

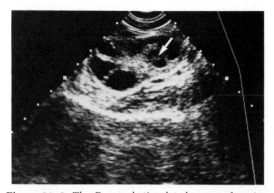

Figure 21–9. The Pergonal-stimulated ovary of an infertile patient. Five centimeters in length the ovary shows the typical replacement of the ovarian cortex by follicles surrounding the more echogenic ovarian medulla. One follicle contains a mural echogenic focus (arrow), the cumulus oophorus, signifying follicular maturity and imminent ovulation.

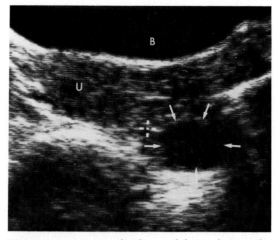

Figure 21–10. Longitudinal transabdominal view of a mature ovarian follicle in a spontaneous cycle. The follicle (arrows), measuring 20 × 22 mm, contains internal echoes, a sign of imminent ovulation. U, uterus, B, bladder.

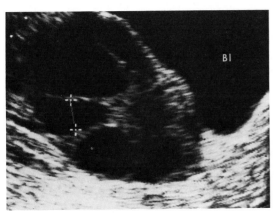

Figure 21–11. Markedly enlarged ovary replaced by septated cystic structures demonstrating geometric packing: the typical appearance of an ovary hyperstimulated by human menopausal gonadotropin (Pergonal). One triangular follicle is marked by *cursors*. Bl, bladder.

The identification of impending ovulation is most important for management of infertility patients. Presence of free fluid in the cul-de-sac may signify that ovulation has already occurred. A corpus luteum, when seen, may be larger or smaller than, but essentially indistinguishable from, a mature follicle. It may contain internal echoes representing hemorrhage and may have smooth or irregular margins. Of greatest significance, however, is that the corpus luteum is a postovulatory structure.[38]

Although routine full-bladder real-time techniques are most frequently used, transvaginal ultrasound is proving to be an accurate, efficient way to monitor sequentially the size and number of developing follicles. Further, transvaginal sonography is useful for guiding percutaneous transvaginal aspiration of follicular fluid. This method may be less painful and traumatic than transvesical or transurethral oocyte harvesting.[11]

ANATOMIC AND PHYSIOLOGIC ABNORMALITIES

One of the most frequently encountered anatomic and physiologic abnormalities is the polycystic ovary. The constellation of obesity, oligomenorrhea, and hirsutism with polycystic ovarian disease comprises the Stein-Leventhal syndrome. It is unusual, however, for all of these features to be pres-ent in any one patient with polycystic ovaries.[33] Although definitive diagnosis of polycystic ovary disease is made by pathologic examination or laboratory data (high luteinizing hormone [LH] values and an increased LH/follicle-stimulating hormone [FSH] ratio with slightly increased androgens), the sonographic appearance of spherical large ovaries containing multiple tiny cysts is suggestive of polycystic ovarian disease. In one study, in most patients with polycystic ovarian disease, the volume of the ovary was abnormally large (mean 14 cc).[19] Cysts are generally 5 to 8 mm in diameter, usually with more than five in each ovary (Fig. 21–12).[34, 61] These features are seen in 35 to 40 percent of cases. In approximately 30 percent of these patients, ovarian volume is within normal limits.[19, 61] In approximately 25 percent, a hypoechoic ovary is noted without definition of discrete individual cysts. Finally, about 5 percent demonstrate an enlarged ovary that is isoechoic with the uterus.[19] It is important for these patients to receive a long-term follow-up, since an unopposed estrogenic environment in amenorrheic patients may increase their risk of endometrial and possibly breast carcinoma.[16]

The majority of follicles in patients taking birth control pills will be small, irregular, and atretic.

Occasionally, an autonomously functioning follicle may be associated with precocious puberty. This condition is usually seen

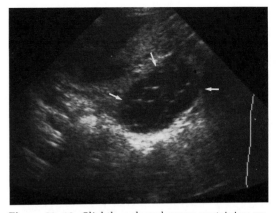

Figure 21–12. Slightly enlarged ovary containing numerous cysts of various sizes separated by septa. This is one sonographic appearance of a polycystic ovary. This hirsute patient was oligomenorrheic and had an elevated luteinizing hormone/follicle-stimulating hormone (LH/FSH) ratio.

in premenarchal girls and has been associated with hypothyroidism.[42]

The McCune-Albright syndrome is also associated with precocious puberty. The ovaries of this small group of patients are large and contain large cysts. This syndrome includes fibrous dysplasia, patchy cutaneous pigmentation, and sexual precocity. Large ovarian cysts have also been reported in some patients with neurofibromatosis.[49]

Turner's syndrome should be suspected in individuals with delayed onset of puberty, primary amenorrhea, and short stature in whom pelvic ultrasonography fails to reveal ovaries. A group with many of the physical characteristics of Turner's syndrome, including short stature, webbed neck, and cubitus valgus, but who have normal ovarian function are patients with phenotypic Turner's syndrome. These patients may have normal karyotypes, and their ovaries appear normal sonographically.[50] Nonvisualization of ovaries because of absent or streak gonads can also be noted in Swyer's syndrome or pure gonadal dysgenesis.

In a study of 13 patients with cystic fibrosis, ovarian cysts greater than 3 cm in size were found in 46 percent of patients. All the cysts were unilateral, unilocular, and transitory.[51]

Other abnormalities reflecting anatomic derangement are ovarian pregnancy (a rare form of ectopic gestation, with approximately 300 cases reported in the literature[6]) and torsion of the ovary.[14]

Sonographic Appearance of Ovarian Masses

Sonographic evaluation of the pelvis in the patient with a suspected mass has several objectives. They include confirming the presence of a mass, determining its origin (e.g., ovarian, uterine), characterizing its internal echoarchitecture, and establishing the presence or absence of related abnormalities such as ascites, obstructive uropathy, and hepatic metastases.

Most often, when attempting a specific diagnosis, a sonographer can develop a small differential based on the echogenicity and echoarchitecture of the lesion (Table 21–1).

Although the differential diagnosis is large, functional or physiologic cysts comprise the majority of lesions in ovulatory women, and these resolve spontaneously within six weeks.[52] Functional cysts should not form when ovulatory activity is lacking.

Cystic Adnexal Masses

Cystic lesions in the adnexa fulfill the same sonographic criteria as cysts of other organs. Lesions are round or ovoid, sharply marginated, and anechoic with distal acoustic enhancement. Frequently, they demonstrate refractive shadows. Most commonly, what is referred to as a cyst is a normal ovarian follicle (Fig. 21–6). The finding should not be termed a "cyst" unless the patient is prepubertal, pregnant, or postmenopausal or the structure is greater than 25 mm in diameter in a menstruating woman.

Several types of adnexal lesions exhibit cystic characteristics, including physiologic or functional ovarian cysts (follicular, corpus luteum, and theca-lutein cysts), cystadenoma, parovarian cysts, endometrioma, and hydrosalpinx.

The most common type of cystic ovarian mass is a physiologic ovarian cyst (Fig. 21–13). Tubo-ovarian abscesses may be anechoic and result from chronic pelvic inflammatory disease. The abscess cavity in-

Table 21–1. TYPICAL SONOGRAPHIC APPEARANCES OF ADNEXAL MASSES*

Completely Cystic	Complex, Predominantly Cystic	Complex, Predominantly Solid	Solid
Physiologic ovarian cyst	Cystadenoma (Ca)	Cystadenoma (Ca)	Adenocarcinoma
Cystadenomas	Dermoid cysts	Dermoid cysts	Solid teratoma (Ca)
Cystic teratomas	Tubo-ovarian abscess	Granulosa cell tumor	Arrhenoblastoma
Ovarian abscess	(Ectopic pregnancy)	(Ectopic pregnancy)	Fibroma
(Parovarian cyst)	(Fluid-filled small bowel)		Lymphomatous metastases
(Hydrosalpinx)			to ovary
(Endometrioma)			Gastrointestinal metastases
(Mesenteric cyst)			to ovary
(Bladder diverticulum)			(Matted omentum)
			(Herniated fat)

*Nonovarian masses that can mimic ovarian masses are denoted within parentheses.
Ca = carcinoma.

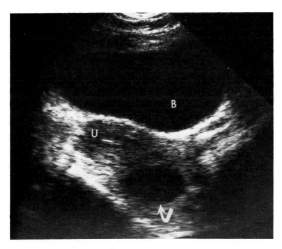

Figure 21-13. Follicular physiologic cyst. There is a 3 × 4.5 cm cyst (arrow) in this 24 year old patient with mild pelvic pain. This longitudinal transabdominal view shows the ovarian cyst posterior to the uterus (U). B, bladder. Six weeks after this study, sonography showed resolution of the cyst.

volves the ovary, and a rim of tissue may be noted bordering the abscess. A fluid-fluid level may also be seen from the layering of pus. Hydrosalpinges, in contrast, frequently demonstrate a tubular rather than a round configuration and do not include the ovary (Fig. 21-14). Cystic lesions unrelated to adnexal structures that may occupy the adnexa are bladder diverticula and mesenteric cysts.

Complex, Predominantly Cystic Masses

Included in this group are masses that are predominantly anechoic but contain septations or solid material. The most common type of complex, predominantly cystic mass is the ovarian epithelial tumor, such as cystadenoma or cystadenocarcinoma. Cystic teratoma (dermoid cyst), tubo-ovarian abscess, endometrioma, and ectopic pregnancy are also in this category.

When large, an ovarian epithelial tumor presents a characteristic sonographic appearance: a well-defined cystic mass with locules delineated by septa. These patients are usually postmenopausal. Mucin-secreting cystadenoma or cystadenocarcinoma may be pelviabdominal in position.[56] The malignant variety should be suspected when there is solid or clumped material and when ascites is associated with the mass. However, the absence of ascites is not a reliable indicator that the mass is benign.

Once a mass of this variety is encountered, one should examine the spaces of the greater peritoneal cavity, including the cul-de-sac, for ascites; the kidneys for obstructive uropathy; the liver to exclude hepatic metastases; and the peritoneal surfaces for peritoneal or omental metastatic deposits. Ultrasound is particularly accurate in detecting ascites; however, only 60 per cent of patients with peritoneal seeding from ovarian carcinoma are identified.[23] Although rare, intrahepatic metastases may be noted in some patients with advanced ovarian carcinoma.[35] Hepatic metastases associated with ovarian carcinoma usually appear as hypoechoic masses with irregular borders. In advanced carcinoma, lesions in the periphery and along the surface of the liver may be noted.

An ectopic pregnancy must be considered when a mass of this type is seen in a woman of childbearing age. Correlation with clinical history and β-hCG levels will aid in differential diagnosis.

Figure 21-14. Pyosalpinx. Transverse (A) and longitudinal (B) scans demonstrating enlarged fluid-filled fallopian tubes (arrows) in a woman with chronic pelvic inflammatory disease. H, head; b, bladder.

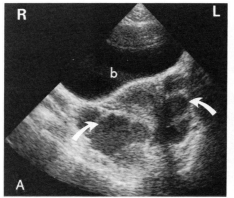
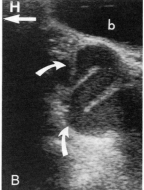

Complex, Predominantly Solid Masses

These lesions are most commonly germ cell tumors, namely, benign cystic teratomas or dermoid cysts. A dermoid cyst presents an interesting sonographic challenge. The sonographic appearance varies from completely cystic to inhomogeneously solid.[48] Most commonly, the lesion presents as a complex, predominantly solid mass containing high-level echoes arising from hair or calcifications within the dermoid cyst. The high echogenicity of these lesions may, on occasion, make it difficult to delineate the mass or differentiate it from surrounding gas-containing loops of bowel.[35] Persistent real-time evaluation of the area with or without a water enema generally demonstrates the changing nature of bowel loops. Transvaginal sonography may also be useful in demonstrating the mass and its multiple components.

Ectopic pregnancy, endometrioma, and ovarian torsion, having variable appearances, must also be considered in this differential diagnosis, depending upon the clinical situation.

Solid Adnexal Masses

Solid tumors of the ovary are rare compared with those having cystic characteristics. Endometrioid tumors, dysgerminomas, and sex cord–stromal tumors are in this group. Also included in the differential diagnosis are nonovarian adnexal abnormalities such as metastases to the ovaries, lymphadenopathy from lymphoma and leukemia, exophytic uterine leiomyomas, contiguous spread of neoplasm from adjacent organs such as rectum, thickened omentum, or mesentery (retractile mesenteritis), and hematoma.

Sonographic Mimics of Ovarian Masses

A variety of structures can mimic ovarian or adnexal masses. Most commonly, fluid or feces-filled loops of intestine may simulate a cystic adnexal mass (Figs. 21–15, 21–16A, B). A differentiating feature is that fluid-

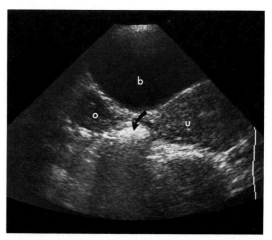

Figure 21–15. The echogenic focus (arrow), with shadowing posteriorly between the uterus (u) and right ovary (o) on this transverse scan, does not represent the "iceberg sign" of a dermoid or fibroma. Gas-filled bowel loops, as here, often occupy this area and may simulate a mass. b, bladder.

filled loops of bowel demonstrate changes with peristalsis. Occasionally, an ileus or closed-loop obstruction may make the distinction less clear. Reverberation echoes from gas in a bowel loop can occasionally be mistaken for the margins of a mass.

A pseudomass from the bladder duplication artifact can occur as a result of a multipath reflection.[24] It is created by the highly curved surface of the urinary bladder. Sound is reflected in a circuitous path back to the transducer, creating, in an abnormal location, an imprecisely defined appearance of the bladder suggestive of an ovoid mass. Rescanning after partial voiding will either change the size of the duplicated bladder artifact or eliminate it completely because of a change in the shape of the bladder.

Masses arising from structures adjacent to the ovaries, such as the uterus, can be difficult to classify. A large leiomyoma of the uterus can present as a mass whose organ of origin is uncertain. Parovarian cysts that arise from the mesovarium can appear to be of ovarian origin.[1] In these circumstances, transvaginal sonography, in providing another anatomic perspective, may help to identify the origin of the abnormality. Pseudomyxoma peritonei and intestinal lipodystrophy can also cause masslike structures in the pelvis that resemble true adnexal masses.

Figure 21–16. Bowel simulating an adnexal mass. A, In this patient evaluated for an adnexal lesion *(arrow)*, a large, poorly echogenic "mass" is seen superior to the uterus. H, head; B, bladder. B, While this simulates a fluid-filled mass by virtue of its apparent posterior acoustic enhancement *(asterisk)*, the rectangular appearance on this transverse scan raises the suspicion that this is indeed shadowing related to bowel gas anteriorly. b, bladder.

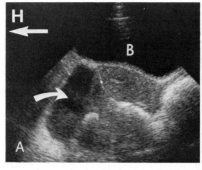
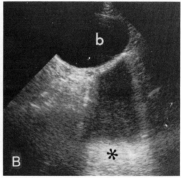

Pathologic Lesions

Non-neoplastic Cystic Lesions of the Ovary

Physiologic changes occur in the ovary that create anechoic structures that appear cystic, namely, follicles and corpora lutea. These should not be confused with functional cysts—which include follicular, corpus luteum, and theca-lutein cysts—and the ovarian remnant syndrome. The appearance of normally developing follicles and corpora lutea have been described.

FOLLICULAR CYSTS. When a mature follicle fails to ovulate or to involute, a follicular cyst results. Although follicular cysts may range in size from 1 to 10 cm in diameter, they cannot be diagnosed until greater than 2.5 cm in diameter, since normal follicles may attain that size. Although large cysts may cause pain related to pressure, hemorrhage, rupture, or torsion, they are rarely symptomatic and usually regress spontaneously. Sonographically, follicular cysts are sharply marginated, thin-walled, unilocular, anechoic structures that are usually unilateral but occasionally bilateral (Fig. 21–13). Since these cysts change with the menstrual cycle, scanning at one or two week intervals or during successive cycles usually demonstrates a change in appearance or regression.

If hemorrhage occurs, internal echoes are noted. These echoes range from low to high level and from focal to diffuse, depending on the extent and age of the bleed. Septations have also been noted.[41]

When seen in postmenopausal women in whom there is no longer significant estrogen activity, the sharply marginated, anechoic mass cannot represent a physiologic cyst. In this group, the differential diagnosis includes simple or inclusion cyst, parovarian cyst, serous cystadenoma or cystadenocarcinoma, mucinous cystadenoma or cystadenocarcinoma, and, less likely, endometrioid carcinoma, clear cell carcinoma, or granulosa cell tumor. Simple or inclusion cysts are postulated to represent fluid collections developing in invaginated and trapped sections of ovarian surface epithelium.[17]

CORPUS LUTEUM CYSTS. Normally, the corpus luteum that forms after discharge of the oocyte from the dominant follicle will involute within 14 days. Excessive bleeding into the corpus luteum or failure of absorption results in a functional corpus luteum cyst. These are generally unilocular, unilateral, and 5 to 11 cm in diameter (Fig. 21–17). These lesions tend to be larger than follicular cysts and more symptomatic. Pain is the predominant clinical finding. They are prone to hemorrhage and rupture. Sonographically, the corpus luteum cyst may be

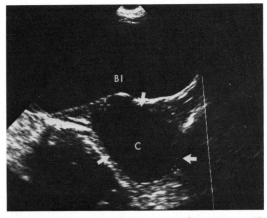

Figure 21–17. A very large corpus luteum cyst (C, *arrows*) is seen in the ovary. These cysts, on occasion, may reach 10 cm and can undergo torsion. Bl, bladder.

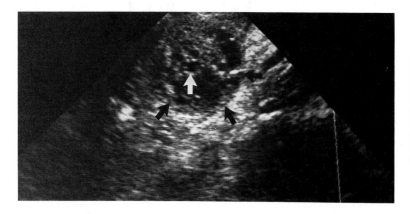

Figure 21–18. Hemorrhagic corpus luteum cyst in a 29 year old patient with severe pelvic pain. A complex, predominantly solid adnexal mass (*black arrows*), containing small cystic areas (*white arrow*) and echogenic material compatible with hemorrhage, is seen transvaginally.

anechoic, but frequently there are low-level internal echoes that may at times fill the lesion (Fig. 21–18). Intermittent bleeding may cause the cyst to appear as a complex adnexal mass not differentiable from others (Fig. 21–19). If rupture occurs, fluid can be seen in the cul-de-sac.

If the ovum is fertilized after ovulation, the corpus luteum continues its development as the corpus luteum of pregnancy. This cyst reaches its maximum size of approximately 6 cm in eight to ten weeks. By 16 weeks, most cysts have resolved. In this early period of pregnancy, these structures elaborate progesterone, which sustains the secretory endometrium. Later in pregnancy, the placenta takes up this role. The corpus luteum of pregnancy may rupture or bleed, causing acute pelvic pain early in pregnancy.[16]

THECA-LUTEIN CYSTS. Theca-lutein cysts, the largest of the functional cysts, are found in association with excessive levels of hCG, generally associated wtih trophoblastic disease. They can also be seen as a complication of drug therapy for infertility (the ovarian hyperstimulation syndrome) and, rarely, in association with normal pregnancy, when they are known as hyperreactio luteinalis.[25, 40]

In contrast to corpus luteum cysts, thecalutein cysts are usually multilocular, bilateral, and very large. Careful evaluation for molar pregnancy must be made when thecalutein cysts are suspected. Theca-lutein cysts can undergo hemorrhage, rupture, and torsion. When associated with the ovarian hyperstimulation syndrome, theca-lutein cysts may be quite symptomatic.

OVARIAN REMNANT SYNDROME. Infrequently, cystic masses may occur in patients who have undergone incomplete oophorectomies. The small amount of residual ovarian tissue may be hormonally stimulated and produce a hemorrhagic functional cyst. The patient may present with dyspareunia and bleeding. Sonographically, an echogenic mass, which can be quite large, may at times be identified.[36]

PAROVARIAN CYSTS. Parovarian cysts, arising from wolffian duct remnants (Gartner's duct) within the mesovarium, are common lesions, accounting for 10 percent of all adnexal masses. They are found in the broad ligament and, like other cystic masses, may undergo hemorrhage, torsion, and rupture. Unlike physiologic ovarian cysts, parovarian cysts show no cyclic changes. These lesions have a wide size range from 1.5 to 19 cm. Although most are anechoic, with the same appearance as cysts found elsewhere in the body, some cysts contain internal echoes due to the presence of hemorrhage.[1] There are no specific sonographic features of un-

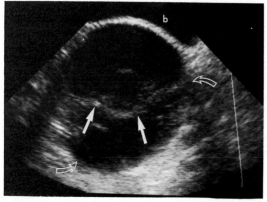

Figure 21–19. Large hemorrhagic cyst (*curved open arrows*) posterior to the bladder (b) with thick internal septation (*arrows*).

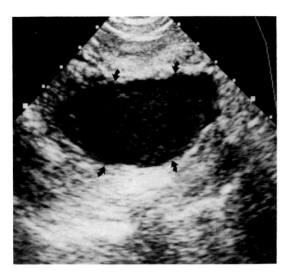

Figure 21–20. Transvaginal sagittal view in a 34 year old infertility patient. A fairly well defined 3.2 × 6.5 cm adnexal mass *(arrows)* containing internal echoes represents an endometrioma. This is a typical appearance.

complicated parovarian cysts. Larger parovarian cysts may resemble serous cystadenomas or endometriomas. Unless a normal ovary is seen in addition to and separate from the cyst, a specific diagnosis is not possible.

ENDOMETRIOMAS. Endometriosis represents ectopic endometrial tissue found in the ovary, fallopian tubes, cul-de-sac, broad ligament, colon, and bladder and, rarely, in remote areas of the body.

The most common form of the disease presents as diffuse tiny endometrial implants involving the pelvic viscera and their ligamentous attachments.[4] These implants respond to hormonal changes and bleed during menses, with local inflammatory reaction leading to adhesions that may impair fertility. Because the implants are too small to be imaged sonographically, this form of the disease is infrequently diagnosed by ultrasound.[12]

Presenting as adnexal or pelvic masses, a more localized form of the disease consists of discrete larger lesions, termed endometriomas or "chocolate cysts." They are generally well-marginated masses with slightly thickened walls and low-level internal echoes (Fig. 21–20).[57] Echoes may be found in the dependent portion of the lesion, and sometimes fluid-debris levels can be noted.[7] Occasionally, endometriomas may contain

foci of more brightly echogenic material, compatible with fresh hemorrhage (Fig. 21–21). Endometriomas may also be anechoic and appear purely cystic.

With endometriosis, prominence of the endometrial echo secondary to endometritis may be seen. In addition, there may be loss of definition of the pelvic structures owing to inflammatory reactions that these lesions incite.

TORSION OF THE OVARY. Torsion of the ovary is most common during the first decades of life. Torsion may also be associated with an ovarian cyst or neoplasm (Fig. 21–22). Additional conditions in which torsion has been reported are pregnancy and the hyperstimulated ovary syndrome.[14] Torsion is a surgical condition in which delay may cause irreversible damage by partial or complete rotation of the ovarian pedicle on its long axis. Various degrees of ovarian arterial, venous, and lymphatic occlusion occur, causing massive congestion of the ovarian parenchyma and hemorrhagic infarction. Clinical findings include severe pelvic pain, anorexia, nausea, and vomiting. A palpable mass and leukocytosis may be present.

Sonographically, the salient finding is a unilaterally enlarged ovary that may appear as a hypoechoic mass (Fig. 21–23). Engorged vessels may appear as small multiple cystic structures of uniform size at the periphery of the enlarged ovary. A dilated uterine tube may also be noted, depending on the site of torsion. The ovary can also resemble a hemorrhagic cyst, and some masses demonstrate

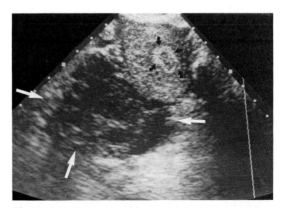

Figure 21–21. 37 year old woman with a long history of intermittent pelvic pain. Transvaginal coronal scan demonstrates a 6 cm hypoechoic complex adnexal mass *(white arrows)*. Echogenic material within the mass is compatible with the hemorrhagic components of a large endometrioma. Very prominent endometrial echoes *(black arrows)* suggest endometritis.

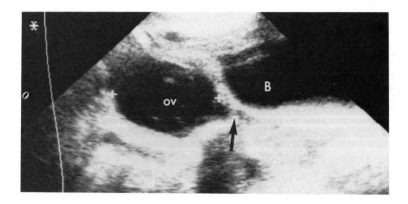

Figure 21–22. Complex ovoid adnexal mass (ov) with some internal echoes demonstrates the "beak sign" (arrow) of torsion. The mass proved to be an ovarian cyst. B, bladder.

a beaklike or curvilinear group of echoes representing the site of torsion. Free fluid in the cul-de-sac is noted in approximately one-third of cases.[14]

OTHER LESIONS. Among these non-neoplastic cystic lesions that may be indistinguishable sonographically, ectopic pregnancy (Fig. 21–24) and pelvic inflammatory disease (see Fig. 21–14) are important diagnostic considerations. Clinical history is frequently of primary importance in arriving at a diagnosis. These abnormalities are addressed in other chapters of this text.

Neoplasms

Ovarian neoplasms are the third most common gynecologic malignancy. Most likely owing to late detection, they have the highest mortality rate and are responsible for almost one-half of the deaths from cancer of the female genital tract. Ovarian malignancy accounts for 6 percent of all cancers in the female and is the fifth most common form of cancer in women, excluding skin cancer.[25] At the time of diagnosis, approxi-

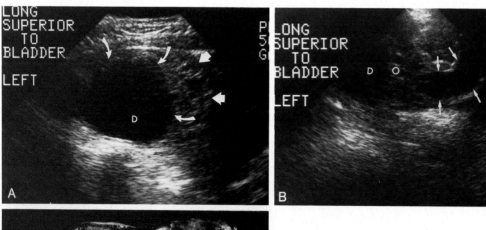

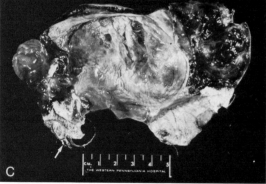

Figure 21–23. Cystic teratoma (dermoid cyst) with torsion. A, Hypoechoic round lesion (curved arrows), a dermoid (D), with a rim of midlevel echogenic ovarian tissue (wide arrows). B, The hypoechoic tubular structure (arrows) is the enlarged uterine tube. O, ovary. C, Pathologic specimen demonstrating the expected mixed tissue components of a dermoid: fatty, solid, and cystic elements. Hair (arrow), frequently found, is seen at the periphery of the lesion.

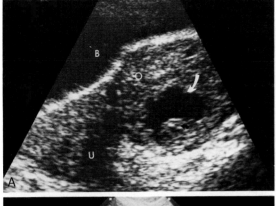

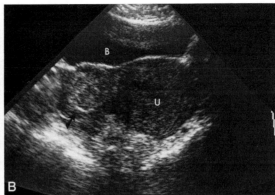

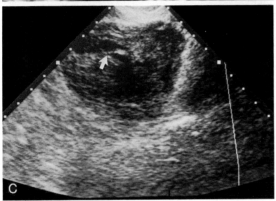

Figure 21–24. *A,* Very rarely occurring in the ovary, the gestational sac of an ectopic pregnancy *(white arrow)* is seen within the enlarged left ovary (O), difficult to differentiate at first from the adjacent uterus (U). Cardiac activity was seen in this unruptured ectopic pregnancy. Transverse transabdominal scan. B, bladder; *(black arrow),* fetus. *B,* Echogenic material *(arrow)* in the right adnexa represents a ruptured ectopic pregnancy in a patient with positive serum β-hCG and no intrauterine gestation. *C,* Ectopic pregnancy. Transvaginal sagittal view shows a 4 × 7 cm complex, predominantly solid adnexal mass. A small, fluid-filled gestational sac *(arrow)* is seen within the mass.

mately two-thirds of patients have distant metastases.

About 80 percent of ovarian tumors are benign, and these occur mostly in young women between the ages of 20 and 45 years. The malignant tumors are more common in older age groups, between 40 and 65 years (Fig. 21–25). Therefore, careful assessment of the postmenopausal ovary is essential. Although an ovary measuring 3 cm × 2 cm × 2 cm may be considered normal in a premenopausal patient, the ovary in a woman who has undergone menopause should measure no more than 2 cm × 1 cm × 0.5 cm.[3] Tables 21–2 and 21–3 present an overview based on the histologic classification of ovarian neoplasms.

Although they may be either predominantly cystic or solid, most malignancies are in the sonographic category of complex lesions. There are but a few differentiating points to determine histology. Only cystadenoma, cystadenocarcinoma, and benign cystic teratoma have sonographic features that may allow for specific differentiation.

Anechoic, sharply marginated lesions have a high likelihood of being benign. In-creasing echogenicity, inhomogeneity, and indistinctness of the margins favor malignancy.[30] Two exceptions to this observation are (1) lesions with very echogenic foci, which are usually benign cystic teratomas, and (2) totally or almost totally echogenic lesions, which tend to represent masses of nonovarian origin or benign lesions.

An attempt should be made to define the extent of a suspected neoplasm based on the International Federation of Gynecology and Obstetrics (FIGO) staging of carcinoma of the ovary (Table 21–4). The specificity of ultrasound in this respect has not been completely defined. In one study of patients with cystadenocarcinoma, ultrasound was highly accurate in demonstrating the primary lesion and in detecting ascites. It was insensitive for detecting prevertebral adenopathy less than 3 cm in size, omental plaques thinner than 1.5 cm, and peritoneal masses 2 cm or less.[58] In another series, the sensitivity of ultrasound in the detection of pelvic masses was 91 percent. It had an accuracy of 81 percent in defining recurrent disease.[47] The sensitivity of ultrasound as a screening technique for ovarian neoplasm has not been

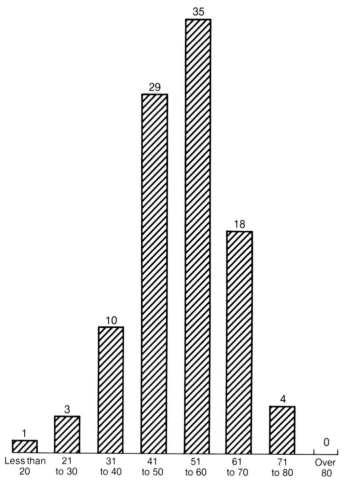

Figure 21–25. Primary ovarian carcinoma: frequency (percentage) as a function of years of age (665 cases). (*From* Zaloudek C: The ovary. *In* Gompel C, Silverberg SG (eds): Pathology in Gynecology and Obstetrics. Philadelphia, JB Lippincott Co, 1985.)

defined. Transvaginal sonography may prove useful in this regard.

Epithelial Tumors

SEROUS TUMORS. Serous cystadenoma and serous cystadenocarcinoma are the most common epithelial ovarian neoplasms. Together, the benign, borderline, and malignant types account for about 30 percent of all ovarian tumors.

Benign serous cystadenomas are large, sharply marginated anechoic masses that are usually unilocular but may contain a lattice of internal thin-walled septations (Fig. 21–26). Papillary projections are occasionally seen, whereas ascites is very uncommon.

Conversely, serous cystadenocarcinomas are usually multilocular lesions containing numerous papillary projections arising from the cyst walls and septations. Echogenic material may be present within locules (Fig.

21–27). Neoplastic excrescences may form on the surface of the cyst and surrounding organs, resulting in a large fixed mass with ascites (Figs. 21–28, 21–29). These tumors may be quite large, over 15 cm in 56 percent of patients in one series.[59]

MUCINOUS TUMORS. Mucinous cystadenoma and cystadenocarcinoma are somewhat less common than the serous forms and account for about 20 percent of all ovarian neoplasms. The benign variants are much more common than the malignant types, in the ratio of approximately 7:1. Occasionally, these lesions can be bilateral, although they are usually unilateral. Mucinous cystadenomas can be huge, up to 50 cm, but are most often 15 to 30 cm, filling the pelviabdominal cavity.[59] Prominent septations are frequently present. Representing mucin, low-level echoes form layers in dependent portions of the lesion (Fig. 21–30).

Table 21–2. OVARIAN NEOPLASMS

Tumors of Surface Epithelium (75% of all ovarian tumors, 95% of malignant ovarian tumors)
  Serous tumors
    Serous cystadenoma
    Serous cystadenocarcinoma
    Adenofibroma and cystadenofibroma
  Mucinous tumors
    Mucinous cystadenoma
    Mucinous cystadenocarcinoma
  Endometrioid carcinoma
  Clear cell adenocarcinoma
  Brenner tumor
  Undifferentiated carcinoma
Germ Cell Tumors (15% of all ovarian tumors; 1% of malignant ovarian tumors)
  Teratoma
    Benign (mature, adult)
      Cystic teratoma (dermoid cyst)
      Solid teratoma
    Malignant (immature)
    Monodermal or specialized (e.g., carcinoid, struma ovarii)
  Dysgerminoma
  Endodermal sinus tumor
  Choriocarcinoma
  Others (embryonal carcinoma, polyembryoma, mixed germ cell tumors)
Sex Cord–Stroma Tumors (10% of all ovarian tumors; 2% of malignant ovarian tumors)
  Granulosa–theca cell tumors
    Granulosa cell tumor
    Thecoma
    Fibroma
  Sertoli-Leydig cell tumor (androblastoma)
  Gonadoblastoma
Metastatic Tumors

From Robbins SL, Cotran RS, Kumar V (eds): Female genital tract. *In* Pathologic Basis of Disease, 3rd Ed. Philadelphia, WB Saunders Co, 1984.

Table 21–4. FIGO STAGING OF CARCINOMA OF THE OVARY

Stage I.	Growth limited to the ovaries
	Ia. Growth limited to one ovary; no ascites
	Ib. Growth limited to both ovaries: no ascites
	Ic. Growth limited to one or both ovaries; ascites present or malignant cells in peritoneal washings
Stage II.	Growth involving one or both ovaries with pelvic extension
	IIa. Extension and/or metastasis to the uterus and/or tubes only
	IIb. Extension to other pelvic tissues
	IIc. Stage IIa or IIb plus ascites or positive peritoneal washings
Stage III.	Growth involving one or both ovaries with intraperitoneal metastasis to the abdomen (including omentum, small intestine, and its mesentery) and/or positive retroperitoneal nodes
Stage IV.	Growth involving one or both ovaries with distant metastasis outside the peritoneal cavity

Note: Stages Ia and Ib are subclassified (i) or (ii) depending upon the absence (i) or presence (ii) of tumor on the ovarian surface and/or capsular rupture.

From Zaloudek C: The ovary. *In* Gompel C, Silverberg SG (eds): Pathology in Gynecology and Obstetrics. Philadelphia, JB Lippincott Co, 1985.

Table 21–3. OVARIAN CANCER: COMPILED STATISTICS

Type of Tumor	Incidence (%)	Bilaterality (%)	5 Year Survival (%)
Serous borderline tumor	10–15	60*	95†
Serous carcinoma	25–35	60*	20
Mucinous borderline tumor	5–10	20*	95†
Mucinous carcinoma	5–10	20*	45
Endometrioid carcinoma	15–30	30*	50
Clear cell carcinoma	4–6	10–30	40
Undifferentiated carcinoma	5–10	55	10
Yolk sac tumor	< 1	< 5	> 50‡
Dysgerminoma	1–2	10–20	90
Immature teratoma	< 1	< 5	> 50‡
Secondary malignant teratoma	< 1	0	15
Granulosa cell tumor	< 5	5	90†
Androblastoma	< 1	5	90

*Approximately half in stage 1.
†Late recurrences common.
‡With appropriate chemotherapy.
From Zaloudek C: The ovary. *In* Gompel C, Silverberg SG (eds): Pathology in Gynecology and Obstetrics. Philadelphia, JB Lippincott Co, 1985.

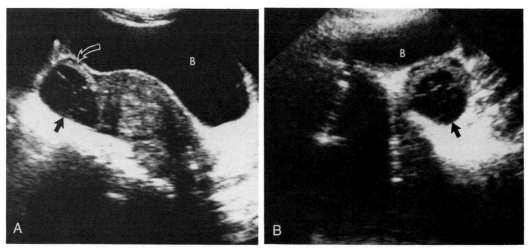

Figure 21–26. Serous cystadenoma. *A,* Transverse view shows a mass *(black arrow)* with a lattice of internal echoes and a rim of ovarian tissue *(curved arrow). B,* Longitudinal view of the same adnexal lesion *(black arrow).* B, bladder.

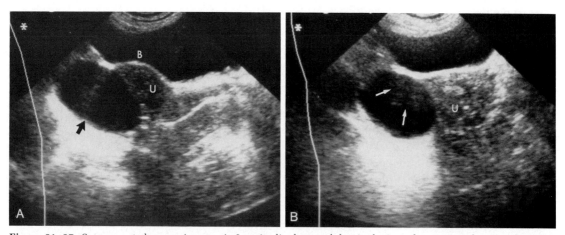

Figure 21–27. Serous cystadenocarcinoma. *A,* Longitudinal transabdominal view shows a predominantly cystic *(black arrow)* adnexal mass posterosuperior to the bladder (B). This mass compresses the uterus (U) and is difficult to separate from it on this view. *B,* Transverse view shows the solid portion as clumped echoes abutting the wall of the mass *(white arrows).* Endometrial echoes are prominent in this postmenopausal patient.

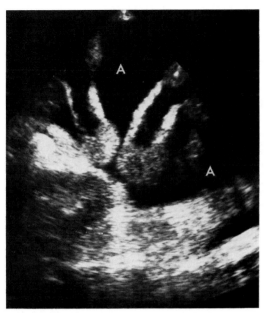

Figure 21–28. Metastatic ovarian carcinoma. Ascites (A) is present. Bowel loops float in the fluid.

Mucinous cystadenocarcinomas are usually large, multiloculated cystic lesions containing echogenic material and papillary projections. They are bilateral in approximately 25 percent of patients (Fig. 21–31). The appearance is similar to serous cystadenocarcinoma, although papillary projections are less common than in the serous

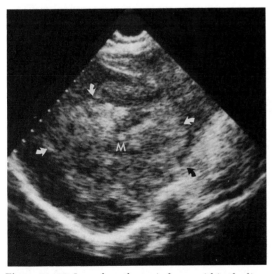

Figure 21–29. Irregular echogenic focus within the liver (arrows) represents metastasis (M) from ovarian carcinoma. Metastases from ovarian carcinoma are usually hypoechoic, but their appearance can be variable.

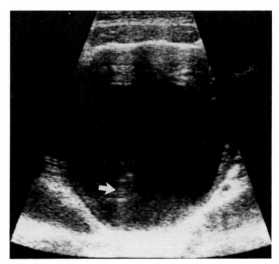

Figure 21–30. Mucinous cystadenoma. Very large cystic adnexal mass with echogenic material layered posteriorly. A small, moundlike projection (arrow) is noted.

type. Metastases from these cystadenocarcinomas or rupture of a malignant tumor gives rise to development of a gelatinous material that may implant on all the serosal surfaces, causing extensive adhesion of the viscera and matting of the abdominal contents. This condition, pseudomyxoma peritonei, may resemble ascites sonographically or manifest itself as grapelike clusters of anechoic spaces filling much of the pelvis and abdomen.[20]

OTHER EPITHELIAL TUMORS. Endometrioid carcinoma accounts for approximately 20 percent of all ovarian cancers.[44] Although benign and borderline forms may occur,

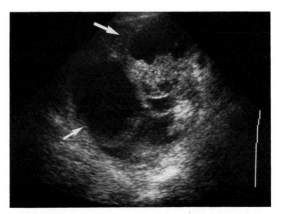

Figure 21–31. Mucinous cystadenocarcinoma of the ovary. In this 47 year old patient with ascites, the large bilobed anechoic adnexal masses (white arrows) with inhomogenous solid components represent clear cell adenocarcinoma (Stage III).

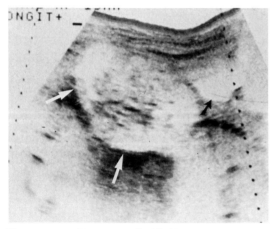

Figure 21–32. Superior to the bladder *(black arrow)* in this 53 year old woman is a large, complex hypoechoic mass *(white arrows)* with a central solid component and cystic areas in the periphery representing necrosis in this endometrioid carcinoma. Static image, transverse transabdominal view with reverse polarity.

most endometrioid carcinomas are true carcinomas. Histologically, this tumor is indistinguishable from endometrial adenocarcinoma of the uterus. Frequently bilateral, it has been described as ranging from cystic with papillary projections to complex solid with areas of necrosis and hemorrhage (Fig. 21–32).[59]

Clear cell carcinoma also presents as a nonspecific, sonographically complex mass (Fig. 21–33). These neoplasms are thought to be of müllerian duct origin and a variant of endometrioid carcinoma.

Brenner tumor is usually benign, occurs at any age, and is uncommon. It ranges in size from 1 to 20 cm. Pathologically, these lesions are generally solid, although occasionally cystic.

Germ Cell Tumors

TERATOMA. Teratomas are divided into three categories: benign, malignant, and monodermal or highly specialized.[44] Most benign teratomas are cystic and clinically termed "dermoid cysts." Dermoids comprise those teratomas in which the ectodermal elements predominate. Cystic teratomas are the most frequently encountered ovarian tumor of childhood but are found at all ages, particularly during the years of active reproduction.

The sonographic appearance of cystic teratomas is extremely variable, although an anechoic mass containing an echogenic mural focus with associated acoustic shadowing, the "dermoid plug," is highly suggestive of a dermoid.[39] Echogenic material is frequently seen in a nondependent portion (Fig. 21–34). The shadowing in a dermoid is frequently due to the presence of hair, although bone or teeth may also account for this finding (Fig. 21–35). If the hair within the lesion floats on top of the fatty material, acoustic shadowing obscures the backwall of the lesion. This has been referred to as the "tip of the iceberg" sign (Fig. 21–36).[15] These lesions can mimic bowel gas and be missed by ultrasound. Malignant teratomas are rare, found chiefly in prepubertal adolescents and young women.

Other lesions, dysgerminomas and endo-

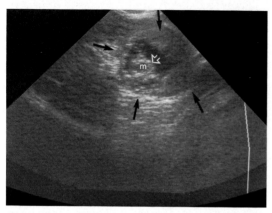

Figure 21–33. Clear cell carcinoma. Transvaginal view of a complex mass *(arrows)* with a central echogenic area *(m, open arrow)*. Sonography identified the mass, although its appearance is otherwise nonspecific.

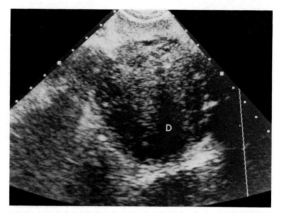

Figure 21–34. Cystic teratoma with a fat-fluid level. This asymptomatic 19 year old patient presented with a palpable adnexal mass. Transvaginal coronal view demonstrates echogenic material anteriorly with a fluid component layering posteriorly, suggestive of the fat-fluid level of a dermoid cyst (D).

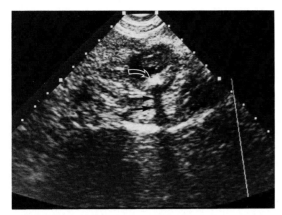

Figure 21–35. Cystic teratoma (dermoid cyst). Coronal transvaginal view in a 27 year old asymptomatic woman shows a 2.8 cm complex adnexal mass with cystic and irregular solid areas. The highly echogenic focus (*open white arrow*) with sharply defined posterior acoustic shadowing (*black arrows*) suggested the diagnosis of a dermoid in this patient.

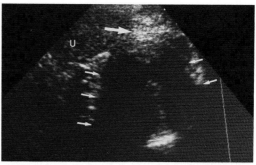

Figure 21–36. Cystic teratoma (dermoid cyst) in a 22 year old woman with pelvic pain. Coronal transvaginal view of the uterus (U) and adjacent adnexa shows an echogenic focus, somewhat vague in outline (*large arrow*), with dense posterior shadowing (*small arrows*), the "iceberg sign," where the bulk of the lesion is obscured by shadowing.

dermal sinus (yolk sac) tumors, both malignant, have been described sonographically as being predominantly echogenic masses that may contain anechoic to hypoechoic areas from hemorrhage or necrosis.[59] Dysgerminoma, the counterpart of the male seminoma, is unilateral and relatively uncommon; however, it accounts for about one-half of malignant germ cell tumors.

Sex Cord–Stromal Tumors

GRANULOSA CELL TUMORS. These lesions are most common in postmenopausal women, with clinical signs of estrogen production often present. The latter leads to endometrial hyperplasia, cystic disease of the breast, breast carcinoma, and endometrial carcinoma. About 10 to 15 percent of patients with estrogen-producing tumors eventually develop endometrial carcinoma.[44] When small, granulosa cell tumors are predominantly echogenic and may resemble leiomyomas, but when large, they have a multiloculated appearance simulating cystadenoma (Fig. 21–37).

THECOMA. Most thecomas (70 percent) occur in postmenopausal women, but the age distribution ranges from 15 to 86 years. The tumor is usually unilateral and benign, with little tendency to undergo malignant degen-

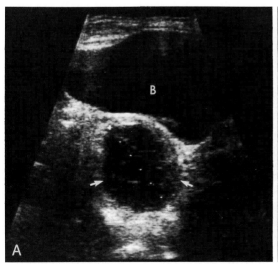

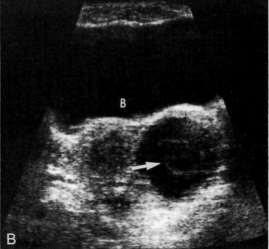

Figure 21–37. Granulosa cell tumor. *A*, Longitudinal transabdominal view shows a multiloculated, predominantly cystic adnexal mass (arrows) posterior to the bladder (B). *B*, transverse view of the same lesion with this central ring of echoes (*arrow*).

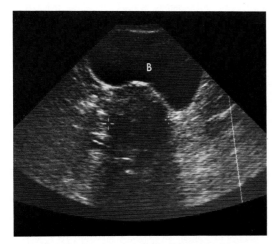

Figure 21–38. Ovarian fibroma. 48 year old woman with an adnexal mass. Longitudinal transabdominal view shows a solid mass *(cursors)* with midlevel echoes and prominent posterior acoustic shadowing. This benign neoplasm may demonstrate homogeneous echogenicity. In this case, no ascites was present. B, bladder.

eration. Sonographically, the lesion is interesting in that it presents a unique pattern of a mass with a prominent acoustic shadow corresponding to the entire extent of the mass, as opposed to a point shadow from calcification or gas.[9, 60]

SERTOLI-LEYDIG CELL TUMORS. These very rare lesions often cause signs of masculinization, although many have no endocrine effect. Three to 20 percent are malignant. The appearance is similar to that of granulosa cell tumors.

FIBROMAS. Fibromas arising in the ovarian stroma account for about 5 percent of ovarian neoplasms and usually affect menopausal or postmenopausal women in their fifth or sixth decade. These lesions tend to be large, in the range of 5 to 10 cm, but may be up to 16 cm in diameter. Ten percent are multiple, with ascites present in 40 percent of patients having tumors greater than 6 cm in diameter. Meigs' syndrome, which consists of associated ascites and pleural effusion, usually on the right, is present with 1 to 3 percent of fibromas. The sonographic appearance of this benign tumor is that of a large adnexal mass, predominantly hypoechoic and with striking attenuation of the sonographic beam (Fig. 21–38).[53] It is important to consider Meigs' syndrome among diagnostic possibilities since this constellation of findings has frequently led to the clinical diagnosis of malignancy, without sufficient documentation.

Metastatic and Direct Extension of Neoplasm

Lymphoma

Lymphoma of the pelvis may occur within the ovaries, most often as a result of dissemination from other sites, or it may represent adnexal lymphadenopathy in extensive pelvic disease. These solid masses are similar to lymphadenopathy in other sites. Generally, the enlarged lymph nodes are hypoechoic and quite trans-sonic. However, because of gas-filled intestine, it is unlikely that the entire tumor volume will be delineated by ultrasound.

Other

The ovary is more often involved by metastatic disease than any of the other pelvic genital organs. Three groups of malignancies account for this and include metastases from other pelvic organs; the upper gastrointestinal tract, including the stomach, biliary tract, and pancreas; and the breast. The term Krukenberg's tumor applies to bilateral metastatic ovarian tumors composed of mucin-producing signet-ring cells, generally of gastric origin (Fig. 21–39). Their sonographic appearance is that of echogenic masses containing variable anechoic spaces. They can also be identical to cystadenocarcinoma of the ovary.[2]

Direct extension of neoplasm from an ad-

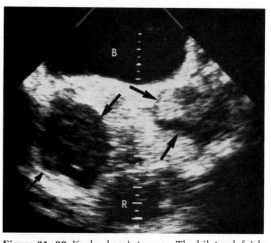

Figure 21–39. Krukenberg's tumors. The bilateral, fairly well defined echogenic adnexal masses *(arrows)* seen on this transverse transabdominal view are metastases to the ovaries from signet-ring cell carcinoma of the stomach. B, bladder; R, rectum.

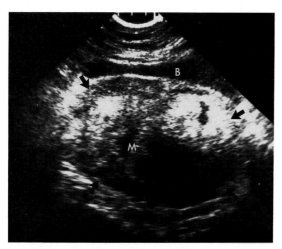

Figure 21–40. Colon carcinoma. Invasion of the pelvic structures, including the ovaries, by this advanced aggressive carcinoma of the colon *(arrows)*. The mass (M) is inhomogeneous but predominantly echogenic. The bladder (B), compressed by the mass, is seen anteriorly.

jacent pelvic tumor must also be considered. Colon carcinoma, in particular, may present as bilateral ovarian tumors (Fig. 21–40).[55] New techniques, including transvaginal and transrectal ultrasound, may prove useful in assessing the extent of a tumor.[27, 28]

References

1. Alpern MB, Sandler MA, Madrazo BL: Sonographic features of parovarian cysts and their complications. AJR 143:157, 1984.
2. Athey PA, Butters HE: Sonographic and CT appearance of Krukenberg tumors. JCU 12:205, 1984.
3. Barber HRK, Graber EA: The postmenopausal palpable ovarian syndrome. Obstet Gynceol 38:921, 1971.
4. Birnholz JC: Endometriosis, an inflammatory disease. Semin Ultrasound, 4:184, 1983.
5. Buttery B, Trounson A, McMaster R, Wood C: Evaluation of diagnostic ultrasound as a parameter of follicular development in an in vitro fertilization program. Fertil Steril 39:458, 1983.
6. Check JH, Chase JS: Ovarian pregnancy with a contralateral corpus luteum: Case report. Am J Obstet Gynecol 154:155, 1986.
7. Coleman BG, Arger PH, Mulhern CB Jr: Endometriosis: Clinical and ultrasonic correlation. AJR 132:747, 1979.
8. Davis JA, Gosink BB: Fluid in the female pelvis: Cyclic patterns. J Ultrasound Med 5:75, 1986.
9. Diakoumakis E, Vieux U, Seife B: Sonographic demonstration of thecoma: Report of two cases. Am J Obstet Gynecol 150:787, 1984.
10. Dornbluth NC, Potter JL, Shepard MK, et al: Assessment of follicular development by ultrasonography and total serum estrogen in human menopausal gonadotropin-stimulated cycles. J Ultrasound Med 2:407, 1983.
11. Feichtinger W, Kemeter P: Transvaginal sector scan sonography for needle guided transvaginal follicle aspiration and other applications in gynecologic routine and research. Fertil Steril 45:722, 1986.
12. Friedman H, Vogelzang RI, Mendelson EB, et al: Endometriosis detection by ultrasound with laparoscopic correlation. Radiology 157:217, 1985.
13. Ganong WF: The gonads: Development and function of the reproductive system. Review of Medical Physiology, 7th Ed. Los Altos, California, Lange, 1975, pp 310–341.
14. Graif M, Shalev J, Strauss S, et al: Torsion of the ovary: Sonographic features. AJR 143:1331, 1984.
15. Gutman PH Jr: In search of the elusive benign cystic ovarian teratoma: Application of the ultrasound "tip of the iceberg" sign. JCU 5:403, 1977.
16. Hall DA: Sonographic appearance of the normal ovary, of polycystic ovary disease and of functional ovarian cysts. Semin Ultrasound 4:149, 1983.
17. Hall DA, McCarthy KA: The significance of the postmenopausal simple adnexal cyst. J Ultrasound Med 5:503, 1986.
18. Hall DA, McCarthy KA, Kopans DB: Sonographic visualization of the normal postmenopausal ovary. J Ultrasound Med 5:9, 1986.
19. Hann LE, Hall DA, McArdle CR, Seibel M: Polycystic ovarian disease: Sonographic spectrum. Radiology 150:531, 1984.
20. Hayashi N, Tamaki N, Yamamoto K, et al: Sonography of pseudomyxoma peritonei. J Ultrasound Med 5:401, 1986.
21. Hull ME, Moghissi KS, Magyar DM, et al: Correlation of serum estradiol levels and ultrasound monitoring to assess follicular maturation. Fertil Steril 46:42, 1986.
22. Ivarsson SA, Nilsson KO, Persson PH: Ultrasonography of the pelvic organs in prepubertal and postpubertal girls. Arch Dis Child 58:352, 1983.
23. Khan O, Wiltshaw E, McCready VR, et al: Role of ultrasound in the management of ovarian carcinoma. J R Soc Med 76:821, 1983.
24. Laing FC: Commonly encountered artifacts in clinical ultrasound. Semin Ultrasound 4:27, 1983.
25. Lawrence PH, Lyons EA, Levi CS: Hyperreactio luteinalis. J Ultrasound Med 2:375, 1983.
26. Lenz S: Ultrasonic study of follicular maturation, ovulation and development of corpus luteum during normal menstrual cycles. Acta Obstet Gynecol Scand 64:15, 1985.
27. Meanwell CA, Rolfe EB, Blackledge G, et al: Recurrent female pelvic cancer: Assessment with transrectal ultrasonography. Radiology 162:278, 1987.
28. Mendelson EB, Bohm-Velez M, Joseph N, Neiman HL: Gynecologic imaging: Comparison of transabdominal and transvaginal techniques. Radiology 166:321, 1988.
29. Mendelson EB, Friedman H, Neiman HL, et al: The role of imaging in infertility management. AJR 144:415, 1985.
30. Moyle JW, Rochester D, Sider L, et al: Sonography of ovarian tumors: Predictability of tumor type. AJR 141:985, 1983.
31. Munn CS, Kiser LC, Wetzner SM, Baer JE: Ovary volume in young and premenopausal adults: US determination. Radiology 159:731, 1986.
32. Nicolini U, Ferrazzi E, Bellotti M, et al: The contri-

bution of sonographic evaluation of ovarian size in patients with polycystic ovarian disease. J Ultrasound Med 4:347, 1985.

33. Orsini LF, Salardi S, Pilu G, et al: Pelvic organs in premenarcheal girls: Real-time ultrasonography. Radiology 153:113, 1984.

34. Orsini LF, Venturoli S, Lorusso R, et al: Ultrasonic findings in polycystic ovarian disease. Fertil Steril 43:709, 1985.

35. Paling M, Shawker T: Abdominal ultrasound in advanced ovarian carcinoma. JCU 9:435, 1981.

36. Phillips HE, McGahan JP: Ovarian remnant syndrome. Radiology 142:487, 1982.

37. Prins GS, Vogelzang RL: Interventional sources of ultrasound variability in relation to follicular measurements. J In Vitro Fert Embryo Transfer 1:221, 1984.

38. Queenan JT, O'Brien JD, Bains LM, et al: Ultrasound scanning of ovaries to detect ovulation in women. Fertil Steril 34:99, 1980.

39. Quinn SF, Erickson S, Black WC: Cystic ovarian teratomas: The sonographic appearance of the dermoid plug. Radiology 155:477, 1985.

40. Rankin RN, Hutton LC: Ultrasound in the ovarian hyperstimulation syndrome. JCU 9:473, 1981.

41. Reynolds T, Hill MC, Glassman LM: Sonography of hemorrhagic ovarian cysts. JCU 14:449, 1986.

42. Riddlesberger M, Kuhn J, Munchshauer R: The association of juvenile hypothyroidism in cystic ovaries. Radiology 139:77, 1981.

43. Ritchie WGM: Sonographic evaluation of normal and induced ovulation. Radiology 161:1, 1986.

44. Robbins SL, Cotran RS, Kumar V: Female genital tract. In Pathologic Basis of Disease, 3rd Ed. Philadelphia, WB Saunders Co, 1984, pp 1142–1155.

45. Rubin C, Kurtz AB, Goldberg BB: Water enema: A new ultrasound technique in defining pelvic anatomy. JCU 6:28, 1978.

46. Sample W, Lippe B, Gyepes M: Gray scale ultrasonography of the normal female pelvis. Radiology 125:477, 1977.

47. Sanders RC, McNeil BJ, Finberg HJ, et al: A prospective study of computed tomography and ultrasound in the detection of staging of pelvic masses. Radiology 146:439, 1983.

48. Sandler M, Silver T, Karo J: Gray scale ultrasonic features of ovarian teratomas. Radiology 131:705, 1979.

49. Shawker TH, Comite F, Rieth KG, et al: Ultrasound evaluation of female isosexual precocious puberty. J Ultrasound Med 3:309, 1984.

50. Shawker TH, Garra BS, Loriaux DL, et al: Ultrasonography of Turner's syndrome. J Ultrasound Med 5:125, 1986.

51. Shawker TH, Hubbard VS, Reichert CM, Guerreiro de Matos OM: Cystic ovaries in cystic fibrosis: An ultrasound and autopsy study. Radiology 152:865, 1984.

52. Spanos WJ: Preoperative hormonal therapy of cystic adnexal masses. Am J Obstet Gynecol 116:551, 1973.

53. Stephenson WM, Laing FC: Sonography of ovarian fibromas. AJR 144:1239, 1985.

54. Taylor KJW, Burns PN, Woodcock JP, Wells PNT: Blood flow in deep abdominal and pelvic vessels: Ultrasonic pulsed-doppler analysis. Radiology 154:487, 1985.

55. Tsukamoto N, Uchino H, Matsukuma K, Kamura T: Carcinoma of the colon presenting as bilateral ovarian tumors during pregnancy. Gynecol Oncol 24:386, 1986.

56. Walsh J, Taylor K, Wasson J, et al: Gray scale ultrasound in 204 proved gynecologic masses: Accuracy in specific diagnostic criteria. Radiology 130:391, 1979.

57. Walsh JW, Taylor KJW, Rosenfeld AT: Gray scale ultrasonography in the diagnosis of endometriosis and adenomyosis. AJR 132:87, 1979.

58. Wicks JD, Mettler FA Jr, Hilgers RD, Ampuero F: Correlation of ultrasound and pathologic findings in patients with epithelial carcinoma of the ovary. JCU 12:397, 1984.

59. Williams AG, Mettler FA, Wicks JD: Cystic and solid ovarian neoplasms. Semin Ultrasound 4:166, 1983.

60. Yaghoobian J, Pinck RL: Ultrasound findings in thecoma of the ovary. JCU 11:91, 1983.

61. Yeh HC, Futterweit W, Thornton JC: Polycystic ovarian disease: US features in 104 patients. Radiology 163:111, 1987.

62. Zacur HA: Ovulation induction with GNRH. Fertil Steril 44:435, 1985.

ECTOPIC PREGNANCY

Roy A. Filly, M.D.*

The first documented autopsy performed in the United States, circa 1638 or 1639, identified an ectopic pregnancy as the cause of death.[1] This disease process has been a continuing problem since then and has probably never been more in the minds of practicing clinicians than it is today. During the 1970s, the number of hospitalizations for ectopic pregnancy more than doubled (Fig. 22–1) (by the mid-1980s, it had easily tripled), and ectopic pregnancy has emerged as a leading cause of maternal death.[2, 3] Fortunately, the risk of death has declined despite the increasing incidence of the disease.

Estimates of the death rate from ectopic pregnancy are approximately one in 1000 cases. However, lest this low death rate calm one's anxiety, it should be noted that ectopic pregnancy carries a relative risk of death ten times greater than that of childbirth and fifty times greater than that of a legal induced abortion.[2, 4] A most troublesome fact is that this disease can result in the death of young women of childbearing age who are, for all intents and purposes, otherwise free of disease and in whom eradication of the ectopic pregnancy ends their current risk.

Ectopic pregnancy has a well-recognized association with infertility. Among women who have had an ectopic pregnancy, the subsequent overall conception rate is ap-proximately 60 percent. Of these, 50 percent are intrauterine and 10 percent are repeat ectopic gestations.[5–7] This association is probably due to the etiologic relationship of tubal scarring to both the implantation of ectopic pregnancies and infertility; 97 percent of ectopic pregnancies are tubal in location (Fig. 22–2).

Misdiagnosed ectopic pregnancies not uncommonly lead to medical malpractice litigation.[8, 9] The latter clearly affects the frequency with which tests are ordered to investigate the possible presence of an ectopic gestation. "Overordering" of tests decreases the prevalence of disease in the test population. Statistically, this will adversely affect the accuracy of a positive prediction of ectopic pregnancy by any test, including ultrasonography.[10, 11]

The above observations document the importance of ectopic pregnancy as a medical entity. Numerous diagnostic strategies have been proposed for the evaluation of patients suspected of harboring an extrauterine gestation (EUG). The following discussion will focus on the utility of ultrasonography in this difficult patient group.

WHO IS AT RISK?

The clinical diagnosis of ectopic pregnancy is not at all straightforward. The "classic" clinical triad of pain, abnormal bleeding, and palpable adnexal mass is not

*This chapter is adapted from Filly, RA: Ectopic pregnancy: The role of sonography. Radiology 162:661–668, 1987, with the permission of the publishers.

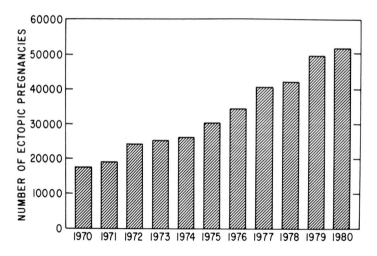

Figure 22–1. Number of hospitalizations for ectopic pregnancy from 1970 through 1980. (*From* Dorfman SF: Obstet Gynecol 62:334, 1983. *Reprinted with permission from* The American College of Obstetricians and Gynecologists.)

commonly present and, when present, may erroneously lead to a diagnosis of ectopic pregnancy. In a review of 154 patients with EUG, pain was present in 97 percent, and abnormal bleeding was noted in 86 percent.[3] Only 61 percent of patients reported "missing" a menstrual period. A pelvic mass was palpated in 41 percent and was equivocally present in 23 percent. No mass was palpable in the remaining patients. The average duration from last menstrual period to surgery was approximately 7.5 weeks. One patient's ectopic pregnancy eluded diagnosis for more

than 17 menstrual weeks. These clinical results are similar to those reported in 1970.[12] The emphasis that clinicians place on history and physical findings varies. However, when an ectopic pregnancy is suspected, the examining ultrasonographer should consistently attempt to document a sequence of observations. Subsequently, the interpretation of findings should not be based on the strength of the clinical history.

Some women are at especially high risk of harboring an ectopic gestation (Table 22–1). The relatively high recurrence risk of

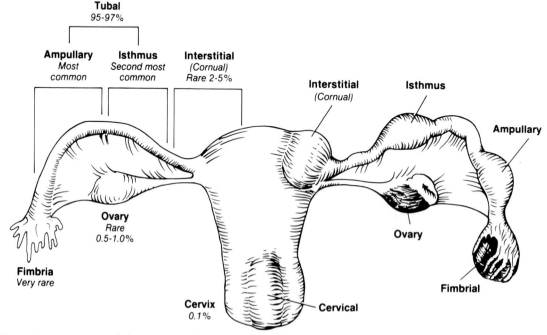

Figure 22–2. Diagram of the common locations of ectopic pregnancy. Note that 95 to 97 percent of ectopic pregnancies occur somewhere along the course of the fallopian tube. (*Modified from* Benson RC: Handbook of Obstetrics & Gynecology, 8th Ed. Los Altos, Lange Medical Publications, 1983; *and from* Schoenbaum S, Rosendorf L, Kappelman N, Rowan T: Gray-scale ultrasound in tubal pregnancy. Radiology 127:757, 1978.)

Table 22–1. FACTORS THAT INCREASE RISK OF ECTOPIC PREGNANCY

Prior ectopic pregnancy
Pregnancy with IUD in place
History of pelvic inflammatory disease
Prior tubal reconstructive surgery
Pregnancy by in vitro fertilization
Pregnancy after laparoscopic tubal coagulation

ectopic pregnancy has already been noted.[5–7] Women with a documented history of pelvic inflammatory disease are at an increased risk of developing ectopic pregnancy. Thirty to 50 percent of women with ectopic pregnancies have a history of acute salpingitis, and chronic salpingitis is histologically documented in a substantial percentage of surgical specimens from ectopic pregnancies.[3, 12, 13]

Women who are pregnant and have an intrauterine contraceptive device (IUD) in place are at an increased risk of ectopic pregnancy (Fig. 22–3).[14] This is not to say that IUDs cause ectopic pregnancy, although some consider this plausible. However, most agree that an IUD is far more effective at preventing implantation in the uterus than it is at preventing implantation in an ectopic location. Thus, a woman *who is pregnant* and has an IUD in place has a substantially greater risk of harboring an EUG than a pregnant woman without an IUD in place.

Other groups of patients, although small, are also at high risk. Certain infertile women with known tubal disease who become pregnant after tubal microsurgery or by in vitro fertilization are at increased risk. One very small group is at exceptional risk.[15] These are women who become pregnant after a laparoscopic tubal coagulation. As expected, the incidence of pregnancy in this group is quite low, but among those unfortunate

women who become pregnant after this attempted procedure to induce permanent sterility, more than one-half have ectopic pregnancies.

Despite the numerous groups at especially high risk of ectopic pregnancy, the only safe rule to remember is as follows: *all women of childbearing age are at risk of harboring an ectopic gestation.* From an ultrasonographic perspective, the following philosophy is highly recommended: the location of a gestation should be firmly established in the first trimester in any pregnant woman who presents for ultrasonography. If the pregnancy cannot be documented as intrauterine, the patient should be considered at risk of an ectopic gestation, and appropriate steps should be taken to determine the patient's status through subsequent testing.

PREGNANCY TESTING

The single most significant advancement in the management of patients suspected of harboring an ectopic gestation has been the appearance of highly sensitive radioimmune assays to detect human chorionic gonadotropin (hCG). The antibodies employed in these tests are specific for the beta subunit of the hormone. Indeed, as will be pointed out, the interpretation of the ultrasonogram is predicated on the results of this test.

In the era when hemagglutination-inhibition tests were employed to chemically confirm pregnancy, a substantial number of patients who were pregnant, but in whom the pregnancy was ectopically located, failed to test positively. This was due to two important factors. First, ectopic pregnancies produce hCG at a slower rate than normally implanted pregnancies.[16] Second, pregnancy

Figure 22–3. Sequential longitudinal articulated-arm B-scan (*A, B*) in a patient with a simultaneous intrauterine contraceptive device (IUD) and an intrauterine pregnancy. The IUD lies within the endometrial cavity and separates the decidua capsularis (DC) from the decidua vera (DV). As a marker of the endometrial cavity, the IUD confirms that sonography can resolve these two separate deciduae even in the absence of intraendometrial blood accumulations. Bl, bladder.

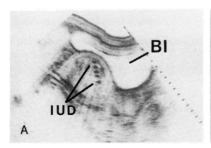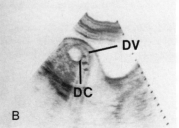

tests of the hemagglutination-inhibition variety were relatively insensitive to the detection of hCG. Thus, one can easily imagine the consternation of the clinician when previously dealing with a suspected case. Neither a positive nor a negative test was particularly helpful. If the pregnancy test was positive, the location of the pregnancy remained in doubt. If the pregnancy test was negative, the patient remained in the group at risk. The latter, extraordinarily difficult patients (i.e., the negative pregnancy test group) were frequently referred for ultrasonography, but this was of little help in managing these patients.[17]

Fortunately for all concerned, the newer radioimmunologic tests can detect extraordinarily small quantities of hCG. By comparison, radioimmunologic tests can detect 1 to 2 mIU/ml of hCG, whereas hemagglutination-inhibition tests detect 1000 to 2000 mIU/ml. It is important that sonographers be aware that more than one standard exists for the measurement of hCG biologic activity.[18] The Second International Standard (2nd IS) was described in the 1960s. Later, a purer standard was defined and is termed the International Reference Preparation (IRP). Both standards are in common use. A given numeric value of hCG in biologic units varies by an approximate factor of two between these standards (i.e., 100 mIU/ml [2nd IS] equals approximately 200 mIU/ml [IRP]). To add to the potential confusion, some laboratories report results in ng/ml.[19] Although this appears to be the preferable method, it is not the accepted standard. Conversion factors are available for changing ng/ml to mIU/ml for both commonly used standards of biologic activity. As a rough guideline, 1 ng/ml = 5 to 6 mIU/ml (2nd IS) and 10 to 12 mIU/ml (IRP). Awareness of the standard employed by the referring clinician's laboratory is of major importance when quantitated levels of hCG are being compared with the sonographic results. These standards are also important for understanding the lower limit of sensitivity in qualitative testing.[20–27] Differences in standards do not affect the interpretation of serial quantitated levels from an individual patient when they are measured in the same laboratory. Remember, patients will likely be referred by clinicians who use different laboratories that may well employ different standards.

Romero and associates found a 0.5 percent false-negative rate among ectopic pregnancy patients when the hCG level was less than 10 mIU/ml (IRP). The false-negative rate increased, as one might suspect, as the lower limit was raised.[25] These results are similar to those of Olson and colleagues, who found a 100 percent sensitivity for ectopic pregnancy when employing a test cutoff level of less than 3 mIU/ml.[26] Longer incubation times are required to achieve greater sensitivity for hCG.[25] Speed may be clinically necessary in some cases of suspected ectopic pregnancy; however, only a few hours of incubation are required to achieve a sensitivity of 30 mIU/ml (IRP).

There is reasonably good evidence that many fetuses of ectopic pregnancies exhibiting very low hCG levels are already dead.[26] The natural history of ectopic pregnancy almost certainly includes those fetuses that implant, die, and are reabsorbed without being clinically recognized. Unfortunately, a clinician cannot count on this probability in any given case.

ULTRASONOGRAPHY

The presence of an elevated hCG level assists the gynecologist in confirming the pregnant state but, at least as an initial screening, does not permit distinction between intrauterine pregnancies (IUPs)—either normal or abnormal—recent spontaneous abortions, and EUGs. Numerous relatively invasive procedures short of laparotomy, such as culdocentesis, laparoscopy, and dilatation and curettage for microscopic evaluation of the endometrium, increase diagnostic accuracy but involve increased risk to the patient.[28] Laparoscopy, although not 100 percent accurate in very early ectopic pregnancies, is the single most accurate method of confirming the presence of an ectopic pregnancy before surgery. However, routine use of laparoscopy in suspected cases of ectopic pregnancy is impractical. This procedure is highly invasive. Furthermore, the prevalence of ectopic pregnancy in a clinically suspected group is relatively low, ranging from 10 to 16 percent.[29–31] Thus, most patients would needlessly undergo a laparoscopic examination. Finally, laparoscopy may lead to the iatrogenic compromise of a normal IUP.[8]

One would like, if possible, to include far

more women with ectopic pregnancy among the group being considered for laparoscopy. Accomplishing this end requires a level of testing interposed between the clinical suspicion of an ectopic pregnancy and the performance of a laparoscopic examination. Gynecologists, at this juncture of the diagnostic work-up, will commonly choose, albeit not exclusively, between culdocentesis and ultrasonography. Culdocentesis, although invasive, is substantially less so than laparoscopy. Aspiration of nonclotting blood from the cul-de-sac, especially if the hematocrit is greater than 15, indicates a high probability that the patient harbors an EUG.[28] Gynecologists commonly proceed directly to laparotomy if the culdocentesis result is positive. Negative aspirations are unreliable for excluding an EUG. This is unfortunate since most suspected pregnancies are not, in fact, extrauterine but instead are normal or abnormal IUPs. This larger patient group will have a negative culdocentesis result. Further testing is then required.

Previous reports emphasize different approaches in the sonographic evaluation of ectopic pregnancy. One group of investigators have attempted to recognize the presence of an ectopic pregnancy on the basis of the adnexal sonographic findings.[30-34] Other groups[23, 35-37] stress that ultrasound's primary utility is its ability to recognize IUPs. Both aspects are important.

The value of demonstrating an IUP in a patient suspected of harboring an EUG is based on the well-established clinical observation that the concomitant occurrence of an IUP and an EUG is rare.[38, 39] In patients who have no special risk factors, the expected rate of concomitancy is extremely low and is usually quoted as one per 30,000 pregnancies.[38] Unfortunately, gynecologists are performing procedures that can alter this frequency.[40, 41] Patients undergoing ovulation induction produce multiple ova per cycle and thus are at greater risk. Such patients have been estimated as having an incidence of combined IUP and EUG as high as one per 7000 pregnancies.[41] One "unlucky" institution recently reported having three such cases in one year.[42] Fortunately, each was recognized by the presence of a living extrauterine embryo.

There is no question that concomitant IUP and EUG occurs and that the incidence is increasing (Fig. 22–4).[38-42] However, it is

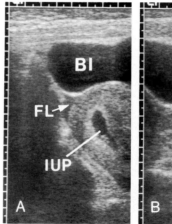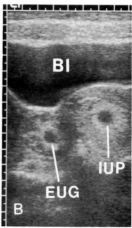

Figure 22–4. Longitudinal (A) and transverse (B) sonograms of a patient with simultaneous intrauterine pregnancy (IUP) and extrauterine gestation (EUG). The intrauterine pregnancy demonstrated a living embryo. A simultaneous extrauterine gestation is extremely improbable, but is becoming somewhat more common with the use of ovulation induction agents. Fortunately, a typical-appearing adnexal mass and pelvic fluid (FL) led to the correct diagnosis. Bl, bladder.

impractical to manage every suspected case of ectopic pregnancy on the basis of a probability of no greater than one in 7000 for concomitancy of an IUP and EUG. This is especially true since the alternative diagnostic pathway includes invasive procedures in virtually every case.

Diagnosis of Early IUP

Sonographic demonstration of an IUP represents extremely valuable evidence against the possibility of an ectopic pregnancy. However, a variety of morphologic observations may be made by the interpreting ultrasonographer when diagnosing an early intrauterine pregnancy (see Chap. 3). Some of these observations are more reliable than others for this purpose. Researchers who first described early intrauterine gestations considered their appearance to be typical. However, more recent observations have disclosed that stimulation of the uterine lining with hormones produced by an ectopic pregnancy can, unfortunately, result in endometrial changes that are quite similar in appearance to those seen with an early IUP.[35-37, 43-48] This stimulation is recognizable in approximately one-half of patients with an ectopic pregnancy (decidual cast,

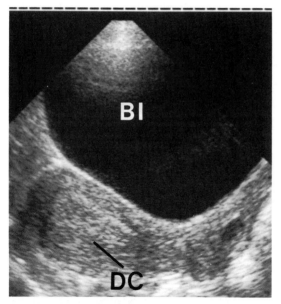

Figure 22–5. Longitudinal sonogram of the uterus in a patient with an ectopic pregnancy. The sonogram shows a large decidual cast (DC) within the uterus. This would not likely be mistaken for an intrauterine pregnancy. Bl, bladder.

Fig. 22–5) and simulates the appearance of an early pregnancy (pseudogestational sac of ectopic pregnancy) in 10 to 20 percent of cases (Table 22–2, Fig. 22–6).[43] This potential for confusion mandates that ultrasonographers be extremely cautious when diagnosing an IUP in patients suspected of harboring an EUG. Specific morphologic criteria should be applied.

Normal IUPs can first be detected with ultrasonography as an intraendometrial fluid collection surrounded by an echogenic margin at approximately five menstrual weeks (three weeks post conception) (Fig. 22–7).[19, 20] By 6.5 weeks, the yolk sac becomes con-

Table 22–2. APPEARANCE OF THE ENDOMETRIAL CAVITY IN 39 PATIENTS WITH PROVEN ECTOPIC PREGNANCY

Normal	21 (54%)
Gestational sac–like	8 (20%)
Prominent central echoes	5 (13%)
Other (including fluid collection not typical of gestational sac and combination of 2nd & 3rd above)	5 (13%)
	—
Total	39

Modified from Marks WM, Filly RA, Callen PW, et al: The decidual cast of ectopic pregnancy: A confusing ultrasonographic appearance. Radiology 133:451, 1979.

sistently visible (Figs. 22–8, 22–9) within the developing gestational sac, and by seven menstrual weeks, an embryo can be consistently detected (Fig. 22–10) (both the yolk sac and an embryo frequently, but not consistently, can be seen 0.5 week earlier than stated).[49, 50] With modern equipment, the fetal heartbeat is visible concurrently with the detection of the embryo or, in some instances, even before the embryo is discretely identified.[49] It is during the brief but important period (5 to 6.5 menstrual weeks) when the pregnancy first becomes visible and definitive signs of an IUP appear (yolk sac or embryo) that one must be cautious not to interpret a pseudogestational sac of ectopic pregnancy as a true IUP.

The recently described "double decidual sac sign" (DDSS) has been suggested as a finding that characterizes an early IUP and reliably discriminates a true gestational sac from the pseudogestational sac of ectopic pregnancy (Table 22–3, Figs. 22–3, 22–6, 22–7, 22–9 to 22–12).[37, 48] The double sac, which consists of two concentric rings surrounding a portion of the gestational sac, is thought to represent the decidual parietalis

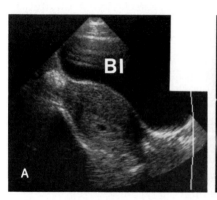

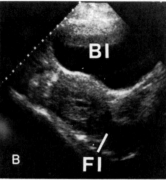

Figure 22–6. *A,* Longitudinal sonogram of a patient suspected of harboring an extrauterine gestation. However, an intrauterine fluid collection surrounded by a double decidual sac is clearly identified, indicating a normal position of the pregnancy. *B,* Conversely, a patient with a similar clinical history shows an intraendometrial fluid collection surrounded by a single rim of echoes. This is a pseudogestational sac of an ectopic pregnancy. Note that this patient also has fluid (Fl) in the cul-de-sac. Bl, bladder.

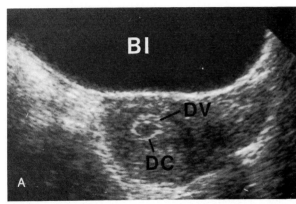

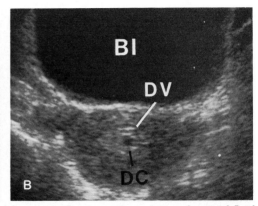

Figure 22–7. Longitudinal *(A)* and transverse *(B)* sonograms of the uterus, demonstrating an intraendometrial fluid collection. A double decidual sac sign, consisting of the concentric rings of the decidua capsularis (DC) and the decidua vera (DV), is seen. Note that no intraendometrial cavity fluid collection is too small to be assessed for this finding. A presumptive diagnosis of an intrauterine pregnancy can be made. Bl, bladder.

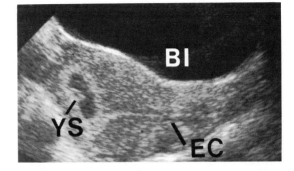

Figure 22–8. Longitudinal sonogram of the uterus, demonstrating an intraendometrial fluid collection. The endometrial cavity (EC) is clearly seen. A yolk sac (YS) is identified within the intraendometrial collection, confirming a true intrauterine pregnancy. Bl, bladder.

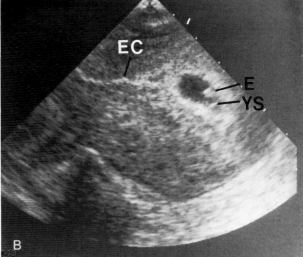

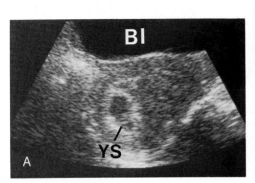

Figure 22–9. Transabdominal *(A)* and intravaginal *(B)* sonograms of a patient suspected of harboring an ectopic pregnancy. On the transabdominal sonogram, a yolk sac (YS) is seen with only moderate confidence. However, on the intravaginal sonogram, not only the yolk sac (YS) but also the embryo (E) is unambiguously identified. Additionally, the embryo demonstrated a heartbeat. Thus, unequivocal demonstration of an intrauterine pregnancy was achieved by the intravaginal sonogram. EC, endometrial cavity.

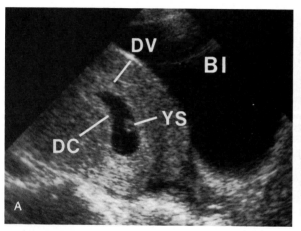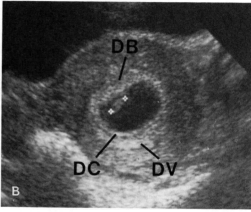

Figure 22–10. Longitudinal *(A)* and transverse *(B)* sonograms of a patient with a differential diagnosis of threatened abortion versus ectopic pregnancy. By this stage of development, all of the features seen in early pregnancy can be noted. These include the double decidual sac sign, consisting of the concentric rings of the decidua vera (DV) and decidua capsularis (DC). Additionally, the yolk sac (YS) and a living embryo *(cursors)* can be detected. Bl, bladder; DB, decidua basalis.

(decidual vera) adjacent to the decidua capsularis (Fig. 22–11). In contradistinction, the pseudogestational sac of ectopic pregnancy is composed of a single decidual layer surrounding an intraendometrial fluid collection and, thus, demonstrates a single echogenic ring (Figs. 22–6, 22–13). Several investigations have been conducted to establish the validity of the DDSS.[29, 36, 48, 51] Although some authors differ in their judgments as to the origin of the double concentric rings,[29, 36, 51] the weight of evidence indicates that this sign is highly reliable in discriminating pseudo- from true gestational sacs. However, *the DDSS does not absolutely exclude a pseudogestational sac nor does it confirm that an IUP is normal* (Table 22–2).[48, 50] Therefore, when employed in patients suspected of harboring an EUG, follow-up examinations may be beneficial.

A most important advancement has occurred in the sonographic evaluation of early

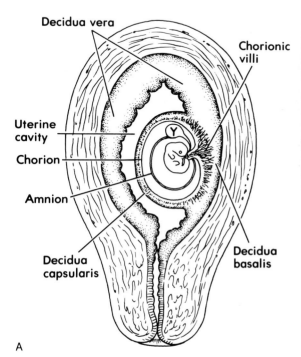

A

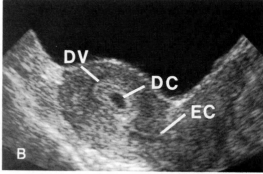

Figure 22–11. *A,* Diagram demonstrating the relationship of the decidua vera and decidua capsularis to the implanted gestational sac. *B,* Longitudinal sonogram of the uterus, demonstrating the double decidual sac sign prior to visualization of either the yolk sac or the embryo. The double decidual sac is composed of the decidua vera (DV) surrounding the decidua capsularis (DC). EC, endometrial cavity.

Table 22–3. ANALYSIS OF INTRAUTERINE FLUID COLLECTIONS IN EARLY PREGNANCY

Final Diagnosis	Ultrasound Diagnosis			Total
	At Risk of Ectopic Pregnancy	*Normal IUP*	*Abnormal IUP*	
Ectopic pregnancy	49	0	1	50
Normal IUP	4	32	0	36
Abnormal IUP	15	9	18	42
Total	68	41	19	128

IUP, intrauterine pregnancy.

From Nyberg DA, Laing F, Filly RA, et al: Ultrasonographic differentiation of the gestational sac of early intrauterine pregnancy from the pseudogestational sac of ectopic pregnancy. Radiology 146:755, 1983.

IUPs: the availability of intravaginal transducers. Such transducers result in a decrease in distance from the transducer face to the endometrial cavity. This enables the sonographer both to use higher frequency transducers and to scan the endometrial cavity in a portion of the beam that is more easily focused. Both advantages result in superior resolution (Fig. 22–9). The widespread use of intravaginal transducers will result in an ability to resolve pregnancies earlier and to confirm more confidently features that reliably distinguish a true pregnancy from the pseudogestational sac of ectopic pregnancy (e.g., DDSS, yolk sac identification, embryonic visualization).

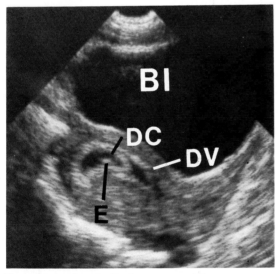

Figure 22–12. Longitudinal sonogram of the uterus. An intrauterine pregnancy can be definitively confirmed by the presence of an embryo (E). However, even after visualization of the embryo, the double decidual sac sign is still readily apparent. The decidua capsularis (DC) and decidua vera (DV) are visualized to advantage because of a small amount of fluid in the endometrial cavity. Bl, bladder.

Evaluation of the Patient At Risk

The results of a prospective study on 219 patients with measurable levels of hCG and a clinical suspicion of ectopic pregnancy are detailed in Table 22–3 and Figure 22–14.[29] Thirty-five of these patients had an ectopic pregnancy, for a period prevalence of 18 percent. When sonography documented the presence of an IUP, the extremely low occurrence rate of concomitant IUP and EUG effectively excluded the diagnosis of ectopic pregnancy. None of the 112 patients with a sonographically visible IUP, by demonstration of either the DDSS (42 patients) or an embryo (70 patients), had an ectopic pregnancy (Table 22–4, Fig. 22–14A). Sonographic visualization of an IUP, therefore, was the most beneficial finding in the exclusion of ectopic pregnancy. When used as a screening test, sonographic documentation

Table 22–4. CONSECUTIVE PROSPECTIVE SONOGRAMS PERFORMED BECAUSE OF A CLINICAL SUSPICION OF ECTOPIC PREGNANCY

Total	219
Lost to follow-up	26
Subtotal	193
Sonographic documentation of IUP	112
Embryo	70
DDSS	42
No sonographic evidence of IUP	81
Follow-up:	
Ectopic pregnancy	35
SAB/IAB	28
Early IUP (not detected with ultrasound)	18

IUP, intrauterine pregnancy; DDSS, double decidual sac sign; SAB/IAB, spontaneous abortion or incomplete abortion.

Modified from Mahony BS, Filly RA, Nyberg DA, et al: Sonographic evaluation of ectopic pregnancy. J Ultrasound Med 4:221, 1985.

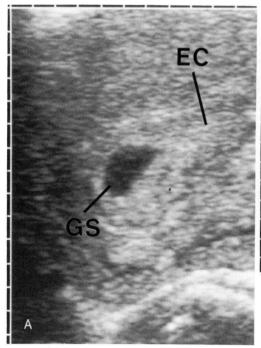
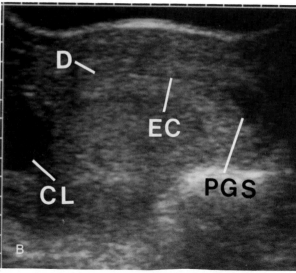

Figure 22–13. *A,* Transverse magnified high-resolution sonogram of a patient with an early intrauterine pregnancy. Notice that the gestational sac (GS) is eccentrically positioned within the endometrial cavity (EC). This is a useful feature for discriminating early pregnancies from the pseudogestational sac of ectopic pregnancy, which commonly fills the entire uterine cavity symmetrically. (See Fig. 22–6B.) *B,* However, like all features designed to distinguish the pseudogestational sac from true intrauterine pregnancies, failures may be anticipated. The pseudogestational sac (PGS) in this transverse magnified high-resolution sonogram of a patient with an ectopic pregnancy is eccentrically positioned within the endometrial cavity (EC). D, decidualized endometrium; CL, corpus luteum cyst.

of an IUP provides the only convincing evidence for the absence of an EUG.

A further analysis of the data from this study documents the utility and accuracy of the DDSS in confirming the presence of an IUP before a stage of development when a yolk sac or embryo can be seen. Special care must be taken to unequivocally document the DDSS. Erroneous interpretation of a pseudogestational sac as an IUP could lead to a false diagnosis and a potentially catastrophic outcome. Subjects whose sonograms did not confirm an IUP immediately entered a high-risk category (43 percent in this study) (Figs. 22–14B, 22–15 to 22–18). Importantly, if the DDSS had not been employed, fewer IUPs would have been initially documented and the risk for ectopic pregnancy in the "no IUP" group would have decreased to 28 percent (only 10 percent higher than the risk at initial presentation).

Characterization of the adnexal findings among the group without a demonstrable IUP improved the ultrasonographic prediction of an ectopic gestation (Fig. 22–14B).

Patients with no visible IUP who in addition demonstrated either an adnexal mass (Figs. 22–19 to 22–22) or cul-de-sac fluid (Fig. 22–23) moved into a category of even greater risk (more than 70 percent with either finding) (Figs. 22–1, 22–4B, 22–5). Combining adnexal findings further improved specificity and positive predictive accuracy (Figs. 22–14B, 22–24). However, each refinement concomitantly reduced sensitivity and the accuracy of a negative prediction. For example, demonstration of a living adnexal embryo (Figs. 22–25 to 22–28) was 100 percent specific for an EUG. Unfortunately, sensitivity dropped to 11 per cent since only four of 35 ectopic pregnancies were so recognized. More recently, improved resolution and intravaginal transducers have enabled confirmation of an adnexal gestation by visualization of a yolk sac independent of embryo recognition (Figs. 22–18, 22–29).

Although sonographic documentation of an adnexal mass or pelvic intraperitoneal fluid in a woman with measurable circulating hCG and no evidence of an IUP substantially increases her risk of harboring an EUG,

Text continued on page 463

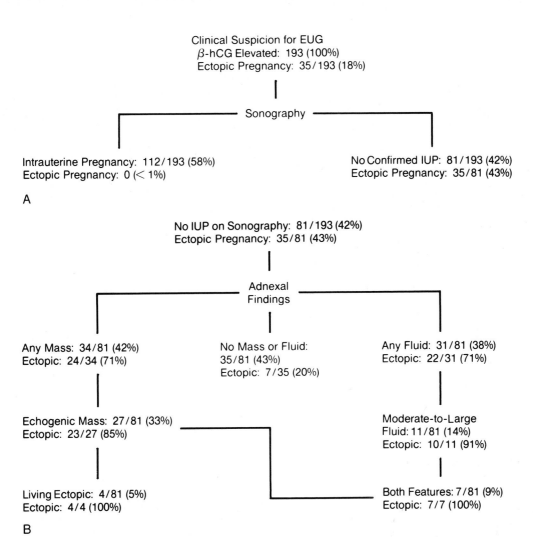

Clinical Suspicion for EUG
β-hCG Elevated: 193 (100%)
Ectopic Pregnancy: 35/193 (18%)

Sonography

Intrauterine Pregnancy: 112/193 (58%)
Ectopic Pregnancy: 0 (< 1%)

No Confirmed IUP: 81/193 (42%)
Ectopic Pregnancy: 35/81 (43%)

A

No IUP on Sonography: 81/193 (42%)
Ectopic Pregnancy: 35/81 (43%)

Adnexal
Findings

Any Mass: 34/81 (42%)
Ectopic: 24/34 (71%)

No Mass or Fluid:
35/81 (43%)
Ectopic: 7/35 (20%)

Any Fluid: 31/81 (38%)
Ectopic: 22/31 (71%)

Echogenic Mass: 27/81 (33%)
Ectopic: 23/27 (85%)

Moderate-to-Large
Fluid: 11/81 (14%)
Ectopic: 10/11 (91%)

Living Ectopic: 4/81 (5%)
Ectopic: 4/4 (100%)

Both Features: 7/81 (9%)
Ectopic: 7/7 (100%)

B

Figure 22–14. *A, B,* Flow charts of a patient's risk for harboring an ectopic pregnancy based on sonographic findings. EUG, extrauterine gestation; IUP, intrauterine pregnancy. (*Modified from* Mahony BS, Filly RA, Nyberg DA, et al: Sonographic evaluation of ectopic pregnancy. J Ultrasound Med 4:221, 1985.)

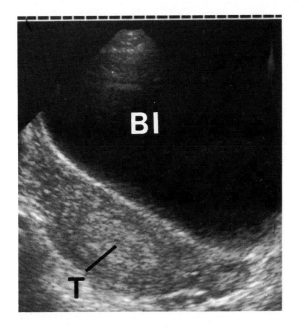

Figure 22–15. Transverse sonogram through the uterus of a patient suspected of harboring an ectopic pregnancy. Instead, the patient had an incomplete abortion. Residual decidual and chorionic tissue (T) is seen within the endometrial cavity. It would be difficult to discriminate this tissue from a decidual cast caused by an ectopic pregnancy. (Compare Fig. 22–5.) However, one can be certain that this is not a normal pregnancy. Thus, this tissue may be safely evacuated and searched grossly and microscopically for chorionic villi. Identification of chorionic villi would confirm an intrauterine pregnancy. If decidua only is discovered histologically, the patient remains in the group at risk for ectopic pregnancy. Bl, bladder.

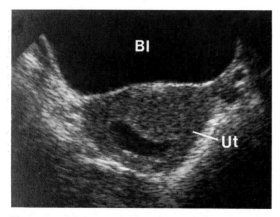

Figure 22–16. Transverse sonogram of the uterus (Ut) in a patient suspected of harboring an ectopic pregnancy. An intrauterine fluid collection surrounded by a single rim of echoes is identified. Thus, a definite diagnosis of intrauterine pregnancy cannot be made. The patient must be considered in the group at risk for ectopic pregnancy. This proved to be an abnormal, nonviable first trimester intrauterine pregnancy. Approximately 30 percent of these fail to disclose a double decidual sac finding. Bl, bladder.

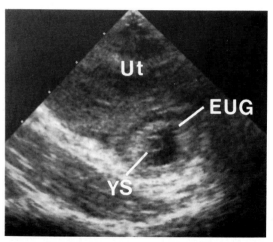

Figure 22–18. Intravaginal sonogram of the mass depicted in Figure 22–17D. As viewed with this newer technology, the thick-walled adnexal cyst demonstrates an unequivocal yolk sac (YS), discriminating this adnexal ring from a corpus luteum and confirming it as an extrauterine gestation (EUG). The uterus (Ut) represents the tissue lying in front of the unruptured ectopic pregnancy. Intravaginal sonography greatly helps to clarify such cases, as illustrated in Figure 22–17.

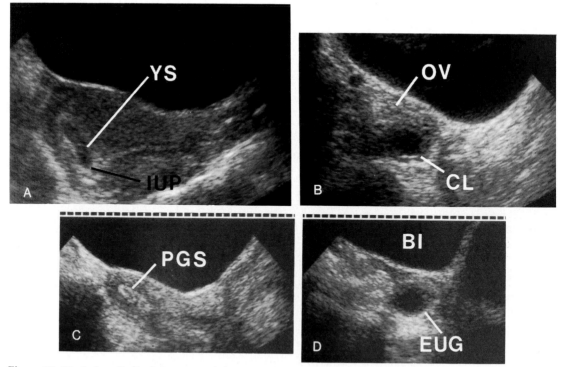

Figure 22–17. A, Longitudinal sonogram of the uterus in a patient suspected of harboring an ectopic pregnancy. An intrauterine pregnancy (IUP) is confirmed by demonstration of a yolk sac (YS). B, In the left adnexa, this patient demonstrates a thick-walled adnexal cystic mass. This may be safely presumed to represent a corpus luteum (CL) in the ovary (OV). C, By contrast, a longitudinal sonogram of the uterus in this patient demonstrates a small intrauterine fluid collection without the definitive morphologic criteria for an intrauterine pregnancy. Indeed, this proved to be a pseudogestational sac (PGS) of ectopic pregnancy. D, In the right adnexa, a thick-walled adnexal cystic mass, quite similar in appearance to that in B, was identified. This mass, however, turned out to be an ectopic gestation (EUG) (see Fig. 22–18). On the basis of the adnexal findings, one could not reasonably discriminate the masses in B and D. It is the identification of the intrauterine pregnancy in A that effectively excludes this patient from the group at risk for ectopic pregnancy. Bl, bladder.

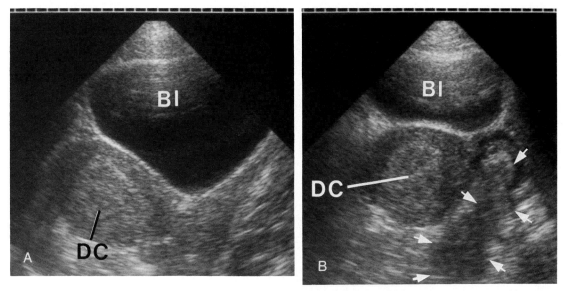

Figure 22–19. Longitudinal (A) and transverse (B) sonograms of a patient with an ectopic pregnancy. There is a large decidual cast (DC) and a vague elliptical echogenic mass in the left adnexa, extending into the cul-de-sac (arrows). A patient who fails to demonstrate an intrauterine pregnancy and also demonstrates an echogenic mass has approximately an 85 percent risk of having an ectopic pregnancy. Masses of this type generally represent a hematosalpinx. Bl, bladder.

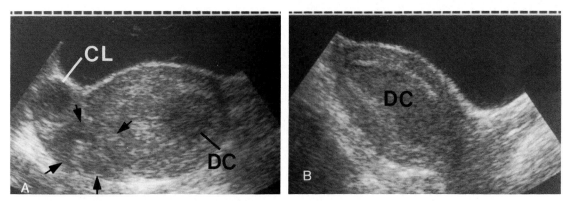

Figure 22–20. Transverse (A) and longitudinal (B) sonograms of a patient with an ectopic pregnancy. A large and somewhat eccentric decidual cast (DC) is seen within the uterus. Decidual casts of this appearance probably "mature" into pseudogestational sacs. No fluid is seen in the cul-de-sac. A relatively typical corpus luteum (CL) is seen in the right ovary. Additionally, an echogenic mass (arrows) is wedged between the right ovary and the uterus. This is a relatively typical location and appearance for an ectopic gestation.

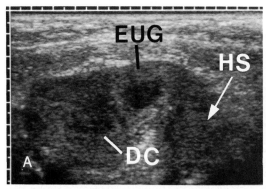

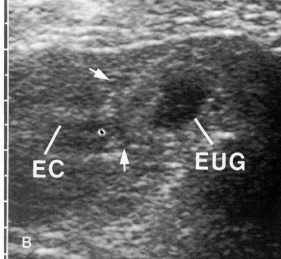

Figure 22–21. *A,* High-resolution transverse sonogram of a patient with an ectopic gestation (EUG) in the cornual portion of the tube. A decidual cast (DC) is clearly identified and marks the endometrial cavity. Distal to the ectopic gestation, an enlarged tube caused by a hematosalpinx (HS) is identified. *B,* Magnified view of *A* demonstrates effacement of the decidualized endometrium *(arrows)* by the cornual ectopic gestation (EUG). This type of ectopic gestation is particularly hazardous because of the extensive vasculature generally associated with pregnancies contained in this portion of the tube. EC, endometrial cavity.

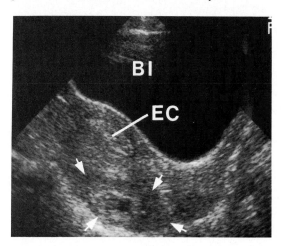

Figure 22–22. Longitudinal sonogram of a patient suspected of harboring an extrauterine pregnancy. There is no evidence of a pregnancy in the endometrial cavity (EC). An echogenic mass *(arrows)* with a lucent center is identified in the cul-de-sac. The cul-de-sac mass is poorly marginated from the posterior wall of the uterus, unfortunately a not uncommon situation. The absence of an intrauterine pregnancy and the presence of an echogenic adnexal mass places the patient at extremely high risk for an ectopic pregnancy (approximately 85 percent). Bl, bladder.

Figure 22–23. Longitudinal sonogram of a patient suspected of harboring an ectopic pregnancy. There is no evidence of an intrauterine pregnancy within the endometrial cavity (EC). A moderate amount of echogenic fluid (Fl) is seen in the cul-de-sac. The absence of an intrauterine pregnancy in the presence of a moderate amount of cul-de-sac fluid places this patient at high risk for an ectopic pregnancy (approximately 90 percent). Bl, bladder.

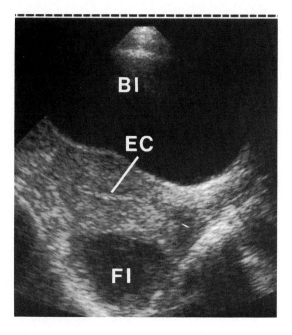

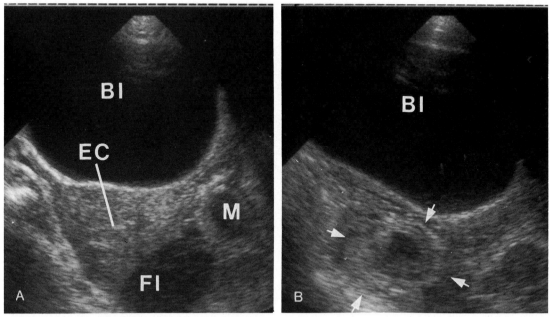

Figure 22–24. Transverse (A) and left longitudinal (B) sonograms of a patient suspected of harboring an ectopic pregnancy. No intrauterine pregnancy is seen within the endometrial cavity (EC). Additionally, a moderate amount of fluid (Fl) is noted in the cul-de-sac, extending into the left adnexa, where a moderately echogenic (arrows) ringlike mass (M) is identified. The combination of moderate fluid, an echogenic mass, and the absence of an intrauterine pregnancy virtually confirms the presence of an ectopic pregnancy. Bl, bladder.

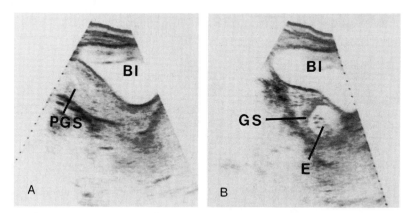

Figure 22–25. Articulated-arm B-scans in midlongitudinal (A) and right longitudinal (B) positions. A pseudogestational sac (PGS) is identified within the uterus. More important, an adnexal gestational sac (GS) with a living embryo (E) was noted, confirming the presence of an ectopic pregnancy. Bl, bladder.

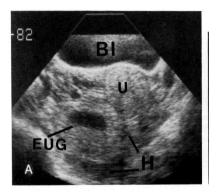

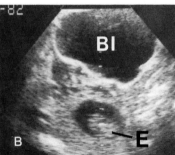

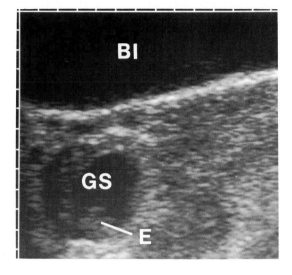

Figure 22–26. Transverse *(A)* and right longitudinal *(B)* sonograms of a patient with moderately severe abdominal pain and a positive pregnancy test. The uterus (U) is partially obscured by contiguous echogenic hemorrhagic fluid (H) and an extrauterine echogenic ringlike mass representing the extrauterine gestation (EUG). These features alone virtually confirm an ectopic pregnancy, but the identification of the living adnexal embryo (E) conclusively documents that the patient has an ectopic pregnancy, which is leaking blood. Bl, bladder.

Figure 22–27. Transverse high-resolution magnified sonogram of a patient suspected of harboring an ectopic gestation. Newer phased-array selectively focused instruments enable the identification of smaller adnexal embryos than was previously possible. In this instance, the embryo (E) and gestational sac (GS) are definitively documented in the right adnexa. High-resolution intravaginal ultrasound scanners will only further augment the ability to demonstrate extrauterine gestations with certainty (see Fig. 22–18). Bl, bladder.

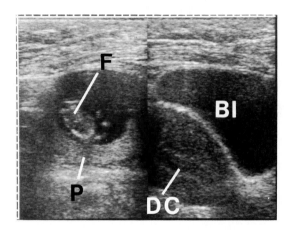

Figure 22–28. Composite, side-by-side, linear array real-time sonograms of a patient suspected of harboring an ectopic pregnancy. Indeed, an extremely large ectopic gestation is seen superior to the fundus of the uterus. A fetus (F), whose biparietal diameter was easily measured, can be identified. Additionally, there is a well-developed placenta (P). Only a decidual cast (DC) is seen within the uterus. Although large and easily seen, such ectopic pregnancies may be misdiagnosed as intrauterine if the ultrasonographer fails to observe a line of demarcation between the ectopic gestation and the uterine fundus. When the sonographer fails to note the separation, the ectopic gestation is mistakenly incorporated into the uterine fundus. This error can be devastating to the patient. Bl, bladder.

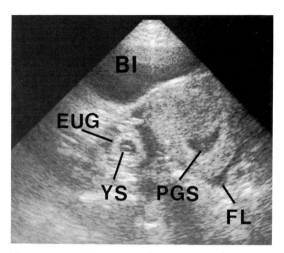

Figure 22–29. Transverse ultrasonogram of a patient suspected of harboring an ectopic pregnancy. A pseudogestational sac (PGS) is seen within the uterus. There is fluid in the cul-de-sac (FL), extending to the right adnexa, where an adnexal ring containing a yolk sac (YS) confirms this mass as an extrauterine gestation (EUG). Just as a yolk sac within an intraendometrial fluid collection confirms an intrauterine pregnancy, a yolk sac within an adnexal mass confirms an extrauterine pregnancy (see Fig. 22–18). Bl, bladder.

the absence of these findings does not exclude an ectopic pregnancy. Twenty percent (7 in 35) of women with a confirmed EUG demonstrated no sonographic evidence of either an adnexal mass or cul-de-sac fluid on initial examination (Fig. 22–30). Indeed, a negative sonogram in such patients did decrease their risk from 43 to 20 percent. However, the patient entered the test with an 18 percent risk. Thus, the only sonographic mechanism that reasonably excludes a patient from the group at risk for EUG is

demonstration of an IUP. If no IUP is demonstrated, a variety of adnexal findings may effectively increase a patient's risk, but the absence of sonographic abnormalities in the adnexal region cannot decrease the patient's risk. The life-threatening nature of this entity necessitates further investigation in these cases.

The Value of hCG Quantitation

In the patient group with a clinical suspicion of EUG, circulating hCG, no sonographically demonstrable IUP, and evidence of either cul-de-sac fluid or an adnexal mass, the potential risk for ectopic pregnancy is sufficiently high (more than 70 percent) that laparoscopy represents a reasonable means of further segregating the falsely suspected case. Of course, patients with documented living ectopic pregnancies could even bypass laparoscopy in favor of laparotomy. Such patients fall into straightforward management groups.

However, patients who fail to demonstrate either an IUP or adnexal pathology (20 percent risk) represent a moderately large and particularly difficult management group. Fortunately, additional noninvasive evidence that will further characterize the patient's risk of EUG can be obtained in an appropriately short time. These women can greatly benefit from quantitation of the level of circulating hCG. The specimen preferably, but not necessarily, should be obtained on the same day as the sonogram. Recall that the reference standard employed by different

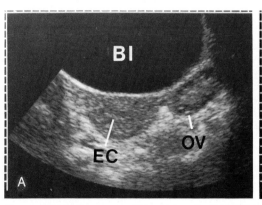

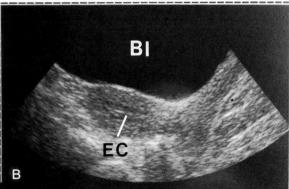

Figure 22–30. Transverse (A) and longitudinal (B) high-resolution sonograms of a patient suspected of harboring an ectopic pregnancy. No intrauterine pregnancy is identified within the endometrial cavity (EC). The adnexa are unremarkable. The left ovary (OV) is clearly identified. There is no fluid in the cul-de-sac. Despite the essentially normal appearance of this pelvis, there is an ectopic pregnancy. It is extremely important to remember that a normal pelvic sonogram does not exclude an ectopic pregnancy. Bl, bladder.

laboratories may result in a reported variation of hCG level as great as 50 percent.

These women have the following differential diagnostic possibilities: they have a normal IUP, but it is too small to be detected sonographically; they have recently spontaneously aborted an abnormal pregnancy (SAB) but still have measurable levels of circulating hCG; or they do indeed have an ectopic pregnancy that is too small to be detected as an adnexal mass and that has yet to produce visible peritoneal fluid. Although quantitation of the hCG level will not unambiguously discriminate between these three possibilities, it can help select the correct management pathway.[20–23]

Evidence indicates that modern sonographic equipment has the capacity to detect all normal singleton gestational sacs when the hCG level exceeds 1800 mIU/ml (2nd IS) (Table 22–5).[20] Furthermore, gestational sac size strongly correlates with quantitative hCG levels in normal singleton pregnancies (see Chap. 3). Alternatively, patients who have recently spontaneously aborted a pregnancy, either completely or incompletely, are unlikely to have an hCG level greater than 1800 mIU/ml. Indeed, only 4 of 39 such patients, in one study, had hCG levels exceeding this limit, and the history in these 4 patients suggested a very recent passage of tissue (Table 22–6).[21]

In contradistinction to these groups, 30 of 68 patients with ectopic pregnancies had hCG levels exceeding 1800 mIU/ml at the time of initial sonographic evaluation (Table 22–6).[22] Thus, if the quantitated hCG level is greater than 1800 mIU/ml (2nd IS), the probability that one is examining a patient with a normal singleton IUP too early to detect with ultrasound is remote. Patients with either a recent SAB or an EUG could have an "empty" uterus and an hCG level greater than 1800 mIU/ml, but when such a

Table 22–5. COMPARISON OF hCG LEVEL WITH SONOGRAPHIC IDENTIFICATION OF EARLY NORMAL GESTATIONAL SACS (ALL BEFORE EMBRYONIC VISUALIZATION)

hCG Level (2nd IS)	Normal IUP (n = 76)	
	No Sac	Sac
< 1800 mIU/ml	19	2*
> 1800 mIU/ml	0	55

IUP, intrauterine pregnancy.
*1750 mIU/ml and 1630 mIU/ml.

Table 22–6. ABSENT INTRAUTERINE GESTATIONAL SAC CORRELATED WITH SIMULTANEOUS QUANTITATIVE hCG LEVELS

hCG Level (2nd IS)	Ectopic (n = 68)	SAB (n = 39)	IUP (n = 19)
> 1800 mIU/ml	30	4	0
< 1800 mIU/ml	38	35	19

SAB, spontaneous abortion; IUP, intrauterine pregnancy.

level is documented, the diagnosis of ectopic pregnancy is strongly favored. The higher the hCG level in a patient without a visible IUP, the more likely is it that one is dealing with a patient who harbors an EUG.

If the quantitated level of hCG is less than 1800 mIU/ml, all three differential diagnostic possibilities remain in effect (Table 22–6), but within 48 hours, the referring physician can further segregate the falsely suspected case from this remaining, most troublesome, patient group. A normal IUP demonstrates an hCG doubling time of approximately two days (with a range of 1.2 to 2.2 days),[24] whereas patients with a recent spontaneous abortion show a substantial decline in their circulating hCG level during an equivalent time course.[19] By contrast, women with ectopic pregnancies tend to show a subnormal increase in circulating hCG over a 48 hour span.[16] Unfortunately, ectopic pregnancies occasionally show hCG "doubling" times similar to those of a normal pregnancy or declining hCG levels similar to those of a spontaneous abortion. When doubt remains, and the clinical status of the patient does not mandate immediate invasive testing, serial hCG levels and repeat sonography may be necessary to further assess the patient's status.

Ultrasonography is a pivotal examination in the evaluation of a patient suspected of harboring an EUG. In most cases, this diagnosis can be promptly excluded with reasonable certainty by the sonographic demonstration of an IUP. Although a definitive sonographic diagnosis of an ectopic pregnancy is uncommon (i.e., documentation of a living extrauterine embryo or a yolk sac), sonography can be employed effectively to assist in determining a patient's risk status. Concomitant measurement of hCG levels can further assist the clinician in risk assessment.

References

1. Estes JW: The practice of medicine in 18th century Massachusetts. N Engl J Med 305:1040, 1981.
2. Dorfman SF: Deaths from ectopic pregnancy, United States. 1979 to 1980. Obstet Gynecol 62:334, 1983.
3. Weinstein L, Morris MB, Dotters D, Christian CD: Ectopic pregnancy—A new surgical epidemic. Obstet Gynecol 61:698, 1983.
4. Lebolt SA, Grimes DA, Cates W: Mortality from abortion and childbirth: Are the populations comparable? JAMA 248:188, 1982.
5. Nagami M, London S, St Amand P: Factors influencing fertility after ectopic pregnancy. Am J Obstet Gynecol 149:533, 1984.
6. Schoen JA, Nowak RJ: Repeat ectopic pregnancy. A 16-year clinical survey. Obstet Gynecol 45:542, 1975.
7. Grant A: The effect of ectopic pregnancy on fertility. Clin Obstet Gynecol 5:861, 1962.
8. James AE, Fleischer AC, Sacks GA, Greeson T: Ectopic pregnancy: A malpractice paradigm. Radiology 160:411, 1986.
9. Berlin L: Malpractice and radiologists. AJR 135:587, 1980.
10. Stempel LE: Eenie, meenie, minie, mo. . . what do the data really show? Am J Obstet Gynecol 144:747, 1982.
11. Phillips WC, Scott JA, Blaszczynski G: How sensitive is "sensitivity"; how specific is "specificity"? AJR 140:1265, 1983.
12. Breen J: A 21-year survey of 654 ectopic pregnancies. Am J Obstet Gynecol 106:1004, 1970.
13. Tancer ML, Delke I, Veridiano NP: A fifteen-year experience with ectopic pregnancy. Surg Gynecol Obstet 152:179, 1981.
14. Lawless M, Vassey M: Risk of intrauterine contraceptive devices. (Letter.) Br Med J 288:1919, 1984.
15. McCausland A: High rate of ectopic prgnancy following laparoscopic tubal coagulation failures, incidence and etiology. Am J Obstet Gynecol 136:97, 1980.
16. Cartwright PS, DiPietro DL: Ectopic pregnancy: Changes in serum human chorionic gonadotropin concentration. Obstet Gynecol 63:76, 1984.
17. Brown TW, Filly RA, Laing FC, et al: Analysis of ultrasonographic criteria in the evaluation for ectopic pregnancy. AJR 131:965, 1978
18. Bangham DR, Storring PL: Standardization of human chorionic gonadotropin, hCG subunits and pregnancy tests. (Letter.) Lancet 1:390, 1982.
19. Batzer FR, Weiner S, Corson SL, et al: Landmarks during the first forty-two days of gestation demonstrated by the β-subunit of human chorionic gonadotropin and ultrasound. Am J Obstet Gynecol 146:973, 1983.
20. Nyberg DA, Filly RA, Mahony BS, et al: Early gestation: Correlation of hCG levels and sonographic identification. AJR 144:195, 1985.
21. Nyberg DA, Filly RA, Filho DL, et al: Abnormal pregnancy: Early diagnosis by US and serum chorionic gonadotropin levels. Radiology 158:393, 1986.
22. Nyberg DA, Laing FC, Filly RA, et al: Ectopic pregnancy: Diagnosis by sonography correlated with quantitative hCG levels. J Ultrasound Med 6:145, 1987.
23. Romero R, Kadar N, Jeanty P, et al: A prospective study of the value of the discriminatory zone in the diagnosis of ectopic pregnancy. Obstet Gynecol 66:357, 1985.
24. Batzer R: Guidelines for choosing a pregnancy test. Contemp Obstet Gynecol 30:57, 1985.
25. Romero R, Kadar N, Copel JA, et al: The effect of different human chorionic gonadotropin assay sensitivity on screening for ectopic pregnancy. Am J Obstet Gynecol 153:72, 1985.
26. Olson CM, Holt JA, Alenghat E, et al: Limitations of qualitative serum β-hCG assays in the diagnosis of ectopic pregnancy. J Reprod Med 28:838, 1983.
27. Berry CM, Thompson JD, Hatcher R: The radioreceptor assay for hCG in ectopic pregnancy. Obstet Gynecol 54:43, 1979.
28. Droegemueller W: Ectopic pregnancy. In Danforth DN (ed): Obstetrics and Gynecology. Philadelphia, Harper & Row, 1982, p 407.
29. Mahony BS, Filly RA, Nyberg DA, et al: Sonographic evaluation of ectopic pregnancy. J Ultrasound Med 4:221, 1985.
30. Lawson TL: Ectopic pregnancy: Criteria and accuracy of ultrasonic diagnosis. AJR 131:153, 1978.
31. Pederson JF: Ultrasonic scanning in suspected ectopic pregnancy. Br J Radiol 53:1, 1980.
32. Maklad NF, Wright CH: Gray scale ultrasonography in the diagnosis of ectopic pregnancy. Radiology 126:221, 1978.
33. Subramanyam BR, Raghavendra BN, Bathazar EJ, et al: Hematosalpinx in tubal pregnancy: Sonographic-pathologic correlation. AJR 141:361, 1983.
34. Schoenbaum S, Rosendorf L, Kappelman N: Grayscale ultrasound in tubal pregnancy. Radiology 127:757, 1978.
35. Weiner CP: The pseudogestational sac in ectopic pregnancy. Am J Obstet Gynecol 139:959, 1981.
36. Nelson P, Bowie JD, Rosenberg ER: Early intrauterine pregnancy or decidual cast: An anatomic-sonographic approach. J Ultrasound Med 2:543, 1983.
37. Bradley WG, Fiske CE, Filly RA: The double sac sign of early intrauterine pregnancy: Use in exclusion of ectopic pregnancy. Radiology 143:223, 1983.
38. Berger MJ, Taymor ML: Simultaneous intrauterine and tubal pregnancies following ovulation induction. Am J Obstet Gynecol 113:812, 1972.
39. Reece EA, Petrie RH, Sirmans MF: Combined intrauterine and extrauterine gestations: A review. Am J Obstet Gynecol 146:323, 1983.
40. Sondheimer SJ, Tureck RW, Blasco L, et al: Simultaneous ectopic pregnancy with intrauterine twin gestation after in vitro fertilization and embryo transfer. Fertil Steril 43:313, 1985.
41. Hann LE, Bachman DB, McArdle CR: Coexistent intrauterine and ectopic pregnancy: A re-evaluation. Radiology 152:151, 1984.
42. Yaghoobian J, Pinck RL, Ramanathan K, et al: Sonographic demonstration of simultaneous intrauterine and extrauterine gestation. J Ultrasound Med 5:309, 1986.
43. Marks WM, Filly RA, Callen PW, et al: The decidual cast of ectopic pregnancy: A confusing ultrasonographic appearance. Radiology 133:451, 1979.
44. Spirt BA, Ohara KR, Gordon L: Pseudogestational sac in ectopic pregnancy: Sonographic and pathologic correlation. JCU 9:338, 1981.
45. Laing FC, Filly RA, Mark WM, et al: Ultrasonic demonstration of endometrial fluid collections un-

associated with pregnancy. Radiology 137:471, 1980.

46. Mueller CE: Intrauterine pseudogestational sac in ectopic pregnancy. JCU 7:133, 1979.

47. Abramovich H, Auslender R, Lewin A, et al: Gestational-pseudogestational sac: A new ultrasonic criterion for differential diagnosis. Am J Obstet Gynecol 145:377, 1983.

48. Nyberg DA, Laing FC, Filly RA, et al: Ultrasonographic differentiation of the gestational sac of early intrauterine pregnancy from the pseudogestational sac of ectopic pregnancy. Radiology 146:755, 1983.

49. Cadkin AV, McAlpin J: Detection of fetal cardiac activity between 41 and 43 days gestation. J Ultrasound Med 3:499, 1984.

50. Nyberg DA, Laing FC, Filly RA: Threatened abortion: Sonographic distinction of normal and abnormal gestation sacs. Radiology 158:397, 1986.

51. Cadkin AV, McAlpin J: The decidua-chorionic sac: A reliable sonographic indicator of intrauterine pregnancy prior to detection of a fetal pole. J Ultrasound Med 3:539, 1984.

Appendix A

Measurements Frequently Used to Estimate Gestational Age and Fetal Biometry

Table 1. CLINICAL PARAMETERS IN ESTIMATION OF GESTATIONAL AGE*

PRIORITY FOR ESTIMATING GESTATIONAL AGE	"ESTIMATED" RANGE FOR 95% CASES
1. In vitro fertilization	less than 1 day
2. Ovulation induction	3–4 days
3. Recorded basal body temperature	4–5 days
4. Ultrasound crown-rump length (CRL)	± .7 weeks
5. First trimester physical examination (normal uterus)	±1 week
6. Ultrasound BPD prior to 20 weeks	+1 week
7. Ultrasound gestational sac volume	± 1.5 weeks
8. Ultrasound BPD from 20 to 26 weeks	± 1.6 weeks
9. LNMP from recorded dates (good history)†	± 2–3 weeks
10. Ultrasound BPD 26 to 30 weeks	+ 2–3 weeks
11. LNMP from memory (good history)	3–4 weeks
12. Ultrasound BPD after 30 weeks	3–4 weeks
13. Fundal height measurement	4–6 weeks
14. LNMP from memory (not good history)	4–6 weeks
15. Fetal heart tones first heard	4–6 weeks
16. Quickening	4–6 weeks

* *Rule* is to always use a more reliable indicator in preference to a less reliable one.

† A "good" history requires knowledge of both LNMP and previous period with regular periods and no use of birth control pills for at least six months prior to the LNMP.

From James D Bowie, MD.

Table 2. VARIABILITY ASSOCIATED WITH FETAL AGE ESTIMATES
DERIVED FROM ANATOMIC PARAMETERS

Parameter	Age Variability							
	Conception	0–6 weeks	6–14 weeks	12–18 weeks	18–24 weeks	24–30 weeks	30–36 weeks	36–42 weeks
Ovulation	±0.1	—	—	—	—	—	—	—
CRL	—	—	±0.4	—	—	—	—	—
BPD	—	—	—	±1.2	±1.7	±2.2	±3.1	±3.2
FL	—	—	—	±1.3 to ±1.9	±1.8 to ±2.6	±2.5 to ±3.1	±3.1 to ±3.7	±3.8 to ±4.2
HC	—	—	—	±1.2	±1.5	±2.1	±3.0	±2.7
AC	—	—	—	±1.7	±2.1	±2.2	±3.0	±3.0
BPD, HC AC, FL	—	—	—	±1.1	±1.4	±1.8	±2.4	±2.3

From Deter RL: Determining fetal age with ultrasound. The Female Patient 11:100, 1986.

Table 3. SAC SIZE VERSUS hCG LEVELS FOR NORMAL PREGNANCIES (n = 56)*

Mean Sac Diameter (mm)	hCG Level (mIU/ml)		
	Predicted†	95% Confidence Limits	
		Lower	Upper
5	1,932	1,026	3,636
6	2,165	1,226	4,256
7	2,704	1,465	4,990
8	3,199	1,749	5,852
9	3,785	2,085	6,870
10	4,478	2,483	8,075
11	5,297	2,952	9,508
12	6,267	3,502	11,218
13	7,415	4,145	13,266
14	8,773	4,894	15,726
15	10,379	5,766	18,682
16	12,270	6,776	22,235
17	14,528	7,964	26,501
18	17,188	9,343	31,621
19	20,337	10,951	37,761
20	24,060	12,820	45,130
21	28,464	15,020	53,970
22	33,675	17,560	64,570
23	39,843	20,573	77,164
24	47,138	24,067	93,325

*2nd International Standard. Note: a value of 100 mIU/ml from the 2nd International Standard (used here) equals approximately 200 mIU/ml from the International Reference Preparation (IRP).

†Log (hCG) = 2.92 + 0.073 (MSD), R^2 = 0.93, P < .001.

From Nyberg DA, Filly RA, Filho DL, et al: Abnormal pregnancy: Early diagnosis by US and serum chorionic gonadotropin levels. Radiology 158:393, 1986.

Table 4. GESTATIONAL SAC MEASUREMENT TABLE

Mean Predicted Gestational Sac (cm)	Gestational Age (weeks)	Mean Predicted Gestational Sac (cm)	Gestational Age (weeks)
1.0	5.0	3.6	8.8
1.1	5.2	3.7	8.9
1.2	5.3	3.8	9.0
1.3	5.5	3.9	9.2
1.4	5.6	4.0	9.3
1.5	5.8	4.1	9.5
1.6	5.9	4.2	9.6
1.7	6.0	4.2	9.7
1.8	6.2	4.4	9.9
1.9	6.3	4.5	10.0
2.0	6.5	4.6	10.2
2.1	6.6	4.7	10.3
2.2	6.8	4.8	10.5
2.3	6.9	4.9	10.6
2.4	7.0	5.0	10.7
2.5	7.2	5.1	10.9
2.6	7.3	5.2	11.0
2.7	7.5	5.3	11.2
2.8	7.6	5.4	11.3
2.9	7.8	5.5	11.5
3.0	7.9	5.6	11.6
3.1	8.0	5.7	11.7
3.2	8.2	5.8	1.9
3.3	8.3	5.9	12.0
3.4	8.5	6.0	12.2
3.5	8.6		

$$\text{Equation: Gestational Age (weeks)} = \frac{\text{Gestational Sac (cm)} + 2.543}{0.702}$$

From Hellman LM, Kobayashi M, Fillisti L, et al: Growth and development of the human fetus prior to the twentieth week of gestation. Am J Obstet Gynecol 103:789, 1969.

Table 5. GESTATIONAL AGE BASED ON CROWN-RUMP LENGTH

Crown-rump length (cm)	Gestational age (wk + d)			Crown-rump length (cm)	Gestational age (wk + d)		
	MacGregor et al	Robinson & Fleming*	Drumm et al†		MacGregor et al	Robinson & Fleming*	Drumm et al†
1.0	7 + 5	7 + 0	6 + 6	3.9	10 + 6	10 + 4	10 + 5
1.1	7 + 6	7 + 1	7 + 1	4.0	10 + 6	10 + 5	10 + 5
1.2	8 + 0	7 + 3	7 + 2	4.1	11 + 0	10 + 5	10 + 6
1.3	8 + 1	7 + 4	7 + 3	4.2	11 + 1	10 + 6	11 + 0
1.4	8 + 1	7 + 5	7 + 4	4.3	11 + 1	11 + 0	11 + 0
1.5	8 + 2	7 + 6	7 + 5	4.4	11 + 2	11 + 0	11 + 1
1.6	8 + 3	8 + 0	7 + 6	4.5	11 + 3	11 + 1	11 + 2
1.7	8 + 4	8 + 1	8 + 0	4.6	11 + 3	11 + 1	11 + 2
1.8	8 + 5	8 + 2	8 + 1	4.7	11 + 4	11 + 2	11 + 3
1.9	8 + 5	8 + 3	8 + 2	4.8	11 + 5	11 + 3	11 + 4
2.0	8 + 6	8 + 4	8 + 3	4.9	11 + 5	11 + 3	11 + 4
2.1	9 + 0	8 + 5	8 + 4	5.0	11 + 6	11 + 4	11 + 5
2.2	9 + 1	8 + 6	8 + 5	5.1	12 + 0	11 + 4	11 + 5
2.3	9 + 1	8 + 6	8 + 6	5.2	12 + 0	11 + 5	11 + 6
2.4	9 + 2	9 + 0	9 + 0	5.3	12 + 1	11 + 5	12 + 0
2.5	9 + 3	9 + 1	9 + 1	5.4	12 + 1	11 + 6	12 + 0
2.6	9 + 4	9 + 2	9 + 2	5.5	12 + 2	11 + 6	12 + 1
2.7	9 + 4	9 + 3	9 + 3	5.6	12 + 3	12 + 0	12 + 2
2.8	9 + 5	9 + 3	9 + 3	5.7	12 + 3	12 + 1	12 + 2
2.9	9 + 6	9 + 4	9 + 4	5.8	12 + 4	12 + 1	12 + 3
3.0	9 + 6	9 + 5	9 + 5	5.9	12 + 4	12 + 2	12 + 3
3.1	10 + 0	9 + 6	9 + 6	6.0	12 + 5	12 + 2	12 + 4
3.2	10 + 1	9 + 6	10 + 0	6.1	12 + 6	12 + 3	12 + 5
3.3	10 + 2	10 + 0	10 + 0	6.2	12 + 6	12 + 3	12 + 5
3.4	10 + 2	10 + 1	10 + 1	6.3	13 + 0	12 + 4	12 + 6
3.5	10 + 3	10 + 1	10 + 2	6.4	13 + 0	12 + 4	12 + 6
3.6	10 + 4	10 + 2	10 + 3	6.5	13 + 1	12 + 5	13 + 0
3.7	10 + 4	10 + 3	10 + 3	6.6	13 + 2	12 + 5	13 + 0
3.8	10 + 5	10 + 3	10 + 4				

*Robinson HP, Fleming JEE: A critical evaluation of sonar "crown-rump length" measurements. Br J Obstet Gynaecol 82:702, 1975.

†Drumm JE, Clinch J, MacKinzie G: The ultrasonic measurement of fetal crown-rump length as a method of assessing gestational age. Br J Obstet Gynaecol 83:471, 1976.

From MacGregor SN, Tamura RK, Sabbagha RE, et al: Underestimation of gestational age by conventional crown-rump length dating curves. Obstet Gynecol 70:344, 1987. *Reprinted with permission from* The American College of Obstetricians and Gynecologists.

Table 6. PREDICTED MENSTRUAL AGES FOR BPD VALUES FROM 2.0 TO 10.0 cm

BPD (cm)	Menstrual Age (weeks)	BPD (cm)	Menstrual Age (weeks)
2.0	12.2	6.1	25.0
2.1	12.5	6.2	25.3
2.2	12.8	6.3	25.7
2.3	13.1	6.4	26.1
2.4	13.3	6.5	26.4
2.5	13.6	6.6	26.8
2.6	13.9	6.7	27.2
2.7	14.2	6.8	27.6
2.8	14.5	6.9	28.0
2.9	14.7	7.0	28.3
3.0	15.0	7.1	28.7
3.1	15.3	7.2	29.1
3.2	15.6	7.3	29.5
3.3	15.9	7.4	29.9
3.4	16.2	7.5	30.4
3.5	16.5	7.6	30.8
3.6	16.8	7.7	31.2
3.7	17.1	7.8	31.6
3.8	17.4	7.9	32.0
3.9	17.7	8.0	32.5
4.0	18.0	8.1	32.9
4.1	18.3	8.2	33.3
4.2	18.6	8.3	33.8
4.3	18.9	8.4	34.2
4.4	19.2	8.5	34.7
4.5	19.5	8.6	35.1
4.6	19.9	8.7	35.6
4.7	20.2	8.8	36.1
4.8	20.5	8.9	36.5
4.9	20.8	9.0	37.0
5.0	21.2	9.1	37.5
5.1	21.5	9.2	38.0
5.2	21.8	9.3	38.5
5.3	22.2	9.4	38.9
5.4	22.5	9.5	39.4
5.5	22.8	9.6	39.9
5.6	23.2	9.7	40.5
5.7	23.5	9.8	41.0
5.8	23.9	9.9	41.5
5.9	24.2	10.0	42.0
6.0	24.6		

From Hadlock FP, Deter RL, Harrist RB, Park SK: The use of ultrasound to determine fetal age—A review. Medical Ultrasound 7:95, 1983.

Table 7. PREDICTED MENSTRUAL AGES FOR HEAD CIRCUMFERENCES

Head Circumference (cm)	Menstrual Age (weeks)	Head Circumference (cm)	Menstrual Age (weeks)
8.0	13.4	22.5	24.4
8.5	13.7	23.0	24.9
9.0	14.0	23.5	25.4
9.5	14.3	24.0	25.9
10.0	14.6	24.5	26.4
10.5	15.0	25.0	26.9
11.0	15.3	25.5	27.5
11.5	15.6	26.0	28.0
12.0	15.9	26.5	28.1
12.5	16.3	27.0	29.2
13.0	16.6	27.5	29.8
13.5	17.0	28.0	30.3
14.0	17.3	28.5	31.0
14.5	17.7	29.0	31.6
15.0	18.1	29.5	32.2
15.5	18.4	30.0	32.8
16.0	18.8	30.5	33.5
16.5	19.2	31.0	34.2
17.0	19.6	31.5	34.9
17.5	20.0	32.0	35.5
18.0	20.4	32.5	36.3
18.5	20.8	33.0	37.0
19.0	21.2	33.5	37.7
19.5	21.6	34.0	38.5
20.0	22.1	34.5	39.2
20.5	22.5	35.0	40.0
21.0	23.0	35.5	40.8
21.5	23.4	36.0	41.6
22.0	23.9		

From Hadlock FP, Deter RL, Harrist RB, Park SK: The use of ultrasound to determine fetal age—A review. Medical Ultrasound 7:95, 1983.

Table 8. RELATIONSHIP BETWEEN CEREBELLAR AND BIPARIETAL DIAMETER

Cerebellar Diameter (mm)	Biparietal Diameter (mm)	+S.E.	−S.E.
15	34.7	38.0	31.5
16	37.2	40.6	34.0
17	39.8	43.2	36.4
18	42.2	45.7	38.8
19	44.6	48.1	41.1
20	46.9	50.5	43.4
21	49.2	52.8	45.6
22	51.4	55.0	47.8
23	53.5	57.2	49.9
24	55.6	59.3	51.9
25	57.6	61.3	53.9
26	59.6	63.3	55.8
27	61.5	65.2	57.7
28	63.3	67.1	59.5
29	65.1	68.8	61.3
30	66.8	70.6	63.0
31	68.4	72.2	64.7
32	70.0	73.8	66.3
33	71.6	75.3	67.8
34	73.0	76.8	69.3
35	74.4	78.2	70.7
36	75.8	79.5	72.1
37	77.1	80.8	73.4
38	78.3	82.0	74.7
39	79.5	83.1	75.9
40	80.6	84.2	77.0
41	81.7	85.2	78.1
42	82.6	86.2	79.1
43	83.6	87.1	80.1
44	84.4	87.9	81.0
45	85.3	88.6	81.9
46	86.0	89.3	82.7
47	86.7	89.9	83.5
48	87.3	90.5	84.2
49	87.9	91.0	84.8
50	88.4	91.4	85.4
51	88.8	91.8	85.9
52	89.2	92.1	86.4
53	89.6	92.3	86.8
54	89.8	92.5	87.2

From McLeary RD, Kuhns LR, Barr M: Ultrasonography of the fetal cerebellum. Radiology 151:439, 1984.

Table 9. NOMOGRAM OF THE TRANSVERSE CEREBELLAR DIAMETER ACCORDING TO PERCENTILE DISTRIBUTION

Gestational age (wk)	Cerebellum (mm)				
	10	25	50	75	90
15	10	12	14	15	16
16	14	16	16	16	17
17	16	17	17	18	18
18	17	18	18	19	19
19	18	18	19	19	22
20	18	19	20	20	22
21	19	20	22	23	24
22	21	23	23	24	24
23	22	23	24	25	26
24	22	24	25	27	28
25	23	21.5	28	28	29
26	25	28	29	30	32
27	26	28.5	30	31	32
28	27	30	31	32	34
29	29	32	34	36	38
30	31	32	35	37	40
31	32	35	38	39	43
32	33	36	38	40	42
33	32	36	40	43	44
34	33	38	40	41	44
35	31	37	40.5	43	47
36	36	29	43	52	55
37	37	37	45	52	55
38	40	40	48.5	52	55
39	52	52	52	55	55

From Goldstein I, Reece A, Pilu G, et al: Cerebellar measurements with ultrasonography in the evaluation of fetal growth and development. Am J Obstet Gynecol 156:1065, 1987.

Table 10. PREDICTED BPD AND WEEKS' GESTATION FROM THE INNER AND
OUTER ORBITAL DISTANCES

BPD (cm)	Gestation (wk)	IOD (cm)	OOD (cm)	BPD (cm)	Gestation (wk)	IOD (cm)	OOD (cm)
1.9	11.6	0.5	1.3	5.8	24.3	1.6	4.1
2.0	11.6	0.5	1.4	5.9	24.3	1.6	4.2
2.1	12.1	0.6	1.5	6.0	24.7	1.6	4.3
2.2	12.6	0.6	1.6	6.1	25.2	1.6	4.3
2.3	12.6	0.6	1.7	6.2	25.2	1.6	4.4
2.4	13.1	0.7	1.7	6.3	25.7	1.7	4.4
2.5	13.6	0.7	1.8	6.4	26.2	1.7	4.5
2.6	13.6	0.7	1.9	6.5	26.2	1.7	4.5
2.7	14.1	0.8	2.0	6.6	26.7	1.7	4.6
2.8	14.6	0.8	2.1	6.7	27.2	1.7	4.6
2.9	14.6	0.8	2.1	6.8	27.6	1.7	4.7
3.0	15.0	0.9	2.2	6.9	28.1	1.7	4.7
3.1	15.5	0.9	2.3	7.0	28.6	1.8	4.8
3.2	15.5	0.9	2.4	7.1	29.1	1.8	4.8
3.3	16.0	1.0	2.5	7.3	29.6	1.8	4.9
3.4	16.5	1.0	2.5	7.4	30.0	1.8	5.0
3.5	16.5	1.0	2.6	7.5	30.6	1.8	5.0
3.6	17.0	1.0	2.7	7.6	31.0	1.8	5.1
3.7	17.5	1.1	2.7	7.7	31.5	1.8	5.1
3.8	17.9	1.1	2.8	7.8	32.0	1.8	5.2
4.0	18.4	1.2	3.0	7.9	32.5	1.9	5.2
4.2	18.9	1.2	3.1	8.0	33.0	1.9	5.3
4.3	19.4	1.2	3.2	8.2	33.5	1.9	5.4
4.4	19.4	1.3	3.2	8.3	34.0	1.9	5.4
4.5	19.9	1.3	3.3	8.4	34.4	1.9	5.4
4.6	20.4	1.3	3.4	8.5	35.0	1.9	5.5
4.7	20.4	1.3	3.4	8.6	35.4	1.9	5.5
4.8	20.9	1.4	3.5	8.8	35.9	1.9	5.6
4.9	21.3	1.4	3.6	8.9	36.4	1.9	5.6
5.0	21.3	1.4	3.6	9.0	36.9	1.9	5.7
5.1	21.8	1.4	3.7	9.1	37.3	1.9	5.7
5.2	22.3	1.4	3.8	9.2	37.8	1.9	5.8
5.3	22.3	1.5	3.8	9.3	38.3	1.9	5.8
5.4	22.8	1.5	3.9	9.4	38.8	1.9	5.8
5.5	23.3	1.5	4.0	9.6	39.3	1.9	5.9
5.6	23.3	1.5	4.0	9.7	39.8	1.9	5.9
5.7	23.8	1.5	4.1				

From Mayden KL, Tortora M, Berkowitz RL, et al: Orbital diameters: A new parameter for prenatal diagnosis and dating. Am J Obstet Gynecol 144:289, 1982.

Table 11. FETAL THORACIC CIRCUMFERENCE MEASUREMENTS*

Gestational age (wk)	No.	Predictive percentiles								
		2.5	5	10	25	50	75	90	95	97.5
16	6	5.9	6.4	7.0	8.0	9.1	10.3	11.3	11.9	12.4
17	22	6.8	7.3	7.9	8.9	10.0	11.2	12.2	12.8	13.3
18	31	7.7	8.2	8.8	9.8	11.0	12.1	13.1	13.7	14.2
19	21	8.6	9.1	9.7	10.7	11.9	13.0	14.0	14.6	15.1
20	20	9.5	10.0	10.6	11.7	12.8	13.9	15.0	15.5	16.0
21	30	10.4	11.0	11.6	12.6	13.7	14.8	15.8	16.4	16.9
22	18	11.3	11.9	12.5	13.5	14.6	15.7	16.7	17.3	17.8
23	21	12.2	12.8	13.4	14.4	15.5	16.6	17.6	18.2	18.8
24	27	13.2	13.7	14.3	15.3	16.4	17.5	18.5	19.1	19.7
25	20	14.1	14.6	15.2	16.2	17.3	18.4	19.4	20.0	20.6
26	25	15.0	15.5	16.1	17.1	18.2	19.3	20.3	21.0	21.5
27	24	15.9	16.4	17.0	18.0	19.1	20.2	21.3	21.9	22.4
28	24	16.8	17.3	17.9	18.9	20.0	21.2	22.2	22.8	23.3
29	24	17.7	18.2	18.8	19.8	21.0	22.1	23.1	23.7	24.2
30	27	18.6	19.1	19.7	20.7	21.9	23.0	24.0	24.6	25.1
31	24	19.5	20.0	20.6	21.6	22.8	23.9	24.9	25.5	26.0
32	28	20.4	20.9	21.5	22.6	23.7	24.8	25.8	26.4	26.9
33	27	21.3	21.8	22.5	23.5	24.6	25.7	26.7	27.3	27.8
34	25	22.2	22.8	23.4	24.4	25.5	26.6	27.6	28.2	28.7
35	20	23.1	23.7	24.3	25.3	26.4	27.5	28.5	29.1	29.6
36	23	24.0	24.6	25.2	26.2	27.3	28.4	29.4	30.0	30.6
37	22	24.9	25.5	26.1	27.1	28.2	29.3	30.3	30.9	31.5
38	21	25.9	26.4	27.0	28.0	29.1	30.2	31.2	31.9	32.4
39	7	26.8	27.3	27.9	28.9	30.0	31.1	32.2	32.8	33.3
40	6	27.7	28.2	28.8	29.8	30.9	32.1	33.1	33.7	34.2

*Measurements in centimeters.

From Chitkara U, Rosenberg J, Chervenak FA, et al: Prenatal sonographic assessment of the fetal thorax: Normal values. Am J Obstet Gynecol 156:1069, 1987.

Table 12. PREDICTED MENSTRUAL AGE FOR ABDOMINAL CIRCUMFERENCE VALUES

Abdominal Circumference (cm)	Menstrual Age (weeks)	Abdominal Circumference (cm)	Menstrual Age (weeks)
10.0	15.6	23.5	27.7
10.5	16.1	24.0	28.2
11.0	16.5	24.5	28.7
11.5	16.9	25.0	29.2
12.0	17.3	25.5	29.7
12.5	17.8	26.0	30.1
13.0	18.2	26.5	30.6
13.5	18.6	27.0	31.1
14.0	19.1	27.5	31.6
14.5	19.5	28.0	32.1
15.0	20.0	28.5	32.6
15.5	20.4	29.0	33.1
16.0	20.8	29.5	33.6
16.5	21.3	30.0	34.1
17.0	21.7	30.5	34.6
17.5	22.2	31.0	35.1
18.0	22.6	31.5	35.6
18.5	23.1	32.0	36.1
19.0	23.6	32.5	36.6
19.5	24.0	33.0	37.1
20.0	24.5	33.5	37.6
20.5	24.9	34.0	38.1
21.0	25.4	34.5	38.7
21.5	25.9	35.0	39.2
22.0	26.3	35.5	39.7
22.5	26.8	36.0	40.2
23.0	27.3	36.5	40.8

Note—$MA = 7.6070 + 0.7645 (AC) + 0.00393 (AC)^2$; $r^2 = 97.8\%$; 1 SD = 1.2 weeks.

From Hadlock FP, Deter RL, Harrist RB, Park SK: Fetal abdominal circumference as a predictor of menstrual age. AJR 139:367, 1982. Copyright 1982, The American Roentgen Ray Society.

Table 13. PREDICTED MENSTRUAL AGE FOR FEMUR LENGTHS

Femur Length (cm)	Menstrual Age (weeks)	Femur Length (cm)	Menstrual Age (weeks)
1.0	12.8	4.5	24.5
1.1	13.1	4.6	24.9
1.2	13.4	4.7	25.3
1.3	13.6	4.8	25.7
1.4	13.9	4.9	26.1
1.5	14.2	5.0	26.5
1.6	14.5	5.1	27.0
1.7	14.8	5.2	27.4
1.8	15.1	5.3	27.8
1.9	15.4	5.4	28.2
2.0	15.7	5.5	28.7
2.1	16.0	5.6	29.1
2.2	16.3	5.7	29.6
2.3	16.6	5.8	30.0
2.4	16.9	5.9	30.5
2.5	17.2	6.0	30.9
2.6	17.6	6.1	31.4
2.7	17.9	6.2	31.9
2.8	18.2	6.3	32.3
2.9	18.6	6.4	32.8
3.0	18.9	6.5	33.3
3.1	19.2	6.6	33.8
3.2	19.6	6.7	34.2
3.3	19.9	6.8	34.7
3.4	20.3	6.9	35.2
3.5	20.7	7.0	35.7
3.6	21.0	7.1	36.2
3.7	21.4	7.2	36.7
3.8	21.8	7.3	37.2
3.9	22.1	7.4	37.7
4.0	22.5	7.5	38.3
4.1	22.9	7.6	38.8
4.2	23.3	7.7	39.3
4.3	23.7	7.8	39.8
4.4	24.1	7.9	40.4

From Hadlock FP, Deter RL, Harrist RB, Park SK: The use of ultrasound to determine fetal age—A review. Medical Ultrasound 7:95, 1983.

Table 14. LENGTH OF FETAL LONG BONES (mm)

Week No.	Humerus Percentile			Ulna Percentile			Radius Percentile			Femur Percentile			Tibia Percentile			Fibula Percentile		
	5	50	95	5	50	95	5	50	95	5	50	95	5	50	95	5	50	95
11	—	6	—	—	5	—	—	5	—	—	6	—	—	4	—	—	2	—
12	3	9	10	—	8	—	—	7	—	—	9	—	—	7	—	—	5	—
13	5	13	20	3	11	18	—	10	—	6	12	19	4	10	17	—	8	—
14	5	16	20	4	13	17	8	13	12	5	15	19	2	13	19	6	11	10
15	11	18	26	10	16	22	12	15	19	11	19	26	5	16	27	10	14	18
16	12	21	25	8	19	24	9	18	21	13	22	24	7	19	25	6	17	22
17	19	24	29	11	21	32	11	20	29	20	25	29	15	22	29	7	19	31
18	18	27	30	13	24	30	14	22	26	19	28	31	14	24	29	10	22	28
19	22	29	36	20	26	32	20	24	29	23	31	38	19	27	35	18	24	30
20	23	32	36	21	29	32	21	27	28	22	33	39	19	29	35	18	27	30
21	28	34	40	25	31	36	25	29	32	27	36	45	24	32	39	24	29	34
22	28	36	40	24	33	37	24	31	34	29	39	44	25	34	39	21	31	37
23	32	38	45	27	35	43	26	32	39	35	41	48	30	36	43	23	33	44
24	31	41	46	29	37	41	27	34	38	34	44	49	28	39	45	26	35	41
25	35	43	51	34	39	44	31	36	40	38	46	'54	31	41	50	33	37	42
26	36	45	49	34	41	44	30	37	41	39	49	53	33	43	49	32	39	43
27	42	46	51	37	43	48	33	39	45	45	51	57	39	45	51	35	41	47
28	41	48	52	37	44	48	33	40	45	45	53	57	38	47	52	36	43	47
29	44	50	56	40	46	51	36	42	47	49	56	62	40	49	57	40	45	50
30	44	52	56	38	47	54	34	43	49	49	58	62	41	51	56	38	47	52
31	47	53	59	39	49	59	34	44	53	53	60	67	46	52	58	40	48	57
32	47	55	59	40	50	58	37	45	51	53	62	67	46	54	59	40	50	56
33	50	56	62	43	52	60	41	46	51	56	64	71	49	56	62	43	51	59
34	50	57	62	44	53	59	39	47	53	57	65	70	47	57	64	46	52	56
35	52	58	65	47	54	61	38	48	57	61	67	73	48	59	69	51	54	57
36	53	60	63	47	55	61	41	48	54	61	69	74	49	60	68	51	55	56
37	57	61	64	49	56	62	45	49	53	64	71	77	52	61	71	55	56	58
38	55	61	66	48	57	63	45	49	53	62	72	79	54	62	69	54	57	59
39	56	62	69	49	57	66	46	50	54	64	74	83	58	64	69	55	58	62
40	56	63	69	50	58	65	46	50	54	66	75	81	58	65	69	54	59	62

From Jeanty P: Fetal limb biometry. (Letter.) Radiology 147:602, 1983.

Table 15. ULTRASOUND FETAL THIGH AND CALF CIRCUMFERENCES
FROM 20 WEEKS' GESTATION TO TERM*

Gestational Age (Weeks)	Fetal Thigh Circumference (cm)	Fetal Calf Circumference (cm)
20	6.5 ± 1.3	4.9 ± 1.5
21	6.3 ± 0.8	4.5 ± 1.0
22	7.8 ± 1.2	6.0 ± 1.3
23	7.9 ± 1.4	6.0 ± 1.3
24	8.3 ± 1.3	6.5 ± 0.9
25	8.6 ± 1.4	6.6 ± 1.4
26	9.2 ± 1.3	7.1 ± 1.1
27	9.6 ± 1.0	7.5 ± 1.2
28	10.3 ± 1.6	8.1 ± 0.6
29	10.5 ± 1.3	8.2 ± 1.7
30	10.5 ± 1.0	8.4 ± 0.7
31	11.3 ± 1.7	8.9 ± 1.7
32	12.0 ± 2.8	9.7 ± 1.0
33	12.4 ± 1.8	9.6 ± 1.1
34	13.5 ± 2.1	10.5 ± 1.1
35	13.9 ± 2.4	10.6 ± 1.0
36	14.1 ± 2.7	11.1 ± 1.5
37	14.2 ± 2.5	11.0 ± 0.9
38	14.8 ± 2.0	11.7 ± 0.6
39	15.3 ± 2.2	11.8 ± 0.6
40	15.7 ± 1.0	12.1 ± 0.8

*Values are expressed as means ± 2 SD.

From Vintzileos AM, Neckles S, Campbell WA, et al: Ultrasound fetal thigh-calf circumferences and gestational age—Independent fetal ratios in normal pregnancy. J Ultrasound Med 4:287, 1985.

Table 16. GESTATIONAL AGE FOR CLAVICLE LENGTH

Clavicle Length (mm)	Gestational Age (weeks and days) Percentile		
	5th	50th	95th
11	8 + 3	13 + 6	17 + 2
12	9 + 1	14 + 4	18 + 1
13	10 + 0	14 + 3	19 + 6
14	11 + 6	15 + 2	20 + 5
15	12 + 5	16 + 1	21 + 4
16	12 + 3	18 + 0	21 + 3
17	13 + 2	18 + 5	22 + 2
18	14 + 1	19 + 4	23 + 0
19	16 + 0	19 + 3	24 + 6
20	16 + 6	20 + 2	25 + 5
21	17 + 4	21 + 1	26 + 4
22	17 + 3	22 + 6	26 + 2
23	18 + 2	23 + 5	27 + 1
24	19 + 1	24 + 4	28 + 0
25	21 + 0	24 + 3	29 + 6
26	21 + 5	25 + 1	30 + 5
27	22 + 4	26 + 0	30 + 3
28	22 + 3	27 + 6	31 + 2
29	23 + 2	28 + 5	32 + 1
30	24 + 0	29 + 4	34 + 0
31	25 + 6	29 + 2	34 + 6
32	26 + 5	30 + 1	35 + 4
33	27 + 4	31 + 0	35 + 3
34	27 + 3	32 + 6	36 + 2
35	28 + 1	33 + 5	37 + 1
36	29 + 0	33 + 3	39 + 0
37	30 + 6	34 + 2	39 + 5
38	31 + 5	35 + 1	40 + 4
39	32 + 4	37 + 0	40 + 3
40	32 + 2	37 + 6	41 + 2
41	33 + 1	38 + 4	42 + 0
42	35 + 0	38 + 3	43 + 6
43	35 + 6	39 + 2	44 + 5
44	36 + 5	40 + 1	45 + 4
45	36 + 3	41 + 6	45 + 3

From Yarkoni S, Schmidt W, Jeanty P, et al: Clavicular measurement: A new biometric parameter for fetal evaluation. J Ultrasound Med 4:467, 1987.

Table 17. COMPARISON OF MEAN POSTPARTUM AND ULTRASONOGRAPHIC FOOT LENGTH WITH STREETER'S PATHOLOGIC DATA (1920)

Gestation week	Streeter's data (mm)	Ultrasonographic foot length (mm)	Postpartum foot length (mm)
11	7	8	
12	9	9	
13	11	10	
14	14	16	
15	17	16	
16	20	21	
17	23	24	
18	27	27	
19	31	28	
20	33	33	33
21	35	35	
22	40	38	
23	42	42	
24	45	44	
25	48	47	48
26	50	51	
27	53	54	52
28	55	58	
29	57	57	57
30	59	61	60
31	61	62	60
32	63	63	66
33	65	67	68
34	68	68	71
35	71	71	72
36	74	74	74
37	77	75	78
38	79	78	78
39	81	78	80
40	83	82	81
41			82
42			82
43			84

From Mercer BM, Sklar S, Shariatmadar A, et al: Fetal foot length as a predictor of gestational age. Am J Obstet Gynecol 156:350, 1987.

Appendix B

Methodology for Fetal Weight Estimation

Table 1. PUBLISHED REGRESSION EQUATIONS FOR SONOGRAPHIC ESTIMATION OF FETAL WEIGHT

Reference	Equation [Log_{10} (Birthweight)] =
Hadlock*	$1.3596 - 0.00386 \, (AC)(FL) + 0.0064 \, (HC) + 0.00061 \, (BPD)(AC) + 0.0424 \, (AC) + 0.174 \, (FL)$
Hadlock†	$1.5115 + 0.0436 \, (AC) + 0.1517 \, (FL) - \dfrac{0.321 \, (AC \, (FL)}{100} + \dfrac{0.6923 \, (BPD \, (HC)}{10000}$
Shepard‡	$-1.7492 + 0.166 \, (BPD) + 0.046 \, (AC) - \dfrac{2.646 \, (AC)(BPD)}{1000}$
Warsof§	$-1.599 + 0.144 \, (BPD) + 0.032 \, (AC) - \dfrac{0.111 \, (BPD)^2 \, (AC)}{1000}$
Roberts‖	$1.6758 + 0.01707 \, (AC) + 0.042478 \, (BPD) + 0.05216 \, (FL) + 0.01604 \, (HC)$

*Hadlock FP, Harrist RB, Sharman RS, et al: Estimation of fetal weight with the use of head, body, and femur measurements. A prospective study. Am J Obstet Gynecol 151:333, 1985.

†Hadlock FP, Harrist RB, Carpenter RJ, et al: Sonographic estimation of fetal weight. Radiology 150:535, 1984.

‡Shepard MJ, Richards VA, Berkowitz FL, et al: An evaluation of two equations for predicting fetal weight by ultrasound. Am J Obstet Gynecol 142:47, 1982.

§Warsof SL, Gohari P, Berkowitz RL, Hobbins JC: The estimation of fetal weight by computer-assisted analysis. Am J Obstet Gynecol 128:881, 1977.

‖Roberts AB, Lee AJ, James AG: Ultrasonic estimation of fetal weight: A new predictive model incorporating femur length for the low-birthweight fetus. JCU 13:555, 1985.

Table 2. NORMAL WEIGHTS* AND STANDARD DEVIATIONS
ACCORDING TO THE SHEPARD FORMULA

	Number of Standard Deviations below the Mean									Mean	Number of Standard Deviations above the Mean								
	2.6	2.4	2.2	2	1.8	1.6	1.4	1.2	1		1	1.2	1.4	1.6	1.8	2	2.2	2.4	2.6
Week 9	43	44	44	44	44	44	44	44	44	45	46	46	46	46	46	46	46	46	47
Week 10	44	44	45	45	45	46	46	46	46	48	50	50	50	50	51	51	51	52	52
Week 11	47	47	48	48	49	50	50	51	51	54	57	57	58	58	59	60	60	61	61
Week 12	52	53	53	54	55	56	57	58	59	63	67	68	69	70	71	72	73	73	74
Week 13	58	60	61	63	64	66	67	68	70	77	84	86	87	88	90	91	93	94	96
Week 14	68	70	72	74	76	79	81	83	85	96	107	109	111	113	116	118	120	122	124
Week 15	81	84	87	90	93	97	100	103	106	122	138	141	144	147	151	154	157	160	163
Week 16	98	102	106	111	115	120	124	129	133	155	177	181	186	190	195	199	204	208	212
Week 17	118	124	130	136	142	148	154	160	167	197	227	234	240	246	252	258	264	270	276
Week 18	142	150	158	166	174	182	190	199	207	247	287	295	304	312	320	328	336	344	352
Week 19	172	183	193	203	214	224	234	245	255	307	359	369	380	390	400	411	421	431	442
Week 20	207	220	233	246	259	272	285	298	311	377	443	456	469	482	495	508	521	534	547
Week 21	245	261	278	294	310	326	343	359	375	456	537	553	569	586	602	618	634	651	667
Week 22	289	309	328	348	368	387	407	427	447	545	643	663	683	703	722	742	762	781	801
Week 23	339	362	386	409	433	456	480	503	527	644	761	785	808	832	855	879	902	926	949
Week 24	392	420	448	475	503	531	559	586	614	753	892	920	947	975	1,003	1,031	1,058	1,086	1,114
Week 25	450	482	514	547	579	612	644	676	709	871	1,033	1,066	1,098	1,130	1,163	1,195	1,228	1,260	1,292
Week 26	514	551	589	626	663	701	738	776	813	1,000	1,187	1,224	1,262	1,299	1,337	1,374	1,411	1,449	1,486
Week 27	583	625	668	711	754	797	839	882	925	1,139	1,353	1,396	1,439	1,481	1,524	1,567	1,610	1,653	1,695
Week 28	656	704	753	802	850	899	948	996	1,045	1,288	1,531	1,580	1,628	1,677	1,726	1,774	1,823	1,872	1,920
Week 29	734	789	844	899	954	1,009	1,064	1,119	1,173	1,448	1,723	1,777	1,832	1,887	1,942	1,997	2,052	2,107	2,162
Week 30	819	880	942	1,003	1,065	1,126	1,188	1,249	1,311	1,618	1,925	1,987	2,048	2,110	2,171	2,233	2,294	2,356	2,417
Week 31	907	976	1,044	1,113	1,181	1,250	1,318	1,387	1,455	1,798	2,141	2,209	2,278	2,346	2,415	2,483	2,552	2,620	2,689
Week 32	999	1,075	1,150	1,226	1,302	1,378	1,454	1,529	1,605	1,984	2,363	2,439	2,514	2,590	2,666	2,742	2,818	2,893	2,969
Week 33	1,092	1,176	1,259	1,342	1,426	1,509	1,593	1,676	1,759	2,176	2,593	2,676	2,759	2,843	2,926	3,010	3,093	3,176	3,260
Week 34	1,188	1,279	1,369	1,460	1,551	1,642	1,733	1,824	1,915	2,369	2,823	2,914	3,005	3,096	3,187	3,278	3,369	3,459	3,550
Week 35	1,280	1,379	1,477	1,575	1,673	1,771	1,870	1,968	2,066	2,557	3,048	3,146	3,244	3,343	3,441	3,539	3,637	3,735	3,834
Week 36	1,366	1,471	1,577	1,682	1,787	1,892	1,997	2,103	2,208	2,734	3,260	3,365	3,471	3,576	3,681	3,786	3,891	3,997	4,102
Week 37	1,441	1,553	1,664	1,776	1,887	1,999	2,110	2,221	2,333	2,890	3,447	3,559	3,670	3,781	3,893	4,004	4,116	4,227	4,339
Week 38	1,499	1,616	1,732	1,849	1,966	2,082	2,199	2,316	2,432	3,016	3,600	3,716	3,833	3,950	4,066	4,183	4,300	4,416	4,533
Week 39	1,525	1,646	1,767	1,888	2,009	2,131	2,252	2,373	2,494	3,099	3,704	3,825	3,946	4,067	4,189	4,310	4,431	4,552	4,673
Week 40	1,514	1,638	1,762	1,887	2,011	2,136	2,260	2,385	2,509	3,131	3,753	3,877	4,002	4,126	4,251	4,375	4,500	4,624	4,748

*Expressed in "estimated grams."

From Jeanty P, Cantraine F, Romero R, et al: A longitudinal study of fetal weight growth. J Ultrasound Med 3:321, 1984. Reprinted with permission of The American Institute of Ultrasound in Medicine, copyright 1984.

Table 3. CALIFORNIA BIRTH WEIGHT/GESTATIONAL AGE

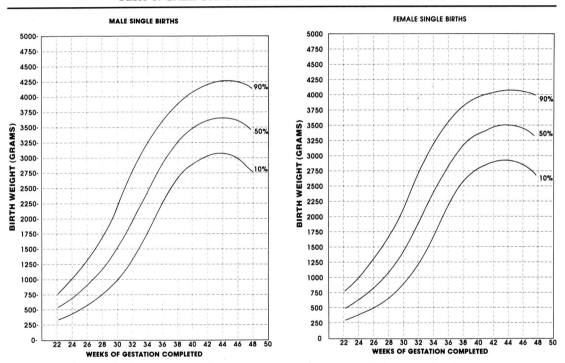

From Williams RL, Creasy RK, Cunningham GC: Fetal growth and perinatal viability in California. Obstet Gynecol 59:624, 1982.

Table 4. ESTIMATES OF FETAL WEIGHT (IN GRAMS) BASED ON ABDOMINAL CIRCUMFERENCE (AC) AND FEMUR LENGTH (FL)

FL (cm)	\ AC (cm) 20.0	20.5	21.0	21.5	22.0	22.5	23.0	23.5	24.0	24.5	25.0	25.5	26.0	26.5	27.0	27.5	28.0	28.5	29.0	29.5	30.0
4.0	663	691	720	751	783	816	851	887	925	964	1006	1048	1093	1139	1188	1239	1291	1346	1403	1463	1525
4.1	680	709	738	769	802	836	871	907	946	986	1027	1070	1115	1162	1211	1262	1315	1371	1429	1489	1551
4.2	697	726	757	788	821	855	891	928	967	1007	1049	1093	1138	1186	1235	1287	1340	1396	1454	1515	1578
4.3	715	745	776	808	841	875	912	949	988	1029	1071	1116	1162	1209	1259	1311	1365	1422	1480	1541	1605
4.4	734	764	795	827	861	896	933	971	1010	1051	1094	1139	1185	1234	1284	1336	1391	1448	1507	1568	1632
4.5	753	783	815	847	882	917	954	993	1033	1074	1118	1163	1210	1259	1309	1362	1417	1474	1534	1596	1660
4.6	772	803	835	868	903	939	976	1015	1056	1098	1142	1187	1235	1284	1335	1388	1444	1501	1561	1623	1688
4.7	792	823	856	889	924	961	999	1038	1079	1122	1166	1212	1260	1310	1361	1415	1471	1529	1589	1652	1717
4.8	812	844	877	911	947	984	1022	1062	1103	1146	1191	1237	1286	1336	1388	1442	1498	1557	1618	1681	1746
4.9	833	865	899	933	969	1007	1046	1086	1128	1171	1216	1263	1312	1363	1415	1470	1527	1585	1647	1710	1776
5.0	855	887	921	956	993	1031	1070	1111	1153	1197	1243	1290	1339	1390	1443	1498	1555	1615	1676	1740	1806
5.1	877	910	944	980	1016	1055	1095	1136	1179	1223	1269	1317	1367	1418	1471	1527	1584	1644	1706	1770	1837
5.2	899	933	967	1004	1041	1080	1120	1162	1205	1250	1296	1344	1395	1447	1500	1556	1614	1674	1737	1801	1868
5.3	922	956	992	1028	1066	1105	1146	1188	1232	1277	1324	1373	1423	1476	1530	1586	1645	1705	1768	1833	1900
5.4	946	981	1016	1053	1091	1131	1172	1215	1259	1305	1352	1401	1452	1505	1560	1617	1675	1736	1799	1865	1933
5.5	971	1005	1041	1079	1118	1158	1199	1242	1287	1333	1381	1431	1482	1535	1591	1648	1707	1768	1832	1897	1966
5.6	995	1031	1067	1105	1144	1185	1227	1271	1316	1362	1411	1461	1513	1566	1622	1679	1739	1801	1864	1931	1999
5.7	1021	1057	1094	1132	1172	1213	1255	1299	1345	1392	1441	1491	1544	1598	1654	1712	1772	1834	1898	1964	2033
5.8	1047	1084	1121	1160	1200	1242	1285	1329	1375	1422	1472	1523	1575	1630	1686	1744	1805	1867	1932	1999	2068
5.9	1074	1111	1149	1188	1229	1271	1314	1359	1406	1454	1503	1555	1608	1663	1719	1778	1839	1902	1966	2034	2103
6.0	1102	1139	1178	1217	1258	1301	1345	1390	1437	1485	1535	1587	1641	1696	1753	1812	1873	1936	2002	2069	2139
6.1	1130	1168	1207	1247	1289	1331	1376	1421	1469	1518	1568	1620	1674	1730	1788	1847	1908	1972	2038	2105	2175
6.2	1160	1198	1237	1278	1319	1363	1408	1454	1501	1551	1602	1654	1709	1765	1823	1882	1944	2008	2074	2142	2212
6.3	1189	1228	1268	1309	1351	1395	1440	1487	1535	1585	1636	1689	1744	1800	1858	1919	1981	2045	2111	2180	2250
6.4	1220	1259	1299	1341	1384	1428	1473	1520	1569	1619	1671	1724	1779	1836	1895	1956	2018	2082	2149	2218	2289
6.5	1251	1291	1332	1373	1417	1461	1507	1555	1604	1655	1707	1760	1816	1873	1932	1993	2056	2121	2188	2256	2328
6.6	1284	1324	1365	1407	1451	1496	1542	1590	1640	1691	1743	1797	1853	1911	1970	2031	2094	2160	2227	2296	2367
6.7	1317	1357	1399	1441	1486	1531	1578	1626	1676	1728	1780	1835	1891	1949	2009	2070	2134	2199	2267	2336	2408
6.8	1351	1391	1433	1477	1521	1567	1615	1663	1713	1765	1819	1873	1930	1988	2048	2110	2174	2240	2307	2377	2449
6.9	1385	1427	1469	1513	1558	1604	1652	1701	1752	1804	1857	1913	1970	2028	2089	2151	2215	2281	2348	2418	2490
7.0	1421	1463	1506	1550	1595	1642	1690	1740	1791	1843	1897	1953	2010	2069	2130	2192	2256	2322	2391	2461	2533
7.1	1458	1500	1543	1588	1633	1681	1729	1779	1830	1883	1938	1994	2051	2110	2171	2234	2299	2365	2433	2504	2576
7.2	1495	1538	1581	1626	1673	1720	1769	1819	1871	1924	1979	2035	2093	2153	2214	2277	2342	2408	2477	2547	2620
7.3	1534	1577	1621	1666	1713	1761	1810	1861	1913	1966	2021	2078	2136	2196	2258	2321	2386	2453	2521	2592	2665
7.4	1573	1616	1661	1707	1754	1802	1852	1903	1955	2009	2065	2122	2180	2240	2302	2365	2431	2498	2566	2637	2710
7.5	1614	1657	1702	1749	1796	1845	1895	1946	1999	2053	2109	2166	2225	2285	2347	2411	2476	2543	2612	2683	2756
7.6	1655	1699	1745	1791	1839	1888	1939	1990	2043	2098	2154	2211	2270	2331	2393	2457	2523	2590	2659	2730	2803
7.7	1698	1742	1788	1835	1883	1933	1983	2035	2089	2144	2200	2258	2317	2378	2440	2504	2570	2638	2707	2778	2851
7.8	1741	1786	1833	1880	1928	1978	2029	2082	2135	2191	2247	2305	2365	2426	2488	2553	2618	2686	2755	2827	2899
7.9	1786	1832	1878	1926	1975	2025	2076	2129	2183	2238	2295	2353	2413	2474	2537	2602	2668	2735	2805	2876	2949
8.0	1832	1878	1925	1973	2022	2073	2124	2177	2232	2287	2344	2403	2463	2524	2587	2652	2718	2785	2855	2926	2999
8.1	1879	1926	1973	2021	2071	2121	2173	2227	2281	2337	2394	2453	2513	2575	2638	2702	2769	2837	2906	2977	3050
8.2	1928	1974	2022	2070	2120	2171	2224	2277	2332	2388	2446	2504	2565	2626	2690	2754	2821	2889	2958	3029	3102
8.3	1978	2024	2072	2121	2171	2223	2275	2329	2384	2440	2498	2557	2617	2679	2743	2807	2874	2942	3011	3082	3155

AC (cm)

FL (cm)	30.5	31.0	31.5	32.0	32.5	33.0	33.5	34.0	34.5	35.0	35.5	36.0	36.5	37.0	37.5	38.0	38.5	39.0	39.5	40.0
4.0	1590	1658	1729	1802	1879	1959	2042	2129	2220	2314	2413	2515	2622	2734	2850	2972	3098	3230	3367	3511
4.1	1617	1685	1756	1830	1907	1987	2071	2158	2249	2344	2442	2545	2652	2764	2880	3002	3128	3260	3397	3540
4.2	1644	1712	1783	1858	1935	2016	2100	2187	2279	2373	2472	2575	2683	2794	2911	3032	3159	3290	3427	3570
4.3	1671	1740	1812	1886	1964	2045	2129	2217	2308	2404	2503	2606	2713	2825	2942	3063	3189	3321	3458	3600
4.4	1699	1768	1840	1915	1993	2075	2159	2247	2339	2434	2533	2637	2744	2856	2973	3094	3220	3352	3488	3630
4.5	1727	1797	1869	1944	2023	2105	2189	2278	2370	2465	2565	2668	2776	2888	3004	3125	3251	3383	3519	3661
4.6	1756	1826	1898	1974	2053	2135	2220	2309	2401	2497	2596	2700	2807	2919	3036	3157	3283	3414	3550	3692
4.7	1785	1855	1928	2004	2084	2166	2251	2340	2432	2528	2628	2732	2840	2952	3068	3189	3315	3446	3582	3723
4.8	1814	1885	1959	2035	2115	2197	2283	2372	2464	2560	2660	2764	2872	2984	3100	3221	3347	3478	3613	3754
4.9	1845	1916	1990	2066	2146	2229	2315	2404	2497	2593	2693	2797	2905	3017	3133	3254	3380	3510	3645	3786
5.0	1875	1947	2021	2098	2178	2261	2347	2437	2530	2626	2726	2830	2938	3050	3166	3287	3412	3542	3677	3818
5.1	1906	1978	2053	2130	2210	2294	2380	2470	2563	2659	2760	2864	2972	3084	3200	3320	3445	3575	3710	3850
5.2	1938	2010	2085	2163	2243	2327	2413	2503	2597	2693	2794	2898	3006	3117	3234	3354	3479	3608	3743	3882
5.3	1970	2043	2118	2196	2277	2360	2447	2537	2631	2728	2828	2932	3040	3152	3268	3388	3513	3642	3776	3915
5.4	2003	2076	2151	2229	2311	2395	2482	2572	2665	2762	2863	2967	3075	3186	3302	3422	3547	3676	3809	3948
5.5	2036	2109	2185	2264	2345	2429	2516	2607	2700	2797	2898	3002	3110	3221	3337	3457	3581	3710	3843	3981
5.6	2070	2143	2220	2298	2380	2464	2552	2642	2736	2833	2933	3038	3145	3257	3372	3492	3616	3744	3877	4015
5.7	2104	2178	2254	2333	2415	2500	2587	2678	2772	2869	2970	3074	3181	3293	3408	3527	3651	3779	3911	4048
5.8	2139	2213	2290	2369	2451	2536	2624	2714	2808	2905	3006	3110	3218	3329	3444	3563	3686	3814	3946	4082
5.9	2175	2249	2326	2405	2488	2573	2660	2751	2845	2942	3043	3147	3254	3366	3480	3599	3722	3849	3981	4117
6.0	2211	2286	2363	2442	2525	2610	2698	2789	2883	2980	3080	3184	3292	3403	3517	3636	3758	3885	4016	4151
6.1	2248	2323	2400	2480	2562	2647	2736	2827	2921	3018	3118	3222	3329	3440	3554	3673	3795	3921	4052	4186
6.2	2285	2360	2438	2518	2600	2686	2774	2865	2959	3056	3157	3260	3367	3478	3592	3710	3832	3957	4087	4222
6.3	2323	2398	2476	2556	2639	2725	2813	2904	2998	3095	3195	3299	3406	3516	3630	3747	3869	3994	4124	4257
6.4	2362	2437	2515	2595	2678	2764	2852	2943	3037	3134	3235	3338	3445	3555	3668	3785	3906	4031	4160	4293
6.5	2401	2477	2555	2635	2718	2804	2892	2983	3077	3174	3274	3378	3484	3594	3707	3824	3944	4069	4197	4329
6.6	2441	2517	2595	2675	2759	2844	2933	3024	3118	3215	3315	3418	3524	3633	3746	3863	3983	4106	4234	4366
6.7	2481	2557	2636	2716	2800	2885	2974	3065	3159	3256	3355	3458	3564	3673	3786	3902	4021	4144	4271	4402
6.8	2523	2599	2677	2758	2841	2927	3016	3107	3200	3297	3397	3499	3605	3714	3826	3941	4060	4183	4309	4439
6.9	2564	2641	2719	2800	2884	2969	3058	3149	3242	3339	3438	3541	3646	3754	3866	3981	4100	4222	4347	4477
7.0	2607	2683	2762	2843	2927	3012	3101	3192	3285	3381	3481	3583	3688	3796	3907	4022	4140	4261	4386	4514
7.1	2650	2727	2806	2887	2970	3056	3144	3235	3328	3424	3523	3625	3730	3838	3948	4062	4180	4300	4425	4552
7.2	2694	2771	2850	2931	3014	3100	3188	3279	3372	3468	3567	3668	3772	3880	3990	4104	4220	4340	4464	4591
7.3	2739	2816	2895	2976	3059	3145	3233	3323	3416	3512	3610	3712	3816	3922	4032	4145	4261	4381	4503	4629
7.4	2785	2861	2940	3021	3105	3190	3278	3369	3461	3557	3655	3756	3859	3966	4075	4187	4303	4421	4543	4668
7.5	2831	2908	2987	3068	3151	3236	3324	3414	3507	3602	3700	3800	3903	4009	4118	4230	4344	4462	4583	4708
7.6	2878	2955	3034	3115	3198	3283	3371	3461	3553	3648	3745	3845	3948	4053	4161	4272	4387	4504	4624	4747
7.7	2926	3003	3081	3162	3245	3331	3418	3508	3600	3694	3791	3891	3993	4098	4205	4316	4429	4545	4665	4787
7.8	2974	3051	3130	3211	3294	3379	3466	3555	3647	3741	3838	3937	4039	4143	4250	4360	4472	4588	4706	4827
7.9	3024	3100	3179	3260	3343	3427	3514	3604	3695	3789	3885	3984	4085	4188	4295	4404	4515	4630	4748	4868
8.0	3074	3151	3229	3310	3392	3477	3564	3653	3744	3837	3933	4031	4131	4234	4340	4448	4559	4673	4790	4909
8.1	3125	3202	3280	3360	3443	3527	3614	3702	3793	3886	3981	4079	4179	4281	4386	4493	4604	4716	4832	4950
8.2	3177	3253	3332	3412	3494	3578	3664	3752	3843	3935	4030	4127	4226	4328	4432	4539	4648	4760	4875	4992
8.3	3230	3306	3384	3464	3546	3630	3716	3803	3893	3985	4080	4176	4275	4376	4479	4585	4693	4804	4918	5034

From Hadlock FB, Harrist RB, Carpenter RJ, et al: Sonographic estimation of fetal weight. Radiology 150:535, 1984.

Table 5. SIMPLIFIED METHOD FOR FETAL WEIGHT ESTIMATES BY HEAD, ABDOMEN, AND LIMB MEASUREMENTS*

14.0 = 493	17.3 = 790	20.6 = 1266	23.9 = 2030	27.2 = 3254
14.1 = 500	17.4 = 801	20.7 = 1285	24.0 = 2059	27.3 = 3301
14.2 = 507	17.5 = 813	20.8 = 1303	24.1 = 2089	27.4 = 3348
14.3 = 514	17.6 = 825	20.9 = 1322	24.2 = 2119	27.5 = 3397
14.4 = 522	17.7 = 836	21.0 = 1341	24.3 = 2149	27.6 = 3446
14.5 = 529	17.8 = 848	21.1 = 1360	24.4 = 2180	27.7 = 3495
14.6 = 537	17.9 = 861	21.2 = 1380	24.5 = 2212	27.8 = 3546
14.7 = 545	18.0 = 873	21.3 = 1400	24.6 = 2244	27.9 = 3597
14.8 = 552	18.1 = 886	21.4 = 1420	24.7 = 2276	28.0 = 3648
14.9 = 560	18.2 = 898	21.5 = 1440	24.8 = 2309	28.1 = 3701
15.0 = 569	18.3 = 911	21.6 = 1461	24.9 = 2342	28.2 = 3754
15.1 = 577	18.4 = 924	21.7 = 1482	25.0 = 2376	28.3 = 3808
15.2 = 585	18.5 = 938	21.8 = 1503	25.1 = 2410	28.4 = 3863
15.3 = 593	18.6 = 951	21.9 = 1525	25.2 = 2445	28.5 = 3919
15.4 = 602	18.7 = 965	22.0 = 1547	25.3 = 2480	28.6 = 3975
15.5 = 611	18.8 = 979	22.1 = 1569	25.4 = 2516	28.7 = 4033
15.6 = 619	18.9 = 993	22.2 = 1592	25.5 = 2552	28.8 = 4091
15.7 = 628	19.0 = 1007	22.3 = 1615	25.6 = 2589	28.9 = 4150
15.8 = 637	19.1 = 1022	22.4 = 1638	25.7 = 2626	29.0 = 4209
15.9 = 647	19.2 = 1037	22.5 = 1662	25.8 = 2664	29.1 = 4270
16.0 = 656	19.3 = 1051	22.6 = 1686	25.9 = 2702	29.2 = 4331
16.1 = 665	19.4 = 1067	22.7 = 1710	26.0 = 2741	29.3 = 4394
16.2 = 675	19.5 = 1082	22.8 = 1734	26.1 = 2780	29.4 = 4457
16.3 = 685	19.6 = 1098	22.9 = 1759	26.2 = 2820	29.5 = 4521
16.4 = 695	19.7 = 1113	23.0 = 1785	26.3 = 2861	29.6 = 4586
16.5 = 705	19.8 = 1129	23.1 = 1810	26.4 = 2901	29.7 = 4652
16.6 = 715	19.9 = 1146	23.2 = 1837	26.5 = 2944	29.8 = 4719
16.7 = 725	20.0 = 1162	23.3 = 1863	26.6 = 2986	29.9 = 4787
16.8 = 735	20.1 = 1179	23.4 = 1890	26.7 = 3030	30.0 = 4856
16.9 = 746	20.2 = 1196	23.5 = 1917	26.8 = 3073	30.1 = 4926
17.0 = 757	20.3 = 1213	23.6 = 1945	26.9 = 3117	30.2 = 4997
17.1 = 768	20.4 = 1231	23.7 = 1973	27.0 = 3162	30.3 = 5069
17.2 = 779	20.5 = 1248	23.8 = 2001	27.1 = 3208	30.4 = 5142

*To estimate fetal weight, add together the biparietal diameter, the mean abdominal diameter, and the femur length in centimeters. Use the table to find the estimated fetal weight in grams. Estimates are within 10% of birth weight 75% of the time.

From Rose BI, McCallum WD: A simplified method for estimating fetal weight using ultrasound measurements. Obstet Gynecol 69:671, 1987. *Reprinted with permission from* The American College of Obstetricians and Gynecologists.

Table 6. NOMOGRAM OF ESTIMATED FETAL WEIGHT IN TWIN GESTATIONS

Gestational age (wk)	5th	25th	50th	75th	95th
16	132	141	154	189	207
17	173	194	215	239	249
18	214	248	276	289	291
19	223	253	300	333	412
20	232	259	324	378	534
21	275	355	432	482	705
22	319	452	540	586	876
23	347	497	598	684	880
24	376	543	656	783	885
25	549	677	793	916	1118
26	722	812	931	1049	1352
27	755	978	1087	1193	1563
28	789	1145	1244	1337	1774
29	900	1266	1395	1509	1883
30	1011	1387	1546	1682	1992
31	1198	1532	1693	1875	2392
32	1385	1677	1840	2068	2793
33	1491	1771	2032	2334	3000
34	1597	1866	2224	2601	3208
35	1703	2093	2427	2716	3336
36	1809	2321	2631	2832	3465
37	2239	2540	2824	3035	3679
38	2669	2760	3017	3239	3894

From Yarkoni S, Reece EA, Holford T, et al: Estimated fetal weight in the evaluation of growth in twin gestations: A prospective longitudinal study. Obstet Gynecol 69:636, 1987. *Reprinted with permission from* The American College of Obstetricians and Gynecologists.

Appendix C

Normal Measurements of the Premenarchal Uterus and Ovaries

Table 1. NORMAL OVARIAN VOLUME*

Age (yr)	No. of Patients	Ovarian Volume (cm³)	
		By Chronologic Age Mean SD	By Bone Age Mean SD
2	5	0.75 ± 0.41	0.78 ± 0.38
3	6	0.66 ± 0.17	0.64 ± 0.18
4	14	0.82 ± 0.36	1.00 ± 0.45
5	4	0.86 ± 0.02	0.95 ± 0.52
6	9	1.19 ± 0.36	1.05 ± 0.65
7	8	1.26 ± 0.59	1.23 ± 0.47
8	10	1.05 ± 0.50	1.29 ± 0.33
9	11	1.98 ± 0.76	1.35 ± 0.71
10	12	2.22 ± 0.69	1.47 ± 0.56
11	12	2.52 ± 1.30	2.45 ± 0.86
12	6	3.80 ± 1.40	3.10 ± 1.29
13	4	4.18 ± 2.30	4.38 ± 2.74

*As determined by ultrasonography in 101 girls from age 2 to 13.
From Orsini LF: Pelvic organs in premenarcheal girls: Real-time ultrasonography. Radiology 153:113, 1984.

Table 2. NORMAL UTERINE DIAMETERS AND VOLUME*

Age (yr)	No. of Patients	Uterine Diameters (mm)				Uterine Volume (cm³)	
		TUL Mean SD	COAP Mean SD	CEAP Mean SD	COAP/CEAP Mean SD	By Chronologic Age Mean SD	By Bone Age Mean SD
2	7	33.1 ± 4.4	7.0 ± 3.4	8.3 ± 2.0	0.84 ± 0.29	1.98 ± 1.58	1.76 ± 0.72
3	8	32.4 ± 4.3	6.4 ± 1.3	7.6 ± 2.2	0.89 ± 0.29	1.63 ± 0.81	1.80 ± 0.74
4	15	32.9 ± 3.3	7.6 ± 1.8	8.6 ± 1.8	0.90 ± 0.22	2.10 ± 0.57	1.97 ± 0.74
5	7	33.1 ± 5.5	8.0 ± 2.8	8.4 ± 1.6	0.95 ± 0.28	2.36 ± 1.39	2.19 ± 1.16
6	9	33.2 ± 4.1	6.7 ± 2.9	7.5 ± 1.8	0.86 ± 0.18	1.80 ± 1.57	1.65 ± 0.93
7	9	32.3 ± 3.9	8.0 ± 2.2	7.7 ± 2.5	1.08 ± 0.26	2.32 ± 1.07	2.81 ± 1.44
8	11	35.8 ± 7.3	9.0 ± 2.8	8.4 ± 1.7	1.05 ± 0.20	3.12 ± 1.52	2.70 ± 1.43
9	11	37.1 ± 4.4	9.7 ± 3.0	8.8 ± 2.0	1.10 ± 0.24	3.70 ± 1.62	2.69 ± 1.83
10	13	40.3 ± 6.4	12.8 ± 5.3	10.7 ± 2.6	1.17 ± 0.31	6.54 ± 3.78	4.66 ± 3.03
11	13	42.2 ± 5.1	12.8 ± 3.1	10.7 ± 2.6	1.22 ± 0.26	6.66 ± 2.87	6.24 ± 3.07
12	6	54.3 ± 8.4	17.3 ± 5.3	14.3 ± 5.2	1.23 ± 0.16	16.18 ± 9.15	8.88 ± 3.65
13	5	53.8 ± 11.4	15.8 ± 4.5	15.0 ± 2.4	1.03 ± 0.15	13.18 ± 5.64	15.55 ± 5.98

*As determined by ultrasonography in 114 girls from age 2 to 13. TUL = total uterine length; COAP = anteroposterior diameter of the corpus; CEAP = anteroposterior diameter of the cervix.
From Orsini LF: Pelvic organs in premenarcheal girls: Real-time ultrasonography. Radiology 153:113, 1984.

INDEX

Page numbers in *italics* refer to illustrations; page numbers followed by "t" refer to tables.